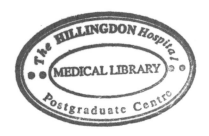

STANDARD ORTHOPAEDIC OPERATIONS

A GUIDE FOR THE JUNIOR SURGEON

For Churchill Livingstone
Publisher: Simon Fathers
Editorial Co-ordination: Editorial Resources Unit
Production Controller: Neil Dickson
Design: Design Resources Unit
Sales Promotion Executive: Kathy Crawford

STANDARD ORTHOPAEDIC OPERATIONS

A GUIDE FOR THE JUNIOR SURGEON

JOHN CRAWFORD ADAMS
MD(London) MS(London) FRCS(England)

Honorary Consultant Orthopaedic Surgeon, St Mary's Hospital, London, UK
Honorary Civil Consultant in Orthopaedic Surgery, Royal Air Force
Formerly Production Editor, *Journal of Bone and Joint Surgery*

CLIFFORD A. STOSSEL
MB BS(London) FRCS(England) FRCS(Edinburgh)

Consultant Orthopaedic Surgeon, Maidstone, UK
Consultant in Charge, Churchill Rehabilitation and Assessment Centre, Maidstone, UK

FOURTH EDITION

CHURCHILL LIVINGSTONE
EDINBURGH LONDON MADRID MELBOURNE NEW YORK AND TOKYO 1992

CHURCHILL LIVINGSTONE
Medical Division of Longman Group UK Limited

Distributed in the United States of America by Churchill Livingstone Inc., 650 Avenue of the Americas, New York, N.Y. 10011, and by associated companies, branches and representatives throughout the world.

First edition 1976
Second edition 1980
Third edition 1985
Fourth edition 1992

ISBN 0-443-04351-5

British Library Cataloguing in Publication Data
A catalogue record for this book is available from the British Library.

Library of Congress Cataloging in Publication Data
Adams, John Crawford.
    Standard orthopaedic operations / John Crawford Adams, Clifford A. Stossel. — 4th ed.
        p.   cm.
    Includes bibliographical references and index.
    ISBN 0-443-04351-5
    1. Orthopedic surgery.   I. Stossel, Clifford A.   II. Title.
    [DNLM: 1. Orthopedics.   WE 168 A214s]
    RD731.A36   1992
    617.3—dc20
    DNLM/DLC
    for Library of Congress   91-36394

WE168 ADA

The publisher's policy is to use **paper manufactured from sustainable forests**

Produced by Longman Singapore Publishers Pte Ltd
Printed in Singapore

Note by Original Author

In general, surgical techniques do not change radically. Much of what was presented in the earlier three editions therefore still stands. Recent advances in orthopaedic surgery have been largely in the fields of joint replacement, fracture surgery and endoscopic surgery. In order to ensure that the book keeps abreast of such advances I have enlisted the help, as co-author, of Mr Clifford Stossel, who trained with me at St Mary's Hospital in London, and afterwards at the Royal National Orthopaedic Hospital. For many years Mr Stossel has been closely involved in the developing techniques of fracture surgery, and particularly with the techniques embraced by the Swiss (A.O.) system. He also has wide experience of joint replacement surgery and of endoscopic techniques. He now brings his expertise and wise counsel to the updating of *Standard Orthopaedic Operations*.

J.C.A.

Preface

As the subtitle indicates, this book is intended as a practical guide for the junior surgeon—in which term we include the orthopaedic surgeon in training and the general surgeon with but a superficial experience of orthopaedics who is confronted from time to time with an orthopaedic problem. The book may also be helpful to those studying for the higher examinations in surgery, to operation room nurses and technicians, and to physiotherapists, occupational therapists and others who wish to become acquainted with the principles of orthopaedic surgical techniques.

The aim has been to provide a more detailed description than is generally available of those routine operations that are commonly delegated to the junior surgeon—operations that he may never have had the opportunity to carry out under supervision or that he may be undertaking alone for the first time. It is often in these standard procedures that the junior surgeon feels the need for guidance. In contrast, the more formidable operations, in which the trainee may expect always to have the supervision of his chief, are covered in less detail or omitted altogether.

Each description is followed by a brief comment designed to indicate any special difficulties or hazards, and the precautions that must be taken to avoid them.

The intention was always that the book should be complementary to the major comprehensive textbooks of operative orthopaedics rather than a substitute for them. Nevertheless it does provide descriptions of virtually all the operations that the orthopaedic registrar or resident is likely to encounter in his day-to-day work, with the exception of the more intricate procedures in such highly specialised fields as scoliosis, hand surgery, and microsurgery.

In general, the emphasis has been on verbal description rather than on profuse illustrations. Nevertheless there are many points that can be illustrated more easily than described, and much attention has been given to the preparation of appropriate illustrations—mostly simple line drawings—wherever they seemed essential to clarify the text.

In most instances we have described only one method of carrying out a given operation—namely the method that we have found most satisfactory over the years. It is recognised, however, that there is often more than one way of achieving a satisfactory outcome, and we would be the last to suggest that the techniques that are presented here are necessarily the best in all circumstances. One of the fascinations of orthopaedic surgery is that there is nearly always room for discussion and for diversity of opinion, even on what might seem the most trivial of topics.

It is our hope that the techniques described here, which have commended themselves to us over a long period, may prove equally satisfactory to future generations of surgeons.

The material in this book is derived overwhelmingly from personal experience and only very little directly from the published descriptions of other authors. Nevertheless on certain points of detail it has been necessary—and indeed proper—to refer to other sources, too numerous to mention individually here. When our description has conformed closely to that of a known originator the source has generally been acknowledged in the text. For tidiness these references are grouped together at the end of the book.

J. Crawford Adams
Clifford A. Stossel

Contents

Introduction

It is well to remember that the operation that the surgeon approaches as a matter of routine—often even casually—may for the patient be a major event of his life. He may have been dreading it for weeks beforehand. He may preserve an outward calm, but often he has a deep apprehension within—a fear of the unknown, a fear of pain, a nightmarish thought that he may be permanently disabled or even die. Unfortunately these qualms are not entirely groundless. Things do go wrong from time to time. Disasters occur: infection, paralysis, ischaemia, occasionally death. The incidence of such complications should indeed be slight, but the threat always exists.

Thus it behoves the surgeon, each time that he operates, to put himself for a moment in the position of the patient. Nothing must go wrong. Even the simplest of operations must be approached in a serious and professional manner. The first rule of surgery must always be foremost in the surgeon's mind—that the operation must not make the patient worse than he was before he submitted himself to it.

If the patient has to come back into hospital for a revision operation because the first one was carried out imperfectly, the surgeon has failed in his duty. Some years ago the senior author made a count of the patients in an orthopaedic ward to discover how many were there for a primary operation and how many had been readmitted for revision or salvage procedures after a previous operation had proved inadequate or had been marred by complications. It was daunting to find that no less than one in four of the patients fell into the second category. Regrettably, many revision operations are occasioned by errors that are wholly avoidable. The moral to which these observations point is expressed in five mono-syllables: *"Get it right first time"*.

How then is the best possible result to be achieved every time that the surgeon operates upon a patient? This question may conveniently be discussed under the following four headings: pre-operative assessment of the patient; planning of the operation; operative technique; and post-operative management.

PRE-OPERATIVE ASSESSMENT OF PATIENT

Even if the proposed operation is a relatively minor one it is important in every case to assess the patient thoroughly, not only from the point of view of the cardiovascular and respiratory systems but also with respect to any special feature that might make operation hazardous. It is these special features that often go unsuspected and may cause serious problems.

For instance, in persons of African stock the presence of abnormal haemoglobin in sickle-cell disease may predispose to agglutination of red cells, especially in conditions of anoxaemia. In women taking contraceptive pills there may be a predisposition to venous thrombosis. In the elderly, anticoagulants used in the prevention or management of deep venous thrombosis may pre-dispose to cerebral haemorrhage. A septic focus, even though it may be remote from the field of operation and consequently unnoticed, may rarely be a source of metastatic infection, especially if the wound is a major one and if foreign material such as acrylic cement or a prosthesis has been implanted. Again, generalised osteoporosis, if unrecognised, may lead to inadvertent fracture of a bone during the course of an operation—as in a case of the authors' in which the shaft of the femur was fractured during the routine manoeuvre employed for reduction of a femoral neck fracture: it later emerged that the patient was suffering from osteoporosis consequent upon a parathyroid adenoma.

These are sufficient examples to indicate that time must be spent not only in routine examination of the various body systems but also in questioning the patient about any circumstance that might have a bearing on the safety of the anaesthetic or of the operation itself.

PLANNING THE OPERATION

When an operation fails to give the best possible result the failure may often be ascribed to incorrect diagnosis or to inadequate planning of the procedure. A hurried assessment of the problem—seemingly perhaps a routine one—without a sufficiently detailed study of the clinical state and of the radiographs has often led the surgeon to

medullary nail, and it may not become apparent until the nail is found to have cut through the soft bone of the greater trochanter that the proximal fragment was too short to afford sufficient grip for a plain nail: a Y-nail or a Zickel device would have been a more appropriate means of fixation.

Another example illustrates how a necessary

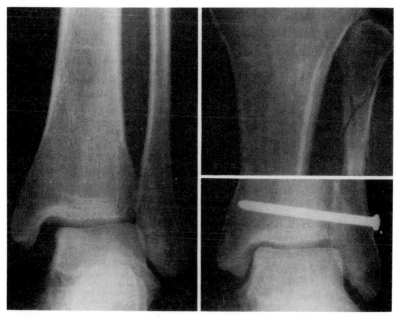

FIGS 1–2. After an injury to the ankle the initial radiographs failed to show any abnormality, but a later film showed lateral subluxation of the talus (Fig. 1), denoting rupture of the inferior tibio-fibular ligament. Wider studies then revealed a high fracture of the fibula (Fig. 2). Fixation of the fibula to the tibia with a screw was carried out (Fig. 2).

undertake a particular operation whereas a more thorough analysis might have suggested the need for a different procedure. For instance, a high fracture of the femoral shaft might at first sight seem suitable for internal fixation by an intra-

operation may be delayed through inadequate investigation and consequent failure to appreciate the correct pathology. A woman had sustained an ankle injury and there was severe disability. The initial radiographs, however, failed to show any abnormality, and the injury was wrongly regarded as a simple strain. When the patient returned later with persistent severe swelling and pain the radiographs now showed well marked lateral subluxation of the talus (Fig. 1), and more comprehensive films revealed a high fracture of the shaft of the fibula (Fig. 2): there had been a rupture of the inferior tibio-fibular ligament, masked at the first examination by spontaneous reduction of the displacement. Had the true nature of the injury been appreciated initially, the correct treatment—to hold the fibula to the tibia with a transverse screw—could have been applied immediately. Suspicion should have been aroused by the severe pain and disability.

If operation is being undertaken to correct a deformity, for instance by wedge osteotomy, it is essential that the degree of the deformity be accurately established by measurements, both clinically and radiologically, so that the amount of correction to be gained—the precise number of degrees—may be planned in advance. Here again the precept *"Get it right first time"* is very relevant.

The advice that emerges from these considerations is, firstly, that clinical examination and appropriate investigations must never be skimped; and secondly, that before each operation the surgeon should sit down quietly with a full knowledge of the clinical state of the patient and with the radiographs before him, to decide whether or not the case is in fact suitable for the operation that he has in mind, and to plan in detail the best method of gaining the objective.

Marking the correct site for operation. Various methods have been suggested to ensure not only that the correct patient is operated upon but that the surgeon embarks on the operation on the correct side and at the correct site. Failure to take adequate precautions does lead from time to time to serious mistakes: cases are on record even of the wrong limb having been amputated. One of the authors himself in his early days of training amputated the wrong toe following ambiguous instructions from his chief.

Such accidents can be prevented with certainty in the following manner. The day before the operation the surgeon himself obtains from the patient his confirmation of the side affected and, in the case of digits, which particular digit or digits are to be operated upon. With an indelible skin pen an arrow is then marked boldly upon the skin surface close to the site of operation to indicate clearly the part that is affected. This procedure has been routine in the authors' practice for many years and it effectively eliminates any possibility of error.

OPERATIVE TECHNIQUE

There is no doubt that manual dexterity as translated into operative skill is to some extent inborn, just as is an aptitude for music or for ball games. There are surgeons who never acquire more than a moderate technical proficiency. Others quickly show an aptitude that with appropriate training and practice evolves into such confident skill that the performance of an operation by such a master is a delight to watch. In orthopaedic surgery a natural flair for things mechanical is a valuable asset. A fondness for Meccano in youth has served many a surgeon in good stead, for just as Meccano is (or was, until its regrettable virtual demise a few years ago) "engineering for boys", so to a large extent orthopaedic surgery is engineering in bone, muscle and tendon—with the difference that restoration of function, not only of form, is the prime objective.

No matter whether or not the young surgeon has a natural aptitude, however, he is unlikely to develop his skill to the full without extreme diligence, study and practical experience under the guidance of a master surgeon.

INSTRUMENTS AND EQUIPMENT

It is not appropriate here to attempt a full description or review of all the equipment available to the orthopaedic surgeon, or even to make selective recommendations. The range of equipment and instruments that are nowadays available is so vast that limitations of space alone would forbid a comprehensive review. Equally importantly, the trainee surgeon for whom this book is intended does not ordinarily have a free choice of the instruments that he will use: in general he must use those that are available in the particular hospital where he works.

Nevertheless it is important to emphasise that an operation should not be embarked upon unless all the apparatus that may be required is available. For instance, before undertaking a nail-plating operation for fracture of the trochanteric region of the femur the surgeon must ensure that a full range of nail-plates of all the standard lengths and angles is available. If a full range is not to hand it is better to defer the operation for a few hours and to send out urgently for further stock. Likewise it is foolhardy to undertake intramedullary nailing of a fractured femur or tibia unless a full set of power-driven reamers is available: hand-driven reamers are not adequate. The patient is entitled to expect that every unit where such operations are to be undertaken should be properly equipped for the purpose.

So far as powered tools are concerned, certain items are necessities, others luxuries. The only powered tools that are essential for general orthopaedic work are a motor saw, a power-driven drill, and a slow-speed drive for medullary reaming. Among the luxuries—more and more regarded as "essential" as surgeons become more sophisticated—are a high-speed drill with dental-type burrs, a reciprocating saw, and an acetabular reamer. Power-operated chisels and powered bone punches are still true luxuries.

Radiographic apparatus is standard equipment for an orthopaedic operation room. For certain operations two machines—one for antero-posterior and the other for lateral radiography—are mandatory. At present not every operation suite is equipped with a mobile image intensifier. It is possible to undertake most orthopaedic operations without one, reliance being placed upon radiographic films: nevertheless in the operative treatment of fractures of the major long bones the saving of time from the use of an image intensifier

is so considerable that in any large accident unit it must be regarded as an essential piece of equipment.

If the surgeon is fortunate enough to have a free choice of equipment he will have to make his selection from a very wide range. He will also have to decide whether to use cobalt-chrome alloy, stainless steel or possibly titanium for his implants. Many patterns of screw, plate, nail and nail-plate are available—most of them entirely adequate for their purpose. The range of fixation devices offered by the Swiss school of surgeons forming the "A.O."* group is outstanding for its precision and versatility, though the cost may be a bar to its adoption as standard equipment.

Good equipment helps; it helps enormously. But in no way does it make up for poor surgical technique. A competent surgeon equipped with only the simplest of tools will enjoy far better results than his ham-fisted colleague who may be equipped at ten times the cost.

SETTING UP FOR THE OPERATION

In orthopaedics more than in most branches of surgery setting up the patient for the operation is of vital importance, and the surgeon who supervises this himself will be well rewarded. Even minor details such as the position of a tourniquet and the pressure to which it is inflated, the position of a limb in respect of postural pressure upon nerves and blood vessels, and the proper placing of the diathermy leads should always be watched. Nothing should go unchecked.

If the patient is to be positioned on the orthopaedic table—as for fixation of a fracture of the neck of the femur—personal supervision by the surgeon is essential: there are so many points of detail to be considered that delegation of this responsibility is most unwise unless an assistant of exceptional experience and skill is available. The surgeon should also himself check the positioning of the radiographic units or image intensifier; otherwise the time will surely come when he calls for a radiograph, only to find that centering of the

* "Arbeitsgemeineschaft Osteosynthesefragen"

beam has been imperfect and that in consequence the film fails to show the essential part.

These remarks apply also to setting up the patient and the apparatus for intramedullary nailing of a fractured long bone. One difficulty here is to position the patient in such a way that easy access is afforded for reduction of the fracture and for insertion of the nail, and at the same time that the limb is accessible for radiography with the image intensifier. In these cases special attachments fitted to the operation table to support the affected limb may prove very useful: examples are described in the relevant sections of this book.

THE USE OF TOURNIQUETS

The use of a tourniquet makes peripheral limb operations very much easier and more precise; and provided that proper precautions are observed the advantages far outweigh the potential hazards.

Types of tourniquet. Long departed are the days of the rubber tube and anchor tourniquet, now seen only in museums. Gone also should be the era of the rubber bandage (Esmarch) tourniquet, which is still found in use occasionally. The Esmarch rubber bandage survives, however, as a useful means of exsanguinating the limb before the occlusive cuff is applied or inflated.

Universally used nowadays is the pneumatic cuff tourniquet. The design of pneumatic tourniquets has improved markedly since the Second World War, and whereas a sphygmomanometer cuff and mercury column will still serve the purpose, the preferred type now is the purpose-made cuff with automatic pressure-maintaining device operated from a small cylinder of liquid gas. With this machine, once the pressure is set at the desired figure the surgeon may operate in the confident knowledge that a sudden failure of the tourniquet—so common a mishap in earlier days—will not occur.

Applying the tourniquet. The important points in applying the pneumatic cuff are, first, that it should be applied in the correct position, and secondly, that it should be applied snugly. A pneumatic cuff may be applied directly to the limb, though some surgeons still prefer to use a protective layer of towelling, plastic foam or gamgee tissue beneath it. The correct sites of application are: in the thigh, high up, close to the groin; in the lower leg, at the thickest part of the calf; in the upper arm, a little above the mid-point of the arm, where the muscles are most bulky. All these sites are those where good muscle bulk acts to protect the underlying nerves. Applying a cuff where nerves are superficial and relatively unprotected—for instance, near the knee—entails a serious risk of nerve damage.

When the pneumatic cuff is being wrapped round the limb it is important that it be applied snugly, without too much slack. If the cuff is applied loosely it may not expand sufficiently on inflation to occlude the arteries.

Exsanguinating the limb. When the cuff has been applied—but not inflated—an Esmarch rubber bandage or Rhys-Davies exsanguinator is applied from the periphery upwards, with moderate tension, to drive the blood in the small vessels proximally. The bandage is applied in spiral fashion, with hardly any overlap. It should extend right up to the lower edge of the tourniquet cuff.

Inflating the cuff. The tourniquet cuff is now inflated to the desired pressure, and immediately thereafter the exsanguinator is removed. The time at which the tourniquet was inflated is recorded.

The correct pressure for a tourniquet depends upon the arterial blood pressure in the limb: ideally the cuff pressure should be higher than this by 30 to 50 millimetres of mercury. Blood pressure is normally higher in the lower limb than in the upper; so a somewhat higher cuff pressure is needed. Naturally, the cuff pressure will need to be appropriately higher in hypertensive patients; in children, on the other hand, a relatively low pressure suffices. The recommended pressures as engraved on most proprietary tourniquet sets are considerably higher than the pressures usually needed: the surgeon's discretion should override these standard markings.

Safe duration of tourniquet compression. No clearcut rule can be laid down concerning the longest time that a tourniquet should be allowed to remain inflated, though it is a reasonably safe working rule to suggest one hour for the upper limb and an hour and a half for the lower limb. Safety does not depend upon time alone: it depends largely upon the pressure of the cuff and the volume of muscle padding. In the early stages of tourniquet compression the danger lies not in ischaemia but in direct pressure upon nerves. The higher the tourniquet pressure, the greater does the risk of nerve damage become. A limb that is very thin is far more vulnerable to injury than one that is well covered with muscle or even with fat. Indeed, in a very thin person tourniquet compression for even half an hour may be sufficient to cause nerve paralysis, whereas in a big muscular individual compression for as long as two hours may be innocuous. The surgeon should thus use his judgement in each individual case, observing the general rule that an hour for the arm and an hour and a half for the lower limb are the outside maximum times allowable, and being prepared to reduce these times, especially if the limb is unduly thin or if an unusually high cuff pressure is required on account of hypertension.

After a tourniquet has been released and the blood allowed to flow for 15 minutes it is safe to inflate the cuff for a second period, though this should not usually exceed half an hour for the arm and three-quarters of an hour for the leg.

The Esmarch rubber bandage tourniquet. The Esmarch rubber tourniquet is no longer used in modern surgical practice. Its occasional use may still be permissible, however, in under-developed areas where modern equipment is not available, and the following guidelines may thus still be apposite.

A major drawback of this type of tourniquet is that the actual constricting pressure applied to the limb is unknown. Unless the bandage is applied intelligently it is almost certain that the pressure will be excessive. As a general rule, only three turns of rubber bandage applied at full stretch by a man of moderate strength exert enough force to occlude the arteries. It is clear therefore that if the whole bandage is applied at full stretch a hugely excessive pressure is brought to bear on the limb: it may easily reach 600 millimetres of mercury or more. A bandage applied injudiciously with full

force may bite into the tissues and do serious damage to nerves, and possibly also to arteries, especially if they are atheromatous. Indeed, because of the relatively small bulk of muscle to protect the nerves and vessels, it is recommended that the Esmarch tourniquet should never be used for the arm.

A further hazard with the Esmarch tourniquet is that, being often hidden from view and not connected by long tubes to a pressure gauge as is the pneumatic tourniquet, it may accidentally be left on and forgotten. Such a disaster is likely to lead to amputation or even to death from tissue damage and consequent renal failure.

The following rules should therefore be strictly observed if this obsolescent type of tourniquet is used. 1) The tourniquet should be applied over a folded towel or cuff of felt or gamgee so that the pressure is evenly distributed. 2) The tourniquet should be applied only over bulky muscle. 3) No more than three turns of the rubber bandage should be applied at full stretch in the first instance: if this proves insufficient to occlude the arteries it is simple to reapply the cuff with a fourth turn. 4) The surgeon should himself routinely supervise the application of the tourniquet, and should personally ensure that the tapes that tie it in position are tied also to a part of the operation table as a precaution against the patient's being inadvertently removed from the table with the tourniquet still in position. 5) A responsible assistant should be detailed to report the tourniquet time every 15 minutes. 6) The duration of compression should never exceed one hour.

Removal of tourniquet. As a general rule it is recommended that the tourniquet be removed before the wound is closed. Significant bleeding points may then be secured and the risk of the formation of a haematoma is greatly reduced. It is true that many surgeons prefer to leave the tourniquet in position until the wound is closed as a matter of routine. But while this may make for neater and cleaner surgery, it is not a policy that can be endorsed. Disastrous haematoma formation resulting from failure to secure sizeable vessels before wound closure is admittedly rare, but it does occur and it may lead to necrosis of the skin and prolonged morbidity. Even one such disaster is one too many, especially since it can so easily be prevented by the precaution of removing the tourniquet before closure.

Contra-indications to use a tourniquet. A tourniquet should not be used on a limb that shows evidence of ischaemia from atherosclerosis. It should be used cautiously, and for the shortest time compatible with the needs of the operation, in cases of sickle-cell disease. It should also be used with great discretion if the patient is unusually thin, because of the risk of damage to the nerves by direct pressure.

THE NON-TOUCH TECHNIQUE

Although the non-touch technique originated by Lane (1914) and advocated again by Fairbank

even in the process of donning gown and gloves: and if this misdemeanour is observed frequently it is obvious that it must be committed unobserved even more often. It was to allow for this kind of human failing that the non-touch technique was designed. Admittedly it is difficult to prove its efficacy in reducing the incidence of wound infection because so many other factors play a part; but the authors are satisfied that it is a worth-while refinement. Moreover, once a surgeon has become accustomed to the technique he usually finds that it makes for neat surgery and adds little if anything to the operating time. There is the further important advantage, in these days of increasingly common infection by the HIV (Aids) virus, that accidental needle-stick injuries and pricks from sharp spikes of bone are largely avoided.

Details of the non-touch technique. Those who follow the non-touch technique assume that

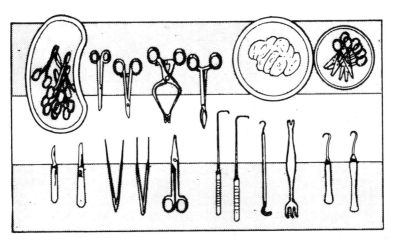

FIG. 3. Instrument table laid out for the non-touch technique. Only the handles of the instruments are touched: the "business ends" of the instruments rest on the central strip and must not be handled.

(1942) has been widely abandoned, the authors believe that it embodies important precautions against inadvertent contamination of the wound. They still employ it and would like to see it readopted by orthopaedic surgeons as standard practice. On many occasions they have watched assistants and nurses contaminate their hands

the gloved fingers are potentially contaminated and they therefore observe the principle that neither the fingers nor anything that has been touched by the fingers must ordinarily be allowed to enter the wound. If at a particular stage of the operation it becomes essential for the hand to enter the wound—as for instance in seating a prosthesis—a fresh over-sized glove is put on over the normal glove for the purpose. (Applying an over-glove is always safer than changing the gloves.) Swabs, packs, ligatures and suture materials are held only with forceps, never by the fingers. Only the point of each instrument is allowed to enter the wound, and that part of the instrument must never be touched by hand.

The instruments for an operation to be performed by the non-touch technique should be set out on a rectangular rather than a kidney-shaped trolley. The cloth draping the top of the trolley is demarcated into three longitudinal strips of about equal width. It is convenient to have the central strip coloured red, the outer strips being white or green. In laying out the trolley the instrument nurse places the handle of each instrument on one of the outer strips and the point rests upon the central strip (Fig. 3). The outer strips of the trolley cover may be touched by hand when instruments are taken from the trolley or replaced upon it, but the central strip is inviolable and must never be touched by hand or by any object that has been handled. After use, each instrument is returned immediately to its proper position on the instrument trolley: no instrument must be left lying about on the operation table or on the patient's body. The instrument nurse must learn to thread and present suture materials and ligatures by long forceps without ever handling them.

CLEAN AIR THEATRES

The development of "clean air" operation rooms in which the incoming air is filtered and rendered virtually free from bacteria has progressed rapidly since the first report of its use by Charnley and Eftekhar (1969) specifically for replacement operations upon the hip. Certainly the principle of operating in a bacteria-free environment has everything to commend it: the surprising thing is that introduction of the technique was so long delayed.

Operating in a clean air environment does, however, bring its own problems. If the system is to be used to fullest effect, the surgical team must be totally enclosed in "space suits" with an exhaust system for the expired air; attendant difficulties of communication arise; and the technique is not easily adapted for operations that demand the use of radiological equipment.

At present clean air rooms are used mainly for joint replacement surgery, but there can be little doubt that their use will be extended to include other major operations upon bone and joint. To some extent the method may be forced upon surgeons by medico-legal considerations.

For further information and discussion on this subject the reader is referred to the papers by Laurence (1983), Lidwell et al. (1982) and Whyte, Hodgson and Tinkler (1982).

POST-OPERATIVE MANAGEMENT

Dressings and splintage. Post-operative management begins when the last skin suture has been inserted. In many centres the surgeon has already left the operation room long before this time, delegating what is a most important part of the treatment—the application of dressings, bandages and plaster-of-Paris splints—to an assistant who may not always be conversant with the details of technique. In the authors' view the surgeon should not only complete the operation himself but he should also personally undertake or supervise the application of dressings and splints. In some operations this last stage in the operative procedure is almost as important as the operation itself.

Much harm can come from careless bandaging and plaster work: position may be lost, over-tight bandaging may obstruct the circulation or imperil a nerve, or on the other hand insufficient tension on the bandage may allow the formation of a haematoma. The authors have seen all these complications from time to time, and have themselves made the mistakes that they are now cautioning against. In one patient, through lack of supervision to the end of the procedure, a knee was so tightly bandaged after lower femoral osteotomy that the foot became partly ischaemic: the situation was saved only in the nick of time and the patient had to endure motor paralysis for several weeks before recovery occurred. In another patient treated by hamstring release for spastic flexion contracture of the knee an attempt was made to gain too much correction in the first plaster splint, with consequent neurapraxia of the sciatic nerve. After operations for Dupuytren's contracture disaster in the form of haematoma or skin necrosis is commonplace, simply because the post-operative management is defective. These are just a few examples of events that may go wrong. The important point to remember is that all such complications are avoidable—but only if the surgeon himself is aware of the hazards and takes the necessary steps personally to see that they are avoided. The young surgeon should always be prepared to learn from the mistakes of others; but he should try to ensure that he is not the model.

Checking of circulation and nerve function. It is always wise to re-examine each patient a few hours after the operation in order to check the state of the circulation and of nerve function. Often a minor adjustment to the dressings or plaster at this early stage may save trouble later.

Period of recumbency. An important precept in post-operative management is that no patient should be confined to bed for longer than is really necessary. The greater proportion of orthopaedic patients should be able to get out of bed soon after the operation, and they should be encouraged to do so. If this is on the day of the operation itself so much the better. There are relatively few operations today that necessitate the patient's being kept in bed for more than a week or two, and with improvements in technique there are likely to be even fewer in the future. Early resumption of activity is particularly important in the elderly. It reduces the period of disability and it almost certainly discourages venous thrombosis and pulmonary embolism.

Sedation. In this connection a brief reference is necessary to the question of sedation of the patient with analgesic and hypnotic drugs. In the authors' view there is a prevalent tendency to oversedate the patient immediately after operation, so that many hours elapse before he is allowed to "come round" sufficiently to appreciate what is going on. After orthopaedic operations heavy sedation is seldom required on account of pain—there are exceptions of course—and it militates against the early resumption of activity which is of such fundamental importance. The authors much prefer that the patient be allowed to come round and to get going within a few hours of the operation.

Physiotherapy. In the early days after operation the assistance of a skilled physiotherapist is an important requirement, especially if a lower limb is the part affected. She is able to impart confidence to the patient and to teach correct methods of walking with crutches or sticks. She should also instruct the patient in appropriate exercises and movements, to be carried out frequently in his or her own time. Under skilled supervision a patient often achieves in a matter of minutes what he believed would be impossible in days or even weeks. Sound advice to a patient recovering from an orthopaedic operation is: "*Don't just lie there; do something*".

CHAPTER ONE

Some Surgical Approaches

In most instances the surgical approach is included in the description of individual operations. Nevertheless there is a need here for a brief survey of the more important exposures, particularly of the deeply placed bones, joints and nerves. Limitations of space dictate that this shall be a selective rather than a comprehensive account.

CONTENTS OF CHAPTER

ANTERIOR EXPOSURE OF SHOULDER

In the anterior approach to the shoulder the delto-pectoral groove is opened, the coracoid process is divided and reflected downwards with the attached muscles, and the subscapularis tendon is divided.

TECHNIQUE

Position of patient. The patient lies supine, with a firm sand-bag under the scapular region of the affected shoulder to thrust it forward. The whole arm is prepared and wrapped in sterile towels covered by a tube of stockingette. Separate draping of the limb in this way allows the surgeon and his assistant to manoeuvre the arm during the operation.

Incision. The main part of the skin incision, about 10 centimetres long, extends downwards and laterally from the coracoid process, following the medial edge of the deltoid muscle. At the proximal end it may if necessary be curved laterally close to the lower border of the outer end of the clavicle (Fig. 4), though in most cases the straight incision suffices. The skin edges are freed from the underlying deep fascia and held apart by retractors.

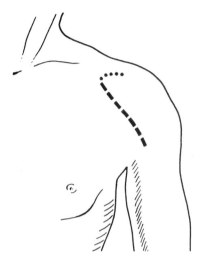

FIG. 4. Anterior exposure of shoulder. The skin incision. The horizontal limb of the incision may be omitted unless wide access is required.

The deep dissection. The deep fascia is incised in the line of the skin incision and the cut edges are turned back in order to identify the delto-pectoral groove—that is, the junction between pectoralis major and deltoid muscles. This groove is marked by the large cephalic vein, which forms a useful landmark. As the two muscles are separated by blunt dissection the vein is retracted medially with the pectoralis major: a few small tributaries entering the vein from the outer side may need to be divided. (If handled with forceps or retractors the normally bulky vein goes into spasm and contracts to a slender strand.)

When the two muscles have been separated in the lower part of the wound attention is directed to the upper part of the deltoid muscle where it is attached to the clavicle. The exposure is much enhanced if the medial part of the muscle origin is separated from the clavicle over a distance of 2 or 3 centimetres. This is best done by scissors after

the muscle has been separated from the underlying tissues by blunt dissection: a small fringe of muscle should be left attached to the bone to aid reconstruction at the end of the operation.

The pectoralis major and the deltoid are separated as widely as possible with a self-retaining retractor, to reveal deep to them the coracoid process with the conjoined coracobrachialis and biceps (short head) muscles attached near its tip and passing vertically downwards into the arm (Fig. 5). The coracoid process is cleared of soft tissue at a point about a centimetre proximal to its tip. The distal part of the coracoid process is then separated with an osteotome.

A holding stitch of strong catgut or silk is passed through the muscle origin immediately distal to the coracoid to allow the muscles to be reflected distally with the attached fragment of coracoid process. Before the muscles can be reflected adequately the fascia that fans out from each side of the muscle origin and from the coracoid process must be divided and the borders of the conjoined muscles clearly defined. As the muscle mass is peeled downwards a few snips with scissors on its deep aspect free slender bridges of areolar tissue. At this point care must be taken not to damage the musculocutaneous nerve, which enters the deep surface of the conjoined muscles. The nerve, which is surprisingly large, should be identified as it passes downwards and laterally from the axilla to enter the coracobrachialis about 7 or 8 centimetres below its origin (Fig. 6). Downward reflection of the muscle must cease when the entrance of the nerve into the muscle is revealed: attempts to reflect the muscle further may lead to stretching of the nerve. Injury to the nerve will, of course, cause paralysis of the coracobrachialis and biceps muscles and of most of the brachialis.

When the coracoid process and the attached muscles have been reflected out of the way the only remaining obstacle in the route to the shoulder is the subscapularis muscle, which in its lateral 2.5 centimetres or so is tendinous. It lies closely upon the anterior capsule of the shoulder and is often partly blended with it. Before the tendon is divided it is important to define its superior and inferior borders. This is done most easily if the muscle is put on the stretch by lateral rotation of the humerus. While an assistant holds the arm in this position the surgeon frees the borders of the subscapularis from adjacent flimsy areolar tissue and passes a blunt-pointed bone lever behind the tendon from above downwards.

To prevent retraction of the muscle belly of subscapularis out of sight when the tendon is divided, holding sutures of strong catgut or silk are inserted proximal to the proposed line of divi-

Closure. Depending upon the nature of the operation to be performed on the shoulder, the capsule may be closed by interrupted sutures or in special circumstances it may be sutured with overlap (see Putti-Platt operation, p. 156). Likewise the subscapularis tendon may be repaired end-to-end or overlapped, as circumstances demand.

The next step in the closure is to approximate the tip of the coracoid process to its base.

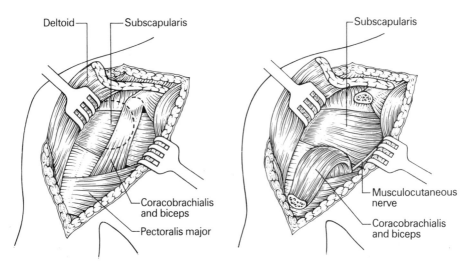

FIGS 5–6. Anterior exposure of shoulder. Figure 5—After separation of the deltoid and pectoralis major the conjoined coracobrachialis and biceps muscles are seen attached to the coracoid process. Deep to them lies the subscapularis, the fibres of which, running horizontally, become tendinous as they approach their insertion into the humerus. The broken line shows the position of the head of the humerus. Figure 6—As the coracobrachialis and short head of biceps are turned downwards, the musculocutaneous nerve is brought into view as it enters the deep surface of the conjoined muscles. Care must be taken to avoid injuring the nerve.

sion. The subscapularis tendon is then divided about 2.5 centimetres proximal to its insertion into the humerus. The proximal (muscular) part of the subscapularis retracts out of the way: the distal part may be retracted laterally with slender hooks or with a holding stitch.

The anterior part of the capsule of the shoulder joint is thus exposed: indeed it is often opened when the subscapularis is divided because the subscapularis tendon may be so closely blended with the capsule that the two are divided together. If the capsule has not already been opened it is incised vertically to whatever extent may be required. Retraction of the capsular flaps exposes the front of the head of the humerus and the anterior rim of the glenoid fossa.

Usually, adequate fixation is attained by sutures through the soft tissues on either side of the bone, but some surgeons prefer to fix it with a screw. Finally the upper edge of the deltoid muscle is reattached to the fringe that remains on the clavicle, and the contiguous edges of deltoid and pectoralis major are tacked together lightly with interrupted absorbable sutures. Nearly always the skin may be closed without drainage.

Comment

The anterior approach to the shoulder is simple and gives good access to the front of the joint. Unless the anatomy has been grossly distorted, as for instance by long-standing dislocation of the shoulder, it does not endanger important blood vessels or nerves, with the possible exception of the musculocutaneous nerve as already mentioned.

In most centres this is the standard approach for stabilisation of the shoulder in recurrent anterior dislocation and for other operations on the front of the joint. It has the disadvantage that the scar often becomes broad and prominent. This matters little in men but may be a disturbing blemish in young women: so much so that in such patients the axillary approach may be considered as an alternative (see below).

ANTERIOR AXILLARY APPROACH TO SHOULDER

An anterior axillary incision has been used for exposure of the shoulder because it is less likely than the delto-pectoral incision to leave an ugly scar. Indeed the scar is largely hidden in the axilla. The method to be described is that of Leslie and Ryan (1962).

TECHNIQUE

Position of patient. The patient lies supine with the upper limb upon a side table. The shoulder is abducted 90 degrees and laterally rotated.

Incision. The incision is vertical. It crosses the mid-point of the anterior axillary fold and is carried 6 or 7 centimetres posteriorly into the axilla (Fig. 7).

The deep dissection. The skin and fascia are undermined widely in a proximal direction so that the skin edges may be easily retracted upwards and laterally. The cephalic vein, marking the delto-pectoral groove, is thus brought into view, and the interval between deltoid and pectoralis major is opened up by blunt dissection, as in the standard anterior approach described in the previous section. The vein is retracted laterally with the deltoid muscle.

In the medial part of the wound the pectoralis major is retracted downwards and medially: to gain sufficient access it may be necessary to separate the tendon of the muscle partly or completely from its insertion on the humerus. The subsequent stages of the exposure follow those of the standard delto-pectoral approach (see above);

they consist in distal reflection of the conjoined coracobrachialis and short head of biceps and division of the subjacent subscapularis close to its musculo-tendinous junction.

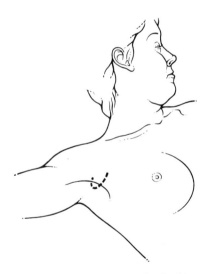

FIG. 7. Axillary approach to the shoulder.
The skin incision.

Closure. If the tendon of pectoralis major has been divided it must be repaired carefully with interrupted sutures. After repair of the subscapularis and coracobrachialis and biceps (or coracoid process) the muscles fall into place and only a few light absorbable sutures are needed to approximate the deltoid and pectoralis major. The skin edges may be drawn together by a subcuticular suture in order that the scar may be as unobtrusive as possible.

Comment

Although this approach to the shoulder is not as direct as the standard anterior approach described in the previous section, it undoubtedly leaves a more satisfactory scar. When a full exposure of the upper part of the joint is not required, therefore, it is to be preferred to the standard anterior approach when appearance is an important factor, as in young women. It probably has its greatest application in the treatment of recurrent anterior dislocation of the shoulder.

ANTERIOR EXPOSURE OF HUMERUS

The humerus may be exposed from end to end through an anterior exposure, and any part of this incision may be used according to requirements (Henry, 1945). Proximally the route is between the pectoralis major and the deltoid. Below the deltoid insertion the route is through the brachialis muscle direct to the humerus.

TECHNIQUE

Position of patient. The patient lies supine, with a rather thick sand-bag behind the lower part of the scapula to thrust the affected shoulder forwards. The whole arm must be prepared and draped, preferably in a stockingette tube.

slightly laterally in the delto-pectoral groove to a point just medial to the insertion of the deltoid (Fig. 8). The distal part of the incision extends vertically downwards from this point along the lateral border of the biceps muscle to the bend of the elbow, whence it descends 3 or 4 centimetres into the forearm, curving slightly medially towards the midline of the limb.

The deep dissection. In the upper half of the exposure the delto-pectoral groove is identified (p. 11) and the fascia over it is divided. The groove is landmarked by the cephalic vein, which should be retracted medially. When the medial border of the deltoid has been cleared as far proximally as its origin from the clavicle, clavicular

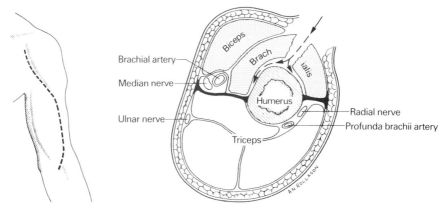

FIGS 8–9. Anterior exposure of humerus. Figure 8—The skin incision. Figure 9—Diagrammatic cross-section near middle of upper arm showing the route of approach, lateral to the biceps and through the brachialis direct to the front of the humerus. Note the position of the radial nerve.

Skin incision. The proximal part of the incision begins in the line of a shoulder strap. It runs downwards from the top of the clavicle to cross the tip of the coracoid process; thence it curves

fibres are severed from the bone in a lateral direction for 3 or 4 centimetres: it is well to leave a small fringe of muscle to aid subsequent reattachment. Separation of the deltoid from the clavicle allows the muscle to be drawn laterally as a large flap, revealing deep to it the greater tuberosity of the humerus and the bicipital tunnel containing the long head of biceps. Distal to this the front of the shaft of the humerus is exposed as far as the deltoid insertion.

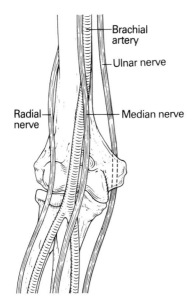

FIG. 10. Disposition of the major arteries and nerves at the front of the elbow region.

To expose the lower half of the humeral shaft the deep fascia is divided a centimetre lateral to the outer border of the biceps muscle and tendon. On this aspect of the arm the brachialis muscle is uncovered by the biceps, and its fibres may be separated by cutting vertically in a postero-medial direction towards the midline of the front of the humerus (Fig. 9). The cut is made straight onto the bone to incise periosteum, which may then be stripped from the anterior half of the bone with an elevator. If the brachialis is incised onto the middle of the front of the humerus as described, the radial nerve is well protected by the outer strip of the brachialis (Fig. 9). If the brachialis were split too far laterally the nerve would be endangered. The exposure is enhanced if the elbow is now flexed in order to relax the flexor muscles, which may then be drawn aside to bring the shaft of the humerus to the surface.

If the vertical incision through the brachialis muscle is continued distally beyond a horizontal line 3 centimetres above the level of the epicondyles of the humerus the elbow joint is opened to reveal the trochlea of the humerus and the coronoid process of the ulna. In this dissection great care must be taken to avoid injury to the median nerve and brachial artery (Fig. 10).

Closure. In the upper part of the wound it is necessary to use strong absorbable sutures to re-unite the medial part of the deltoid origin to the clavicle. In the remainder of the wound the muscles fall easily together once the elbow is extended, and only a few light sutures are needed. The skin is closed with or without drainage as circumstances require.

Comment

This is a useful and straightforward exposure applicable either to the whole length of the humerus or to any part of it. It is appropriate for operations upon the neck or head of the humerus, and lower down for fixation of humeral shaft fractures by plating or bone grafting. It is less appropriate for open intramedullary nailing of the shaft of the humerus, which is better done through a posterior approach. Provided proper care is exercised there is little danger to nerves or vessels.

In the lower half of the exposure the radial nerve might be damaged either by cutting through the brachialis muscle too far laterally or by over-vigorous retraction of the lateral muscles by bone levers passed round the back of the humerus. In the upper part of the wound work on the bone should be confined so far as possible to the anterior half of the humeral shaft. If it is desired to work round the lateral aspect of the shaft to the back, stripping of the bone should be done strictly subperiosteally with a well curved elevator.

In the extreme lower end of the wound, where the skin incision enters the forearm, the radial artery is in some danger if the incision is made injudiciously (Fig. 10); special care is needed in opening the deep fascia so that the vessels may be seen and protected.

POSTERIOR EXPOSURE OF HUMERUS

The route to the humerus from behind is through the triceps muscle: the long head and the lateral head are separated and the medial or deep head is incised in the midline of the arm.

TECHNIQUE

Position of patient. The patient may be prone or, preferably, in the lateral position with the affected limb uppermost and resting on a platform placed over the body (Fig. 11). The authors prefer the lateral posture because it allows the elbow to be flexed more readily: this is important especially for intramedullary nailing.

Incision. The incision is a vertical one in the midline of the arm. It begins 4 or 5 centimetres below the back of the acromion process and

The deep dissection. The deep fascia is opened first in the upper part of the arm. Here again the loose fleshy mass of the long head of triceps should first be identified and the fascia incised vertically along its outer border. As the incision proceeds distally the V-shaped gap where the long head and the lateral head of the triceps meet and blend comes into view. In the distal part of the arm the two bellies are intimately blended.

When the deep fascia has been split throughout the whole length of the wound the superficial part of the triceps—the blended long and lateral heads—is divided longitudinally to separate its two component parts (Fig. 13). This division has to be made with due regard for the structures that lie deep to the muscle plane—namely the radial nerve and the profunda vessels. These run obliquely downwards and outwards, and in its groove behind the arm the nerve gives off large motor

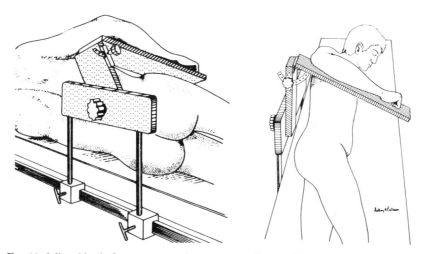

FIG. 11. Adjustable platform to support the upper arm, elbow and forearm for operations upon the posterior aspect of the humerus.

extends if necessary to the olecranon (Fig. 12). In the upper part of the arm it lies over the lateral border of the long head of the triceps. This muscle is easily identified because it lies as a loose fleshy wad along the medial half of the back of the arm and is easily grasped between finger and thumb: this characteristic looseness distinguishes it from the lateral head of the triceps and from the deltoid, which feel much less mobile.

branches to the lateral and medial heads of the triceps which must be preserved. The nerves and vessels should be mobilised and drawn safely out of the way while the medial or deep head of the triceps is split vertically in the midline of the arm right to the bone (Fig. 13). It only remains to strip the periosteum on each side of the incision to gain a full exposure of the posterior aspect of the humeral shaft.

Closure. Light absorbable sutures should be used to coapt the divided edges of the long head and the lateral head of the triceps. This is the only muscle layer that needs to be sutured. The skin is closed, usually without drainage.

basic incision may be used for exposure of the radial nerve in the middle of the arm. It is an approach that is simple and straightforward, though great care must be taken to avoid injury to the radial nerve and to its muscular branches. It

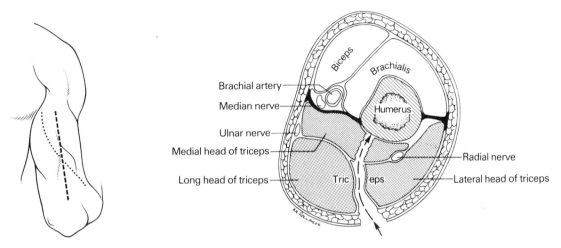

FIGS 12–13. Posterior exposure of humerus. Figure 12—The skin incision. The line of the radial nerve is indicated. Figure 13—Diagrammatic cross-section a little below the middle of the upper arm, showing the route of approach between the lateral head and the long head of the triceps and through the medial or deep head direct to the back of the bone. The radial nerve, crossing the back of the humerus obliquely downwards and laterally, lies immediately deep to the blended lateral and long heads of the triceps. Great care is needed to avoid injuring the nerve.

Comment

The posterior exposure of the humerus is used mainly in dealing with fractures in the mid-part of the bone. It is the most convenient approach for intramedullary nailing of the humerus. The same

should be noted also that in the upper part of the wound, in its medial corner, the ulnar nerve and the brachial artery, lying in relation to the medial part of the medial or deep head of the triceps, may come into view and must be carefully protected.

ANTERIOR EXPOSURE OF RADIUS

The whole length of the radius may be exposed from the front by the approach described by Henry (1945). The technique entails stripping of the anterior fibres of the supinator muscle from the front of the radius, the posterior interosseous nerve being thus protected where it lies within the muscle. Lower down, the route is between the brachioradialis laterally and the flexor carpi radialis medially.

TECHNIQUE

Position of patient. The patient lies supine with the limb resting upon the arm table. The elbow should be slightly flexed. If a tourniquet is used it should be placed high on the upper arm.

Incision. The incision begins 5 centimetres proximal to the anterior flexor crease of the elbow, just lateral to the biceps tendon. It follows the outer border of the biceps tendon into the forearm and thence extends in a straight line towards the styloid process of the radius (Fig. 14). The skin edges are freed from the underlying fascia for a short distance on each side of the incision.

insertion of the tendon, exposes the upper part of the radial shaft. Just lateral and distal to that point fibres of the supinator muscle, wrapped round the radius from behind, reach the front of the bone. With an elevator the supinator is peeled away from the anterior and lateral aspects of the radius

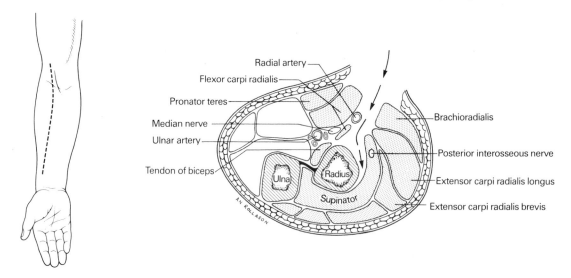

FIGS 14–15. Anterior exposure of radius (Henry 1945). Figure 14—The skin incision. Figure 15—Diagrammatic cross section through proximal part of forearm. The posterior interosseous nerve is protected by stripping the supinator muscle, within which the nerve lies, from the anterior aspect of the radius, beginning just lateral to the insertion of the biceps tendon.

The deep dissection. After division of the deep fascia the first step is to mobilise and retract laterally the wad of three muscles that lies along the lateral border of the forearm: these muscles are the brachioradialis, the extensor carpi radialis longus and the extensor carpi radialis brevis (Fig. 15). This wad of muscles is strikingly mobile, so that it may easily be grasped between the fingers and thumb and moved from side to side. The muscle wad is tethered by a leash of vessels that extends laterally from the upper part of the radial artery close below the elbow. This leash is easily identified beneath the deep fascia and may be ligated and divided: the mobile wad of muscles may then be drawn laterally.

The key to the starting point of the dissection down to bone is the tendon of the biceps. This should be followed down to its insertion into the bicipital tuberosity of the radius. At the outer side of the tendon at this point is a small bursa, and an incision through this, immediately lateral to the

(Fig. 15). The posterior interosseous nerve, embedded in the supinator as it passes towards the back of the forearm, is displaced with the muscle and is thus held out of harm's way so long as retraction is gentle.

Distal to the supinator the shaft of the radius is clearly exposed between the flexor carpi radialis in front and the wad of strap-like muscles (brachioradialis and extensors carpi radialis, longus and brevis) behind. The exposure is enhanced by pronation of the forearm, which carries the pronator radii teres medially.

Comment

This exposure, of which any particular part rather than the whole may be used according to requirements, is widely used for routine operations upon the radius, and particularly for the plating or bone-grafting of fractures. It is also useful for intramedullary nailing.

The bugbear of all approaches to the upper third of the radius is the risk of damage to the posterior interosseous nerve where it lies in the supinator muscle, and distal to this where it ramifies at the back of the forearm. The nerve is very susceptible to bruising, as for instance by over-vigorous retraction. Extreme care and gentleness are therefore required when the supinator is being stripped from the front of the radius and when it is drawn postero-laterally with bone levers or retractors.

The radial artery lies close to the medial edge of the wound. The proximal part of the artery, immediately below its origin from the brachial artery at the medial side of the biceps tendon, is relatively superficial and may be damaged by careless incision of the deep fascia in the proximal part of the wound. Danger to the artery is averted if the skin and fascial incisions are strictly lateral to the biceps tendon, and if the deep fascia in particular is divided with due caution.

POSTERIOR EXPOSURE OF PROXIMAL HALF OF RADIUS

The upper part of the radius may be approached from behind by a route that lies between the ulna and the group of extensor muscles that arise from it and from the interosseous membrane.

Incision. The incision begins at the lateral epicondyle of the humerus and extends obliquely downwards and medially across the back of the upper forearm, following the lower border of the

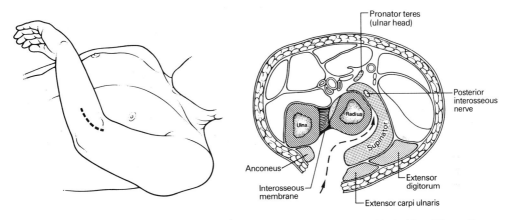

FIGS 16–17. Posterior exposure of proximal end of radius. Figure 16—The skin incision. Figure 17—The route is between the anconeus and the extensor carpi ulnaris and, more distally, between the ulna and the extensor carpi ulnaris. The interosseous membrane then guides the operator to the shaft of the radius.

TECHNIQUE

Position of patient. The patient lies supine with the affected forearm supported across the chest (Fig. 16). To stabilise the limb in this position it is convenient to attach a small weight to the wrist with a soft bandage and to suspend the weight over the side of the table. A tourniquet may be used on the upper arm.

anconeus muscle to its insertion into the ulna. The incision then sweeps vertically downwards over the subcutaneous aspect of the ulna (Fig. 16).

The deep dissection. Deep fascia is opened throughout the length of the incision and the interval is developed between the anconeus and the extensor carpi ulnaris and, more distally, between the shaft of the ulna and the extensor carpi ulnaris. This muscle is stripped from the bone as far as the interosseous membrane, and the adjacent extensor muscles (extensor digitorum and extensors carpi radialis longus and brevis) are stripped from the interosseous membrane in a dissection that proceeds laterally until the shaft of the radius is reached (Fig. 17). The periosteum of the radius may then be incised vertically and the posterior aspect of the bone exposed to view.

Comment

This exposure avoids injury to the posterior interosseous nerve by following a plane deep to the nerve and to the muscles that its terminal branches supply. It is appropriate for bone plating or for bone-grafting of fractures. It does not offer any advantage over the anterior approach, which the authors prefer.

EXPOSURE OF SHAFT OF ULNA

The postero-medial aspect of the ulna is subcutaneous throughout its whole length; the bone may therefore be exposed by a direct approach between the flexor muscles anteriorly and the extensors posteriorly. Periosteum is incised longitudinally and peeled back with an elevator.

SIMULTANEOUS EXPOSURE OF SHAFTS OF RADIUS AND ULNA

Although it is easily possible to reach the shafts of both forearm bones from the posterior approach to the radius already described above, nevertheless when both bones have to be operated upon it is usually wiser to expose each bone independently through a separate incision. In cases of fracture, the use of separate incisions reduces the risk of cross union between the two bones.

EXPOSURE OF BRACHIAL PLEXUS ABOVE CLAVICLE

It is seldom that the whole of the brachial plexus has to be explored: usually the exploration is concerned mainly with the uppermost trunk of the plexus or with the lowest trunk.

TECHNIQUE

Position of patient. The patient lies supine, with a firm sand-bag behind the shoulder of the affected side to thrust it forwards, with the head turned towards the opposite side, and with the arm abducted (Fig. 18).

Incision. For exploration of the whole plexus a "lazy L" incision is used. The vertical component of the incision extends from the region of the mastoid process to the medial half of the clavicle: it thus lies over the sternocleidomastoid muscle.

The horizontal limb curves laterally to end about 5 centimetres below the lateral half of the clavicle (Fig. 18). The incision is deepened to the sternocleidomastoid and pectoralis major muscles and the triangular flap of skin is reflected backwards together with the superficial fascia.

The deep dissection. First the external jugular vein is identified and ligated above the clavicle. The posterior belly of the omohyoid muscle is identified and removed. The transverse cervical vessels are ligated at the medial and lateral extremities of the wound and the intervening parts of the vessels are removed. Medial retraction of the sternocleidomastoid muscle is enhanced if necessary by separation of its clavicular head from the clavicle.

The scalenus anterior muscle should next be sought. Its fibres slope downwards and slightly outwards towards their insertion into the upper margin of the first rib. In the deep angle between

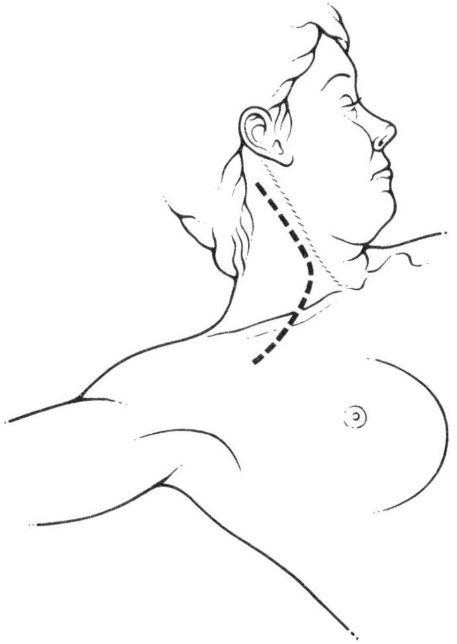

FIG. 18. Exposure of supraclavicular part of brachial plexus. The skin incision.

may be divided near its attachment to the first rib, with care to avoid injury to the phrenic nerve and on the left side to the thoracic duct. The trunks of the brachial plexus may now be identified and traced proximally or distally as required.

Distal extension of dissection deep to clavicle. If necessary the components of the brachial plexus, together with the subclavian vessels, may be followed into the arm by excision of the central part of the clavicle (Fig. 19). Before the bone is divided all soft tissues must be stripped circumferentially from it, and in this manoeuvre it is essential to keep close to the bone.

Closure. The wound is closed in layers, with care to ensure a smooth repair of the platysma. If desired, the skin incision may be closed by subcuticular sutures.

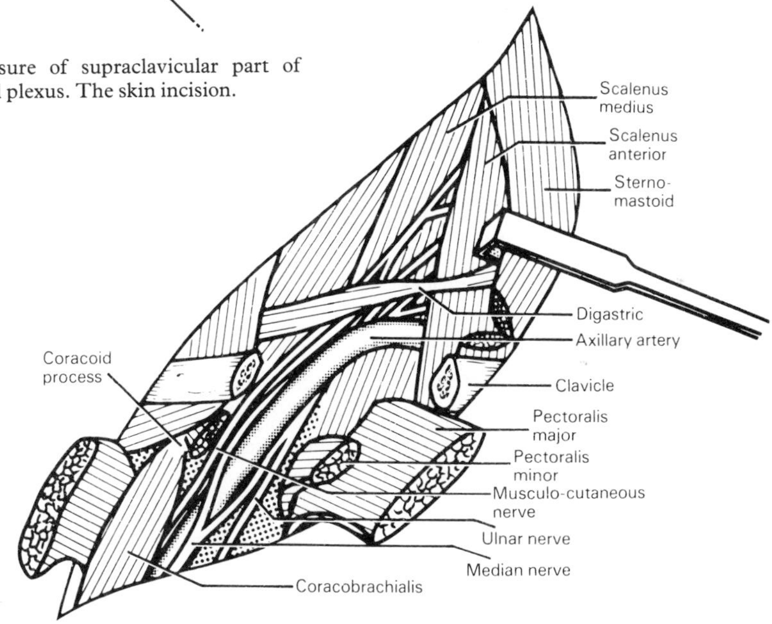

FIG. 19. Simplified diagram of the brachial plexus, with its more important anatomical relationships. The central part of the clavicle has been removed to allow the nerve trunks to be followed into the axilla.

the scalenus anterior and the sternocleidomastoid the pulsatile internal jugular vein may be identified. If necessary—particularly for exposure of the lowest trunk of the plexus—the scalenus anterior

Comment

The skin incision may be modified according to the extent of the exploration that is required. If this is concerned mainly with the uppermost trunk of the plexus a straight oblique incision extending from the mastoid process to the mid-point of the clavicle may suffice. If the lowest trunk alone is to be explored a horizontal incision just above the clavicle may be preferred in the interest of an unobtrusive scar. The need for a delicate technique in order to avoid injury to the main vessels, nerve trunks, thoracic duct and pleura hardly requires emphasis. It is all too easy to pierce the dome of the pleura, with consequent pneumothorax.

EXPOSURE OF BRACHIAL PLEXUS BELOW CLAVICLE

The infraclavicular part of the brachial plexus lies within the axilla deep to the pectoralis major muscle.

TECHNIQUE

Position of patient. The patient is positioned in the same manner as for exposure of the supra-clavicular part of the plexus (p. 20).

Incision. The incision extends from the mid-point of the clavicle downwards and outwards towards the lateral extremity of the anterior wall of the axilla, just medial to the coracoid process (Fig. 20). If necessary the incision may be extended down the antero-medial aspect of the upper arm.

The deep dissection. After incision of the deep fascia the upper and lower borders of the pectoralis major muscle are identified where the fibres converge towards the humerus. The muscle is divided near its insertion and reflected medially, with care to preserve the lateral and medial anterior thoracic nerves. The pectoralis minor muscle may likewise be divided close to its attachment to the coracoid process and reflected medially: again care must be taken to preserve its nerve supply

(the medial anterior thoracic nerve). The component parts of the brachial plexus, together with the major vessels, may now be identified. If neces-

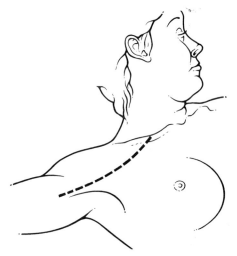

FIG. 20. Exposure of axillary part of brachial plexus. The skin incision.

sary the exposure may be extended above the clavicle (see previous section), and if complete exposure is required the mid-part of the clavicle may be excised (Fig. 19).

Closure. The deep muscles are repaired and the skin is closed with interrupted eversion sutures.

EXPOSURE OF RADIAL NERVE IN ARM

Proximal to the lower border of the teres major muscle the radial nerve is exposed as part of the brachial plexus (see above). The following description relates to exposure of the nerve distal to the axilla, where it courses round the back of the humerus towards the outer side.

TECHNIQUE

Position of patient. The patient lies in the lateral posture with the affected limb uppermost. The elbow is flexed 90 degrees. It is best to support the forearm on an adjustable platform over the body (Fig. 21).

Incision. The skin incision is postero-lateral. If the whole length of the nerve in the arm is to be exposed the incision begins just distal to the postero-lateral angle of the acromion process and follows the posterior border of the deltoid muscle skin flaps are reflected and the deep fascia is incised in the line of the skin incision.

The deep dissection. In the middle of the arm the lateral head of the triceps is identified (Fig. 23)

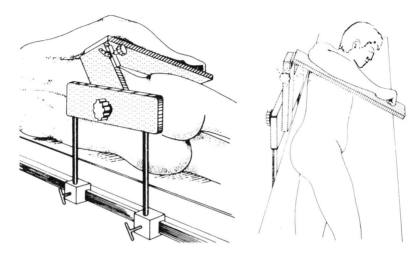

FIG. 21. Adjustable platform to support the upper limb for exposure of the radial nerve.

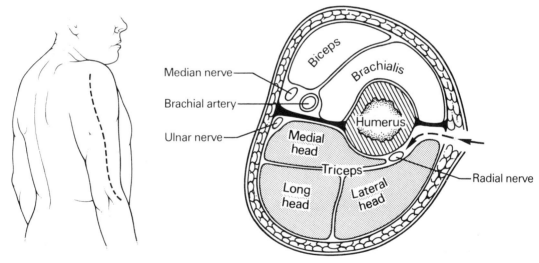

FIGS 22–23. Exposure of radial nerve. Figure 22—The skin incision. Figure 23—The lateral head of the triceps is detached from the humerus and retracted medially and posteriorly. The nerve is thus revealed in its groove at the back of the humerus.

as far as its insertion. Thence it extends vertically down the arm, following the lateral margin of the triceps, to a point 2 centimetres anterior to the lateral epicondyle of the humerus (Fig. 22). The and its anterior margin defined. The muscle is then reflected from its attachment to the humerus and displaced posteriorly until the radial nerve is displayed in its groove at the back of the humerus.

Once the nerve has been located in this position it is easily traced proximally as far as the inferior fold of the axilla and distally as far as may be necessary.

Closure. The muscles fall back into place, and only a few light catgut sutures are required to hold the deeper tissues. The skin is closed without drainage.

EXTENSION OF EXPOSURE TO DISPLAY POSTERIOR INTEROSSEOUS NERVE

When the radial nerve has been exposed in the arm it is easily traced distally to the point of origin of its terminal divisions in front of the lateral epicondyle of the humerus, and the posterior interosseous nerve may be followed round the radius to the back of the forearm. The skin incision is prolonged distally from the front of the lateral epicondyle for about 10 centimetres towards the styloid process of the radius. The nerve is followed anterior to the lateral intermuscular septum, where it lies beneath the brachioradialis, to the point where it enters the supinator muscle at the front of the upper end of the radius. It may be followed through the supinator muscle in its groove round the lateral aspect of the radius by dividing the overlying muscle fibres.

EXPOSURE OF POSTERIOR INTEROSSEOUS NERVE AT BACK OF FOREARM

The posterior interosseous nerve, the main terminal branch of the radial nerve, enters the antero-lateral part of the supinator muscle in the upper forearm and winds obliquely downwards

TECHNIQUE

Position of patient. The patient lies supine with the affected limb resting upon the arm platform.

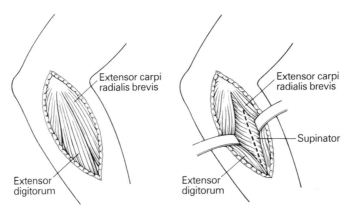

FIGS 24–25. Exposure of posterior interosseous nerve in forearm. Figure 24—The interval between the mobile wad of muscles (of which extensor carpi radialis brevis is the most posterior member) and the relatively fixed extensor digitorum is defined and opened from below. Figure 25—The supinator muscle exposed by retraction laterally of extensor carpi radialis brevis and medially of extensor digitorum. The line of the posterior interosseous nerve within the supinator is shown.

and backwards round the upper part of the radius within the supinator muscle. Near the lower edge of the supinator the nerve lies directly over the back of the radius.

The elbow is flexed 90 degrees and the forearm is held in pronation so that the extensor aspect of the forearm faces upwards. A tourniquet may be used on the upper arm.

Incision. The skin incision begins at the lateral epicondyle of the humerus and follows the back of the radius in a line directed towards the styloid process of the radius. The lower end of the incision extends to about the junction of the uppermost third and the middle third of the forearm.

The deep dissection. The deep fascia is incised from below upwards to expose the interval between the extensor carpi radialis brevis and the extensor digitorum (Fig. 24). This plane is easily located because the extensor carpi radialis brevis is one of the three muscles that together form a mobile wad that shapes the lateral contour of the forearm. This wad, of which the extensor carpi radialis brevis is the most posterior member, is easily moved from side to side when grasped between finger and thumb whereas the extensor digitorum is relatively fixed. The interval between

these two muscles is developed first in the lower part of the wound.

Higher up the muscles are blended and may have to be separated with scissors. The muscles are drawn apart with a self-retaining retractor to expose the oblique fibres of the supinator muscle deep to them (Fig. 25). The posterior interosseous nerve is most easily found 5 or 6 centimetres distal to the head of the radius, precisely over the back of the radial shaft. Since the nerve is enclosed within the supinator muscle the fibres of the muscle must be separated by blunt dissection with round-nosed scissors. This manoeuvre must be carried out gently lest the nerve be damaged: the layer of muscle covering the nerve is very thin.

Once the nerve has been identified the exposure may be extended proximally and distally along the course of the nerve by dividing the superficial fibres of the supinator.

EXPOSURE OF MEDIAN AND ULNAR NERVES

The whole length of the median and ulnar nerves may be exposed through a single incision along the medial side of the limb. Alternatively, the median nerve may be separately exposed in the forearm through an incision near the midline.

EXPOSURE OF WHOLE LENGTH OF MEDIAN NERVE WITH ULNAR NERVE

TECHNIQUE

Position of patient. The patient lies supine with the arm abducted upon the side table and laterally rotated.

Incision. The skin incision follows the medial border of the biceps muscle from the axilla to the junction of the upper two-thirds and lower third of the upper arm. Thence it curves slightly medially towards the medial epicondyle of the humerus, and from there it extends over the medial part of the anterior forearm in a straight line terminating at the radial side of the pisiform bone

(Fig. 26). The skin edges are reflected to expose the deep fascia, which is incised in the same line as the skin incision.

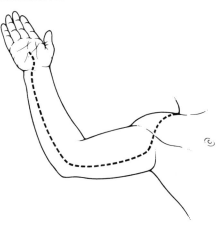

FIG. 26. Exposure of whole length of median and ulnar nerves. The skin incision. Only part of the incision, depending upon the site of the lesion, is used at any one operation.

Exposure in the upper arm. Both the median nerve and the ulnar nerve are superficial in the upper arm and their exposure does not present any difficulty. The median nerve lies in close relationship with the brachial artery in the groove between the medial border of the biceps muscle and the brachialis muscle (Fig. 27). It crosses the elbow into the forearm just medial to the biceps tendon (Fig. 10).

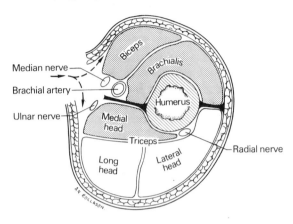

FIG. 27. Exposure of median and ulnar nerves in upper arm. Both nerves lie superficially and at first close together. At the level shown they are separated by the medial intermuscular septum.

The ulnar nerve, which as it leaves the axilla is in close relationship with the brachial artery and the median nerve, diverges from them as it descends in the arm, following a straight course between the axilla and the medial epicondyle of the humerus. In the mid-arm it lies in close relationship to the antero-medial edge of the triceps, and lower down it lies behind the medial intermuscular septum (Figs 10 and 27).

Exposure in the forearm. The ulnar nerve is exposed without difficulty. The dissection may be begun distally by developing the interval between the flexor carpi ulnaris (which gains insertion into the pisiform bone) medially and the flexor digitorum superficialis laterally. This interval is then followed proximally into the upper forearm. The ulnar nerve lies upon the flexor digitorum profundus, close to its medial edge and in close relationship to the flexor carpi ulnaris. Having been found distally, the nerve is easily traced throughout its length in the forearm.

The median nerve may be exposed by lifting the flexor digitorum superficialis forwards and outwards, when the nerve will be found adherent to the under surface of the muscle mass. Alternatively, the lateral skin edge may be raised as far as the midline of the forearm. The nerve is then identified in the lower forearm where it lies strictly in the midline deep to the palmaris longus, when this is present. The nerve is then traced proximally, where it lies deep to the flexor digitorum superficialis. The radial origin of this muscle, composed of fibres running downwards and medially, must be divided; more proximally, the pronator teres, which crosses the nerve obliquely downwards and outwards, should be separated from its insertion into the radius. Near the elbow the deep ulnar head of the pronator teres must also be divided where it lies over the nerve.

EXPOSURE IN FOREARM OF MEDIAN NERVE ALONE

If the median nerve alone is to be exposed the skin incision should be made in the mid-line of the forearm. The nerve is identified just proximal to the wrist, where it lies deep to the palmaris longus, strictly in the mid-line of the limb. Thence it may be traced proximally as already described.

ANTERIOR EXPOSURE OF HIP

The anterior approach to the hip is often named after Smith-Petersen, who described it in 1949. The approach is through intermuscular planes— superficially between the sartorius medially and the tensor fasciae latae laterally, and more deeply between the ilio-psoas medially and the rectus femoris laterally. The exposure is enhanced by detachment and distal retraction of the origin of the rectus, allowing the front of the capsule of the hip joint to be fully revealed.

TECHNIQUE

Position of patient. The patient lies supine, the affected hip being thrust forward slightly by a sand-bag placed under the buttock.

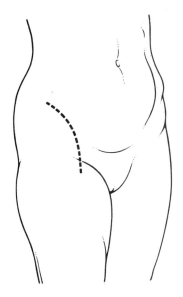

FIG. 28. Anterior exposure of hip.
The skin incision.

Incision. The skin incision follows the line of the crest of the ilium forwards from a point at the junction of its anterior and middle thirds. Upon reaching the anterior superior iliac spine the incision is angled to run vertically downwards towards the outer border of the patella, ending about 8 centimetres below the anterior superior spine (Fig. 28). Underlying fatty tissue is cleared to expose the deep fascia.

The deep dissection. Immediately distal to the anterior superior iliac spine the deep fascia of the upper thigh is split in the direction of its fibres, to reveal the gap between the sartorius and the tensor fasciae latae muscles. Sartorius may be detached from the bone by sharp dissection and retracted medially. The antero-medial edge of the tensor fasciae latae is identified and retracted laterally.

Attention is now directed to the crest of the ilium, where the fascia that covers the external oblique muscle of the abdomen is continuous with the fascia over the tensor fasciae latae muscle. This membrane is incised over the crest and reflected medially and laterally by sharp dissection close to the bone. Over the lateral corner of the crest the knife may be slid down upon the lateral face of the ilium, separating the tensor fasciae latae muscle and part of the gluteus medius from their origins. The muscles are retracted far laterally and the space between them and the wing of the ilium is plugged with a gauze pack. On the medial side of the ilium the iliacus muscle may be similarly detached from the front part of the inner face of the ilium and held away from the bone with a gauze pack.

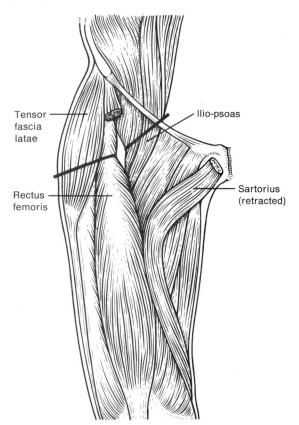

FIG. 29. The anterior muscles of the hip. In the anterior exposure the route is, firstly, between the sartorius and the tensor fasciae latae, and, more deeply, between the ilio-psoas and the rectus femoris.

The dissection is now carried distally through the area immediately distal to the anterior superior iliac spine (Fig. 29), where there is a thickish layer of fibro-fatty tissue. This is cleared away by dissection with scissors, to expose in the floor of the space the upper part of the rectus femoris muscle arising from the ilium by the direct head attached to the anterior inferior iliac spine and the reflected head attached near the superior lip of the acetabulum. The muscle is detached from these origins and reflected distally. Clearance of fatty tissue deep to the rectus origin and medial to the ilio-psoas now reveals the outer surface of the capsule of the hip joint. According to the requirements of the operation, the capsule may be opened by an H-shaped incision or it may be excised.

Dislocation of hip. If the nature of the operation to be performed necessitates dislocation of the head of the femur from the acetabulum the dislocation is best achieved by flexion and lateral rotation. Before dislocation is attempted, however, any obvious obstruction to extrusion of the femoral head must be removed. In osteoarthritis the head is often invested by osteophytes projecting from the anterior and superior margins of the acetabulum. These should be chiselled away. Dislocation may be aided by a skid or lever inserted between the femoral head and the acetabulum. The temptation to apply a strong rotation force on the thigh to disengage the head from the acetabulum must be resisted. Even moderate force may fracture the shaft of the femur, especially if the bones are rarefied, as in the elderly.

Of course, if the planned operation is to include removal of the femoral head it may be simpler to divide the femoral neck with an osteotome or a reciprocating saw before the femoral head is removed. It may then be removed piecemeal if necessary. By this prior division of the femoral neck the risk of spiral fracture of the femoral shaft from forced rotation is eliminated.

Closure. The fascia over the external oblique muscle of the abdomen and that over the tensor fasciae latae muscle are united over the crest of the ilium with interrupted sutures of strong catgut. The rectus femoris is restored to its natural position and held by sutures through the soft tissues. Sartorius and tensor fasciae latae are united immediately distal to the anterior superior iliac spine. The skin is closed by interrupted or continuous sutures. A polythene tube for suction drainage may be left in position in the deep layers of the wound if desired.

Comment
The anterior exposure of the hip may be varied in the extent to which the tissue planes are opened up, according to the requirements of the operation. For instance, if the operation is to be limited to obtaining a piece of synovial membrane for histological examination the exposure may be much less extensive than that described above; whereas for reconstructive operations such as arthroplasty or arthrodesis the full exposure is required.

This exposure is used less often now than it was a decade or two ago. In the years that followed immediately upon the Second World War it was made popular by Smith-Petersen, who used it mainly for cup arthroplasty. That operation is now seldom performed, and the anterior approach does not lend itself well to replacement of the femoral head or to total replacement arthroplasty. Nevertheless it still has an important place, particularly for routine exposure of the hip to obtain material for biopsy, for intra-articular arthrodesis, and for open reduction of congenital dislocation. Better exposure of the acetabulum for replacement arthroplasty is obtained through the antero-lateral or the postero-lateral incision.

ANTERO-LATERAL EXPOSURE OF HIP

In the antero-lateral exposure of the hip the interval between the tensor fasciae latae muscle and the gluteus medius is developed to reveal the antero-lateral aspect of the hip capsule. The acetabulum is approached by dislocating the hip in lateral rotation.

TECHNIQUE
Position of patient. The patient may lie supine on the operation table. A small sand-bag may be placed under the buttock of the affected side to rotate the trochanter slightly forwards. Some surgeons practise this approach with the patient

in the lateral position: others have the patient set up on the orthopaedic table (McKee and Watson-Farrar, 1966).

Incision. The incision forms an angle open anteriorly. Its upper limb begins 2.5 centimetres behind the anterior superior spine of the ilium and extends obliquely backwards to the tip of the greater trochanter. The lower limb of the incision extends vertically downwards from the greater trochanter for 6 to 8 centimetres (Fig. 30). The skin flaps are mobilised from the underlying deep fascia, which is cleared of adherent adipose tissue.

the hip joint now comes into view with, immediately above it, the reflected head of the rectus femoris muscle. The reflected head and the anterior part of the capsule may be excised or, if the capsule is to be preserved, it may be opened by an H-shaped incision and flaps turned proximally and distally.

If work is to be done on the acetabulum it is necessary to dislocate the hip by rotating the limb laterally. Before this is attempted the surgeon must be sure that the capsule has been adequately freed or excised, and that osteophytes projecting from the anterior margin of the acetabulum have

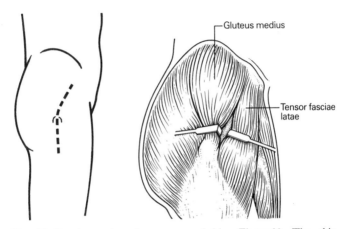

FIGS 30–31. Antero-lateral exposure of hip. Figure 30—The skin incision. Figure 31—The tensor fasciae latae (anteriorly) and the gluteus medius lie close together on the wing of the ilium but are easily separated nearer the greater trochanter.

The deep exposure. When the deep fascia has been incised the interval between the tensor fasciae latae muscle anteriorly and the gluteus medius posteriorly is identified immediately proximal to the antero-superior corner of the greater trochanter. This interval is widened by separating the fibres with dissecting scissors and is pursued proximally. Towards the crest of the ilium the two muscles are blended more closely and have to be separated by sharp dissection with scissors (Fig. 31). The space between the muscles is opened up by stripping part of the muscle origins from the outer aspect of the wing of the ilium. Nearer the trochanter, the gluteus minimus is also partly raised from the bone and retracted posteriorly. In the lower half of the wound the capsule of

been trimmed away; otherwise dislocation may be impeded. In any case only moderate lateral rotation force should be applied to the femur: excessive force entails a risk of fracturing the shaft of the femur, especially if the bone is rarefied. If dislocation seems difficult it may be aided by a broad sharp bone lever or skid insinuated between the joint surfaces. Easier still, if the proposed operation includes discarding the femoral head, is to divide the femoral neck with an osteotome or saw before dislocation is attempted and to remove the femoral head either entire or piecemeal.

Once dislocation has been achieved full lateral rotation of the limb, with lateral retraction of the proximal part of the femur with a bone hook, allows a good exposure of the acetabulum.

Closure. If the capsule has been preserved the flaps are approximated with two or three fine catgut sutures, after which the separated muscles are likewise approximated with interrupted sutures. The skin is closed with deep tension sutures and skin edge sutures. Suction drainage is optional: it is used or not according to individual circumstances and the surgeon's preference.

Comment

The antero-lateral approach to the hip has the advantage that muscles are separated rather than divided. It is used extensively for total replacement arthroplasty of the hip. Nevertheless many surgeons prefer the postero-lateral exposure for hip arthroplasty, claiming better access thereby to the upper end of the femur for fitting of the femoral head prosthesis, with the facility also to protect the sciatic nerve from injury.

The antero-lateral exposure is also appropriate for biopsy of the synovial membrane, for anterior wedge osteotomy to correct deformity in slipped femoral epiphysis, and for open reduction of an intracapsular fracture of the neck of the femur.

POSTERIOR (POSTERO-LATERAL) EXPOSURE OF HIP

The posterior exposure of the hip has been practised at least since Langenbeck's description of it in 1874. The method became popular after Kocher's classic description in 1892. The modification of Kocher's method used most commonly at the present time is that described by Gibson in 1950 or the variation of Gibson's technique described by McFarland and Osborne in 1954. A somewhat more limited exposure devised by Austin Moore (1957) is also used commonly for hip replacement operations.

Position of patient. The patient lies in the true lateral position with the affected hip uppermost. It is convenient to have a bridge-like platform which rests upon the lower part of the table, upon which to support the affected leg (Fig. 32). The platform is about 15 centimetres high and thus it ensures that the limb rests conveniently in a horizontal position. The sound limb may lie extended beneath the platform or, better still if the joints are fully mobile, the hip and knee may be flexed 90 degrees and secured in that position by strapping:

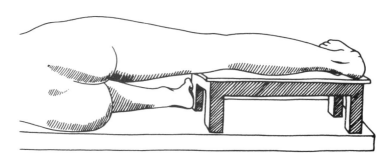

FIG. 32. Position of limbs for postero-lateral exposure of hip. The affected limb rests horizontally upon a simple platform. The unaffected limb lies beneath the platform or, preferably, it may be flexed at the hip and knee as shown here, in order to stabilise the pelvis.

THE GIBSON TECHNIQUE

In this technique the hip joint is displayed from the back, the gluteus medius muscle is detached from the greater trochanter and the hip is dislocated by lateral rotation to give a full end-on view of the acetabulum and of the femoral head.

this ensures greater stability of the pelvis (Fig. 32).

Incision. The upper part of the skin incision is oblique. It extends from a point on the iliac crest 6 centimetres in front of the posterior iliac spine to the top of the anterior margin of the greater trochanter. From this point the lower part of the incision extends vertically downwards for 8 to 10 centimetres (Fig. 33).

The deep dissection. With the skin edges retracted the fascia lata is cleaned in the lower half of the wound. It is then incised vertically in the line of its fibres and the splitting of this layer is pursued proximally with scissors into the gluteal muscle mass. Here the plane of cleavage is either between the anterior border of gluteus maximus and the tensor fasciae latae muscle or through anterior fibres of the gluteus maximus (Fig. 34).

stay sutures which are used to reflect the muscles posteriorly (Fig. 36): in this way the gemelli and the obturator internus are used to protect the sciatic nerve. The gluteus medius, cut from the trochanter close to the bone, is reflected proximally and forwards, revealing beneath it the gluteus minimus. This muscle is similarly detached from the trochanter and turned forwards.

The whole of the superior and posterior parts of the capsule of the hip joint are now clearly displayed. The capsule is incised vertically close behind the greater trochanter and the incision is extended to the superior part of the capsule.

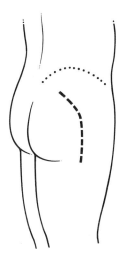 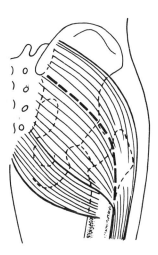

FIGS 33–34. Postero-lateral exposure of hip. Figure 33—The skin incision. Figure 34—The gluteus maximus is split in the direction of its fibres. The dotted outline shows the underlying bony landmarks.

The mass of tissue formed by the gluteus maximus and its distal aponeurotic prolongation is retracted posteriorly, a manoeuvre that is made easy by the large trochanteric bursa which lies immediately deep to the muscle. It may be convenient now to insert a large self-retaining retractor, thus displaying the gluteus medius muscle and more distally the short transverse lateral rotator muscles of the hip—namely from above downwards the piriformis, the superior gemellus, the obturator internus, the inferior gemellus and a broad fleshy muscle, the quadratus femoris (Fig. 35). These muscles, except for the last named which need not be disturbed, are detached from the greater trochanter after the insertion of

Through this incision curved bone levers may be placed round the femoral neck, one above and the other below. The head and neck of the femur, and the margin of the acetabulum, are thus clearly revealed. To expose the hip further the posterosuperior part of the capsule and synovial membrane may either be excised or, if capsule is to be preserved, flaps outlined by an H-shaped incision may be reflected.

Dislocation of hip. If intra-articular work is contemplated the hip must be dislocated. Before dislocation is attempted, any large osteophytes projecting from the margin of the acetabulum and closely investing the femoral head should be chipped off with a chisel; otherwise they may make dislocation difficult or impossible. Once these obstructions have been removed dislocation is achieved by flexing the hip 90 degrees and then

If there is resistance to dislocation with the femur intact, it is easier to divide the femoral neck through its middle and then to remove the severed head separately, either as a whole or piecemeal.

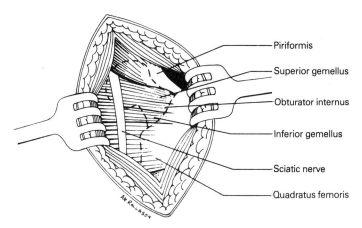

FIG. 35. The short transverse lateral rotator muscles deep to the gluteus maximus. Note that the sciatic nerve lies deep to the piriformis but upon the superficial aspect of the obturator internus, gemelli and quadratus femoris. The position of the femoral head is shown by the interrupted line.

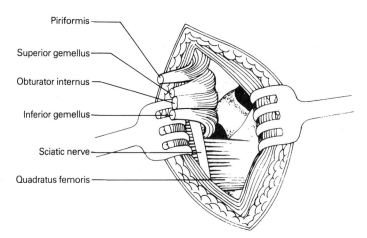

FIG. 36. The piriformis, obturator internus and gemelli have been divided close to the greater trochanter and reflected backwards. In this way they protect the sciatic nerve. The capsule of the joint has been excised. The femoral neck is thus exposed.

rotating it laterally so that the foot comes to lie near the opposite iliac crest, its sole directed upwards towards the axilla.

If the proposed operation entails discarding the femoral head it is not essential to dislocate the upper end of the femur in one piece as described.

Closure. If capsule has been preserved the incisions through it are repaired by three or four absorbable sutures. Gluteus medius is re-attached by mattress sutures. Piriformis and the conjoined gemelli and obturator internus are re-attached near their insertions with the stay sutures already holding them. The gluteal aponeurosis and fascia lata must be closed meticulously with strong interrupted absorbable sutures. The muscle fibres more proximally lie naturally in position and call for only light sutures. In closure of the skin it is recommended that deep tension sutures be first inserted and then the skin edge sutures, which may be interrupted or continuous. Suction drainage from the deeper layers may be provided if considerable oozing is feared.

The McFarland-Osborne Modification

The main disadvantage of the Gibson exposure is the detachment of the gluteus medius and gluteus minimus muscles from the greater trochanter.

flake of the lateral aspect of the greater trochanter with the conjoined muscle mass to ensure continuity of the fibres. When the muscle mass with the flake of bone has been separated from the trochanter it is slid forwards by a bone lever inserted under it. This is made easy by the fact that gluteus medius and vastus lateralis meet at an angle which is open forwards (Fig. 37). In all other respects the McFarland-Osborne exposure is the same as that of Gibson.

Comment

The full Gibson exposure, or preferably the McFarland-Osborne modification of it, is useful when reconstructive work necessitates a full view

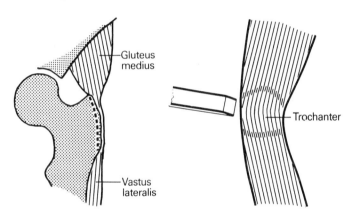

FIG. 37. McFarland-Osborne exposure of hip. Note that the gluteus medius muscle is prolonged over the trochanter as an aponeurosis to become continuous with the vastus lateralis. The two muscles form an angle that is open anteriorly. The musculo-aponeurotic layer is raised from the trochanter with a sliver of bone and displaced forwards.

Even though the muscles be sutured firmly back into position abductor power tends to be weakened. This difficulty is overcome by the modified technique described by McFarland and Osborne (1954), who pointed out that the fibres of the gluteus medius are continuous over the greater trochanter with the origin of the vastus lateralis. Instead of detaching the gluteus medius from the trochanter, therefore, they separated this continuous muscle layer from the underlying bone after defining the posterior border of the gluteus medius and incising along this edge down to the trochanter (Fig. 37). They recommended raising a

of both the front and the back of the acetabulum. It is ideal for major work such as open reduction of a traumatic dislocation of the hip, especially in a difficult late case with extensive fibrous adhesions; it is appropriate also for replacement and screw fixation of a large posterior fragment of acetabulum displaced in a posterior fracture-dislocation of the hip. The exposure is, however, rather more extensive than is necessary for prosthetic replacement of the femoral head or for total replacement arthroplasty. The restricted postero-lateral exposure of Austin Moore (see below) is adequate and more appropriate for those procedures.

POSTERO-LATERAL EXPOSURE OF HIP

This incision was developed by Austin Moore (1957) for use in prosthetic replacement of the femoral head, though it had been described much earlier by Osborne (1931). It was referred to by Moore as the Southern approach, partly because it utilised the lower part of the Kocher exposure and partly because of its origination by him in the southern states of America. It is essentially similar to the Kocher and Gibson procedures, with the important differences that the gluteus medius and minimus muscles are not detached from the greater trochanter and that the hip is dislocated by medial rotation instead of by lateral rotation.

TECHNIQUE

Position of patient. The patient is placed in the true lateral position as described for the Gibson approach (p. 30).

Incision. The incision is the same as that described for the Gibson approach (Fig. 33) except that it need not begin so far proximally. Its upper limit may be half way between the crest of the ilium and the greater trochanter, but in an obese patient it will have to extend somewhat more proximally.

The deep dissection. The gluteal aponeurosis is split vertically in the lower half of the wound, over the greater trochanter and upper end of the femoral shaft (Fig. 34), and the split is extended proximally in the line of the skin incision, separating the anterior fibres of the gluteus maximus or opening the interval between the gluteus maximus and the tensor fasciae latae. The gluteal mass is retracted backwards and held with a self-retaining retractor.

Deep to the gluteus maximus areolar tissue conceals the piriformis muscle and the short transverse lateral rotators of the hip (gemelli and obturator internus with quadratus femoris below), which are disposed horizontally behind the greater trochanter. This areolar tissue is sponged away and the muscles are cleaned (Fig. 35). The muscles become more prominent if the assistant rotates the limb medially. The sciatic nerve may be identified where it lies upon the superficial surface of the quadratus femoris, obturator internus and gemelli: it passes deep to the piriformis. Stay sutures are inserted near the attachments of the gemelli and obturator internus to the trochanter, and the muscles are divided close to their insertion and reflected backwards (Fig. 36). The piriformis may be similarly reflected but this is not always necessary. Gluteus medius and minimus above and quadratus femoris below are left undisturbed. Backward reflection of the short transverse muscles protects the sciatic nerve.

The posterior part of the capsule of the hip joint is thus exposed and should be incised close to the greater trochanter. The capsule and synovial membrane may be excised or not according to the demands of the proposed operation. If the capsule is not to be excised an H-shaped incision is made and the flaps are turned back to reveal the posterior aspect of the neck of the femur.

Dislocation of hip. If an assistant now rotates the hip slightly to and fro the demarcation between femoral head and acetabular margin becomes more clearly evident. Often large osteophytes will be found protruding from the acetabular margin: these should be separated with a chisel. When capsule and osteophytes have been thoroughly cleared the hip is ready for dislocation. This is accomplished by flexing the hip through 90 degrees and rotating the thigh medially, with care not to apply excessive force lest the femur be fractured. Dislocation may be aided by a strong curved lever introduced into the joint between the head of the femur and the acetabulum. If there is some resistance to dislocation and if the head of the femur is to be discarded (for instance in replacement arthroplasty), it is convenient to divide the femoral neck before the head is dislocated. The head may then be removed with a corkscrew and curved lever, or it may be taken out piecemeal. To expose the acetabulum more fully the femoral shaft may be rotated a little more medially and retracted forwards with a bone hook.

Closure. The first step in the closure of the wound is to re-attach the short transverse muscles either near their original point of insertion or in such a way that they will best obliterate any potential dead space. One or two sutures to hold each muscle suffice. Next the gluteal aponeurosis is sutured carefully with interrupted absorbable sutures: this is an important layer and a secure suture line is essential. Before the skin edge sutures are inserted it is well to use four or five deep tension sutures traversing skin and muscle. As a general rule the authors prefer not to drain the wound, but in certain circumstances suction drainage from the deeper layers is appropriate.

Comment

This is one of the most useful of all the approaches to the hip. It is particularly suitable for prosthetic replacement of the femoral head and for total replacement arthroplasty. The technique is simple and it does not harm important structures. Since the gluteus medius and greater trochanter are left undisturbed there is no risk of impairment of abductor power.

POSTERO-LATERAL EXPOSURE OF SHAFT OF FEMUR

In this standard approach to the shaft of the femur the route lies between the posterior aspect of the quadriceps muscle in front and the biceps muscle and tendon behind (Fig. 39).

Incision. With the knee slightly flexed the lateral intermuscular septum is palpated as it extends proximally from the lateral condyle of the femur, about 2 centimetres in front of the biceps tendon.

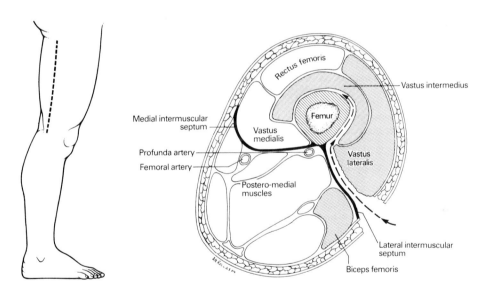

FIGS 38–39. Postero-lateral exposure of femur. Figure 38—The skin incision. Figure 39—The route lies between the vastus lateralis and the biceps femoris, which are separated by the lateral intermuscular septum. It is easy to peel the vastus lateralis from the front of the septum and then to strip it from the femur.

TECHNIQUE

Position of patient. It is convenient to have the patient in the true lateral position with the affected limb uppermost and with the knee and calf resting upon a bridge-like platform (Fig. 32).

The septum is marked on the surface by a shallow furrow immediately behind the mid-lateral line of the thigh. The skin incision lies immediately behind this line, between it and the biceps femoris, which in the lower part of the thigh is easily palpated near its insertion into the fibula (Fig. 38).

The proximal and distal limits of the incision depend upon the particular part of the femur that is to be exposed and upon the required length of the exposure.

The deep dissection. The fascia lata is divided longitudinally immediately anterior to the lateral intermuscular septum. The vastus lateralis muscle is thus exposed, and by blunt dissection it may be separated from the anterior surface of the inter-muscular septum. In this way the dissection proceeds medially, between the vastus lateralis in front and the intermuscular septum and biceps femoris muscle behind, until the linea aspera of

four corners of the wound to display the bone over as long a distance as may be necessary (Fig. 40).

Closure. The muscles fall naturally into place and only light absorbable sutures are needed to approximate them. The fascia is repaired with interrupted sutures and the skin is closed, usually without drainage.

Comment

This is the best approach for routine operations upon the femoral shaft. The risk of subsequent knee stiffness is less than it is after exposure of the

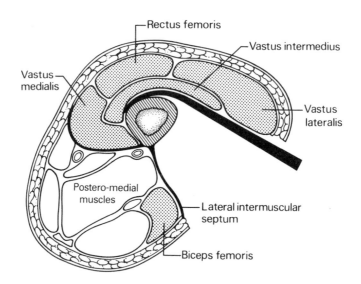

FIG. 40. Curved bone levers hooked over the front of the femur are used to lift the vastus lateralis and the vastus intermedius out of the way, thus exposing a wide expanse of the femoral shaft.

the femur is reached (Fig. 39). In this dissection perforating branches of the profunda femoris artery are encountered: if necessary they may be clamped and divided.

Curved bone levers are now inserted behind the vastus lateralis and hooked over the front of the femur to lever the muscle forwards. The periosteum may then be incised longitudinally and stripped from the lateral aspect of the femur. Bone levers are re-inserted deep to the periosteum at the

femur by the antero-lateral route. The perforating vessels may demand attention: they may often be preserved but may be ligated if necessary.

This incision, extended down to a point immediately proximal to the lateral femoral condyle, offers a convenient route to the popliteal fossa from the outer side. Dissection with blunt scissors is made between the lateral intermuscular septum and the tendon of the biceps to reach the posterior aspect of the lower end of the femur.

LATERAL EXPOSURE OF UPPER END OF FEMUR

This exposure is an adaptation of the standard postero-lateral approach to the shaft of the femur described above (p. 35). It gives a true lateral view of the trochanteric and subtrochanteric regions of the femur. It is used routinely for fixation of fractures of the neck of the femur or of the trochanteric region.

TECHNIQUE

Position of the patient. The patient lies supine on the operation table. Alternatively, when the nature of the proposed operation demands it, the patient may be positioned on the orthopaedic table with the feet strapped to the foot-plates and the sacral area supported upon the pelvic rest.

Incision. The incision is a vertical one upon a line extending distally from the lateral aspect of the greater trochanter. It is in fact the upper part of the line described in the previous section for postero-lateral exposure of the shaft of the femur. Its length will depend upon the requirements of the operation.

Exposure of bone. The surface of the fascia lata is cleared of fatty tissue for a centimetre or two on each side of the line of the skin incision in order to facilitate subsequent suture. A vertical slit is made through the fascia lata in the lower part of the wound and the slit is extended upwards with scissors. In the upper part of the wound fascia gives place to the tapering muscle belly of tensor fasciae latae. This is also split proximally in the direction of its fibres.

The edges of the fascia are retracted to reveal beneath it the glistening surface of the vastus lateralis muscle. It is better not to divide this muscle in the line of the skin and fascial incisions but to seek its posterior border and to lift this forwards with a curved bone lever, the tip of which is hooked over the front of the femoral shaft to hold the muscle forwards (Figs 41 and 42). A second bone lever may be similarly inserted in the lower part of the wound. A vertical cut straight onto the bone releases the remaining fibres of the

vastus lateralis and exposes the lateral aspect of the femur: this may be cleared further by stripping the periosteum.

The exposure may be extended as far proximally or distally as may be required. Generally there is little bleeding except from branches of the circumflex artery at the upper extremity of the wound.

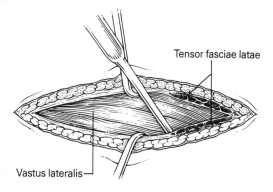

FIG. 41. Seeking the posterior edge of the vastus lateralis after incision of the fascia lata and tensor fasciae latae muscle.

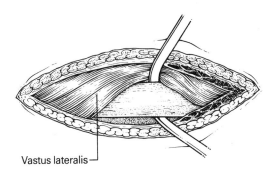

FIG. 42. The vastus lateralis muscle has been levered forwards to expose the femur.

Closure. The posterior edge of the vastus lateralis is tacked lightly in place by two or three absorbable sutures far back in the wound, deep to the posterior flap of fascia lata. The fascia lata itself, and more proximally the tensor fascia latae muscle, are repaired with interrupted sutures. The skin is closed by deep tension sutures and skin edge sutures. Drainage is usually not required.

Comment

It is important that the integrity of the vastus lateralis be disturbed as little as possible. If it is divided in the line of the skin and fascial incisions there is a risk that adhesions may bind it to the fascia lata, with consequent impairment of knee movement. Reflection of the vastus from its posterior edge, as described, is therefore much to be preferred.

ANTERO-LATERAL EXPOSURE OF SHAFT OF FEMUR

In this approach to the femur the route lies between the rectus femoris and the vastus lateralis muscles; deep to them it traverses the vastus intermedius (Fig. 44).

TECHNIQUE

Position of patient. The patient lies supine. The operation is commonly done without a tourniquet, but it is possible to employ a tourniquet if the following modified technique of application is

tourniquet cuff is applied to the upper thigh, proximal to the transfixion pin.

Incision. The skin incision is on a line that extends from the anterior superior spine of the ilium to the lateral border of the patella (Fig. 43). The length of the incision and its position on this line depend upon the extent of the exposure required and upon the level of the lesion for which operation is being undertaken. For the purpose of description it is assumed that the whole length of

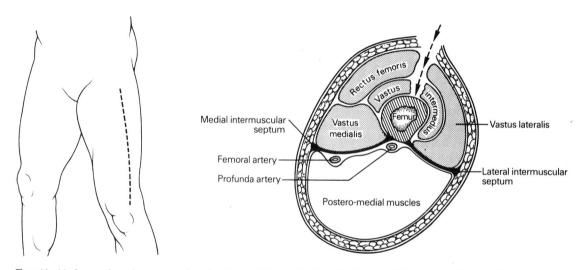

Figs 43–44. Antero-lateral exposure of shaft of femur. Figure 43—The skin incision. Figure 44—The route lies between the rectus femoris and the vastus lateralis, and then through the substance of the vastus intermedius direct to the front of the femur.

used. First a long thick Steinmann pin is thrust antero-posteriorly through the soft muscle mass (tensor fasciae latae and gluteus medius) between the crest of the ilium and the tip of the greater trochanter. The purpose of the pin is to retain the tourniquet high up in the groin. Protective padding of felt or towelling is first applied and the

the femoral shaft is to be exposed, although this is seldom necessary in practice.

The deep dissection. After division of skin and deep fascia the underlying muscles are identified. In the proximal part of the wound, immediately below the anterior superior iliac spine, the diverging fibres of sartorius and tensor fasciae latae form an inverted V. Distal to this the fibres of rectus femoris and vastus lateralis converge to unite in V fashion, but the seam between them is clearly definable throughout most of the length of the thigh, lying approximately in the line of the skin incision.

First the seam between rectus femoris and vastus lateralis is incised either with a knife or by scissors from above. Rectus femoris is retracted medially and vastus lateralis laterally. Deep to this muscle layer the silvery glistening surface of vastus intermedius comes into view, the fibres running vertically downwards.

At this stage care must be taken to identify and preserve a bundle of blood vessels and nerves that passes obliquely downwards and outwards upon the surface of vastus intermedius 8 or 10 centimetres below the anterior superior iliac spine. The artery in this bundle arises from the circumflex artery and is destined to supply the vastus lateralis. Likewise the nerve, originating from the femoral nerve, passes outwards to the vastus lateralis, which it supplies. This neurovascular bundle may be easily mobilised from the fatty tissue that surrounds it and held out of harm's way during the subsequent stages of the operation.

The line of incision through the vastus intermedius is vertical and is approximately at the junction of the outer third and the inner two-thirds of the muscle mass (Fig. 44). The muscle is incised straight onto the antero-lateral aspect of the femur (Fig. 44). In the lower part of the wound the suprapatellar pouch extends proximally for 6 or 7 centimetres above the upper margin of the patella. If the pouch is not to be opened due care must be taken when the muscles are incised in this region.

Exposure of the femur is completed by dividing the periosteum, raising it from the bone, and retracting it on each side with well curved bone levers passed round and behind the femur.

Closure. The periosteal layer does not require suturing. Vastus lateralis and rectus are reunited with interrupted catgut sutures. The skin is closed with deep tension sutures and interrupted or continuous skin edge sutures. Usually drainage is not required.

Comment

The main advantage of this approach is its simplicity. The patient is in a convenient position and the operation is comfortable for the surgeon. On the other hand the incision has the major disadvantage that it may promote adherence of the quadriceps muscle to the underlying bone, with consequent restriction of knee movement which may yield only slowly to intensive exercises continued over many months. For this reason the postero-lateral exposure is generally to be recommended in preference to it.

EXPOSURE OF ANTERO-MEDIAL SURFACE OF TIBIA

Although the antero-medial surface of the tibia is subcutaneous it is better to incise the skin over muscle rather than directly over the bone.

TECHNIQUE

Position of patient. As a rule the patient should lie supine. It is quite practicable, however, to expose the antero-medial surface of the tibia with the patient in the lateral position if the affected leg is the one nearer to the table. It is even possible to make the exposure with the patient prone, by flexing the knee to its full extent. A tourniquet may be used on the upper thigh, but if the exposure is to be made for the purpose of obtaining a bone graft the use of a tourniquet is not recommended*.

Incision. The incision is a vertical one placed over muscle rather than over the bone (Fig. 45).

* Since the taking of a graft is a small step in what is often an elaborate and time-consuming operation, a tourniquet used during the stage of removing the graft may be forgotten and inadvertently left in position until the conclusion of the main operation. Many limbs have been crippled from this cause, and since a graft can very easily be taken without the use of a tourniquet, it is safer to omit it in this circumstance.

Usually the main part of the incision is placed one centimetre lateral to the anterior crest of the tibia. Proximally it should not extend higher than the level of the tibial tubercle: its distal extent will

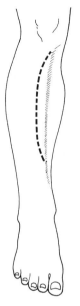

FIG. 45. Exposure of antero-medial aspect of tibia. The skin incision.

depend upon the requirements of the operation. The upper and lower extremities of the incision may be curved slightly medially to cross the anterior crest of the tibia; but there must be no sharp angulation lest the viability of the flap be prejudiced.

The skin flap thus outlined is held lightly by skin hooks and reflected medially in the subcutaneous plane as far as the postero-medial border of the tibia. The flap is held back by slender bone levers inserted round the postero-medial border of the tibia, their curved blunt points being kept close to the bone. Periosteum is incised vertically down to bone mid-way between the anterior and postero-medial borders. Near the ends of the incision the periosteum is incised transversely, so that the anterior and posterior periosteal flaps may be raised with an elevator to expose the raw cortex of the tibia.

Closure. Usually it is impossible to close the periosteum completely. It is best to tack the periosteal flaps with light catgut sutures spaced widely apart and to be content with coaptation that is far from complete.

Comment
Although the antero-medial surface of the tibia is exposed very easily this approach is not recommended for the application of a plate or bone graft, which should usually be applied to the lateral surface of the tibia in order that it may be well covered by muscle. Nevertheless the antero-medial exposure is used frequently, and it is the method of choice when the operation is undertaken for the purpose of obtaining a bone graft from the tibia.

It is important that the incision, and therefore the scar, be placed over muscle rather than directly over the bone, because a scar that is over the bone may become adherent, with consequent discomfort. In the usual type of case in which the patient lies supine it is most convenient to make the incision over the anterior muscles, as described; but if the circumstances of the operation demand that the patient lie in the lateral position it is more convenient and equally satisfactory to place the incision over the calf muscles, behind the postero-medial border of the tibia, and to turn the skin flap forwards.

EXPOSURE OF LATERAL SURFACE OF TIBIA

The lateral surface of the tibia is easily reached by stripping the anterior muscles outwards and backwards, through an incision that lies slightly lateral to the anterior crest of the bone.

TECHNIQUE

Position of patient. The patient should preferably lie supine. Alternatively, if the circumstances of the operation demand it, he may be in the lateral position with the affected limb uppermost. A tourniquet may be used on the upper thigh.

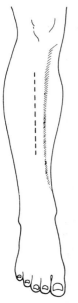

FIG. 46. Exposure of lateral surface of tibia. The skin incision.

Incision. The incision is a vertical one over muscle, one centimetre lateral to the tibial crest (Fig. 46). Near the crest fascia is incised to allow access to the plane between the lateral surface of the tibia and the tibialis anterior muscle arising from it. Periosteum is incised just behind the anterior crest of the tibia and stripped from the bone with an elevator, together with the tibialis anterior muscle. Well curved bone levers are inserted behind the postero-lateral margin of the tibia at the upper and lower ends of the wound to hold the muscles back and thus to give access to the lateral cortex of the tibia.

Closure. The muscles fall readily back into position, and a few light catgut sutures to repair the periosteum are all that are required. The skin is closed with interrupted eversion sutures.

Comment

As with the antero-medial exposure it is important that the scar be placed over muscle rather than over bone. This approach should always be used in preference to the antero-medial exposure for the plating or grafting of fractures. A good covering of muscle prevents a plate from bulging the skin, as it often does when screwed to the antero-medial surface of the tibia; and in the case of bone grafting a covering of healthy muscle is desirable in order to promote early revascularisation of the graft.

EXPOSURE OF POSTERIOR SURFACE OF TIBIA

The posterior route to the tibia lies first between the posterior border of the fibula and the flexor hallucis longus muscle, and more deeply between the fibula and interosseous membrane laterally and the tibialis posterior medially (Fig. 47).

TECHNIQUE

Position of patient. The patient lies prone. A tourniquet may be used on the upper thigh.

Incision. A vertical incision is made just behind and parallel with the postero-lateral border of the fibula. The skin edges are raised from the under-lying fascia for a short distance on either side to reveal a whitish line which marks the junction of the postero-lateral intermuscular septum with the deep fascia.

The deep dissection. The deep fascia is incised vertically just behind the postero-lateral intermuscular septum. The interval between the septum and the calf muscles is opened up in order to reach and expose the posterior surface of the fibula. This aspect of the bone is covered by the flexor hallucis longus muscle, which should be stripped away with an elevator. The dissection then proceeds on the medial surface of the fibula where the tibialis posterior muscle is stripped from the bone and, more medially, from the interosseous membrane (Fig. 47).

When the tibia has been reached by working antero-medially along the interosseous membrane the periosteum is incised vertically and stripped from the posterior aspect of the bone, together

the wound. Thus mobilised, it may be retracted forwards out of the way, or in some cases a section may be discarded.

Closure. The muscles fall back into place and it is necessary only to repair fascia and the skin. Usually drainage of the wound is not required.

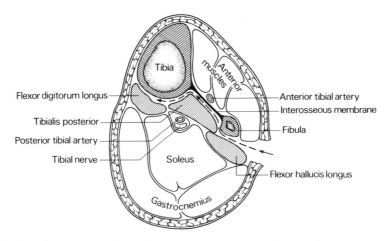

FIG. 47. Posterior exposure of tibia. Diagrammatic cross-section showing the route of approach between the fibula and the flexor hallucis longus, then between the fibula and the tibialis posterior, and finally between the interosseous membrane and the tibialis posterior.

with the flexor digitorum longus muscle. The postero-medial muscles are retracted medially by levers passed subperiosteally round the back of the tibia.

In this dissection the posterior tibial vessels and the tibial nerve lie behind the tibialis posterior and are protected by it. The anterior tibial vessels, lying in the anterior compartment of the leg, are protected by the interosseous membrane (Fig. 47).

If it is found that the fibula, which in patients requiring this approach is often deformed from mal-union of a fracture, gets in the way it may be divided at the proximal and distal extremities of

Comment

This is a useful approach to the tibia when exposure from the front or side is prohibited by extensive scarring or by recent infection in the area. It seems to have been too little used in the past.

The key to the exposure is first to clear the posterior surface of the fibula and then to work round its medial side, keeping close to the bone, until the interosseous membrane is reached: this guides the elevator safely across the gap between fibula and tibia to strike the postero-lateral angle of the tibia. From this point the posterior surface of the tibia is easily exposed subperiosteally.

POSTERO-LATERAL EXPOSURE OF LOWER END OF TIBIA

Perhaps rather surprisingly, the back of the lower tibia and ankle joint are exposed more easily through an incision lateral to the calcaneal tendon than by a medial incision (Fig. 49).

TECHNIQUE

Position of patient. The patient may be prone or in the lateral position with the affected limb uppermost, according to preference. If a tourniquet is used it should be placed on the upper thigh.

Incision. The incision is a vertical one between the posterior margin of the fibula and the lateral margin of the calcaneal tendon (Fig. 48). Its lower limit should be within a centimetre or so of the tuberosity of the calcaneus, and the incision may be from 7 to 10 centimetres long according to

In the lower part of the wound part of the back of the tibia is found exposed, distal and lateral to the flexor hallucis longus. From this point the muscle may be displaced medially to expose the bare tibial cortex (Fig. 49).

Closure. Little or no repair of the deeper structures is required and reliance is placed mainly on interrupted skin sutures.

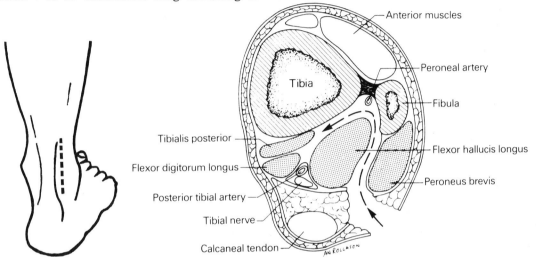

FIGS 48–49. Exposure of back of lower tibia and ankle. Figure 48—The skin incision. Figure 49—The approach is lateral to the calcaneal tendon, between the flexor hallucis longus and the medial surface of the fibula. Flexor hallucis longus is retracted medially.

requirements. The skin edges are retracted with hooks and the calcaneal tendon is drawn medially. Beneath the fascia, in the interval between the calcaneal tendon and the fibula, the lower fibres of the flexor hallucis longus are seen arising from the fibula: they slope obliquely downwards and medially. Care should be taken that the peroneus brevis muscle is not mistaken for the flexor hallucis: it lies in the lateral corner of the wound and its fibres, becoming tendinous, are directed vertically downwards towards the back of the lateral malleolus.

Comment

This approach is useful when the back of the lower tibia has to be reached in operations for replacement of a displaced fragment after a posterior marginal fracture of the tibia, or for exposure of the ankle from behind. The posterior tibial vessels and the tibial nerve are well out of the way, but care is needed to avoid damage to the peroneal artery and veins, which lie close to the medial aspect of the fibula (Fig. 49).

EXPOSURE OF FIBULA

The lower half of the fibula may be exposed between the extensor muscles anteriorly and the peroneal muscles posteriorly, where for a distance of several centimetres above the lateral malleolus the fibula is subcutaneous. If the proximal part or the whole length of the fibula is to be exposed, however, the route is between the peroneal muscles anteriorly and the soleus muscle posteriorly. The description that follows applies to exposure of the whole length of the fibula.

TECHNIQUE

Position of patient. The patient is placed in the lateral position with the affected limb uppermost. The underneath (sound) limb lies fully extended. The knee of the affected limb should be slightly flexed in order to relax the biceps tendon.

muscle as it nears its insertion. The nerve is mobilised a short distance proximally, and the groove in which it lay is used as the starting point for division of the deep fascia distally. This groove marks the plane of separation between the peroneus longus muscle anteriorly and the soleus muscle behind. The nerve is then mobilised distally as it slopes downwards and forwards across the outer aspect of the neck of the fibula. Here it is covered by a bridge of peroneus longus muscle which should be divided. At about this point the

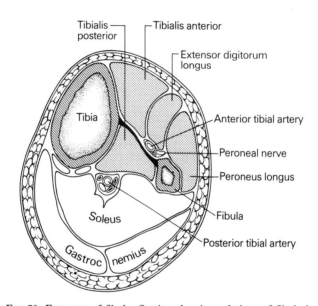

Tibialis posterior
Tibialis anterior
Extensor digitorum longus
Tibia
Anterior tibial artery
Peroneal nerve
Peroneus longus
Soleus
Fibula
Posterior tibial artery
Gastroc nemius

FIG. 50. Exposure of fibula. Section showing relations of fibula in upper third of leg. Note the close proximity to the bone of the anterior tibial artery and the peroneal nerve.

Incision. The proximal part of the incision begins 5 to 7 centimetres proximal to the head of the fibula and follows the tendon of the biceps femoris to the back of the fibular head. The incision then descends vertically downwards to the back of the lateral malleolus. The skin edges are reflected a short distance anteriorly and posteriorly.

The deep dissection. The dissection begins proximally, where it is essential first to identify and define the common peroneal nerve. The nerve is located where it lies behind the head of the fibula and deep to the tendon of the biceps femoris

nerve divides into its three terminal branches, namely the recurrent tibial nerve, the anterior tibial nerve and the musculocutaneous nerve. The mobilised loop of nerve is drawn forwards out of the way while the peroneal muscles are stripped from the fibula and retracted forwards with the nerve.

Once the nerve has been dealt with the opening of the plane between the soleus and the peroneal muscles is continued distally (Fig. 50). In the lower half of the leg it is important to keep the dissection close to the bone: it is best to incise the periosteum vertically and to make the separation of muscle from bone subperiosteally. The reason for this is that the peroneal artery and veins descend in close proximity to the medial aspect of the fibula and may easily be damaged if the muscles are stripped injudiciously.

Comment

Clearly, this exposure of the fibula will seldom be required in its entirety, but any part of it may be used according to requirements. It is a straightforward exposure but it demands care because of the hazard to the common peroneal nerve and its branches above, and to the peroneal artery and veins below. It is important that any exposure of the head or neck of the fibula should always be preceded by identification and gentle mobilisation of the common peroneal nerve.

EXPOSURE OF SCIATIC NERVE

The sciatic nerve may be exposed throughout the whole of its length in the buttock and thigh, or any part of the exposure may be used as required.

TECHNIQUE

Position of patient. The patient lies prone. The whole limb should be draped in a tube of stockingette so that the knee may be flexed and extended as required. It is not practicable to use a tourniquet.

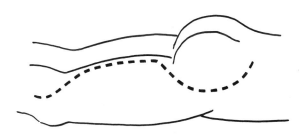

FIG. 51. Exposure of sciatic nerve. The skin incision.

Incision. The skin incision begins over the crest of the ilium 5 centimetres in front of the posterior superior iliac spine. It follows the anterior border of the gluteus maximus as far as the greater trochanter. After descending along the posterior border of the greater trochanter it curves backwards to join the midline of the limb at the inferior fold of the buttock (Fig. 51). Thence it descends vertically in the posterior midline of the thigh, deviating laterally in the lower part of the thigh towards the head of the fibula.

The deep dissection. It is easiest to find the nerve just distal to the fold of the buttock. Here the nerve lies deep to the long head of the biceps femoris muscle, which overlaps it from the medial

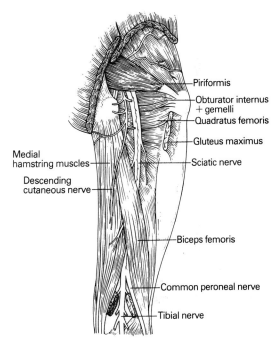

Piriformis
Obturator internus + gemelli
Quadratus femoris
Gluteus maximus
Sciatic nerve
Medial hamstring muscles
Descending cutaneous nerve
Biceps femoris
Common peroneal nerve
Tibial nerve

FIG. 52. The course of the sciatic nerve at the back of the thigh. Part of the gluteus maximus has been cut away.

side. From this point the nerve may be traced proximally by lifting the gluteus maximus backwards and detaching it from its insertion into the femur and the fascia lata. Working proximally, the surgeon thus reflects the gluteus maximus posteriorly and medially, allowing the nerve to be followed upwards to its point of emergence from the pelvis through the greater sciatic notch, where it lies deep to the piriformis muscle.

If the nerve is to be exposed in the thigh it may best be identified immediately distal to the buttock fold where it lies deep to the long head of the biceps femoris, as already described. From this point the nerve is easily traced distally. It lies beneath the long head of the biceps femoris, which crosses it very obliquely from the medial to the lateral side (Fig. 52).

To find the nerve in the lower third of the thigh it is a simple matter to identify the common peroneal branch of the nerve where it lies deep to the tendon of the biceps a little above the head of the fibula. This nerve may be traced proximally to the point where the main sciatic trunk divides into its terminal divisions, and above that the main nerve may be traced as far as is necessary.

EXPOSURE OF COMMON PERONEAL NERVE

Exposure of the common peroneal nerve is closely related to that of the upper end of the fibula, the description of which should be consulted (p. 43).

Proximally the nerve lies immediately deep to the biceps tendon, emerging distally to cross the lateral aspect of the neck of the fibula.

EXPOSURE OF POPLITEAL FOSSA FROM BEHIND

This exposure may be used for access to the posterior aspect of the lower femur or upper tibia or to the major vessels and nerves.

TECHNIQUE

Position of patient. The patient is placed prone, with a soft support under the dorsum of the ankle to give moderate flexion of the knee and thus to relax the gastrocnemius muscle. A tourniquet may be used on the upper thigh.

Incision. A mid-line vertical incision is often used but it is perhaps better to make the incision slightly serpentine at the point of knee flexure to minimise possible bow-stringing if the scar contracts. The incision may extend 7.5 to 10 centimetres above the joint level (the joint line is 1 centimetre above the top of the fibula) and an equal distance down the calf. The skin edges are drawn laterally and medially and the fascia is opened.

The deep dissection. At the upper end of the wound the V-shaped gap between the medial and lateral heads of the gastrocnemius muscle is sought. Below this, surprisingly proximally, the

muscle heads blend, and the site of their union is marked by a groove. This groove is further marked by a vertical superficial vein (short saphenous vein) and, deep to the fascia, by the sural nerve. A freshly gloved finger may be inserted

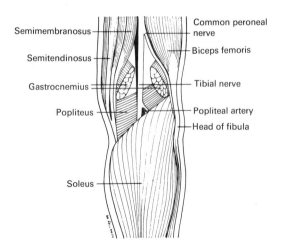

FIG. 53. Exposure of popliteal region from behind. Diagram shows the structures exposed by reflection of the gastrocnemius.

deep to the conjoined muscle bellies of gastrocnemius to lift the muscle from the deeper structures. The medial and lateral bellies of the gastrocnemius are then separated by a vertical incision in the groove between them: if preferred, this incision in the muscle seam may be made with blunt-nosed scissors.

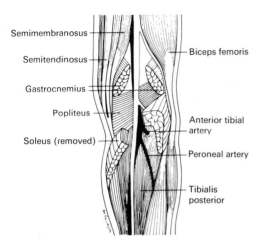

Semimembranosus

Semitendinosus

Gastrocnemius

Popliteus

Soleus (removed)

Biceps femoris

Anterior tibial artery

Peroneal artery

Tibialis posterior

FIG. 54. Disposition of the structures deep to the soleus.

When the gastrocnemius bellies have been retracted medially and laterally the tibial nerve and the popliteal artery deep to it are seen lying upon the popliteus muscle, the oblique fibres of which slope downwards and medially (Fig. 53). Near the lower margin of the popliteus the nerve and artery pass deep to the proximal margin of the soleus, where musculo-aponeurotic fibres bridge its fibular and tibial origins. The edge of this bridge also slopes downwards and medially. The main artery and nerve may be exposed deep to the soleus by dividing the muscle vertically in the mid-line. In this way the popliteal artery may be traced to its point of division into posterior tibial and anterior tibial arteries about 3 centimetres distal to the level of the fibular head (Fig. 54). A little below this the posterior tibial artery gives off the large peroneal artery at a Y-shaped fork. At this point the peroneal artery differs little in size from the main continuation of the posterior tibial artery.

If the back of the extreme upper end of the tibia is to be exposed, the popliteus muscle must be mobilised by transecting it near its medial end by a vertical incision down to bone and incising along its upper and lower borders nearly as far as the mid-line of the limb: the muscle may then be reflected laterally as a flap.

EXPOSURE OF TIBIAL NERVE

The tibial nerve may be exposed in its whole length by splitting the posterior calf muscles. Its lowest third may be exposed from the medial side of the leg without splitting the calf.

TECHNIQUE

Position of patient. For the full exposure the patient should lie prone. The instep should be supported on a large sand-bag so that the knee rests slightly flexed. For the limited exposure of the lower third of the nerve it is equally convenient to have the patient in the lateral position: the unaffected leg, which is uppermost, is held forward out of the way and the knee on the affected side is flexed to just short of the right angle.

The exposure. For the exposure of the whole length of the nerve a vertical incision is made in the mid-line of the leg from the popliteal fossa to the junction of the upper two-thirds and the lowest third of the calf. From that point the incision curves towards the medial side and is prolonged downwards to end midway between the medial malleolus and the calcaneal tendon (Fig. 55). In the popliteal fossa the nerve is found by separating the two heads of the gastrocnemius muscle as described above. It is followed down to the point where it disappears deep to the upper edge of the soleus muscle. This muscle is then split vertically in the mid-line as far as the musculo-tendinous junction. In the lower end of the wound the nerve is identified where it lies behind the posterior tibial vessels in the interval between the medial malleolus and the calcaneal tendon. From this point it is traced proximally deep to the soleus muscle, where the exposure becomes continuous with that in the upper two-thirds of the leg. The nerve can be mobilised deep to the remaining overlying bridge of soleus and calf tendon and these structures need not necessarily be divided.

For the limited exposure of the nerve in the lowest third of the leg a postero-medial incision is

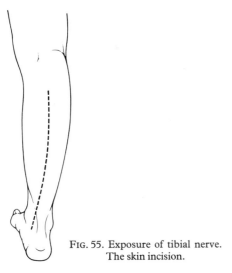

FIG. 55. Exposure of tibial nerve.
The skin incision.

used. The incision should begin in the interval between the medial malleolus and the calcaneal tendon, lying rather nearer to the tendon than to the malleolus (Fig. 55). From this point the incision extends proximally and slightly anteriorly to end just behind the postero-medial border of the tibia at the junction of the upper two-thirds and the lowest third of the leg. In the lower part of

the wound the nerve is easily identified where it lies behind the posterior tibial vessels and in front of the tendon of flexor hallucis longus (Fig. 56). From this point the nerve is traced proximally, the medial margin of the soleus being detached from its origin on the tibia to allow retraction of the

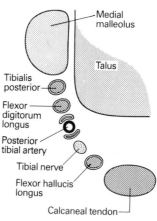

FIG. 56. Relationships of tendons, vessels and nerves at the postero-medial aspect of the ankle. The tibial nerve lies between the vascular bundle and the tendon of flexor hallucis longus.

muscle laterally. Distally the nerve may be traced into the medial part of the foot as far as is necessary.

Closure. The muscles fall back into place and may be held by a few interrupted absorbable sutures. The skin is closed without drainage.

EXPOSURE OF SURAL NERVE

The sural nerve is one that is commonly used for nerve grafting: although it is not a large nerve quite a long piece of it may be easily removed and a number of strands may be laid side by side as a "cable" graft to bridge the gap between the freshened and clean-cut stumps of the recipient nerve. The consequent loss of sensibility in the postero-lateral aspect of the lower leg and over the outer part of the heel is generally regarded as insignificant or at least acceptable, though Seddon (1975) had some misgivings, particularly since the insensitive area sometimes includes part of the weight-bearing skin of the heel.

The nerve is superficial in the lower three-quarters of the calf. Distally it lies just lateral to the calcaneal tendon, and more proximally it lies in the sulcus between the two heads of the gastrocnemius muscle.

TECHNIQUE

This description relates to removal of part of the nerve for use as a graft.

Position of patient. The patient should preferably lie in the prone position, though the exposure can readily be made with the patient in the lateral position with the donor leg uppermost. A tourniquet may be used on the upper part of the thigh.

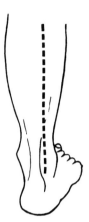

FIG. 57. Exposure of sural nerve. The skin incision.

Incision. The incision begins at the level of the lateral malleolus at a point between this bony prominence and the calcaneal tendon, about one centimetre lateral to the tendon. Thence it extends vertically upwards in a line that joins the point of commencement to the mid-point of the popliteal fossa (Fig. 57). The length of the incision depends upon the length of nerve required for use as a graft. If a relatively short length is required only the lower part of the full incision is made.

Identification of nerve. It should be remembered that in the distal part of its course the nerve lies very superficially, superficial to the deep fascia. It lies alongside the small saphenous vein, a fact that is useful in identification. The nerve is not large—perhaps 2.5 or 3 millimetres in diameter, or a little larger than the standard guidewire used in nailing

a femoral neck fracture. It is best to identify the nerve distally and then it is a simple matter to trace it proximally, where the nerve still lies in a superficial plane until it perforates the deep fascia in the upper part of the calf.

Alternative technique: use of nerve stripper. In order to avoid a long incision it is permissible to identify the nerve distally through a short incision and to divide the nerve at that distal level and introduce it through the ring of a stripping instrument which is then passed subcutaneously up the calf to strip the nerve over the required length. A second small incision is then made through which to divide the nerve proximally.

Closure. After release of the tourniquet and occlusion of any bleeding vessels, the skin alone needs to be sutured, without drainage.

POST-OPERATIVE MANAGEMENT

The calf is supported in a crepe bandage for 10 or 12 days until the sutures are removed. A little walking may be permitted at an early stage.

Comment

The mistake that is sometimes made by surgeons exposing this nerve for the first time is to incise too deeply—that is, through the deep fascia. The nerve will not then be found because it will be retracted with one or other edge of the divided deep fascia. Points to remember are that the nerve is virtually just under the skin, that it lies quite close to the calcaneal tendon on its outer side, and that it is accompanied by the small saphenous vein.

CHAPTER TWO

Basic Orthopaedic Techniques

This chapter is devoted to descriptions of procedures that are commonplace in orthopaedic surgery and which are appropriate—perhaps with modifications—to more than one part of the body. In this way much repetition will be avoided in the subsequent chapters dealing with regional sites.

CONTENTS OF CHAPTER

THE USE OF CHISELS, OSTEOTOMES AND GOUGES

Osteotomes and chisels have very distinct functions. An osteotome, being symmetrically tapered, is used for driving straight into a bone or for dividing it (Fig. 58). It is appropriate only for cutting bone that is fairly soft, especially cancellous bone or the long bones of children. If the shaft of a long bone has to be divided in an adult it is usually best to weaken the cortex by multiple drill holes before the osteotome is applied.

Chisels are used for working the surface of a bone—for instance in taking shavings or in smoothing off irregularities to make the surface flat to receive a plate or bone graft. A chisel is bevelled only on one side, and it is important that it be held in the correct way for the function desired. For instance, in taking shavings from a flat surface the bevelled side should be held towards the bone, as shown in Figure 59. For smoothing a convex surface, on the other hand, it is more convenient to direct the flat surface against the bone; likewise for cutting a notch or groove in a bone (Figs 60 and 61).

Gouges are more suitable than chisels for working on rounded concavities such as the acetabulum. A narrow gouge is useful for making a notch as the starting point for a drill, or for countersinking a screw. It is also useful for scooping out cancellous bone from the ilium for bone grafting.

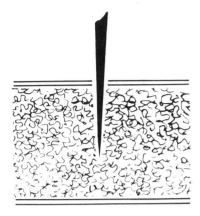

FIG. 58. Cutting soft bone with an osteotome.

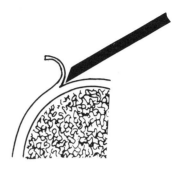

FIG. 60. Shaping a convex surface with a chisel. Note direction of the bevel.

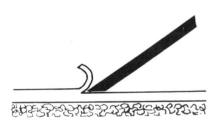

FIG. 59. Using a chisel to trim a flat surface. Note direction of the bevel.

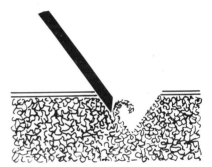

FIG. 61. Cutting a V-notch with a chisel. Note direction of the bevel.

OSTEOTOMY

Osteotomy is the general term for division of a bone. It may be required to correct angular deformity or to produce compensatory angulation; or secondly, it may be needed to correct rotatory deformity. Thirdly, the bone may be divided in order to shift one fragment in relation to the other. Finally, it may be done to shorten a bone or occasionally to lengthen a bone. These functions are denoted by such titles as wedge osteotomy, rotation osteotomy and displacement osteotomy. The actual principles of dividing the bone are similar in each case.

OSTEOTOMY OF A LONG BONE IN A CHILD

In young children the cortex of the long bones is relatively soft, and even the femur can be divided quite easily by a sharp thin osteotome. Sometimes it is equally convenient or more convenient to begin the division with a fine-pointed bone cutting forceps. When this is used an attempt should not be made to cut the bone right through in one bite. Such an attempt is liable to crush or splinter the bone. Instead, the sharp points of the instrument should be used to work their way in with numerous small bites, the first doing little more than scratch the surface and the subsequent ones cutting deeper and deeper.

OSTEOTOMY OF CANCELLOUS BONE IN A CHILD

In a site such as the iliac crest or the calcaneus, where the bone is spongy throughout, osteotomy is a simple matter and should be effected with a sharp thin osteotome (Fig. 58). If a wedge is to be removed a chisel is useful for truing up the sides of the wedge (Fig. 61): a chisel used with the bevelled surface towards the bone is more accurate than an osteotome in shaping a flat surface (Fig. 59).

OSTEOTOMY OF A LONG BONE IN AN ADULT

In the case of a strong bone such as the femur or tibia it is usually impracticable to divide the bone straight through with an osteotome. The same applies even to the bones of the upper limb unless the patient is slender or the bone rarefied. Mechanical aids such as a saw (p. 56) or powered drill (p. 54) are clearly best for the division of tough adult bone. If the osteotomy is to be done

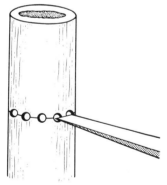

FIG. 62. Osteotomy of cortical bone facilitated by multiple drill holes.

by hand, however, the easiest way is to make multiple drill holes close together in the line of the proposed osteotomy, and then to divide the remaining bridges of bone with the osteotome (Fig. 62).

OSTEOTOMY OF CANCELLOUS BONE IN AN ADULT

In adults, as in children, cancellous bone is easily cut with a sharp osteotome.

WEDGE OSTEOTOMY

Wedge osteotomy is used to correct or to create angulation of a bone. It is usual to excise a wedge of the appropriate size and then to close the gap, thus angulating the bone. Finally, the fragments are usually fixed internally with staples or with a plate and screws to ensure stability. This is the "closing wedge" technique (Fig. 63), and is usually the method of choice.

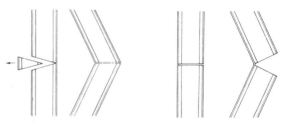

FIGS 63–64. Wedge osteotomy by the closing wedge technique (Fig. 63) and by the opening wedge technique (Fig. 64).

As an alternative, it is sometimes permissible to divide the bone straight across and to angulate it, thus opening a wedge (Fig. 64): sometimes the wedge-shaped gap may be filled with a graft. The opening wedge technique has the merit that length is preserved, but at the cost of less stability and perhaps slow union.

PRELIMINARY STUDIES

Before wedge osteotomy is undertaken the surgeon should be sure of the exact dimensions of the wedge that is to be removed. The angle of the wedge should be determined from clinical studies and from measurements on the radiographs. When the optimal angle has been determined it is often convenient to make a template or pattern of the correct angle from thin metal and to have this sterilised so that it can be used as a guide at the time of operation.

TECHNIQUE

The technique to be described applies to wedge osteotomy of a long bone by the closing wedge technique. The bone is exposed at the appropriate level and the soft tissues are retracted, usually by curved bone levers passed round the bone, two on each side. The desired length of bone is thus clearly presented in the field of operation. The

multiple drill holes and chisel if the bone is hard. It is nearly always best to leave a small strip of cortex intact at the apex of the wedge, to act as a hinge: certainly the periosteum at this point should be left undisturbed. This helps to ensure stability. When the wedge of bone has been cleanly removed a check is made to ensure that the gap thus created is of the required dimensions. The wedge-shaped gap is then closed by forcibly

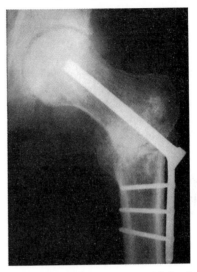

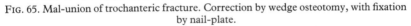

FIG. 65. Mal-union of trochanteric fracture. Correction by wedge osteotomy, with fixation by nail-plate.

correct level for the osteotomy is then determined. This is often critical, and if the surgeon is in any doubt about the correct starting point it is best to take a radiograph after a guide wire or drill has been driven part way into the bone as a marker.

Once the correct level has been established it is necessary next to determine the correct position for the base of the wedge. From pre-operative studies it will be known whether this should face anteriorly, posteriorly, medially or laterally, or in some intermediate direction. The line of osteotomy may now be marked on the bone surface by scratching with a scalpel or by light cuts with an osteotome. The width of the base of the wedge that will subtend the required angle has to be calculated according to the thickness of the bone concerned: here the template may prove useful.

The sides of the wedge are now shaped by dividing the bone either by osteotome and chisel if the bone is soft, or by a powered saw or by

angulating the bone. This should be done with care to prevent displacement of the fragments.

When the gap has been closed and the cut surfaces are in contact appropriate means should be selected to fix the fragments. A plate with four screws is often the simplest method. Sometimes two or three metal staples are appropriate, especially in soft bone such as that of the upper end of the tibia or of the tarsus. At the upper end of the femur a nail-plate with screws is often the method of choice (Fig. 65).

POST-OPERATIVE MANAGEMENT

In most cases some form of external support, usually a plaster-of-Paris splint, is advisable. If internal fixation is rigid, however, it may be possible to dispense with splintage—as for example after osteotomy of the upper end of the femur fixed by a strong nail-plate.

DRILLING BONE

Almost always, bone is drilled with twist drills held either in a hand-operated engineer's brace or in a power-driven chuck. For small holes in soft bone an awl or a guide wire is sometimes used instead of a drill.

DRILLING BY HAND

Drilling by hand does not present any special difficulties. It is easy to penetrate even hard bone provided the drill is sharp. For the smaller sizes of drill (up to 5 or 6 millimetres), however, hand drilling has no advantage over power drilling and it has one important disadvantage, namely that the drill is more likely to be accidentally broken in the bone. Breakage seems to occur through inadvertent angulatory force on the slowly revolving drill point: with the more rapidly revolving power drill this accident hardly ever occurs. Breakage is, however, less common today than it was in the past, because the metal used for manufacture is more resistant.

When the larger sizes of drill are being used (for instance between 9.5 and 12.5 millimetres) hand drilling has a distinct advantage over power drilling, because only slow revolutions are required and the hand drill offers more delicate control than even a slow speed power-operated drill. These remarks apply particularly to enlargement of a pre-existing hole. In this situation very slow turning is required, and a drill held in a simple hand chuck on a T-handle may prove to be the best instrument.

TECHNIQUE

Hand drilling is almost the simplest of all procedures on bone, and little description is required. The first main essential is to check the size of the drill that has been fitted to the brace. A personal check is to be preferred to a report from a third party. The next point of detail is to establish and locate the correct starting point for the drill. If the drill holes are to be prepared for screwing on a plate or nail-plate this presents no problem; if the plate is held against the bone the holes automatic-

ally locate the drill point in the correct position. If there is nothing thus to locate the drill it is apt to slide across the bone as soon as it begins to turn. To prevent this it is best to make a small starting notch with a narrow gouge or awl; or a special drill sleeve may be used. If the drill hole is to traverse the bone obliquely it is best first to drill transversely until the drill has penetrated a few millimetres, and then to redirect the drill in the desired direction (Fig. 66).

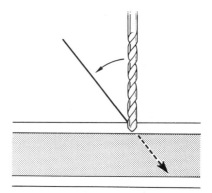

FIG. 66. When drilling at a tangent to a bone it is best first to introduce the drill at a right angle, and then to change to the required direction when the drill point has entered the cortex.

Pressure applied to the drill to force it through the bone should always be well controlled, so that when the drill emerges at the far side of the bone it is not driven on with a sudden jerk into the tissues, with possible serious damage to a vital structure. It is wise always to have one hand resting upon the patient's body to steady the drill, so that when the point penetrates the bone it is prevented from shooting forwards into the tissues. Usually it is clear from the feel of the drill when the point is about to emerge from the distal cortex of a bone. Drilling should then proceed very slowly and pressure upon the drill should be reduced.

To extract the drill it is best to continue to rotate it forwards while pulling upon the brace. This is more successful than attempting to rotate the drill in the reverse direction, which may have the effect only of loosening the grip of the chuck.

POWER DRILLING

It matters little whether the drill is driven by electric power or by compressed air. The first principle is that whereas fairly high speeds are appropriate for drilling with the smaller drills (up to 5 or 6 millimetres), slow revolutions are essential when it comes to drilling a large hole, say in the region of 12.5 millimetres.

TECHNIQUE

Many of the technical points made in the previous paragraphs apply equally to power drilling. The drill point should preferably be applied to the bone with the motor running; and here again, as in hand drilling, it is best to form a starting notch with a gouge or awl before the drill is applied to the bone, unless the position of the hole is located by a plate or other appliance. With a power drill it is particularly important that the onward pressure be controlled at all times by supporting the hand against the part of the patient's body that is being drilled. This is the only safeguard against inadvertent damage to important structures by sudden penetration of the drill.

When a large hole is to be drilled through cortical bone with a power drill great care must be exercised, and the advisability of using a hand drill in preference to the powered instrument should always be considered. Slow revolutions are essential, and even with a slow speed power drill damage may be done if the cutting edge suddenly bites into a brittle piece of cortex. With a hand drill the extra resistance can be felt, but with a power drill the torque is such that a fragment of bone may be broken off before the drill can be checked.

RETRIEVAL OF A BROKEN-OFF DRILL POINT

Whereas some drills are virtually unbreakable others tend to be brittle and—especially when used in a hand brace—may be broken within the bone. The distal end of the drill, that is the point, is then left behind in the bone when the main part of the drill is withdrawn. This presents a difficult situation unless by lucky chance enough of the broken drill is left protruding to allow it to be gripped and pulled out by forceps or pliers. If the broken piece cannot be retrieved in this way one of several methods may be adopted. If the drill has penetrated only one cortex and is lying in the medullary canal, it may be best to enlarge the hole in the proximal cortex to about twice its original size in order to allow a slender forceps to be passed through to grip the drill fragment and pull it out. If on the other hand the drill had already penetrated the far cortex or almost so before breaking, it is better to hammer it right through the bone with a punch and then to retrieve it from the far side.

If retrieval of a broken drill proves to be difficult it may often be wise to leave it in the bone rather than to prejudice the strength of the bone by continued attempts at removal. This is especially so in an elderly patient. Most drills are now made from stainless steel, which remains relatively inert in the body. Their removal is thus less imperative than it was when drills were made from carbon steel.

MEASURING THE DEPTH OF A DRILL HOLE

To determine the length of screw required to fix a plate or bone graft to the shaft of a bone the depth

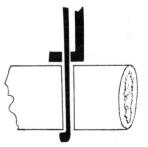

FIG. 67. Principle of the Crawford Adams depth gauge for estimation of screw length.

of the drill hole in the recipient bone must be measured. This is done with a depth gauge, which in principle is a blunt probe with a step near its tip which is engaged on the distal cortex after the probe has been passed through the drill hole

(Fig. 67). A plunger is then brought down onto the proximal cortex of the bone, and the thickness of the bone is read off on a scale engraved upon the instrument (Adams 1943).

For notes on the A.O. system of internal fixation see page 66.

SAWING BONE

Bone may be sawn either by hand or by machine. Machine sawing is by far the more rapid method, and with the development of refined machine tools it has largely superseded hand sawing except in certain situations. Some experience is required, however, in the handling of machine saws if accidents are to be avoided.

SAWING BONE BY HAND

Hand saws vary in size from the traditional amputation saw, which resembles a carpenter's tenon saw, to small instruments with fine detachable blades.

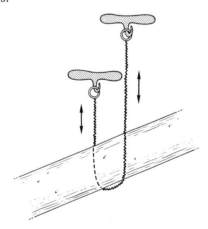

FIG. 68. Gigli saw.

A special variety of hand saw is that known as the Gigli saw, commonly used in the past but now seldom used where power saws are available. The Gigli saw is a flexible wire with cutting teeth arranged spirally round its circumference. To operate it the saw is passed round the deep surface of the bone. One end is held in each hand and the saw is worked with a reciprocal action (Fig. 68). Skill in the use of the Gigli saw takes a little time to acquire: in inexperienced hands the saw tends to stick or jam.

The main advantage of the Gigli saw is that it may be used in a confined space, and especially where the bone to be divided is deeply placed and cannot be delivered to the surface—a difficulty that is encountered, for instance, in the operation of innominate osteotomy.

THE USE OF MACHINE SAWS

The original power-operated saw was a rotating blade on an arbor held in the chuck of a high speed motor. This type, the rotating circular saw, is now hardly ever used, because of the danger of its "running away" and damaging soft tissues or even an assistant's fingers. It has given place to the oscillating saw, which does not revolve but oscillates in a small arc of a circle. It is thus much safer than a rotating circular saw. This type of blade may also be used on an end-cutting saw.

Another development is the reciprocating blade saw in which a miniature straight blade reciprocates in the manner of an ordinary hand saw but at much greater speed.

USING THE CIRCULAR SAW

As already noted, rotating circular saws should be used only in those rare circumstances when an oscillating saw is not available.

The first step is to select a saw blade of the correct diameter for the work in hand. It must be large enough to cut to the required depth, it being borne in mind that the blade will not sink in deeper than is permitted by the steel collar on the arbor. The blade commonly used for cutting longitudinally down the cortex of a bone is about 4 centimetres in diameter. A blade of much smaller diameter, perhaps 2.5 centimetres, is to be preferred for cutting the end of a graft crosswise. Circular saw blades have a very limited life. They quickly become blunt or bent out of the true. It is best therefore to insist upon using a new blade for each operation.

The next essential is to check that the saw blade has been secured on the arbor the correct way round. The blades are disposable, and when it is fitted to the arbor by inexperienced staff the blade may be placed upside down, so that the teeth are directed backwards instead of forwards: a blade used in this way cuts extremely poorly, if at all. As viewed from the side of the chuck, the teeth of the saw should project forwards in a clockwise direction (Fig. 69): if they are seen to be directed in an

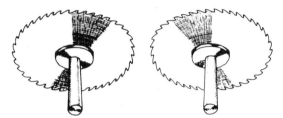

FIG. 69. Correct (left) and incorrect mounting of saw blade on the arbor.

anticlockwise direction the blade has been assembled wrongly and must be changed. At the same time that this feature is checked the surgeon should also ensure that the blade has been secured very tightly on the arbor: otherwise it may loosen during sawing and fly apart.

For a description of the technique of using the rotating saw the example will be taken of making a longitudinal cut down the shaft of a tibia, for instance in removing a bone graft. First the bone is exposed over a sufficiently wide area, by incision and stripping of the periosteum. This leaves a clean surface of raw bone ready for sawing. The next important point is that all swabs, packs and loose folds of draping towels must be moved well clear of the operation area: it is all too common for a saw blade to become tangled up in dressings or towels, which in an instant are gathered into a ball before the saw can be stopped. In this way the patient's skin may be inadvertently cut. It must also be emphasised that all assistants should hold their fingers and hands well out of the line of the saw; otherwise accidental damage may occur.

For the actual cutting of bone the saw blade is applied to the bone surface while revolving at full speed: it is a mistake to apply it to the bone and

then to start the motor. It hardly needs to be said that at this stage, and in fact throughout the sawing process, the motor must be gripped extremely firmly, and in such a way that the surgeon is ready to forestall any tendency of the saw blade to run along the surface. A vice-like rigid grip is the best key to safety.

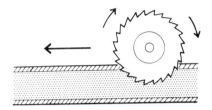

FIG. 70. When a rotating saw is used the cut should always be made from right to left.

In making a long cut down the length of the bone the saw should always be entered at the right hand end and moved along to the left (Fig. 70). Once the blade has sunk through the cortex it is better to leave it at full depth throughout the cutting process. Worked from right to left, it will bite into the bone; whereas if an attempt is made to cut from left to right the saw will tend to run out of the bone. With practice it is possible to cut many centimetres in a straight line in only a few seconds.

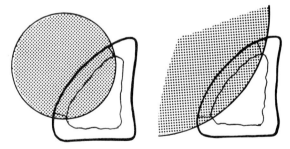

FIGS 71–72. Diagrams to show the advantage of a small blade (Fig. 71) for cutting the end of a tibial graft. A large blade tends to cut into the angles of the tibia, thus weakening it (Fig. 72).

For cutting the cortex of a tibia crosswise—as for instance in freeing the ends of a tibial graft—a small saw blade should be used so that it may be sunk to moderate depth without encroaching upon the corners of the bone (Figs 71 and 72). In making these transverse cuts the surgeon should place a folded towel over the bone, on which to rest his wrists while making the saw cuts. Here again a vice-like grip is essential, because the saw blade has a great tendency to run out of the bone, lacerating the skin flaps and becoming wrapped up in the draping towels.

USING THE OSCILLATING SAW

The oscillating saw, now used almost universally in preference to the rotating saw, presents less hazards because the arc through which the blade oscillates is small (Fig. 73): the teeth may come

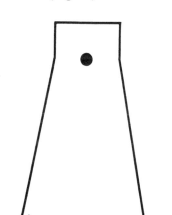

FIG. 73. Oscillating saw.

into contact even with skin or soft tissue without doing harm, so long as the tissue is mobile enough to move to and fro with the teeth. The technique of cutting bone with an oscillating saw is thus rather different from that used for a rotating saw. Cutting is achieved by pressing the blade vertic-

ally against the bone, section by section, rather than by moving it along the bone continuously.

USING THE RECIPROCATING SAW

The reciprocating saw (Fig. 74) is very useful for cutting bone in awkward situations where it may be impossible to gain access for a rotating saw. It may thus be used in many situations where formerly a Gigli saw was the only practicable method. Blades of a variety of sizes and shapes are available, and the first detail of technique is to

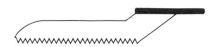

FIG. 74. Reciprocating saw.

select the blade appropriate to the work. Sawing is very simple. The only precaution of major importance is to ensure that the saw is not thrust too far into a deep wound, with risk of damage to soft tissue. The wound edges should be retracted sufficiently to enable the tip of the saw blade to be kept under direct vision throughout the sawing process. The body of the saw does not need to be moved longitudinally: all that is necessary is to apply steady pressure to engage the teeth of the saw in the bone. The reciprocations of the blade are sufficient to divide even a strong cortical bone in a matter of seconds. It is important, however, that the blade be in good sharp condition. These blades have only a limited life, and a blade that is becoming worn must be discarded and replaced in good time.

CUTTING BONE WITH THE HIGH SPEED BURR

Burrs of the type used in dental surgery, rotating at very high speed usually in a turbine-driven compressed air motor, are useful for fine work upon bone, particularly upon the small bones of the hands and feet. A range of burrs is available, some used for cutting, others for drilling. For cutting, the revolving burr is used rather in the manner of a fine knife. It is pressed sideways

against the bone to be cut, and it may be moved gently to and fro in a longitudinal direction to help to clear the cutting teeth of bone dust. Heavy sideways pressure upon the burr should be avoided because the shank may easily be broken.

Most cutting burrs may also be used for drilling soft bone, simply by exerting end pressure upon the instrument.

THE USE OF SCREWS

Screws may best be regarded as temporary bone sutures: they hold bones together or hold appliances to the bone until natural healing has occurred. They cannot be expected to serve these purposes permanently. If natural healing fails to occur, a screw will eventually loosen or break.

Screws are made usually from cobalt-chromium alloy, from special (18/8 SMo) stainless steel or from titanium alloy. They may be plain or, more often, self-tapping (with fluted points). Lag screws and cancellous screws are also commonly used (Fig. 75). The heads may have a plain slot to take an ordinary screwdriver, or a cruciform recess of Phillips pattern to receive the Phillips screwdriver. The screws designed for the A.O. system have a hexagonal recess for which a matching screwdriver is required.

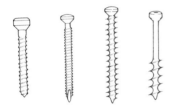

Fig. 75. Plain screw; self-tapping screw; cancellous screw; lag screw.

From the point of view of fixation with screws, bone may be regarded as being of two kinds: hard and soft. The cortex of the long bones in adults is hard. All cancellous bone, the cortex of flat bones, and the cortex of the long bones in young children, are soft. Hard bone, like metal, will not accept a screw unless the drill hole made to receive it is tapped with matching threads. Soft bone, like wood, will take a screw without tapping and often without pre-drilling. This means in practice that in order to drive a screw into adult cortical bone a hole equal in diameter to the core diameter of the screw must always be drilled, and the hole must either be tapped or a self-tapping screw must be used. In cancellous bone, on the other hand, the receiving hole may be undersized and threads need not be cut; thus a plain rather than a self-tapping screw may be used if desired.

If a bone onlay—for instance a cortical graft—is to be screwed to the recipient bone the hole in the onlay should be drilled out to match the overall diameter of the screw. This allows a sliding fit, and thus ensures that when the screw is tightened the onlay is compressed against the underlying bone (Fig. 76). The same principle applies when

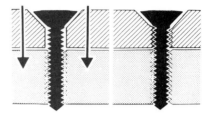

Fig. 76. Correct (left) and incorrect methods of screwing a bone graft to the host bone. The graft should always be drilled out to allow a sliding fit for the screw, so that when the screw is tightened the two bones are compressed together. The same principle applies when broken fragments of bone are screwed together.

two bone fragments are to be screwed together: the deeper fragment should be drilled to the core diameter of the screw whereas the superficial fragment should be drilled to allow a sliding fit.

COUNTERSINKING

Most screws have tapered heads designed for countersinking, and metal plates and other appliances are supplied with recessed holes to receive the screw heads. When bone is to be screwed to bone, it is usual to countersink the mouth of the drill hole, to ensure that the head of the screw is not unduly prominent. This is an important precaution if the screw head is to lie close under the skin. Recessing should be done with a countersink made to match the particular screws that are to be used, but in the absence of such an instrument an adequate recess may be made with a larger drill, or even with a narrow gouge.

Screwing a Plate to Cortical Bone with Self-tapping Screws

TECHNIQUE

First the bone is drilled to the required depth (in the case of a long bone, usually through both cortices), the drill being equal in diameter to the core diameter of the screw. (In very hard bone it may be necessary to drill the mouth of the hole out half a millimetre or so wider in order to allow the self-tapping threads of the screw to bite.) The depth of the hole is then measured with a depth gauge (Fig. 67), and a screw of the correct length is chosen. The screw is introduced on a self-holding screwdriver and driven in until about half the screw is engaged. The self-holding screwdriver is then removed and an ordinary screwdriver, appropriate to the pattern of screw, is substituted. The screw is driven on until it is fully engaged. It should be tightened with a firm but not excessive final twist: too much force can easily strip the thread in the bone and render the screw virtually useless.

Caution. Growth of bone into the self-tapping flutes of the screw may make the screw difficult to remove, especially in the case of a chrome-cobalt screw. Such screws should not generally be used if it is likely that their removal will be required later. Subsequent removal is easier if the screw selected is long enough to allow the fluted part to project outside the bone.

For the use of A.O. screws and plates see page 66.

SCREWING A PLATE TO CORTICAL BONE WITH A PLAIN SCREW

TECHNIQUE
The procedure is the same as described for a self-tapping screw except that threads must be pre-tapped to receive the screw. First a hole is drilled of the same diameter as the core diameter of the screw. The appropriate tap is then introduced and turned steadily by hand to cut the threads. The tap is removed, the depth of the hole is measured, and a screw of the correct length is inserted and driven in with the appropriate screwdriver.

SCREWING A PLATE OR BONE GRAFT TO CANCELLOUS BONE

TECHNIQUE
The softer the bone, the greater is the care needed to preserve a grip of the screw threads: it is all too easy to strip the threads in the bone by exerting only moderate force. It is important therefore that the primary hole in the bone should not be larger than the core diameter of the screw. Indeed, in soft bone it is often wise deliberately to drill an undersized hole: the screw will enlarge the track as it is driven in. The second important point is that the torque used in driving the screw should be light: twisting should be stopped as soon as the screw head is felt to be "home". It is recommended that special screws be used for cancellous bone. Cancellous screws have deeply cut threads and a relatively small core diameter in relation to the overall diameter (Fig. 75).

REMOVING A SCREW

Present-day screws are made from inert metal and in most cases it is not necessary or even desirable that they be removed. When special circumstances arise in which removal of a screw is

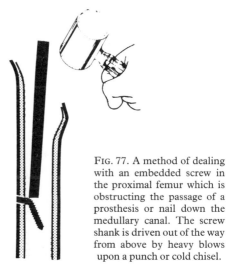

FIG. 77. A method of dealing with an embedded screw in the proximal femur which is obstructing the passage of a prosthesis or nail down the medullary canal. The screw shank is driven out of the way from above by heavy blows upon a punch or cold chisel.

required, the operation is usually simple but it may be exceptionally difficult. Only the difficult problem need be discussed here.

The most difficult cases are those in which the tip of a self-tapping cobalt-chromium screw has lain in cortical bone for a considerable time—for instance, a screw holding a nail-plate to the shaft of the femur. Because bone tends to grow into the flutes of the self-tapping point, the screw may refuse to turn. As more and more force is applied the screw eventually breaks: the head twists off the shank. This complication may present a serious dilemma: what is to be done with the buried screw shank?

Of course, shearing of the screw head allows the plate or other appliance that it was holding to be removed, and in most cases, this objective having been achieved, it is safe and indeed wise to leave the broken screw remnant undisturbed. The more difficult problem arises when the screw fragment is in the way of some other appliance that is to be fitted—for instance an intramedullary nail or the stem of a hip prosthesis. Something must then be done to get the fragment out or to bend it out of the way. To extract the fragment is usually very difficult and time-consuming: it entails cutting a channel alongside the screw. A trephine of such a diameter as to slide easily over the screw is the best instrument for this purpose, though even with this it is a slow and laborious process to cut through hard cortical bone, because the fine teeth of the trephine repeatedly become blocked with bone dust. An alternative is to use a fine dental burr on a high speed drill, but this may remove a sizeable area of bone before the screw is liberated: the bone is correspondingly weakened and may be at risk of fracture. Unless it is quite essential that the screw remnant be removed, therefore, it is often wisest and quickest, when fitting an intramedullary nail or a hip prosthesis, to bend the fragment out of the way by heavy blows upon a cold chisel or other long-handled semi-sharp instrument inserted down the medullary canal from above (Fig. 77).

(For notes on the A.O. techniques see page 66.)

THE USE OF NAILS AND PINS

The terms nail and pin are sometimes used synonymously; the distinction between them is arbitrary, a nail being generally regarded as a strong rigid appliance whereas a pin is much more slender and often to some extent flexible.

Nails and pins are used somewhat less frequently now than they were in the past. To some extent they have been superseded by screws, especially in the smaller ranges of size; for a screw has threads to give a positive grip whereas there is nothing other than friction to prevent a smooth nail from sliding in the bone. Some pins are indeed threaded over part of their length or perhaps over the whole length, and these come into the borderline between screws and pins.

The main present-day uses for stout nails are: 1) for fixation of fractures of the neck of the femur; and 2) in the form of intramedullary nails, for fixation of the long bones whether after fracture or after operative removal of tumours, cysts, etc; or to aid arthrodesis.

Pins of more slender proportions are used: 1) in the form of Steinmann pins for transfixing a long bone for the purpose of applying skeletal traction; 2) in the application of an external fixator; and 3) for fixation of bone fragments, as for instance in the treatment of slipped upper femoral epiphysis, fracture of the lower end of the fibula, unstable fracture of a metacarpal shaft, and certain fractures and dislocations of the clavicle: pins used for these purposes are often threaded or partly threaded.

These applications of nails and pins are referred to in greater detail in the relevant sections of this book. The only technique to which further reference is required here is that of transfixing a long bone with a Steinmann pin for the purpose of applying traction.

INSERTION OF STEINMANN PIN FOR SKELETAL TRACTION ON LOWER LIMB

General anaesthesia or local anaesthesia may be used. If a local anaesthetic is used it is necessary to infiltrate the skin at the proposed sites of insertion and of exit of the pin, and then to infiltrate the deeper layers down to and including the periosteum. This procedure allows the bone to be penetrated without significant discomfort. Depending upon the purpose for which traction is required, the pin may be inserted 1) through the upper end of the tibia immediately distal to the tibial tubercle, 2) through the lower end of the tibia, or 3) through the calcaneus.

Plain Steinmann pins may be used, but Denham pins, which are threaded over part of their

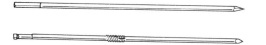

FIG. 78. Plain Steinmann pin and (below) threaded Denham pin.

length (Fig. 78), offer the advantage that sliding of the pin in the bone is prevented.

TECHNIQUE: TRANSFIXION OF UPPER END OF TIBIA

The correct site for transfixion of the upper end of the tibia is at a level immediately distal to the tibial tubercle and 2.5 centimetres behind the anterior border of the tibia. The pin is inserted from the lateral to the medial side (Fig. 79)

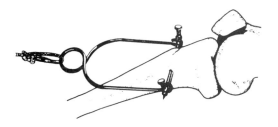

FIG. 79. Transfixion of upper end of tibia by Steinmann pin for skeletal traction. Drawing shows correct position of pin.

After draping and sterilisation of the locally shaved skin a small stab cut is made with a fine-pointed knife blade immediately over the proposed point of entry of the pin. The knife cut facilitates entry of the point of the pin and reduces the risk of contamination of the pin as it enters. The pin, held in a hand chuck, is then thrust forwards until it strikes the lateral surface of the tibia. It is important at this stage to line the pin up in the correct axis: it must be at right angles to the long axis of the limb as a whole and it should be strictly in the coronal plane—that is, with the limb lying in the neutral position and the patella directed forwards the pin should be horizontal (parallel with the floor).

When the pin has thus been lined up, by a to-and-fro twisting movement it is made to enter the bone and is driven steadily on until it is felt to emerge through the medial cortex. At this point it is a necessary precaution to ensure that a finger of the surgeon's counterthrusting hand is not in the line of the advancing pin; otherwise if the pin were to emerge suddenly the finger could easily be pierced. If a threaded pin such as the Denham pin is used in preference to a Steinmann pin, it is, of course, necessary to drive it in by rotating it to advance the threads in the bone.

When the point of the pin has emerged from the bone the pin is driven on with a steady rotary action until it bulges the skin at the point of emergence. The skin is pressed over the point of the pin so that the pin may be driven on through the skin and out on the medial side of the leg for a convenient distance. The pin holder is then removed.

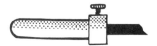

FIG. 80. Domed shield fixed over end of Steinmann pin to protect against injury. The shield is held in place by a set screw.

The points of entrance and emergence are sealed by a plastic occlusive spray or by collodion, gauze dressings are applied over the pin ends, and the area is supported by a lightly applied crepe bandage. The appropriate stirrup may then be slipped over the ends of the pin for the purposes of traction. Finally the point of the pin and usually the blunt end as well are protected by domed shields secured by set screws (Fig. 80).

TECHNIQUE: TRANSFIXION OF LOWER END OF TIBIA

Again the pin is inserted from the lateral side to emerge at the medial side. It should enter the tibia immediately in front of the fibula at a level about 4 or 5 centimetres above the tip of the medial malleolus. This ensures that the pin is well clear of the ankle joint. The technique is essentially similar to that described for transfixion of the upper end of the tibia. Again the important point is to line up the Steinmann pin correctly before it enters the

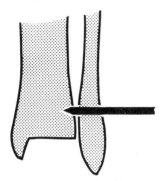

FIG. 81. Transfixion of lower end of tibia by Steinmann pin for skeletal traction. Diagram shows position and direction of pin, which passes in front of the fibula.

bone, so that it is strictly at right angles to the long axis of the limb as a whole and is also in the coronal plane (Fig. 81).

TECHNIQUE: TRANSFIXION OF CALCANEUS

In this technique, as in the previous two procedures, the Steinmann pin may be entered from the lateral side. The site for insertion of the pin is on or just behind the mid-point of a vertical line joining the tip of the lateral malleolus to the lower border of the heel (Fig. 82). This ensures that the

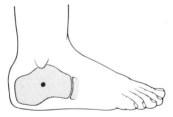

FIG. 82. Site for insertion of calcaneal pin.

pin, driven strictly at right angles to the axis of the limb, emerges well clear of the posterior tibial vessels.

Comment

A transfixion pin through the upper end of the tibia or through the lower end of the tibia is appropriate for sustained traction for up to 8, 10 or 12 weeks provided the pin has been inserted in the correct axis. If it has been inserted incorrectly, not truly at right angles to the axis of the limb, a plain Steinmann pin will tend to pull sideways if traction is continued for any length of time. (The use of a threaded pin obviates this difficulty.)

The authors recommend that traction through a calcaneal pin should be only of short duration— not more than a few hours. It is thus best reserved for applying traction during an operation such as intramedullary nailing of the tibia. Unaccountably, prolonged traction through the calcaneus seems more prone than tibial traction to promote pin track infection, which occasionally progresses to more widespread osteomyelitis of the calcaneus. Fortunately there is hardly any situation in which calcaneal traction has a distinct advantage over lower tibial traction for prolonged use, and therefore the latter should be preferred.

A further point to note in connection with skeletal traction through a Steinmann pin is that when a stirrup is used over the pin ends it should be a loose fit on the pin and should not be clamped to it by the set screws that are often provided in the collars of the stirrup. If the stirrup grips the pin too tightly movements of the stirrup tend to rotate the Steinmann pin in the bone and thus gradually to loosen it. When set screws are provided in the stirrup collars they should be removed lest some enthusiastic attendant, finding the set screws loose, should be tempted to tighten them on to the pin.

REMOVAL OF A STEINMANN'S TRACTION PIN

A Steinmann's pin that has been used for some time for traction purposes may usually be removed without anaesthetic.

The protruding part of the pointed end of the pin is carefully cleaned with detergent, with care to scrape away any dried exudate that may be adherent to it. The pin is then wiped with alcohol (surgical spirit). The squared end of the pin is gripped very securely in a hand chuck, and with a sharp rapid twist and a pull it may be extracted in a matter of two or three seconds without significant discomfort to the patient. Gauze dressings and a crepe bandage are applied over the site of the pin track.

Removal of a partly threaded pin such as a Denham pin entails rotating it in an anticlockwise direction. This can be done by locking it in the chuck of a hand drill and reversing it. Often the pin can be extracted painlessly without any anaesthetic.

THE USE OF STAPLES

U-shaped metal staples provide a useful method of internal fixation of bone in certain situations. One of their great merits is their simplicity. Staples are available in a wide range of gauge, length and width.

Sites suitable for staples. Staples are particularly applicable for the fixation of soft bone. A common example is their use for holding the tarsal bones apposed after osteotomy or as an aid to tarsal arthrodesis. Stapling is also a standard

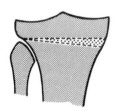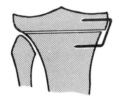

FIG. 83. Offset staple used for fixation after upper tibial osteotomy.

method of fixation after wedge osteotomy of the upper end of the tibia for genu varum or genu valgum. The bone at this site is mainly cancellous, with only a thin cortex, and multiple staples offer the most convenient form of fixation (Fig. 83).

Staples may also be used to coapt the fragments after osteotomy at other sites, but the method is seldom used for the fixation of adult cortical bone because the tracks for the limbs of the staple must be pre-drilled: in such a situation a plate fixed with screws is usually to be preferred—if only because the fixation is stronger.

Special instruments are now available to hold and control the staple and, if necessary, to angle its limbs as a precaution against penetration of the adjacent joint (Fig. 83).

TECHNIQUE

While the bone fragments that are to be fixed together are held in close apposition the correct size of staple is estimated. In general, wide staples give a better grip than narrow ones, but the width that can be used is often restricted by the proximity of adjacent joints or other structures. Likewise a long staple is to be preferred to a short one, provided sufficient depth of bone is available. When the correct staple has been selected a staple starter of matching size is hammered in to prepare the holes for the legs of the staple. This instrument is withdrawn and the staple, held in a staple-holding clamp, is driven in at the prepared site (Fig. 83). Hollow punches are available for driving the staple fully home. In most situations two or three staples are usually inserted to ensure adequate stability.

THE USE OF WIRE

Malleable wire, usually of stainless steel, is used frequently both in operations on bone and in soft-tissue operations.

USE OF WIRE IN OPERATIONS UPON BONE

The main function of wire in bone operations is to secure bone fragments together or to secure muscle, tendon or ligament to bone. Wire is perhaps used less often now than it was in the past for the internal fixation of fractures: better methods have been found. Nevertheless circumferential wiring still has a place in the treatment of long spiral fractures, particularly of the femur or tibia. For this purpose heavy wire, in the order of gauge 22 (standard wire gauge) is required. Wiring—

particularly of butterfly fragments—is often combined with intramedullary nailing.

An alternative to circumferential wiring is the use of self-locking nylon bands (Partridge and Evans, 1982). These incorporate small studs on the under surface of the band, to permit some vascular flow beneath the band even after tightening.

Wire sutures are used for attaching tendon or muscle to bone in a variety of situations. Common examples are re-attachment of the quadriceps tendon to the upper pole of the patella in repair of traumatic avulsion: and attachment of the triceps muscle to the stump of the olecranon after excision of the olecranon process for comminuted fracture.

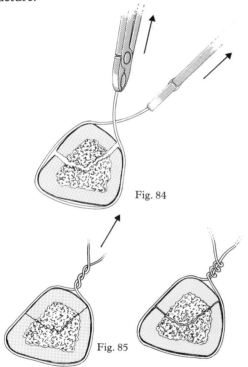

Fig. 84

Fig. 85

FIGS 84–85. Correct and incorrect techniques of tightening a wire. Figure 84—The wires are tensed as twisting is begun, so that one wire does not wrap around the other. Figure 85—At each half-twist a strong pull is maintained on the wire ends. If this is not done one end of the wire simply winds round the other (right) and the wire will break.

Tightening a wire. In tightening a wire with pliers it is a mistake simply to twist the two ends. This tends to wind one end of the wire round the other (Fig. 85) and eventually leads to breakage. To avoid this and to ensure an even twist the wire ends should first be gripped together in the pliers and then pulled towards the operator before the twisting force is applied (Figs 84–85).

TECHNIQUE: CIRCUMFERENTIAL WIRING FOR FRACTURE

The affected bone is exposed as described elsewhere to display the fracture site. The fractured bone ends are cleared as much as is necessary to allow full reduction of the displacement, so that the fracture surfaces are in intimate contact in the anatomical position. The fragments are held reduced by one or two bone-holding forceps clamping the fragments together. In all these manoeuvres soft tissues and periosteum are stripped as little as possible from the bone in order so far as possible to preserve the blood supply to the cortex.

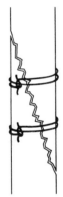

FIG. 86. Oblique fracture of a long bone secured with two circumferential wires.

With a sharply curved instrument a track is made round the periphery of the bone to transmit the wire. The track should be close to the bone but need not necessarily be deep to the periosteum. A loop of wire of a gauge suitable for the purpose is passed round the bone on an eyed wire passer designed specially for the purpose. It is recommended that the wire be looped round the bone twice before being drawn taut and finally twisted up tight with pliers (Fig. 86). In this manoeuvre the twisted wire should be drawn towards the operator before each new twist with the pliers is given. Twisting without preliminary pulling is liable to break the wire.

As a rule circumferential wiring should be carried out at two sites, one near the proximal end of the spiral fracture and the other near the distal end. In a very long spiral fracture of a large bone such as the femur wiring may be carried out at three sites.

TECHNIQUE: WIRING OF MUSCLE OR TENDON TO BONE

A tourniquet may be used but the surgeon must be prepared to release it before the wire sutures are tightened, to allow the muscle to be drawn down to the bone without tension.

First the area of bone to which it is intended that the muscle or tendon should adhere is scarified by light cuts with an osteotome if the surface is not already raw. Next, fine drill holes are made through the cortex of the bone transversely or obliquely, with a drill not more than 1.5 millimetres in diameter. Three to six holes usually suffice, depending upon the size of the muscle or tendon that is to be anchored. The end of the muscle or tendon is freshened to promote adherence and brought down close to the bone. Wire sutures of appropriate gauge are then prepared. It is often convenient to use mattress sutures, each traversing two adjacent drill holes and being tied over the muscle or tendon after it has been drawn well down (Fig. 87). Each drill hole may be used

to transmit two or even three wires. The wire sutures are usually reinforced by further catgut sutures through the soft tissues.

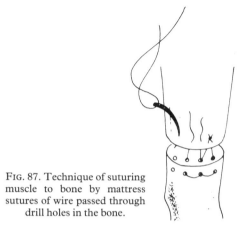

FIG. 87. Technique of suturing muscle to bone by mattress sutures of wire passed through drill holes in the bone.

USE OF WIRE IN OPERATIONS ON SOFT TISSUE

Fine stainless steel wire used for internal sutures has the advantages that it does not provoke an inflammatory reaction in the tissues, that it is strong, and that the knots will not slip. It finds its main application in tendon suture. It may also be used for aponeurotic layers where the integrity of the suture line is of prime importance—as for instance in repair of the gluteal aponeurosis after postero-lateral exposure of the hip. Some surgeons also use stainless steel wire for suture of the skin.

NOTES ON THE A.O. SYSTEM

The A.O. group was formed in Switzerland in 1958 by Martin Allgöwer, Maurice E. Müller, Robert Schneider and Hans Willenegger. A.O. stands for Arbeitsgemeineschaft Osteosynthesefragen. This translates into English as the Association for the Study of Internal Fixation of Fractures, known by the initials ASIF.

The objective of the group is not to encourage surgeons to operate on fractures. It is to ensure

that if a surgeon decides that operation is the best way of treating a fracture, the method chosen will have been well planned and supported by sound scientific reasoning. The development of the techniques has resulted in the production of special instruments and implants. These are combined into sets to make each operation self-contained.

The methods used for fracture fixation are taught at special instructional courses held in many countries. A centre for instruction, together with a research institute, has been built at Davos in Switzerland.

To further research, accurate documentation and reporting of results is necessary. A centre to gather and assess results has been established at Berne in Switzerland.

Instruments and Implants of the A.O. System

DRILLING

The accurate drilling of bone can be achieved only if the site of drilling is stabilised. The A.O. system has drill guides, or sleeves, to prevent a drill from moving at the start of drilling (Fig. 88). The serrated teeth of the drill sleeve are pushed firmly into the periosteum or bone to prevent slipping of the drill.

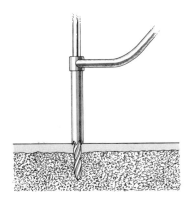

FIG. 88. A.O. drill sleeve, used to locate the drill for penetrating bone.

Drill sleeves used with plates either centre the drill in the hole, or place the drill to one end of a slotted hole to allow dynamic compression. The drill sleeves supplied for this use are in pairs on one instrument that is marked with the drill size, tap size and screw size with which it should be used.

The green coloured drill sleeve has a central drill hole. The orange sleeve has an offset drill hole. A screw inserted through the offset hole compresses the fracture when it is tightened fully.

To ensure that the plate movement is in the correct direction to compress the fracture, the arrow on the top of the orange drill sleeve must point towards the fracture.

THE USE OF CORTICAL SCREW TAPS

Taps of three lengths are available. It is important to use a tap that is long enough. If an unthreaded part of the tap shaft is tightened into the bone the tap is liable to break. A small unthreaded piece of metal may then be left behind and its removal may be difficult.

The cutting thread on each of the larger taps is incomplete around the circumference of the tap. The long groove or flute is to allow bone debris to be removed. If the groove becomes blocked the tap will not fit properly and may even break. The groove should therefore be cleared by means of the sharp hook. Clearing the sharp corners of the cutting thread with a swab should be avoided because fibres from the swab may be carried into the bone when the tap is turned.

Rules for operating the tap. Observance of the following rules will make for clean and rapid tapping of screw holes. 1) Tap the hole by hand. Power tapping is too fast; it is difficult to feel when the tap breaks through the far cortex; and there is danger of dragging soft tissue back when the tap is withdrawn. 2) Twist the tap handle with thumb and forefinger. 3) The tap centre-line must coincide with the hole centre-line. 4) Cut the first few threads in each cortex carefully. 5) Never force the tap. 6) Tap to the outside of the far cortex. 7) Withdraw the tap carefully. 8) Irrigate the holes. 9) Feel for the quality of the bone.

A.O. SCREWS

Each screw has a head, a core and a thread. The distance from one thread to the next in the line of the core is the pitch. The thread form of A.O. screws is of a special design based on the fact that they are used with pre-tapped holes to produce more acceptable thread/bone interface stresses when tightened. The thread is more "fin-like" than is usually the case on self-tapping screws, and it is buttressed for easier driving and greater holding power.

Cancellous screws have a much coarser thread than cortical screws. In other words, the ratio of effective thread depth to core diameter is greater.

head and the conical countersink of standard plates, and to allow angulation of the screws when they are used in conjunction with dynamic compression plates.

Screw heads with hexagon slots, although

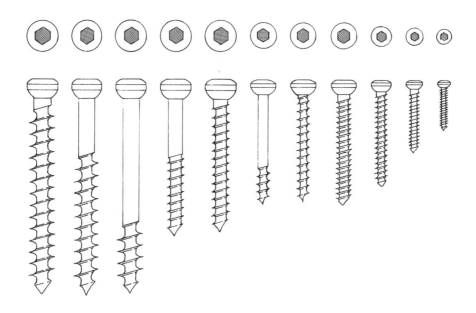

FIG. 89. Range of A.O. screws. Note the hemispherical heads, with hexagonal slots necessitating a special screwdriver.

They are made in various thread lengths. The series 216 screws have 16 millimetres threaded; the series 217 have 32 millimetres threaded; and the series 218 screws are threaded throughout their length.

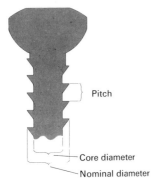

FIG. 90. Longitudinal section of A.O. cortical screw to show the shape of the thread.

The heads of A.O. screws have a hemispherical shape to reduce contact stresses between screw

slightly deeper than cross-slotted screws, allow the screw to be fully tightened without thrust on the driver. After tightening, placing the driver in the slot will subsequently give the direction of the screw centre-line.

Screw size. The *nominal size* of a screw is the diameter across the tip of the threads. The *core diameter* is the diameter of the central cylindrical core around which the helical thread is formed. The *drill diameter* is the size of the pilot hole required in the bone before the thread is formed by the tap. It must be at least equal to the core diameter to allow the tap to be introduced without causing micro-fracture. The *effective thread depth* is the difference between the nominal radius of the screw and the radius of the pilot drill. The *shank diameter* is the diameter of the plain (unthreaded) portion of cancellous and malleolar screws.

CARE OF DEPTH GAUGE

It is important that regular care be given to depth gauges used to estimate the length of screws required after drilling cortical bone. Accidental bending of the stem of the gauge prevents its effective use, as shown in Figure 91. Similarly, care must be taken to ensure that the tip of the gauge is not worn, with consequent difficulty in hooking it positively over the deep cortex (Fig. 91).

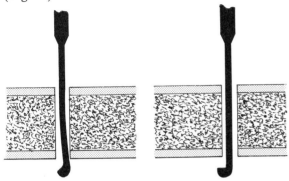

FIG. 91. *Left*—A depth gauge may become defective on account of bending of the stem and wear of the tip. *Right*—The defects corrected.

LAG SCREW TECHNIQUE

A lag screw is threaded in only part of its length—that is, in the part away from the head. The shank is plain, and is equal in diameter to the core diameter of the screw. The plain shank allows the tension in the screw during tightening to pull two fragments together if the thread grips only the far

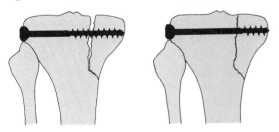

FIG. 92. Incorrect and correct use of a lag screw for fixation of detached medial condyle of tibia. The threaded part of the screw should engage only the distal fragment, so that the fragments are drawn together.

fragment. A fully threaded screw may also be used as a lag screw to provide interfragmentary com-

pression. In this technique a gliding hole is drilled in the bone nearest to the screw head, so that the screw thread will not hold on the bone around this hole. When a hole drilled in the far cortex is tapped, insertion of the screw closes the bone fragments together with compression (Fig. 94).

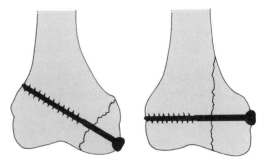

FIG. 93. Correct use of lag screw for condylar fracture of femur.

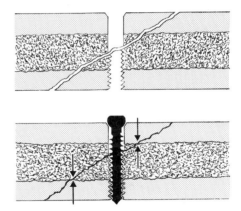

FIG. 94. Correct method of coapting fragments when a fully threaded screw is used. The hole in the near cortex is drilled out to allow a sliding fit. When the screw is driven home the fragments are thus drawn together.

THE USE OF THE COUNTERSINK

When a screw is driven directly into bone the shape of its head is such that only a small area is in contact with the bone. The use of a countersink increases this area and spreads the force of compression.

If countersinking is excessive the hole may be so greatly deepened that the screw head is in danger of sinking into the medulla of the bone. If this threatens, a washer may be used to avoid the danger. A washer may also be used to spread the force if the bone into which a screw is inserted is very soft.

SCREWDRIVERS

Four screwdrivers are included in modern A.O. sets. All have hexagonal heads. The one for the cannulated screw is drilled right through the centre of the shaft. In using this the surgeon must take care to ensure that the guide wire used is not so long as to come right through the driver and penetrate the palm when the screw is inserted.

In patients who have had a small fragment screw or mini-fragment screw inserted years ago, the radiographs must be studied carefully before screw removal to determine whether the screw head is of the old cruciform type. One of the old-type screwdrivers would then be needed. These older type cruciform-headed screws are still in stock in some hospitals. The shallower depth of the cruciform head is, in fact, preferred by some surgeons for fixing shallow fragments in intra-articular fractures.

REMOVAL OF BROKEN SCREWS

Despite correct insertion of screws, unexpected forces or destruction of bone may cause overloading, with possible breakage of a screw.

For each larger size of screw there is a set of removal tools. A centre stem may be used to guide a crown drill to enlarge the hole over a buried broken screw. If the screw has broken at the bone surface, the centre pin is removed and the crown drill is used directly around the broken screw shaft to make enough space for the screw extractor to be applied.

THE USE OF THE SHARP HOOK

The sharp hook is used to clear the threads of drills and taps of bone debris, which may interfere with their function and lead to overheating or instrument breakage. It may also be used to remove soft tissue from the slots of screw heads before screw removal, and to tease soft tissue from plates so that they may be easily lifted from the bone when all the screws have been removed.

THE USE OF DYNAMIC COMPRESSION PLATES

Dynamic compression plates are available in two sizes. The larger size, for use with cortical screws, has the end holes enlarged to receive cancellous screws. Cancellous screws cannot be used through any of the other holes.

In each hole of the plate the crescent of the hole away from the centre of the plate has a sloped surface. When a screw is tightened into it the screw head bears against this sloping surface, forcing the plate along the bone. When the plate is already fixed to the other side of the fracture, tightening of the screw compresses the fracture by 1 millimetre. This, however, does not give any indication of the compression force applied, or even of whether it will close the fracture gap. By using each of the holes in sequence, it is possible to gain more distance of compression. Before the next screw is tightened home the previous one must be temporarily released. Used in this way, compression plating can give a maximal compression distance equal in millimetres to the number of holes used for compression.

Plate bending. The thin plates of the small fragment and mini-fragment series can be bent with small pliers. The larger plates need a bending press. When a long plate is held in the press jaws, the use of a bending iron allows a twist to be applied. The shape for bending a plate may be prepared by the use of a malleable strip.

Any plate should be bent as few times as possible before application in order to prevent damage to its surface, which could lead to corrosion, and to prevent early fatigue failure.

Plates applied to a concave surface should be slightly under-bent to give better distribution of the compression. They should be fixed to the bone first through the end holes and subsequently through adjacent holes, working towards the middle of the plate. Each screw should be fully tightened before the next hole is drilled.

Transverse or short oblique fractures of the humerus, radius or ulna may be fixed by a plate that is slightly over-bent in order to distribute more evenly the axial compression across the fracture site. A plate contoured exactly to the shape of the bone and placed under tension will induce compression only in the cortex immediately adjacent to the plate. The plate should first be contoured to the bone surface and then slightly over-bent at its central, solid portion that will overlie the fracture site: it must not be bent through a screw hole.

THE ARTICULATED COMPRESSION/DISTRACTION DEVICE

The articulated compression/distraction device (Fig. 95) has a load guide when full compression or distraction is applied. Before the red section is covered, the force is 80 kiloponds. This is a technical term for the application of a force of 80 kilograms acting on the plate.

apply compression of up to 80 kiloponds across the fracture. While this compression is maintained the remaining holes for screws on this side of the fracture are drilled, tapped and fitted with screws of the correct length.

Use in distraction. If the articulated device is fitted to the plate with the swinging foot reversed, it can be used to distract a fracture (Fig. 95). The foot then bears against the side of the end hole of the plate nearest to the fracture. The use of the spanner on the nut on the screw's thread thus provides distraction of the fracture. Distraction may be required either to allow more accurate reduction of the fracture, or to provide for the insertion of a bone graft, for instance from the iliac crest. When either of these functions has been achieved the distraction force may be released and the foot of the loosened apparatus reversed. Compression can then be applied. This technique is useful for insertion and compression of a bone

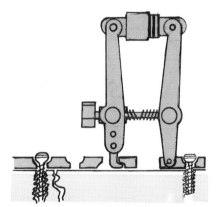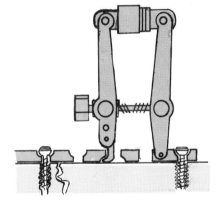

FIG. 95. The A.O. articulated compression device used for compression (*left*) and distraction (*right*). To compress a fracture the plate is screwed in position on one side of the fracture and the foot of the compression device is screwed to the other fragment with the lug, facing away from the fracture, in the end hole of the plate. With compression applied, screws are inserted through the remaining holes of the plate. To distract a fracture the direction of the lug is reversed.

The plate is first fixed to the bone on one side of the reduced fracture. The lug of the drilling template is then placed in the end hole at the other end of the plate. Through the template the near cortex is drilled. The hole is tapped to receive a cortical screw. The articulated device is then screwed to the bone with an 18 millimetre screw. The swinging foot of the device is placed in the end hole of the plate at the side away from the fracture. A spanner is then used to tighten the appliance to

graft when much of the diameter of the bone has been lost, particularly in the distal end of the tibia.

PRECAUTIONS IN THE USE OF THE A.O. SYSTEM

The principles of the techniques for the use of the A.O. system are now well established. In using the system, however, the surgeon may find that the equipment available includes items which are no longer in the current catalogue.

Mention has been made elsewhere of the cruci-form head screws used in years gone by, and of the need to be equipped with the appropriate driver if removal of such screws is intended.

Confusion may also arise from the change in the diameter of the 206 series screw from 3.5 to 4.0 millimetres. Screws of this series have a pitch of 1.75 millimetres, in both the 3.5 and 4.0 milli-metre range. For the 3.5 millimetre screw the instruction was to use a 2 millimetre drill and the corresponding tap, which exactly matched the thread of the screw. The third edition of the small fragment set manual, published in 1988, advises the use of the 3.5 millimetre tap for the 4 milli-metre screw. New production of the 3.5 milli-metre tap will be labelled 4.0 millimetres. This indicates the size of screw for which it is to be used. In future years the diameter of the tap may be increased to 4.0 millimetres. This would make it over-size for any remaining 3.5 millimetre 206 series screws found in sets.

TAKING A GRAFT FROM THE TIBIA

The tibia is usually the best donor site when a cortical graft is required. Such a graft is strong enough to give reasonable stability, especially when it is fixed in position with screws; and in addition it provides a stimulus for the growth of new bone in and about it. When a graft is taken correctly the tibia suffers little disability and sub-sequent fracture is rare.

TECHNIQUE

The graft is usually taken from the medial (subcu-taneous) surface of the bone. It may be cut as wide as three-quarters of the width of the bone surface provided that the anterior and posterior angles of the shaft are left intact (Fig. 96). It is essential that these angles be preserved; otherwise there is a serious risk of subsequent fracture.

Position of patient. Usually it is most convenient to take the graft with the patient lying supine. If the patient has to be prone for the purpose of the main part of the operation for which the graft is required, it is still feasible to obtain a tibial graft by flexing the knee acutely. If it is necessary that the patient lie in the lateral position, it is best to take the graft from the underneath leg—that is, the side on which the patient is lying—the hip and knee on that side being flexed 90 degrees.

It is recommended that the graft be taken with-out the aid of a tourniquet. When the taking of a graft is only a small incident in a long operation it is very easy, while concentrating on the main part of the operation, to overlook the donor leg and

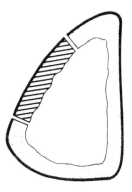

FIG. 96. When a cortical graft is cut from the tibia it is important to leave the corners of the bone intact: otherwise the strength of the tibia is seriously im-paired.

inadvertently to leave the tourniquet in position for too long—perhaps until the main part of the operation is completed. Moreover in this particu-lar procedure the absence of a tourniquet does not make the operation appreciably more difficult.

Incision. The incision is placed over muscle rather than over the bone itself in order to avoid a scar that is adherent to the bone. If the patient is supine or prone the main (vertical) part of the incision is lateral to the crest of the tibia over the antero-lateral muscles, but it curves medially to cross the bone at top and bottom (Fig. 97). If the patient is in the lateral position it is more convenient to place the vertical part of the incision behind the posterior border of the tibia over the calf; again the incision curves across the bone at top and bottom. In either case the length of the incision depends upon the length of graft required.

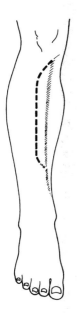

FIG. 97. Taking a tibial graft. The skin incision.

Exposure of cortical surface of tibia. The skin flap thus outlined is reflected medially or forwards as the case may be to expose the periosteum over the medial surface of the tibia. This is incised vertically down to bone in the midline of the proposed graft. Cross cuts are made at top and bottom of the vertical incision. The periosteal flaps thus outlined are scraped to each side with an elevator; the periosteal reflection should extend close to the borders of the tibia. Slender well curved bone levers are inserted beneath the periosteum round the anterior border of the bone and round the posterior border. The points of the levers are kept close to the bone. These four bone levers, one at each corner of the wound, serve to keep the periosteal flaps retracted so that the cortical surface of the tibia is fully exposed in the area of the proposed graft.

Cutting the graft. First the outline of the graft is marked on the surface by lightly striking the bone with an osteotome, the measurements being checked with a rule. Longitudinal cuts are then made with a motor saw to sever the sides of the graft from the donor bone. If the saw is of the rotating type the cut must always be made from right to left: otherwise the saw blade will run out of the cut (Fig. 70). The circular blade should be of medium size, usually about 40 millimetres in

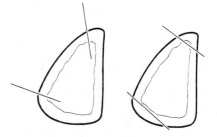

FIG. 98. Taking a tibial graft. *Left—* Diagrammatic cross-section of tibia showing the correct plane of the saw cuts. *Right—* Unless the triangular shape of the tibia is borne in mind it is all too easy to saw off the corners of the bone, with potentially disastrous consequences.

diameter. The blade should penetrate the whole thickness of the cortex at one cut. For the anterior cut the blade should be slanted parallel with the lateral cortex of the tibia, and for the posterior cut it should be parallel with the posterior cortex (Fig. 98). If this rule is not observed the corners of the bone may inadvertently be cut off. The longitudinal cuts should be about 5 millimetres longer than the proposed length of the graft; otherwise the ends of the graft may not be fully separated from the donor bone because of the curve of the saw blade.

In order to cut the ends of the graft transversely a blade of small diameter (about 20 millimetres) is substituted. If a rotating saw is used it is essential that the motor be gripped very firmly for these transverse cuts; otherwise the blade is very likely to "run away", with risk of cutting the skin edges.

When the cuts on the four sides of the graft have thus been completed the graft should already be free. If so, it is easily levered out with a thin osteotome. If it is still adherent at one or more points the cuts must be run over again with the saw where the graft is still held; or alternatively it may be sufficient to free any small remaining bridges with an osteotome.

Finally, the graft is lifted out and placed in a shallow dish. It may be covered with a moist pack but need not be immersed in saline.

Closure. Haemostasis must be secured before the wound is closed. This seldom presents a problem, but occasionally bleeding points in the medulla may need to be sealed with the diathermy.

It will usually be found impossible to close the periosteum fully with close sutures. Nevertheless the edges should be approximated by three or four widely spaced absorbable sutures. The skin is closed with eversion sutures, without drainage.

POST-OPERATIVE MANAGEMENT

Any blood remaining in the cavity left by removal of the graft should be squeezed out by firm pressure over a pad of gauze so that the skin surface is slightly concave into the bone defect. Firm pressure by soft gauze dressings and crepe bandages is required to prevent the formation of a haematoma. Usually the dressing need not be disturbed until the sutures are removed after 10 to 14 days.

TAKING A GRAFT FROM THE FIBULA

Fibular bone is not ideal for grafting because it tends to be brittle and because the surface is seldom wide enough to allow drilling for screws without serious loss of strength. Nevertheless there are circumstances in which fibular bone is the graft of choice—for instance for replacement of a radius that has been excised on account of a primary neoplasm. Since the fibula is not significantly concerned with weight bearing, its whole thickness may be taken and if necessary almost its whole length. The lower end should be preserved, however, unless the ankle is to be arthrodesed.

TECHNIQUE

Position of patient. The patient may be supine, prone or in the lateral position depending upon the nature of the main operation for which the graft is required. A tourniquet is not required and is not to be recommended.

Incision. The skin incision is vertical over the lateral aspect of the bone: its length depends upon the length of the graft required. The bone is exposed between the peroneal muscles in front and the soleus behind (see p. 44). When the bone has been exposed the periosteum is incised longitudinally throughout the length of the incision and stripped from the whole circumference of the bone. To some extent this may be done with a periosteal elevator, but in places sharp dissection is required; on the deep surface of the bone a rib stripper or a small retractor of Langenbeck type may be used. In stripping the periosteum it is important to keep close to the bone: neglect of this precaution may endanger the peroneal artery or other sizeable vessels that may cause troublesome bleeding.

When the required length of bone has been stripped over its whole length and circumference, the bone is divided at the appropriate points proximally and distally to yield the required length of graft. The fibula is not easily cut with bone-cutting forceps or osteotomes: it tends to splinter too easily, the graft then being spoilt. It may be cut with a motor-saw, preferably with a reciprocating blade (see p. 58), or with bone nibbling forceps used in such a way that the bone is penetrated in small bites.

When the graft has been cut at each end it is free; it is lifted out and placed in a shallow dish. When haemostasis has been secured the wound is closed without drainage.

POST-OPERATIVE MANAGEMENT

A firm crepe bandage is applied over gauze dressings and may be left undisturbed until the sutures are removed. Exercises for the ankle and foot should be practised.

Comment

If the upper end of the fibula is to be removed special care must be taken to identify and preserve the common peroneal nerve as it winds from behind forwards round the neck of the bone (see p. 44).

TAKING A GRAFT FROM THE ILIUM

The wing of the ilium is the best source of cancellous bone. It may be obtained in the form of slivers or chips, or it may be taken as a block which may include one cortex or both cortices. Techniques for taking bone both from an anterior approach and from behind will be described.

Techniques of Cutting Grafts from Anterior Part of Ilium

The patient may be in the supine, the lateral or the prone position, depending upon the requirements of the main operation for which the graft is to be obtained. Most commonly the patient is supine, and in that case it is convenient to take the graft from the antero-lateral prominence of the ilium, immediately behind the anterior superior spine. If chips or slivers are required, the crest and adjacent part of the wing of the ilium afford good supplies. If an elongated block of bone is needed (as for filling an extensive defect in a long bone) it is best obtained from the iliac crest. On the other hand, if a flat rectangular or square block is needed together with its cortex, the wing of the ilium a little below the crest is to be preferred, the crest being left intact.

TECHNIQUE: SLIVER OR CHIP GRAFTS

A straight skin incision joins two points on the iliac crest like the string of a bow, one just behind the anterior superior spine and the other 7 to 10 centimetres behind this, the actual length of the incision depending on the quantity of bone required (Fig. 99). The skin edges are retracted and the underlying fascia and muscle are divided in the line of the skin incision right down to bone.

With a periosteal elevator muscle and periosteum are stripped from the bone over a short distance on each side of the incision. In the same line as the

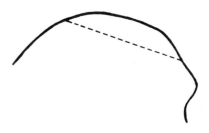

FIG. 99. Taking sliver grafts from the ilium. The line of incision.

skin and muscle incisions, the bone is divided right through both cortices with an osteotome, so that a crescentic portion of the wing of the ilium is separated from the main body of the bone, remaining attached only by a hinge of soft tissue

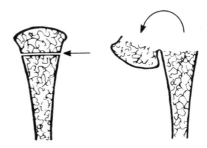

FIGS 100–101. Taking sliver grafts from the ilium. Figure 100—Cross-section of ilium showing line of osteotomy. Figure 101—The "lid" turned over to expose the two cut surfaces.

on its proximal and deep aspects (Fig. 100). (The crest may be well controlled by a Verbrugge forceps—A.O. 398.80). A blunt bone lever is inserted through the site of osteotomy and the hinged piece of bone is forced medially and turned over through 180 degrees so that its cut surface now faces proximally, lying adjacent to the cut surface of the main part of the ilium (Fig. 101). It is steadied in this position by bone hooks, one at each end. Suitable slivers or chips of cancellous bone may now be scooped out both from the main body of the ilium and from the everted "lid" with a narrow gouge inserted at the cut surface. Bone may be excavated in this way until a mere shell of iliac wing and crest remains.

In the reconstruction, the bone flap is turned back into position so that the cut surfaces of bone are accurately apposed, and retained by strong catgut sutures through muscle and deep fascia. The skin is sutured without drainage.

TECHNIQUE: ELONGATED BLOCK GRAFT

The skin incision begins just behind the anterior superior spine of the ilium and arches backwards, following the outline of the iliac crest: its length is dictated by the length of graft required. The in-

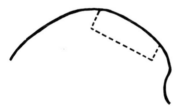

FIG. 102. Taking a block graft from the iliac crest. Outline of graft.

cision is deepened to bone, and the crest of the ilium is isolated by clearing away muscle attachments by sharp dissection, with the knife kept close to the bone. The outline of the proposed graft is marked upon the bone surface with a sharp instrument (Fig. 102). The graft, consisting of the entire thickness of the iliac crest, is then cut free from the main body of the ilium by a series of cuts through both cortices with a sharp thin osteotome.

In the closure of the wound, the muscles stripped from the inner and outer tables of the iliac crest are sutured together with closely spaced mattress sutures. The skin is closed, usually without drainage.

Pre-drilling the graft. If the graft is designed to fill a gap in a long bone and to be fixed in position by an intramedullary nail passing down its centre, it is useful to prepare the track for the nail with a long drill before the graft is cut. First a

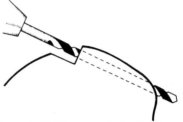

FIG. 103. Drilling a graft longitudinally before its removal.

notch is cut at one end of the proposed graft as a starting point for the drill, which is then directed as accurately as possible down the thickest part of the iliac crest (Fig. 103). The graft is then cut free, and if necessary trimmed along the edges in such a way that the drill hole is central.

TECHNIQUE: RECTANGULAR BLOCK GRAFT

The principle is to leave the crest of the ilium intact and to excise the requisite block of bone just distal to it, leaving a "window" in the wing of the ilium (Fig. 104). A flat or a slightly curved block of bone may be obtained according to requirements, by selecting the appropriate part of the wing of the ilium as the donor site (Fig. 105).

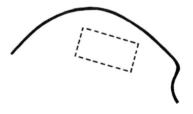

FIG. 104. Taking a rectangular block graft from the ilium. Outline of graft.

Only the outer aspect of the ilium need be exposed. The skin incision is parallel with the crest of the ilium but 1 centimetre below it. Fascia and muscle are incised in the line of the skin incision, and the muscle is stripped proximally and distally to expose a wide area of the wing of the ilium. The outline of the proposed graft is marked on the bone surface by light cuts with an osteotome (Fig. 104). The four sides of the graft are then cut, the osteotome penetrating through the whole thickness of the ilium, but with care not to drive it more than a millimetre or two beyond the inner cortex. When the graft has been thus isolated from the body of the bone it remains attached only by the iliacus muscle on its deep aspect. One edge of the graft is levered out with the osteotome and the muscle can then be stripped easily from the deep face of the graft, which is lifted out and placed in a shallow dish ready for use.

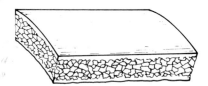

FIG. 105. Rectangular block graft after removal. It includes both cortices of the ilium.

In the repair of the soft tissues it is good practice to suture the deep muscle (iliacus) to the superficial muscle mass by mattress sutures inserted through the window in the ilium. This helps to prevent haematoma. The wound is then closed in layers. Because of the extensive stripping of muscle from the bone, suction drainage for 24 hours is recommended.

TECHNIQUES OF CUTTING GRAFTS FROM POSTERIOR PART OF ILIUM

When the patient is to be in the supine position for the main grafting operation, it is clearly most convenient to obtain grafts from the anterior part of the ilium, as described above. But if the nature of the grafting operation dictates that the patient be prone or in the lateral posture, it is equally appropriate to take grafts from the back of the ilium near the region of the posterior superior iliac spine.

The skin incision, about 10 centimetres long, runs obliquely downwards and medially, with its centre over the posterior superior spine of the

ilium (Fig. 106). (If grafting is being undertaken for spinal fusion, a prolongation of the spinal incision running downwards and laterally may be

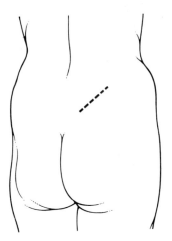

FIG. 106. Taking a posterior iliac graft. The skin incision.

used, as described on page 134.) The incision is deepened through the subcutaneous fat to expose the gluteal aponeurosis—the tough fibrous layer covering the gluteus maximus and bounded

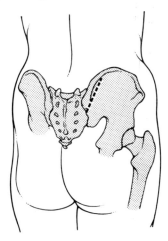

FIG. 107. Posterior aspect of ilium and posterior superior spine. The line of incision in the gluteal aponeurosis is shown.

medially by the crest and medial edge of the wing of the ilium where it forms the posterior superior spine. The incision through the aponeurosis is made obliquely from above downwards and medially, close to the everted crest of the iliac bone (Fig. 107).

Deep to the gluteal aponeurosis are muscle fibres of the gluteus maximus, arising from the wing of the ilium, close up against the crest and posterior superior spine. The muscle, together with the periosteum to which it is attached, is stripped downwards and outwards with a periosteal elevator to expose as much raw bone of the posterior third of the wing of the ilium as is required.

This exposure serves to permit the taking of abundant graft material whether this be in the form of multiple slivers, a long piece from the iliac crest and posterior iliac spine, or a rectangular block of bone from the wing of the ilium. The technique for each of these procedures is analogous to that for taking similar grafts from the anterior part of the ilium, as described in the previous section (p. 76).

Comment

No special problems are presented in the taking of iliac grafts. The operation is, however, often complicated by the formation of a haematoma and by consequent delay in healing, and steps must be taken to prevent this.

First, haemostasis at the time of operation must be meticulous; and second, the deeper layers of the wound must be closed very carefully, and sufficient deep mattress sutures should be used to ensure that no potential dead space remains. Suction drainage is advisable if there has been considerable stripping of muscle from the bone, but reliance should be placed more on haemostasis and on careful suture of the deep layers than upon drainage of the wound.

Patients often complain of considerable pain in the operation area after removal of an iliac graft. This may necessitate rest in bed for a few days. Nevertheless walking may be resumed as soon as pain allows.

BONE GRAFTING

Bone grafting is infinitely variable, and no description could fit every occasion. The principles will therefore be illustrated by descriptions of three techniques: 1) onlay cortical bone grafting for ununited fracture of a long bone; 2) sliding bone graft; 3) circumferential sliver grafting (Phemister 1947) for ununited fracture of a long bone; and 4) cancellous chip grafting for filling of a cavity or defect.

ONLAY CORTICAL BONE GRAFTING FOR UNUNITED FRACTURE OF A LONG BONE

In this operation a stout cortical graft is screwed to the recipient bone, bridging the fracture (Fig. 108). This type of bone graft gives rigidity, as well as providing a stimulus for the formation of new bone about the fracture.

TECHNIQUE

Selection of site for graft. First the most suitable surface upon which to apply the graft must be determined. As a general rule it is inadvisable to apply the graft to a subcutaneous surface: a submuscular surface is to be preferred, partly for cosmetic reasons and partly because a graft in contact with muscle is more likely to be quickly revascularised than is one that is covered by fat and skin alone. Another factor that has a bearing on the siting of the graft is extensive scarring of

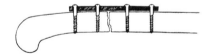

FIG. 108. Cortical onlay bone graft.

the skin and subcutaneous tissues. Whenever possible, it is better to place the graft in an unscarred area. For instance, in the case of the tibia the preferred site for grafting is usually the lateral surface deep to the antero-lateral muscle mass; but if there is extensive scarring in this area it is preferable to apply the graft to the posterior surface.

Exposure. Exposure of the bone follows the usual practice as outlined in Chapter 1. It has to be remembered that soft tissues and bone may be extensively matted together around the site of fracture, and it is usually wise first to expose normal bone above and below the fracture. It is then easy to follow the bone towards the fracture. In this way the risk of damaging an important structure due to distortion of the anatomy is reduced to the minimum. At the completion of the exposure the bone should be fully displayed over a length a little longer than the proposed graft, the soft tissues being retracted by four curved bone levers, two at each side.

Preparing the bed for the graft. If apposition and alignment of the fragments are acceptable it is unnecessary to clear the fracture surfaces, and the bone work may be restricted solely to that aspect of the bone upon which the graft is to be laid. The recipient surface must be made flat over an area as long and as wide as the proposed graft. A chisel is used for this purpose, with its bevelled side against the bone. Although a certain amount of cortex usually has to be removed in the smoothing process, it is a mistake to remove more than about half the normal thickness of cortex: a substantial thickness must be left intact in order to provide a firm base for the graft (Fig. 109).

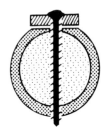

FIG. 109. Cross-sectional diagram showing fixation of graft to host bone by screw. Note the amount of cortex removed to form a flat bed for the graft.

Preparation of graft. A cortical bone graft, usually from the tibia, is obtained in the manner described on page 72. Care should be taken to ensure that the graft is of the correct dimensions, and it is often convenient to drill four holes for the fixation screws before the graft is lifted from its bed. If any further trimming to size is required this is now carried out with the motor saw. Finally the medullary aspect of the graft is smoothed flat by shaving away irregular cancellous bone with a chisel.

Application and fixation of graft. The graft is laid in position upon its bed. If it does not seem to be in close contact with the bed along its whole length adjustments may have to be made either to the bed or to the cancellous surface of the graft to ensure that an accurate fit is secured. The graft is then held lightly apposed to the recipient bone by two bone-holding forceps, one above the fracture and the other below it. If the graft has been pre-drilled before its removal from the tibia it now

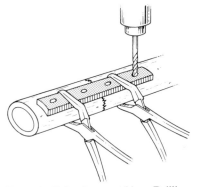

FIG. 110. Onlay bone grafting. Drilling the screw holes in the recipient bone.

only remains to drill holes in the recipient bone equal in diameter to the core diameter of the screws to be used (Fig. 110). If the graft has not yet been drilled, appropriate holes are drilled through the graft and recipient bone together, and the holes in the graft are subsequently enlarged to the overall diameter of the screw to allow a sliding fit. As a rule the holes in the graft should be countersunk to receive the screw heads, but this is not essential if the graft will be covered by a good thickness of muscle. The correct length for each screw is determined by a depth gauge (Fig. 67) and the four screws are driven home.

Closure. Whenever possible a good covering of muscle should be drawn over the graft and lightly held with absorbable sutures. The skin is closed, usually without drainage.

POST-OPERATIVE MANAGEMENT

At the conclusion of the operation gauze dressings are applied and held firmly but not too tightly with a crepe bandage. Over this a well padded plaster is applied. The possibility of marked swelling of the limb must be borne in mind, and the surgeon must be ready to split the plaster, bandage and dressings if there is any sign of embarrassment of the circulation. After two weeks the initial plaster is removed, and after removal of the sutures a new lightly padded and well moulded plaster is applied. This is retained until the fracture is united.

SLIDING BONE GRAFT

A sliding bone graft may be used to bridge an ununited fracture, especially of the tibia. A section of intact cortical bone is cut from the bone above the fracture and slid downwards so that it bridges the fracture (or in appropriate cases the graft may be slid upwards). An advantage of the sliding graft is that the necessity to take bone from another site is avoided. The technique to be described relates to the tibia, which is by far the commonest site for this method of grafting.

TECHNIQUE

Position of patient. The patient lies supine. A tourniquet should be used on the upper thigh.

Incision. A longitudinal incision is made over the front of the tibia (see p. 39). Two-thirds of the incision is above the level of the fracture and one-third below.

Procedure. The tibial cortex is exposed by incising the periosteum and carefully reflecting it with an elevator. The bone is then marked off 10 centimetres above the fracture and 5 centimetres below it. The width of the bone graft must be less than the whole width of the subcutaneous surface of the tibia, to preserve the strength of the anterior and posterior borders. The graft is outlined on the bone, tapering slightly from above downwards (Fig. 111). The taper ensures that the width of the saw cuts is taken up as the graft is moved downwards, promoting a tight fit of the graft in its bed.

A mechanical (oscillating) saw is used to cut out the graft. The saw-blade is angled appropriately in order to undercut the graft (Fig. 112). This ensures that the graft will not sink into the

medullary cavity when it is screwed into place. It also prevents harmful encroachment upon the anterior and posterior borders of the tibia, which must be preserved to avoid undue weakening of the bone (see Fig. 113).

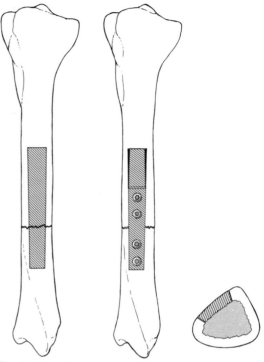

FIGS 111–113. Sliding bone graft. Figure 111—Outline shows slightly tapered graft, two-thirds above the fracture and one-third below the fracture. Figure 112—Upper part of graft slid down and secured in position across the fracture. Figure 113—The graft shown in cross section.

When the two-thirds portion of the graft above the fracture has been cut out it is lifted free, with any attached medullary bone carefully kept intact. The one-third portion below the fracture is similarly freed, and the main portion is slid into position to bridge the fracture. Two drill holes are made through the graft above the fracture and two below the fracture, and the appropriate screws are driven home (Fig. 112). The smaller fragment of freed bone is placed in the remaining defect above the main graft. If, because of its smaller width, it tends to drop into the medullary cavity it may be reversed so that the wider end is a snug fit, and driven upwards so that the narrower end is supported by the slope of the transverse cut at the proximal end.

Closure. The periosteum is closed separately, and the skin is repaired in the routine manner.

POST-OPERATIVE MANAGEMENT

A full length plaster is applied. The grafted bone has no great mechanical strength and it must be fully protected from weight-bearing until union is sound.

CIRCUMFERENTIAL CANCELLOUS SLIVER GRAFTING FOR UNUNITED FRACTURE

This technique for the treatment of ununited fractures of the major bones was popularised by Phemister (1947), but similar methods had been used earlier. The essential principle is that multiple thin slivers of cancellous bone are laid about the fracture round a great part of its circumference, beneath the periosteum (Fig. 114). The fracture itself is not disturbed. Fixation may be provided externally by a plaster splint, but many surgeons now combine cancellous sliver grafting with internal fixation by an intramedullary nail when the site of fracture is suitable for this.

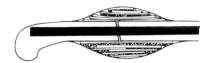

FIG. 114. Circumferential sliver grafts with reinforcement by intramedullary nail.

TECHNIQUE

Exposure. The comments made in the section on cortical bone grafting (p. 78) apply here also. In contrast to cortical bone grafting, in which the graft is applied only to one aspect of the bone, the aim in cancellous sliver grafting is to lay the grafts round as much of the circumference of the bone as can conveniently be reached from one incision. Occasionally it is in order to make two incisions to allow grafting of a greater surface area.

Preparation of the recipient bone. If internal fixation by intramedullary nailing is to be used this should be done before the bone grafts are applied.

The technique of medullary nailing is described on page 84.

When the fracture site has been exposed together with a short length of each fragment adjacent to the fracture, soft tissues and as much of the periosteum as can be identified are stripped peripherally round the area of the fracture by a combination of sharp dissection and separation with an elevator. The surface of the bone thus exposed is rawed by light cuts with a chisel to promote increased vascularity.

Obtaining the bone grafts. The method of cutting cancellous sliver grafts from the ilium was described on page 75. A plentiful supply of slivers should be obtained, each 2 or 3 centimetres long.

Applying the grafts. The grafts are laid snugly about the fracture, each sliver lying longitudinally and in close contact with the bone. Where the bone is well covered by muscle further slivers may be laid to form a second and a third layer, but where the bone is subcutaneous the grafts should be applied sparingly to avoid too much disturbance of the normal contour. A considerable quantity of slivers is required, so that at the conclusion of the operation they form a collar of spongy bone round a good part of the circumference. The grafts are held in place by suture of the overlying periosteum and muscles.

Closure. If a large quantity of bone slivers has been inserted there may be some difficulty in closing the skin edges. It is wrong to attempt to close them under tension. It is better to relieve the tension by chiselling away exuberant callus from the recipient bone, or when practicable by excision of redundant or expendable soft tissue.

POST-OPERATIVE MANAGEMENT

A firm crepe bandage is applied over gauze dressings. In most cases the limb is protected by a full-length plaster splint, which is changed at two weeks to allow removal of the sutures. The plaster is retained until the fracture is united. When rigid fixation by an intramedullary nail has been secured, external support is unnecessary and the plaster may be omitted.

CANCELLOUS CHIP GRAFTING OF BONE CAVITY

Cancellous bone chips or slivers may be used to obliterate a cavity created by excision of a bone cyst or other benign local destructive lesion. Chip grafting may also be used for filling defects consequent upon osteomyelitis, but modifications of the technique may be required in order to secure viable skin cover (see p. 107).

TECHNIQUE

Exposure. As in cortical grafting, it is better to expose the affected bone through a muscle plane rather than through a subcutaneous approach.

Preparation of cavity. When the area of bone containing the cavity has been displayed a wide opening is made into the cavity by removing part of the overlying cortex. The window so created should be large enough to enable the whole interior of the cavity to be brought into view. The contents of the cavity will vary according to the nature of the condition. If solid, the contents are removed piecemeal; if liquid, they are evacuated by suction. Next the interior wall or lining of the cavity is curetted very thoroughly either with a simple curette or by chisels and gouges; occasionally a rotary rasp in a power-driven chuck may be preferred. The scrapings are thoroughly washed out by saline irrigation and suction. Specimens from the interior of the cavity and from the lining wall are sent for histological examination.

Insertion of grafts. Bone chips or slivers obtained from the ilium in the manner described on page 75 are placed in the cavity and packed together firmly but not too tightly. If the supply of chips is exhausted before the cavity is completely obliterated it may sometimes be possible to raise a flap of muscle adjacent to the cavity and to suture it within the mouth of the cavity to obliterate the remaining dead space.

Closure. In closure of the wound it is important whenever possible to cover the opening in the bone with a good layer of muscle. The skin is then closed, preferably without drainage.

POST-OPERATIVE MANAGEMENT

If the defect in the bone is small and does not significantly impair its strength soft dressings only are required. If the defect is judged to be a cause of serious weakness of the bone, with risk of pathological fracture, the limb is best protected in a full-length plaster splint for two or three months until the bone has consolidated.

CANCELLOUS CHIP GRAFTING FOR DEFECT RESULTING FROM OSTEOMYELITIS

In chronic osteomyelitis it is often necessary to excavate the diseased bone in order to eradicate the infection (see p. 105). This may leave a large cavity and the bone is correspondingly weakened, with risk of pathological fracture. Filling such a cavity with bone chips is attended by the hazard of recurrent infection. In order to reduce the risk to the minimum it is therefore important that bone-grafting be delayed until sound healing has been secured by a first-stage operation that entails the removal of all diseased bone and the elimination of dead space either by filling the defect with a flap of muscle or by applying split-skin grafts directly to the wall of the cavity, as described on page 106.

FIXATION OF BONE FRAGMENTS BY PLATING

Plating is used mainly for fresh fractures or after osteotomy. A plate fixed with screws may be regarded as a rigid but temporary bone suture. No plate can be relied upon to hold bones together or to hold a prosthesis to a bone indefinitely. Indeed, in general it may be said that a plate will hold only for two or three months. After that, if natural healing of the bone has not occurred, there is an increasing risk as time goes on of fracture of the plate, or of loosening or shearing of the screws.

Many types of plate have been devised: all are the same in principle except for compression plates, which will be described below. Basically, a plate is simply a strip of metal with a series of holes for fixation screws. The many different shapes, contours and thicknesses that are available do not constitute significant differences of one plate from another. The main essential is to select a plate that is strong enough and of appropriate size for the particular purpose for which it is to be used. It goes without saying that the plate must be of inert material, which for practical purposes means that it must be made from special stainless steel, from cobalt-chromium alloy or from titanium. At some centres non-metallic plates, made from carbon fibre and acrylic, are being used on the ground that, being semi-elastic rather than rigid, they may permit the formation of more abundant callus. The use of such plates must, however, be regarded as experimental at present (Tayton *et al.* 1982). For fixing bone fragments a plate with less than four screw holes is hardly ever of use; nor is it necessary except in rare instances to use a plate with more than six screws.

TECHNIQUE

Whenever the site of operation allows, the use of a tourniquet is recommended.

Exposure. The remarks made on exposure in relation to cortical bone grafting (p. 79) apply also to plating of long bones. As a general rule a plate should not be applied to a subcutaneous surface of the bone but should be buried under muscle. For instance, in the tibia it is preferable whenever possible to apply the plate to the submuscular lateral surface or to the posterior surface rather than to the subcutaneous medial surface.

Preparation of recipient bone. The periosteum is incised and stripped to each side over a length a little greater than that of the proposed plate: excessive stripping of the bone is to be avoided lest the blood supply be prejudiced. Anatomical reduction of the fragments is achieved under direct vision, and if necessary the fragments are

held in position by bone-holding forceps or by a bone clamp. Special care is needed to ensure that the rotational position of the fragments is correct: this can usually be determined from the matching denticulations of the fracture surfaces. Usually the plate is applied direct to the cortex, which in a fresh fracture does not require further preparation.

Application and fixation of plate. When all is ready the plate is applied in position and held tightly to the bone by a suitable clamp or forceps. A final check is then made to ensure that the bone fragments are correctly lined up and that the plate is in the same longitudinal axis.

Screw holes equal in diameter to the core diameter of the screws to be used are then drilled; usually they should penetrate both cortices of the bone. If plain rather than self-tapping screws are to be used it is next necessary to tap the holes to cut the appropriate threads. The length of screw required is determined for each hole by a depth gauge (Fig. 67). Each screw is introduced on a self-holding screwdriver, which is changed for a normal screwdriver when about half the screw is engaged. The force used in the final tightening of the screws must be judged carefully according to the strength of the recipient bone: it is important not to apply so much torque that the threads in the bone are stripped.

Upon completion of the plating procedure, the muscle layer is sutured back into position over the plate and the wound is closed, usually without drainage.

Compression plating. The principle of compression plating is that during application of the plate the bone fragments are forced together strongly so that even the smallest gap between the fragments is eliminated. The method was first advocated by Danis of Belgium in 1949. It did not gain favour at the time, but in its revised form as advocated by the Swiss school and by others it has attracted wide acceptance, and several distinct methods of achieving compression have been devised.

Briefly, the mode of application of one such plate is as follows. First the plate is screwed firmly to one of the bone fragments—this may be either the proximal or the distal fragment according to convenience. A screw-operated tensioning device is then screwed to the other fragment and the two fragments are drawn up tightly together by turning the tensioning screw. While compression is thus maintained screws are driven home through the remaining holes of the plate. The tensioning device is then removed. In the remaining stages the technique of compression plating is the same as for the application of a simple plate.

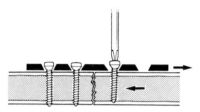

FIG. 115. Principle of the slotted-hole compression plate. Because of the shape of the holes and of the screw heads, tightening the screw (inserted at the end of the slot) forces the bone fragments together (arrows).

A rather simpler device for achieving compression is now more often used. The plate is pierced with slots rather than round holes. It is screwed to one fragment in the ordinary way, but in securing the other fragment the surgeon introduces the screws at the very edge of each slot, at the end away from the fracture. Then, by virtue of the shape of the slots and of the screw heads, tightening the first screw forces it, and with it the bone, against the opposing fragment (Fig. 115).

POST-OPERATIVE MANAGEMENT

A plate applied to only one aspect of a bone can seldom give enough rigidity to resist strong angulatory forces. Some plates are worse in this respect than others, but in many cases it is wise to give additional protection in the form of a plaster-of-Paris case. If very rigid fixation has been gained, however, the use of additional external support may be omitted.

Comment

Plates are easy to apply and have an important place in the treatment of fractures, as also in the fixation of bone fragments after osteotomy. In most cases union occurs readily. Occasionally, however, union is slow and a small gap persists between the fragments. Indeed, the plate may sometimes seem to hold the fragments apart, with consequent delay in union, or even non-union. It was because of this disadvantage of plain plates that compression plates were devised. Even with compression plates, however, the problem has not been solved completely: failure of union still occurs from time to time. Further long-term studies will be required before firm conclusions can be drawn on the relative merits of simple plating and compression plating, as also on the merits, if any, of using semi-flexible non-metallic plates.

(For notes on use of A.O. dynamic compression plates, see page 70.)

INTRAMEDULLARY NAILING

Intramedullary nailing, properly performed, is the most rigid form of internal fixation of bone (Laurence *et al.* 1969). The method was made popular for the treatment of fresh fractures—especially those of the femoral shaft—by Kuntscher during the Second World War (Böhler 1948). The principle was, however, well known long before that time: similar methods had been used by Lambotte (1913) of Antwerp and by Hey Groves (1918) of Bristol during the First World War. These pioneers were handicapped by lack of a suitable inert metal, and it was the development of special stainless steels that made nailing more practicable.

Intramedullary nailing is now used not only for the treatment of fresh fractures of long bones but also for delayed union and non-union. It is also used for congenital pseudarthrosis of the tibia in early childhood, and for providing fixation after osteotomy for correction of deformity or after excision of diseased segments of bone (for instance a bone cyst or giant-cell tumour). In these latter cases nailing is usually combined with bone grafting.

INTRAMEDULLARY NAILING FOR FRESH FRACTURES

Intramedullary nailing is appropriate for the fixation of certain fractures of any of the major long bones. It is used particularly for the femur, the tibia and the humerus. The technique is applicable also to fractures of the forearm bones, though it is not used extensively for fractures of the radius because this bone does not offer a convenient site for entrance of the nail.

In general, the fractures that are most suitable for fixation by an intramedullary nail are those of the middle two-thirds of the shaft. Fractures near the ends of the long bones are not always suitable for nailing because the short fragment may not give sufficient grip to the nail. Additional fixation may, however, be provided by one or two cross screws transfixing the bone and the nail (locking nail). Increasing use is being made of this modification, especially in nailing of the femur and of the tibia.

As to the pattern of fracture, the most suitable for nailing is a transverse fracture or a short oblique fracture. Some degree of comminution is acceptable, but a grossly comminuted fracture may be unsuitable for intramedullary nailing.

Fractures of the long spiral type are often unsuitable for nailing, but sometimes a combination of circumferential wiring and intramedullary nailing may be appropriate.

If intramedullary nailing is to give its full advantage it is important that a nail of adequate thickness be used. A thick nail in a properly reamed medullary canal affords complete rigidity against angulatory movement and also prevents rotation. A thick nail is particularly advantageous in the femur and tibia because it allows full weight bearing without external protection and without fear of bending or breaking of the nail. In adults an appropriate thickness for a femoral nail is 15 or 16 millimetres and for a tibial nail 13 or 14 millimetres.

If it is possible to secure full reduction of the fracture by manipulation, with or without traction, nailing can be performed without exposure of the fracture itself by driving the nail over a guide wire from the end of the bone. On the other hand, if adequate reduction cannot be achieved by closed methods it becomes necessary to expose the fracture and to reduce the fragments to the anatomical position under direct vision. Two basic techniques of nailing are therefore to be described: 1) closed nailing; and 2) open nailing.

Closed Nailing

TECHNIQUE

Position of patient. For nailing of the femur the patient should be in the lateral position; of the tibia, supine with the knee flexed; of the humerus, in the lateral position; of the ulna, supine with the forearm across the chest; for the radius, as for ulna. A tourniquet may be used for nailing of the tibia and of the forearm bones, but it is hardly practicable to use a tourniquet for nailing of the femoral shaft or of the humerus.

Reduction. The first essential is to obtain full reduction of any displacement that may be present. In a transverse or short oblique fracture this may be possible by manipulation alone, but in many fractures a combination of manipulation and mechanical traction is required. Some means must therefore be improvised for applying and maintaining traction. This will usually entail the use of a Steinmann pin or Kirschner wire to transfix the distal segment and thus to provide a grip for the traction cord. The progress of reduction should be checked by the image intensifier or by radiographic films. If there is failure to secure adequate reduction closed nailing must be abandoned in favour of the open method (p. 89).

Sites of insertion of nail. The recommended sites for insertion of a nail in the major long bones are as follows: humerus, lower end (olecranon fossa);

ulna, upper end; radius, lower end (dorsum); femur, upper end; tibia, upper end.

Insertion of guide wire. When adequate reduction has been achieved the next step is to pass a suitable guide wire from the proposed point of entry of the nail through the full length of the medullary canal. Only a short incision is required over the point of entry. The soft tissues are retracted to expose the end of the bone. The cortex is broached at the point of entry, usually with an awl or narrow gouge. It is well to pass a rigid instrument such as a screwdriver or a Steinmann pin on a suitable chuck part way down the medullary canal before the flexible guide wire is introduced: this sets the guide wire on the right course.

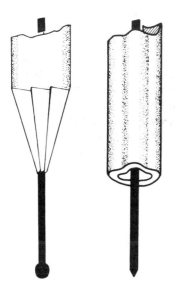

FIGS 116–117. An olive-tipped guide wire is used to guide the reamers (Fig. 116), so that in the event of a reamer's breaking the broken fragment may be retrieved. In contrast, a plain guide wire is used for guiding the nail (Fig. 117), so that there is no obstruction to removal of the wire when the nail has been driven home.

The first guide wire, designed to centre the reamer in the medullary canal, should be of the olive-tipped type—that is, with a small knob at the tip, the purpose of which is to retrieve the head of

the mechanical reamer should it break off during the reaming process (Fig. 116). Without this bulbous tip the broken reamer head would be lost in the medullary canal and its retrieval would present great difficulty. The guide wire should pass easily down the medullary canal by hand pressure and a twisting movement imparted through the hand chuck. By pre-measurement of the total length of the guide wire and measurement of the amount still protruding, the length within the bone is repeatedly ascertained. The aim should be to pass the wire almost to the extremity of the medullary canal. The position of the wire is checked by the image intensifier or by radiographic films.

Reaming of medullary canal. Flexible reamers of graded sizes are laid out ready for use in order of increasing diameter. A check should be made to ensure that reamers are not unduly worn and perhaps therefore less than the marked diameter. Reaming should be begun with a small reamer— one that is judged to be sufficiently narrow to cut its way easily down the canal. Only moderate pressure should be applied upon the rotating reamer: it is best to allow the reamer to cut its way slowly. Attempts to hurry matters may lead to jamming of the reamer or splitting of the bone. The reamer should penetrate to the full length of the guide wire, but care should be taken not to drive it too far and to damage the adjacent joint.

When the first reamer has done its work it is withdrawn without stopping the motor: it is easier to withdraw the machine while it is revolving. The reaming process is repeated with successively larger reamers until the canal has been enlarged to the desired size. It is usually wise to avoid further enlargement of the canal when a particular reamer has had to work very hard to cut its way through. As a rule this size should be accepted as the optimal size for the nail.

Selection of nail. The thickness of the nail should usually be equal to the diameter of the final reamer. As already noted, a nail of 15 or 16 millimetres diameter is often appropriate for the femur, and one of 13 or 14 millimetres is often correct for the tibia. For the humerus a nail 10 millimetres in diameter is usually adequate, and for the forearm bones, 6 or 7 millimetres may be suitable. The size chosen must, however, depend upon the build of each individual patient.

The correct length of the nail should be determined from the length of the guide wire that is within the bone. As a double check it is a good plan to measure also the limb segment externally—that is, the length from the point of entry of the nail to the opposite end of the bone. As a general rule the nail selected should be long enough to occupy almost the entire length of the bone. Usually it should penetrate to within a few millimetres of the adjacent articular surface, though of course it is important to avoid over-penetration so that the joint is entered.

The general rule about length may have to be varied in the case of the femur. It has to be remembered that the femoral shaft is bowed for-

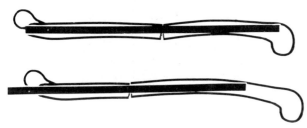

FIGS 118–119. In femoral nailing, a nail that follows the natural curve of the bone should normally be used. The insertion of a straight nail into the curved shaft of the femur may present difficulties. If the fracture is near the middle of the shaft, slight angulation at the fracture may allow a full-length nail to be accommodated (Fig. 118). But if the distal curved fragment is long, a full-length nail often cannot be accommodated and it may become jammed (Fig. 119) or penetrate the anterior cortex. A three-quarters length nail should therefore be used. In all femoral nailing a curved nail is to be preferred to a straight nail.

wards, and in using the standard Kuntscher type nail the surgeon is driving a straight nail, with hardly any flexibility in the larger sizes, into a curved track. (A curved nail is clearly to be preferred for the femur: such nails are available, but they are not always included in the standard equipment at every hospital.) If the fragments are about equal in length the curve in either fragment is not sufficient to obstruct a straight nail (Fig. 118), but if one fragment is long, and the bone hard, the nail may easily become impacted if

an attempt is made to drive it the full distance (Fig. 119). It is therefore suggested that if a straight nail is to be used for a femoral shaft fracture above the mid-point of the femur the nail should be so chosen that it penetrates only about two-thirds or three-quarters of the length of the medullary canal: in other words, an attempt should not be made to penetrate the whole length of the long, curved lower fragment.

The length of the nail should always be so calculated that, when it has penetrated to the required level, the base of the nail should be flush with the surface bone at the point of entry, or a few millimetres deep to it (Fig. 120). It is a mistake to leave the nail protruding from the recipient bone (Fig. 121).

Driving the nail. Before the nail is driven in it is essential that the initial olive-tipped guide wire be removed. This is important because otherwise the bulbous tip of the wire would prevent its being withdrawn after the nail has been driven over it (Fig. 117). In some cases the guide wire may be dispensed with at this stage, but usually it is wise to have the wire in position to guide the nail, and therefore the olive-tipped wire should be replaced by a plain wire. When this has been done the nail is passed over it so that its point enters the reamed channel.

At this stage it is important to orientate the nail so that the extraction slot will come to lie in an accessible position—a great convenience if removal of the nail should ever be required. The nail is now driven on into the canal with moderately heavy blows from a split hammer sliding over the guide wire. The nail should be felt to drive on with each blow: if obvious resistance is felt something may be wrong. To check that all is well repeated views of the progress of the nail should be taken with the image intensifier. In this way any impending misdirection of the nail can be forestalled.

During the driving of the nail counter-pressure should be applied at the distal extremity of the limb. This helps to prevent distraction of the fragments at the fracture site, a possibility that always exists in closed nailing. Again, repeated observations with the image intensifier will show if distraction is occurring and will allow preventive measures to be taken. Distraction can usually be prevented by adequate counter-thrust upon the distal end of the limb, but if serious distraction occurs in spite of this it may be necessary to expose the fracture and to prevent the fragments from being distracted by gripping them with a suitable bone clamp, or even by temporarily screwing on a plate.

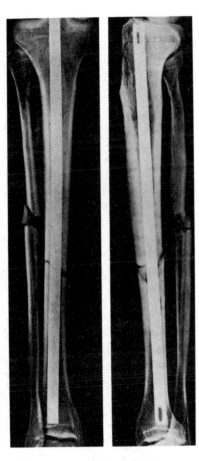

FIG. 120. Radiograph showing an intramedullary nail of adequate thickness and correct length, used for fixation of a tibial fracture.

If all goes well, the nail is driven on until only about 2 centimetres remain outside the bone. At this stage it is important to observe the position of the distal end of the nail with the image intensi-

fier. Repeated observations in this way allow the nail to be driven close up to the adjacent joint but not to penetrate the subchondral bone. If the length of the nail has been calculated correctly, when it has been hammered in to this optimal position the head of the nail should just have disappeared within the bone at the point of entry.

The use of cross screws. If fixation is not already rigid (as for instance if one of the fragments is short) it is well to use a nail with perforations

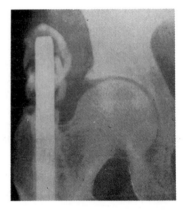

FIG. 121. Too much of this nail was left protruding above the greater trochanter. A painful bursa developed.

designed to take one or two cross screws (locking screws) close to the end of the nail. The cross screws are to be so placed that they transfix both cortices of the bone as well as the plate. The cross screws may be located freehand, or a special radiographic locating device may be used.

Closure. If a tourniquet has been used it should be removed before closure is begun. The wound is closed with interrupted sutures, without drainage.

POST-OPERATIVE MANAGEMENT

If good fixation has been obtained with a stout nail gripping an adequate length of each main fragment, soft dressings only are required and external support from plaster-of-Paris may be avoided. The patient is allowed to lie free in bed, and early movements of all the limb joints are encouraged. In the case of nailing of the femur or tibia, weight bearing may be permitted as soon as the soft tissues have healed. If the fracture is a long spiral one, however, only partial weight bearing should be permitted until about six to eight weeks after operation; otherwise slight telescoping upon the nail is liable to occur.

Comment

Closed nailing is often difficult because of the need to obtain adequate reduction and to maintain it while the nail is introduced. It should not be attempted unless proper equipment is available, and in particular graded flexible reamers operated by a slow-speed motor.

Other important rules are to check the position of the guide wire radiographically before reaming is begun; to ream slowly without attempting to hurry the reamer on by too much force; to use serial reamers with not more than 1 millimetre increase in diameter between successive reamers; to ream down to the full length of the medullary canal; to be careful to select a nail of the correct thickness and length; to remove the olive-tipped guide wire and replace it by a plain one before the nail is driven in; and to check carefully the progress of the nail by repeated viewing with the image intensifier.

It has happened occasionally that a nail has become impacted and jammed, so that it resists both driving on and removal—a serious dilemma. This happens most often in the case of the femur, where impaction may occur despite the surgeon's ensuring that the nail corresponds in thickness to the diameter of the reamed channel. The usual reason for such impaction is that the surgeon is attempting to drive a straight nail into a curved femoral canal. Clearly, for the femur it is desirable that a nail that is curved to match the natural curve of the femur should be used. If this is not available the precautions that have already been mentioned (Figs 118–119) should be strictly observed.

OPEN NAILING

The general principles of open intramedullary nailing are the same as those for closed nailing, but certain modifications may be introduced by virtue of the fact that the fracture surfaces are exposed to direct vision.

TECHNIQUE

Position of patient. The positioning of the patient is the same as for closed nailing.

Exposure of fracture site. The fracture site is exposed through the most convenient approach consistent with satisfactory placing of the scar from the point of view of function. In general, the best approaches for mid-shaft fractures are as follows: femur, postero-lateral approach; tibia, antero-lateral approach; humerus, posterior approach; ulna, direct approach; radius, anterior approach (see Chapter 1).

To expose the fracture it is best first to expose normal bone on each side and then to work centrally towards the fracture site. In this way the risk of damaging some important structure, misplaced by distortion of the normal anatomy, is reduced to a minimum.

When the fracture site has been fully displayed the bone ends are cleared of fibrin and blood clot so that the surfaces may be fitted together accurately. If the fracture is a long oblique or spiral one longitudinal traction may be required to aid reduction. When perfect reduction has been secured appropriate means are found to hold the fragments firmly in the reduced position. According to circumstances a bone-holding forceps, a bone clamp (Charnley type) or a Lowman's clamp may be found the most appropriate.

Reaming of medullary canal. As a general rule reaming of the medullary canal follows the principles laid down in the previous section: that is, a suitable entry hole is first made and through this an olive-tipped guide wire is directed down the medullary canal to its far extremity. Over this guide wire sucessive reamers, each 1 millimetre greater in diameter than its predecessor, are driven in with the slowly revolving motor until a channel of the required size has been made.

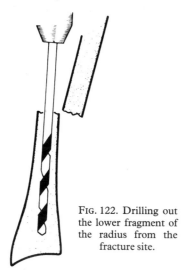

FIG. 122. Drilling out the lower fragment of the radius from the fracture site.

Retrograde reaming. With the fracture site exposed at operation, however, there is an alternative method of reaming: each fragment may be

instruments. This alternative technique is not applicable to every bone: indeed its only major application is to the shaft of the femur. Here this so-called retrograde method of reaming presents certain advantages. Thus if a guide wire or long drill is driven up the proximal fragment of the femur from the fracture site it can be made to find its own way through the greater trochanter, and in consequence a formal exposure of that area is avoided; all that is necessary is to make a stab incision over the point of the emerging guide wire or drill. This saves time and it ensures that the opening in the greater trochanter is made at the correct point. Likewise reaming of the distal fragment of the femur may be easier if the reamers can be introduced at the site of fracture.

Reaming from the fracture site is not readily applicable to the tibia because a guide wire and reamer driven proximally from the fracture site are unlikely to emerge at the correct point of entry for the nail at the front of the intercondylar ridge of the tibia. Retrograde reaming of the humerus is hardly practicable because the point of entry of

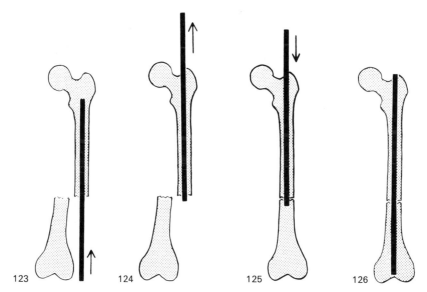

FIGS 123–126. Retrograde nailing of femur. Figure 123—Nail inserted in proximal fragment at fracture site. Figure 124—Nail driven out through greater trochanter to allow fragments to be brought into apposition. Figure 125—Fragments apposed: nail engaged in distal fragment. Figure 126—Nail driven down into distal fragment.

reamed separately, the guide wire and reamers being introduced through the fracture surfaces, which are suitably displaced to allow entry of the

the nail in the olecranon fossa is critical, and a guide wire or drill entered at the site of fracture and driven distally is unlikely to emerge at the correct point. In the radius and in the ulna retrograde reaming sometimes offers advantages. In those bones reaming with a long rigid drill fitted to a hand brace is often easier than reaming with flexible reamers over a guide wire (Fig. 122).

Selection and driving of nail. A nail of the correct thickness and length is chosen according to the criteria laid down in the previous section (p. 86). There are two methods of driving the nail: 1) the direct method; and 2) the retrograde method (Figs 123–126). In most cases the direct method is to be preferred, but in the case of fractures of the shaft of the femur retrograde nailing may give advantages.

Direct nailing. In direct nailing the nail is introduced at the site of election as outlined in the previous section. First, as in closed nailing, a plain guide wire is substituted for the olive-tipped guide wire before the nail is introduced. At the same time the surgeon must check by direct inspection of the fracture that full anatomical reduction has been maintained. The fragments must be held rigidly together with a suitable bone-holding forceps or clamp while the nail is driven in. A check must also be made that there is no rotational deformity. Ideally this is assured by fitting the fracture surfaces together so accurately that the ridges and depressions on each fragment interdigitate with each other. If in a transverse fracture there is any doubt about the correct position as regards rotation reliance must be placed on clinical inspection of the limb as a whole.

With the fracture surfaces thus held rigidly together the nail is driven in as described in the previous section. As it passes the fracture site it is important to check that the fragments are not driven apart. To help to prevent distraction, counter-thrust should be applied to the distal part of the limb. As the tip of the nail nears the far extremity of the bone repeated check views are taken with the image intensifier to ensure that the nail is driven on exactly to the optimal depth.

Retrograde nailing. Retrograde insertion of the nail is applicable mainly to fractures of the shaft of the femur; occasionally to fractures of the ulna.

The nail is entered at the site of fracture and is first driven proximally along the prepared track in the proximal fragment (Fig. 123) until it emerges from the proximal end of the bone. It is brought out sufficiently to allow the fracture surfaces to be engaged in accurate apposition (Figs 124–125), and is then driven down into the distal fragment (Fig. 126). As in direct nailing, the position of the nail should be checked repeatedly with the image intensifier, especially as it nears full penetration.

Closure. The wounds are closed in layers, usually without drainage.

POST-OPERATIVE MANAGEMENT

This is the same as for closed nailing (p. 88).

Comment

Open nailing is required more frequently than closed nailing because it is often impossible to gain adequate reduction by closed methods. It is a less satisfying procedure than closed nailing because it converts a closed fracture into an open one, with consequent risk of infection, slight though this should be if proper precautions are observed. Gentle handling of the tissues is of prime importance, and it should be a rule that the fingers should never be inserted into the wound except after a sterile over-glove has been freshly applied.

Other important requirements are to excise badly bruised and devitalised tissue and to prevent haematoma formation by ensuring full haemostasis and by obliteration of all potential dead space. The hazards mentioned in the preceding section on closed nailing (p. 89) should also be noted in connection with open nailing.

LOCKING NAILS

Surgeons have for a long time been accustomed to using cross screws to anchor a nail either at the proximal or at the distal end, passing the screw through the extraction slot or drilling the nail across at the appropriate point. The principle of cross screwing has also long been an essential feature of the Huckstep nail (p. 335). In recent years the principle has been adopted more widely by manufacturers for nails of traditional pattern, one or two transverse holes being provided at each end of the nail. A nail so drilled has become known by the term "locking" or "interlocking" nail. The main purpose of cross screws is to prevent rotation of the nail in the bone. They also enhance the grip of the nail, especially in a rather short fragment.

LOCATING DISTAL HOLES IN INTRAMEDULLARY NAILS

This often poses a difficult problem. It is easiest with the Huckstep nail, for which a rigid jig may be fixed to the nail. To ensure accurate alignment the jig is first assembled to the nail by finger tightening. Drills are passed through the distal holes in the jig to ensure easy alignment, and then the jig is tightened with the spanner supplied.

With other types of locking nails, inserted closed, more difficulty is encountered. The proximal ends of the nails are not rigid enough to allow a fixed jig system to locate the screw holes accurately at the distal end of the nail. Radiological assistance may thus be needed, and devices for definitive location of the holes radiologically are now available. Even then, accurate location may not be easy because great care must be taken to avoid excessive radiation. If necessary the distal incision should be extended. A larger hole can then be drilled in the lateral cortex of the bone so that the hole in the nail can be seen. Once the first hole has been located the appropriate guide can be used to find the second hole at the distal end. If undue enlargement of the bone cortex has been necessary, better fixation may be achieved by the use of a washer to support the head of the screw.

INTRAMEDULLARY NAILING FOR UNUNITED FRACTURES

Intramedullary nailing is very valuable in the treatment of non-union of a long bone fracture. It is usually combined with cancellous sliver grafting (Phemister 1947), but probably in a high proportion of cases nailing alone is sufficient to promote union, as reported by Christensen (1973).

TECHNIQUE

The technique of nailing does not differ in any significant respect from that of nailing for a fresh fracture. If the fragments are in satisfactory position and alignment it may be unnecessary to disturb the site of fracture. Often, however, there is dense sclerosis of the fracture ends with total obliteration of the medullary canal over a short distance on each side of the fracture. This may prevent the passage of a guide wire. Even so it may not be necessary to take the fracture apart, for it may be possible to restore the medullary canal by the use of a long drill introduced at the proposed point of insertion of the nail. If the fracture is not accessible to direct drilling, however, it may occa-

sionally be necessary to clear and separate the fracture ends and to restore continuity of the medullary canal by drilling from the fracture surfaces.

When a suitable medullary canal has been restored in the region of the fracture the fragments are reduced accurately and held in position by a bone-holding forceps or a suitable clamp, and the full length of the medullary canal is then reamed out to size over an olive-tipped guide wire. Nailing is then completed in the manner described for nailing of a fresh fracture.

In most cases the surgeon will elect to combine medullary nailing with cancellous sliver grafting by the Phemister technique. This was described on page 81. In cases of non-union with longstanding infection there is also sometimes a place for excision of diseased bone and its replacement—either at the same operation or later—by a block of cancellous bone from the iliac crest, as described by Nicoll (1956): an intramedullary nail is then driven in, to traverse the graft as well as the recipient bone fragments (Figs 127 and 128).

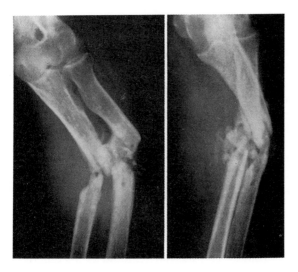

FIG. 127. Non-union with long-standing infection of the forearm bones after unsuccessful plating of the open fractures.

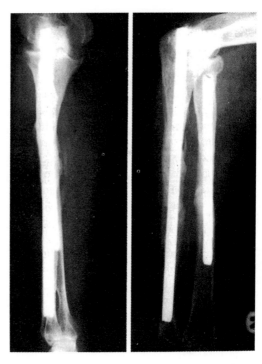

FIG. 128. Early union after excision of infected bone, cancellous block grafting of the defects and fixation by intramedullary nails.

POST-OPERATIVE MANAGEMENT

As with nailing of a fresh fracture, the aim should be to avoid external splintage in a plaster-of-Paris case. As a general rule, splintage should be unnecessary if a sufficiently stout nail has been inserted and if the bone fragments are each long enough to afford a satisfactory grip for the nail. If for some reason fixation is not sufficiently rigid, then external support from a plaster splint will be required.

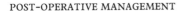

APPLICATION OF EXTERNAL FIXATOR

External fixation allows stabilisation of a fracture without operation at the fracture site. It is preferred to internal fixation when the fracture is compound, with soft-tissue damage. External fixation may also allow active use of the fractured limb at an early stage.

Choice of fixator. Although in the past two-bar (bilateral) fixators joined to pins that transfix the bone fragments through and through have been widely used, they are no longer generally recommended because they almost inevitably transfix and anchor muscles and thus interfere with function. In most instances, therefore, a single-bar (unilateral) fixator should be used (Fig. 129).

Many types of fixator are now available, from the original improvised device in which transfixion pins were simply anchored to side bars with acrylic cement, to modern sophisticated apparatus that tends to be versatile but often unduly complex. Three types will be described here, as examples.

GENERAL PRINCIPLES OF APPLICATION

Site of application. The fixator should be so sited that the pins or screws are clear of all muscles. In the tibia the subcutaneous (antero-medial) surface is the obvious site. In the femur the postero-lateral aspect is appropriate, the pins being inserted between the extensor and the flexor muscles—that is, between the vastus lateralis in front and the biceps femoris behind (Fig. 39). In the humerus the lateral aspect, between the flexor and the extensor muscles, should be chosen.

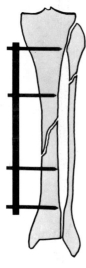

FIG. 129. Diagram showing the principle of external fixation. Threaded pins grip each fragment rigidly and are anchored by clamps to the external bar.

Incisions. Incisions about 2 centimetres long should be used in preference to stab incisions. A pin may not be well centred in a stab incision and pressure necrosis, with risk of infection, may occur. In the case of the femur there is much to be said for using a longer incision in order to lift the vastus lateralis from the lateral intermuscular septum and thus to ensure that the pins do not traverse the muscle.

Insertion of pins and application of fixator bar. It is important that before the fixator is applied the bone fragments be secured in good alignment. Since external fixation is mostly applied in cases of open fracture it is often possible to align the fragments under direct vision, and ideally they should be held temporarily by a suitable clamp—for instance the Charnley bone clamp—while the fixator is applied.

The aim should be to insert the two central pins quite close to the fracture—but in healthy bone—and the peripheral pins at a suitable distance away—say 5 to 8 centimetres depending upon the length of bone that is available. The pins must be inserted through previously made drill holes: the correct size of drill is 4.5 millimetres if the usual 5 millimetre Schanz pin is to be used.

One of the two central pins should be inserted first. Through the skin incision the bone is located by a drill sleeve or cannula with trocar. When this has been well positioned the trocar is removed and both cortices of the bone are penetrated by the drill, inserted through the sleeve. The drill and the sleeve having been removed, the fixator pin, the leading end of which should be threaded, is inserted on a hand chuck. The pin must just penetrate the far cortex of the bone but should not protrude more than a few millimetres.

With the first pin in position the fixator bar is applied in the appropriate position and loosely clamped to the pin. The bar, or clamps placed upon it, may thus be used to guide the insertion of subsequent pins, which are similarly inserted into prepared drill holes. Four pins are usually adequate for the tibia or humerus, but six may sometimes be preferred for the femur.

Finally, after a further check that the bone fragments are correctly aligned, the bar is clamped or cemented rigidly to all the pins, just clear of the skin surface.

Closure. The incisions are sutured snugly about the pins, with care to ensure that there is no pressure of the pin against the skin edge at any point.

Care of skin. While the fixator and screws are in place, care must be taken to ensure that the skin is not under tension where it is adjacent to the screws. Any crusts at the screw entry sites must be cleaned away daily with a swab dipped in a suitable antiseptic such as mercurochrome.

THE ORTHOFIX FIXATOR

The Orthofix device (Fig. 130) is applied to one side of the bone. The screws inserted into the bone are conical. The screws for cancellous bone have a coarse thread and require a 3.2 millimetre drill for the preparatory hole. The cortical screws require a 4.5 millimetre drill.

The central bar or shaft of the fixator allows sliding to adjust length when the locking nut is loosened. It does not allow angulation or rotation. At each end of the body there is a universal joint that allows for adjustment of the angle between

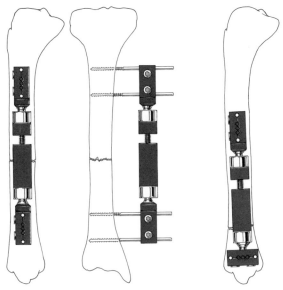

Fig. 130. *Left*—Orthofix external fixator in place for fixation of mid-shaft tibial fracture. *Right*—Use of distal T-piece for fracture near ankle.

the fragments. When correct alignment has been gained, the universal joint at each end is locked by a cam on a bush. If the cam is rotated beyond 180 degrees the joint is loosened; so this degree of rotation must not be exceeded. To prevent over-tightening, the torque wrench supplied in the instrument set should be used.

The screws are guided into the bone by a jig. At each end the jig's universal joint has a slightly smaller range of movement than those of the fixator itself. If the jig can be aligned then the fixator can be. Special alignment forceps are available for use on the ends of the fixator to give leverage to aid fracture reduction.

Once they are inserted, the conical screws cannot be undone without loosening in the bone. If a screw has been inserted too far it must be com-

pletely removed and reinserted at an adjacent site. The screws depend for their hold on the bone's being intact from one end of the screw to the other. If the bone is split between the two screw insertions the screw is deflected: it may separate the fragments, distort and break.

It is usual to use three screws at each end for the femur, and two screws at each end for the tibia.

Removal. When union is complete, the fixator itself and the cortical screws can be removed without anaesthetic, provided great gentleness is used. If the extractor is knocked sharply onto a screw the jarring causes pain and the patient's confidence will be lost.

Use of the fixator in leg lengthening. The Orthofix fixator is adaptable for use in leg lengthening. A threaded lengthener can be inserted through the centre of each cam, so that when the body locking nut is released the leg can be lengthened, usually by 1 millimetre a day, simply by screwing out the lengthener.

In the technique of callotasis, or callus stretching, the fixator is first applied and the bone is divided at the cortex alone around its circumference by multiple shallow drill holes and the gentle use of an osteotome: care is taken not to divide the medullary bone. After two or three weeks, when callus is beginning to form, lengthening may be started. The stretched callus fills in the gap fully in both planes. If check radiographs during the course of lengthening show that the callus is being broken, the lengthening is discontinued or even reversed until the callus bridge is restored.

Chondrodiastasis. The technique of chondrodiastasis is used to lengthen children's bones when the epiphysis is intact. A right-angled piece is inserted at one end of the Orthofix fixator and, through it, cancellous screws are inserted into the epiphysis. Lengthening is started at once and is obtained by distraction of the epiphysis.

Maintaining gained length. In leg lengthening, when the required lengthening has been achieved, the body locking nut is tightened and the apparatus is retained for several weeks until radiographs show the bone to be consolidated.

The lengthener device may be used in reverse to close the gap at a fracture site when there has been significant loss of bone.

THE A.O. FIXATOR, LARGE SIZE

This fixator is widely adaptable for the control even of multiple fragments, but it is rather more cumbersome for use on simple fractures than the Orthofix device.

Usually pins are passed right through the bone. Clamps are then applied to the pins. The clamps are tightened onto a longitudinal bar. The clamps permit different angulation of each pin on the bar, thus allowing for angled fragments to be held.

If there is difficulty in gaining satisfactory alignment of the fragments, the longitudinal bar may be replaced by two shorter bars with a double-hinged joint between them.

The system also allows large "butterfly" fragments to be manipulated into place and held firmly. This may necessitate the use of a third bar, forming a three-dimensional frame. By loosening the clamps for the pins which hold this bar, it can be moved in three planes so that accurate reduction of the fragments can be achieved.

THE A.O. FIXATOR, SMALL SIZE

This system has four parts and is very adaptable. It is used particularly for fractures of the clavicle, humerus, forearm, hand and foot.

A threaded pin 2.5 millimetres in diameter is inserted into the bone at each chosen site. The pins are then attached to 4-millimetre bars by special clamps, and the bars are joined together by further clamps.

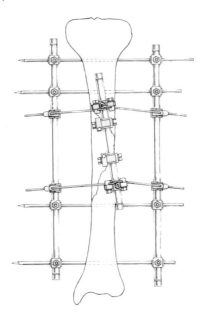
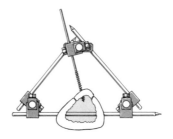

FIG. 131. Plan and end views of the A.O. large external fixator used to fix a comminuted fracture with large "butterfly" fragment.

Lengthening or compression is applied by closing a special clamp to the bar. The screw thread that passes through it is then used to move a clamp through which a pin passes when it has been loosened from the bar. After adjustment it is re-tightened onto the bar.

An advantage of the system is that the pins can be sited at choice to avoid vital structures. As many as necessary can be used, and additional longitudinal bars used for bracing can make up a very strong structure.

TECHNIQUES OF TENDON SUTURE

Tendon suture may be required either to reunite the ends of a tendon that has been divided or ruptured, or to join one tendon to another in the course of tendon grafting or tendon transfer operations. Three main methods are employed: 1) end-to-end suture; 2) interlacing or splicing; and 3) side-to-side suture. End-to-end suture is appropriate for joining the ends of a divided tendon, and it has an occasional place in tendon grafting or tendon transfer operations when the junction has to be made in a confined space such as a tendon sheath, or when there is not sufficient length of tendon to allow any overlap. The interlacing or splicing technique is used commonly in tendon grafting or tendon transfer operations when there is sufficient length to allow overlap of the tendon ends and when the tendon will not be confined within a sheath. It leaves a more bulky mass of tissue than does end-to-end suture and therefore it must be effected in a subcutaneous or intermuscular plane where there is plenty of room. Side-to-side suture is used mainly to restore continuity after tendon lengthening by Z-cut.

TECHNIQUE: END-TO-END SUTURE

End-to-end union is promoted by a suture of stainless steel wire which is buried almost entirely within the substance of the tendon. Fine wire made specially for the purpose, with a straight needle swaged to each end, should be used. The wire may be either a single strand or a braided multi-strand wire.

Adjustment of tension. The aim should be to unite the tendon ends in such a way that the tendon is of normal length. Except in cases of recent injury, however, it is often a difficult matter to judge the tension correctly. A useful guide is to relax the muscle as completely as possible by appropriate positioning of the joints, and then to make the tendon junction under just sufficient tension to take up all the slack.

Preparing the ends for suture. When the correct tension has been determined it is a good plan to anchor the tendon stumps in proximity to each other by impaling each stump upon a fine straight needle that transfixes adjacent tissue or a small piece of sterilised cloth (Fig. 132). In this way the tendon ends are prevented from retracting, and the end-to-end suture may be carried out in com-

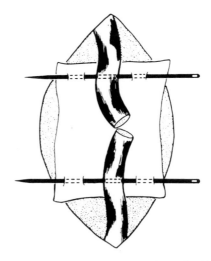

Fig. 132. Transfixion of tendon ends with suture needles upon a square of calico to hold them apposed for suture.

fort. Immediately before the suture is made, the ends that are to be joined should be freshened by cutting away a tiny thickness of the surface with a very sharp blade.

The suture. In order to gain a secure grip on the tendon ends the sutures should extend 8 to 10 millimetres away from the freshened surface of each stump. Two sutures are used, one for each stump. Each suture is inserted in the manner shown in Figure 133. The needle enters at one cut surface and is first directed longitudinally in the tendon substance. Emerging at the surface 8 to 10 millimetres from the site of the tendon junction, it is then looped round to transfix the tendon transversely, as shown. With a further loop the needle then enters the opposite lateral surface and is directed longitudinally to emerge again at the cut surface. A second identical suture is inserted in the same manner in the opposing tendon stump. As the sutures are carefully drawn together before

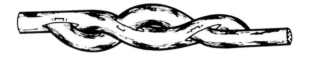

be made in the recipient tendon, one a few millimetres distal to the other and at right angles to it (Fig. 135). If there is considerable overlap of the tendon ends a third slit may be made at right angles to the second to give a longer splice and

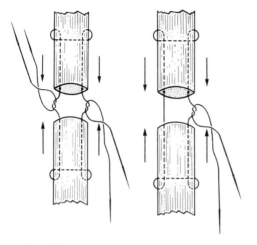

FIGS 133–134. Two methods of end-to-end suture of a tendon.

FIG. 135. Interlacing suture of tendon.

thus greater strength. When the slits have been made in the recipient tendon the other tendon end is drawn through with mosquito forceps with just sufficient tension to take up the slack. To aid adhesion the surface of the interlacing tendon may be scarified where it lies within the slits in the recipient tendon. At each point of intersection the two tendon ends are then sutured with fine stainless steel wire, the ends being buried within the tendon substance.

tying the tendon stumps are bunched together to bring the cut surfaces into close contact. The wires are then tied and the knots are concealed between the tendon ends. An alternative method of directing the sutures is shown in Figure 134.

TECHNIQUE: SUTURE WITH OVERLAP AND INTERLACING

The interlacing technique resembles the splicing of rope. Overlap of at least 2 centimetres is desirable. The junction must be made at a site where the formation of adhesions is not likely to be a serious problem, and where the tendon is free from constriction from surrounding tissues.

Interlacing the tendons. If the tendon ends to be joined are of equal thickness it is immaterial which end is pierced with slits to receive the other. If the tendons are of unequal thickness, however, it is best to make slits in the thicker tendon and to pass the thinner one through. As a rule two slits should

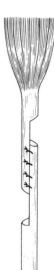

FIG. 136. Side-to-side suture used in tendon lengthening.

Burying the ends of the tendon stumps. Unless the rawed ends of the tendon stumps can be enveloped in muscle (for instance a lumbrical muscle in the case of a tendon junction in the palm), each end must be tucked out of the way by burying it within the substance of the opposing stump. To do this a slit must be made in the surface of the tendon that is to receive the raw stump. The end of the stump is then pushed into the slit so that it lies within the substance of the recipient tendon, and anchored there with a fine suture of wire or catgut (Fig. 135). Again the suture ends should be buried in the tendon.

TECHNIQUE: SIDE-TO-SIDE SUTURE

Side-to-side suture is straightforward. Simple interrupted sutures of absorbable material or of stainless steel wire are used along each cut edge. This technique may be used, for instance, after tendon lengthening by a Z-cut technique (Fig. 136).

Comment

The most important essential in tendon suture is a delicate technique. Any unnecessary trauma to the tendon surfaces must be avoided because it may lead to the formation of adhesions which restrict the free gliding of the tendon. The tendon ends must therefore be handled with extreme care so that the surface is not damaged by toothed instruments or crushed by the pressure of coarse forceps. Likewise it is important that the tendon surface be not allowed to dry. The surface must be kept constantly moist either with blood or by occasional sponging with saline.

The tension under which the tendon ends are joined is fairly critical. Excessive tension may lead to contracture whereas excessive laxity may prejudice power or function. It is not always easy to judge the correct tension with the patient anaesthetised and the limb exsanguinated with a tourniquet. In general, the tendency is to effect the suture with too much slack. Usually it is best to place the joints in a position to relax the muscle concerned and then to make the junction with just sufficient tension to ensure that all slack is taken up.

TECHNIQUES OF ATTACHING TENDON TO BONE

In tendon transfer operations or tendon grafting operations it is often necessary to attach the end of the tendon to bone at the point of insertion. The three basic methods of making the attachment are: 1) suture through adjacent soft tissues; 2) looping through a tunnel in the bone and suture of the tendon to itself; and 3) insertion into a tunnel and anchorage by suture or by transfixion with a wire.

TECHNIQUE: SUTURE TO ADJACENT SOFT TISSUES

This simple method does not give a positive insertion into the bone, but the fixation may be adequate if some stretching of the tissues at the site of insertion is not of material significance.

TECHNIQUE: LOOPING THROUGH TUNNEL

A tunnel is drilled through the recipient bone approximately at right angles to the line of the incoming tendon. The tendon is then looped through the tunnel and folded back on itself to be sutured 10 or 15 millimetres proximal to the site of insertion (Fig. 137). This technique gives good

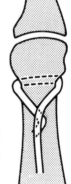

FIG. 137.   Attachment of tendon to bone by loop-through-tunnel technique.

fixation of tendon to bone. It uses up a considerable length of tendon, however, and it is practicable only when adequate tendon length is available.

TECHNIQUE: ANCHORAGE WITHIN TUNNEL

At certain sites it is convenient to drill a hole through the recipient bone at the site of insertion of the tendon and to pass the tendon end into the

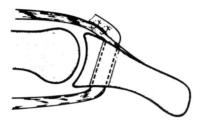

FIG. 138. Attachment of tendon to bone by insertion through tunnel and suture to soft tissue on far side.

drill hole. If there is sufficient length the tendon may be drawn right through the drill hole and sutured to periosteum or other soft tissue at the distal side (Fig. 138). This method is appropriate,

for instance, for anchoring a reconstructed flexor tendon of a finger to the distal phalanx (see p. 239). If the tendon cannot be passed right through the bone it may be anchored by sutures through the periosteum at the proximal end of the

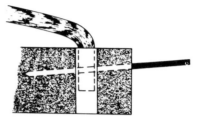

FIG. 139. Attachment of tendon to bone by insertion into tunnel and transfixion with Kirschner wire.

drill hole; or the tendon and drill hole may be transfixed by a Kirschner wire passed at right angles to them (Fig. 139), the wire being removed after five or six weeks when the junction may be assumed to be reasonably secure.

SUTURE OF DIVIDED NERVE

When a peripheral nerve has been freshly divided a decision must first be made whether to undertake primary suture or whether secondary suture is more appropriate. Seddon (1975) strongly favoured secondary suture rather than primary repair in virtually every case, but there has been a trend in recent years towards primary suture whenever the conditions are suitable. In general, it may be said that primary suture may be undertaken if the division has been caused by a clean sharp object, such as a fragment of glass or a razor, and takes the form of a linear incised wound, provided always that adequate operation theatre facilities are available, that a surgeon experienced in nerve repair is at hand and that not more than eight hours have elapsed since the injury. Primary suture is generally to be preferred in the case of nerves severed in the hand, especially since these slender structures are much more easily identified in the freshly injured hand than in the later stages when the nerves may be embedded in dense scar tissue. Primary suture also has a relatively favourable prognosis in children.

In all other cases, and of course when the patient first presents after an interval, secondary suture is required.

PRIMARY NERVE SUTURE

The main essential in nerve suture is that the ends should be brought together without excessive tension. It is also important so far as possible to ensure that the two ends of the nerve are correctly orientated in relation to each other: this gives the greatest opportunity for the divided nerve bundles (fasciculi) to meet and unite with their opposite numbers.

TECHNIQUE

Whenever it is practicable the operation should be done in a bloodless field. The skin wound may be appropriately extended proximally and distally in order to expose the nerve trunks some little distance each side of the point of division.

Mobilisation of nerve ends. Relaxation of the nerve, with consequent ability to bring the ends together without tension, may be achieved to a limited extent by flexion of the adjacent joint. If this alone is successful in allowing the nerve ends to be brought together easily, further mobilisation is not required; but in most cases it will be found advisable to mobilise the proximal stump of the nerve, or if necessary both proximal and distal ends (see p. 102), to allow the nerve to be carefully stretched. In the case of the ulnar nerve, transposition to the front of the elbow gives additional relaxation.

It is important not to attempt to gain too much by joint flexion and mobilisation of the nerve. It is a mistake to try to suture a nerve under strong tension. Beyond a certain critical point, it is better to restore continuity by nerve grafting rather than by direct suture under tension (see below).

Trimming of cut surfaces. Ideally, each cut surface should be flat, and the cut edge of the epineurium or sheath should be level with the nerve fasciculi. In a clean wound of the type that is being discussed this may already be the case, but there is a tendency for the fasciculi to pout out above the level of the cut edge of the sheath. If this is so, the fasciculi should be trimmed level with a new razor blade.

Technique of nerve suture. Very fine instruments and fine suture material are required. Greater accuracy can be achieved if the surgeon wears a magnifying loupe.

If the pattern of the fasciculi on the cut surfaces of the nerve can be discerned it may be possible to establish the correct orientation of the two parts by matching up opposing bundles. If this cannot be done, reliance must be placed on the natural lie of the nerve ends. Any obvious twisting must be avoided.

The first two sutures are the important ones. These are placed at diametrically opposed points on the circumference of the nerve. Very fine (6/0) suture material should be used. The suture unites only the edges of the epineurium (Figs 140 and 141). These first two sutures are left long so that the ends may be used to steady the nerve and later

to rotate it to allow suture of the deep surface. A series of further closely spaced sutures is inserted between the two primary sutures, first on the

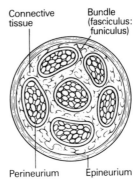

FIG. 140. Diagrammatic cross-section of nerve, showing nerve fasciculi or bundles, perineurium and epineurium.

superficial aspect of the nerve and then, after rotation of the nerve through 180 degrees, on the deep aspect.

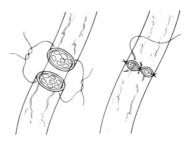

FIG. 141. Suture of nerve trunk. The first sutures secure the epineurium at opposite points on the circumference of the nerve.

Closure. If a tourniquet has been used it should be removed before the wound is closed, so that one may be sure that bleeding is not occurring within the nerve sheath. After adequate haemostasis has been secured the wound is closed in layers, with care to ensure that the flexed position of the adjacent joint (to relax the nerve) is maintained.

POST-OPERATIVE MANAGEMENT
This is described on page 103.

REPAIR BY MICROSURGICAL TECHNIQUE

The use of a microsurgical technique allows the repair of severed nerves with much greater precision than could be achieved by the naked eye, even when aided by a loupe. In particular, it enables individual fasciculi or groups of fasciculi to be coapted by perineural suture. In appropriate cases it may be practicable to excise scar tissue from between the fasciculi after local excision of the epineurium, thus releasing the fibres from strangulation. Care must be taken, however, not to be over-ambitious: more harm than good may result from excessive intervention, because of further scar tissue formation. It should be noted, also, that in the case of a small nerve such as a digital nerve there is nothing to be gained from undertaking anything more radical than careful coaptation of the epineurium.

SECONDARY NERVE SUTURE

Ideally, secondary suture of a nerve should be the definitive part of a two-stage procedure. At the first stage the nerve should have been explored and, being found divided but not amenable to primary suture, the ends should have been approximated by two sutures, one at each side of the nerve, and these should have been so placed as to preserve the correct orientation of the cut ends relative to each other. Definitive secondary suture is then carried out three weeks later, or as soon after that as the skin wound is fully healed without infection.

It often happens, however, that diagnosis of the nerve lesion is delayed for one reason or another, and when the patient first presents himself for examination the primary wound may be already healed without anything having been done to the nerve. In this latter type of case the nerve ends may be retracted and embedded in scar tissue, and secondary repair may be correspondingly more difficult.

TECHNIQUE

There are three steps in the secondary repair of a nerve: 1) mobilisation of the nerve ends; 2) resection of the end bulbs; and 3) the nerve suture itself (Fig. 142). Magnification should be used when available; or, if the necessary expertise is at hand, a full microsurgical technique may be employed.

Mobilisation. It is essential that healthy nerve fasciculi be brought together without undue tension. As noted above, some relaxation of the nerve

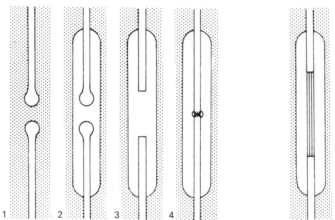

FIGS 142–143. Technique of nerve suture (diagrammatic). Figure 142—
1. End bulbs embedded in scar. 2. Mobilisation. 3. Resection of end bulbs.
4. Suture. Figure 143—Nerve graft by multiple strands.

can be obtained by flexion of the adjacent joint, though it is wrong to rely upon this for more than very slight gain in length because when the joint is straightened again harmful stretching may occur.

Further reduction in the gap between the nerve ends can be gained by mobilisation of the nerve proximally or distally, or both. But the length that can be gained is limited: it is seldom more than 5 centimetres and often less, depending upon the particular nerve affected.

It is important that any mobilisation of the nerve be carried out with great care, to ensure that the accompanying small blood vessels are preserved: for it is all too easy to bring about ischaemia of the nerve, with consequent impairment of function, if mobilisation is pursued too radically. If the gap that will need to be bridged after trimming of the end bulbs exceeds 5 centimetres (less in some nerves) consideration should be given to the advisability of nerve grafting in preference to direct suture under excessive tension.

Resection of end bulbs. Before suture is undertaken the bulbous ends of the divided nerve must be resected to expose healthy nerve bundles. The resection is done with a new razor blade. The first cut is made at the junction of end bulb with nerve trunk, but if healthy fasciculi do not pout out with the first cut further slices of scarred nerve are cut away until healthy bundles are exposed. The fresh ends are then brought together for suture.

Nerve suture. The technique of uniting the nerve ends by circumferential suture of the epineurium is the same as that described for primary suture (p. 101). As with primary nerve suture, there are advantages to be gained from the use of a microsurgical technique.

POST-OPERATIVE MANAGEMENT

If it has been necessary to flex one or more of the joints in order to relax the nerve and thus to avoid undue tension at the suture line, the limb should be supported in a plaster-of-Paris splint with the joints concerned suitably flexed. The initial plaster is removed after three weeks, when the sutures are removed. Further serial plasters are then applied at intervals of ten days, with less joint flexion on each occasion, until by the end of two months or so the neutral position is regained and the plaster is discarded.

If nerve suture has been achieved without tension at the suture line splintage is needed only for a much shorter period, and without much flexion: or it may be omitted altogether.

NERVE GRAFTING

If the gap between the nerve ends cannot be closed without excessive tension, resort may be had to nerve grafting. The donor nerve varies according to circumstances: often the sural nerve is used, and as this is not a large nerve several strands may be required in bridging a major nerve trunk (Fig. 143).

Length of graft. In nerve grafting any tension should be avoided. With the joints in the neutral position the gap between the trimmed nerve ends is measured, and 10 per cent is added: this gives the minimum length of graft required (Millesi 1983).

The nerve suture. Except in the case of small nerves, for which epineural suture may be adequate, a microsurgical technique offers clear advantages in nerve grafting because it enables individual fasciculi or groups of fasciculi to be joined to the graft by perineural suture. After excision of epineurium locally, fasciculi can be dissected out and trimmed and sutured at different levels: the grafts thus lie more snugly in place. Since there is no tension, one or two sutures for each bundle or group of bundles suffices.

DECOMPRESSION OF PERIOSTEUM AND BONE IN ACUTE OSTEOMYELITIS

The condition to which this operation applies is acute haematogenous osteomyelitis, usually occurring in the metaphysial region of a long bone in a child.

Reference to the pathology as shown diagrammatically in Figures 144–146 will underline the obvious desirability of making the diagnosis at the earliest stage of the disease, when prompt treatment by antibiotics may obviate the need for operation. Once this stage has passed, and marked constitutional upset and exquisite tenderness well localised to a point over the metaphysis of the long bone suggest the development of an abscess, operation should be undertaken with only sufficient delay to establish an effective level of antibiotic in the blood stream. The operation entails tissues and of the periosteum itself. The periosteum is incised vertically right through to the bone. The usual finding is that there is a collection of pus under tension beneath the periosteum; pus escapes as soon as the incision is made. The subperiosteal pocket is cleaned out thoroughly by suction and swabbing, to allow inspection of the underlying bone. In a florid case there will be

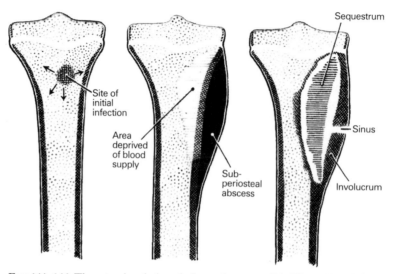

FIGS 144–146. The natural evolution of a focus of osteomyelitis. Figure 144—Initial lesion in the metaphysis. Figure 145—Pus has escaped to the surface of the bone and formed a subperiosteal abscess. Part of the bone has lost its blood supply from septic thrombosis of vessels. Figure 146—The devitalised area eventually separates as a sequestrum. Meanwhile new bone (involucrum) is formed beneath the stripped-up periosteum; it is perforated by sinuses through which pus escapes. This is the stage of chronic osteomyelitis. With prompt treatment the disease can often be arrested at the stage shown in Figure 144.

incision of the periosteum to drain pus pent up beneath it, and in some cases drainage of the medulla of the bone by appropriate drill holes. Early operation relieves pain and allows identification and typing of the organism; and in a favourable case it promotes healing without sequestrum formation.

TECHNIQUE

The affected bone is exposed over a length that extends a little above and a little below the point of greatest tenderness. Preferably the incision should lie over a muscle-covered surface of the bone rather than over a subcutaneous surface. As periosteum is approached it will often be found that there is considerable oedema of the overlying signs of pus exuding through the rather spongy bone. Because pus may be collecting within the bone some surgeons recommend that one or two drill holes 3 or 4 millimetres in diameter be made through the spongy cortex of the bone to enter the medulla; but this is a matter of some controversy. Pus may or may not be encountered, but so long as loose shavings of bone created by the drilling are removed, drilling should not be harmful: if pus is present within the bone then it is clearly important that it be evacuated.

Before closure a solution of the appropriate antibiotic drug should be instilled in the area of operation. In the ordinary acute case it is recommended that the skin be closed by interrupted sutures, without drainage.

POST-OPERATIVE MANAGEMENT

The affected limb should be immobilised in a plaster-of-Paris splint to ensure complete rest and thus to provide the best conditions for healing. When the plaster is dry it is bivalved to allow periodic inspection of the wound area. The patient should be confined to bed with the affected limb elevated. Systemic antibiotics are given in high dosage, and once the nature of the infecting organism and its sensitivity to antibiotic drugs have been determined from culture of the pus, definitive antibiotic therapy with the most appropriate drug can be established. Up to this point, antibiotic therapy is empirical, usually comprising a combination of fusidic acid and erythromycin. If treatment has been instituted early and if the organism is sensitive to the antibiotics available, primary healing may nearly always be expected.

ERADICATION OF DISEASED BONE IN CHRONIC OSTEOMYELITIS

In chronic osteomyelitis there may be recurrent flares of infection or chronic purulent discharge from a sinus. Whether the disease be haematogenous or post-traumatic, successful operation entails the removal of diseased bone and the obliteration of cavities, either by filling them with soft tissues or by direct skin grafting of the walls of the cavity, which is thus exteriorised. Moreover, any fragments of dead bone or of foreign material must be removed; otherwise discharge is likely to persist after operation.

TECHNIQUE

Exposure. The site of the incision must depend largely upon local conditions and must take account of scarring and adherence of skin, the site of any discharging sinus and the availability of muscle with which to fill a cavity that is found in the bone. So far as is possible the incision should be made through healthy non-adherent skin, but it may often be convenient to excise the sinus track with an ellipse of skin. In general, it is preferable to approach the bone through muscle planes rather than where the bone is subcutaneous. After incision of the skin any sinus should be followed down to the bone and its walls excised in the process. The exposure should be ample in order to allow thorough exploration of the affected area and excision of all diseased bone.

Removal of sequestrum. In a proportion of cases of chronic osteomyelitis, persistent purulent discharge is due solely to the existence of a sequestrum locked in a cavity in the bone. By definition a sequestrum is dead bone, and since it lies loose in a cavity, virtually suspended in pus, there is no mechanism by which it can be absorbed. On the other hand, when such a sequestrum is removed the operation is nearly always followed by primary healing of the wound.

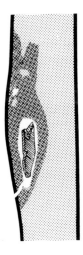

FIG. 147. A sequestrum locked in a cavity in sclerotic bone. Note the sinus leading to the surface. Removal of the sequestrum and obliteration of the cavity are necessary if healing is to be assured.

Usually a sequestrum can be demonstrated radiologically, though sometimes special projections or tomographs may be required to reveal it.

Removal of a sequestrum is often easy but sometimes difficult. The most useful guide to its location—other than the radiograph—is the sinus track. If this is followed from the surface through the deeper tissues it will be found to lead to the cavity containing the sequestrum, though the route may be tortuous rather than direct. When the cavity has been located, all that is necessary is to unroof it sufficiently to allow the sequestrum to be extracted. Once the sequestrum has been encountered there can be no question of its identity. It is a hard, rather rough piece of bone of irregular outline and it lies totally loose within its cavity, coated with pus (Fig. 147).

After removal of the sequestrum it is best if possible to obliterate the cavity by inserting into it a flap of muscle as described in the succeeding paragraphs.

Excision of diseased tissue. When the bone is reached one or more sinuses may be found leading down to cavities within it. The bone may be sclerotic, and under the surface it may be honey-combed with small cavities and areas of granulation tissue. The principle is to excise all this diseased mass of bone, leaving a cavity with healthy well vascularised walls. To help to obliterate dead space it is often appropriate to cut away overhanging bone and thus to make the cavity larger but relatively shallow—a process known as "saucerisation". Of course, in shaping out the cavity in this way due regard must be given to the strength of the remaining bone. Although in many cases a considerable quantity of bone substance has to be removed, as much as possible of bone that is healthy must be left, to preserve strength.

Obliteration of cavity with muscle flap. If the residual cavity is broad and shallow, overlying soft tissues may fall into it and obliterate dead space without further intervention. Often, however, the cavity is too deep to be obliterated in this way. In that event the aim should be to fill the cavity with a flap of muscle, if the site of the osteomyelitic process permits this. In the thigh and in the upper part of the lower leg, as in the upper arm and upper part of the forearm, it is fairly easy to find a suitable muscle from which to form a flap. In the lower part of the lower leg it is impracticable to fill the cavity with muscle because muscle bellies have given place to tendons. Whenever possible the flap of muscle should be based proximally, to ensure that it retains an adequate blood supply. If it is impossible to fashion a proximally based flap, however, a distally based flap may be used. The

flap should not be greater in length than three times its width at the base. Clearly, the closer the base of the flap is to the cavity that is to be filled, the better.

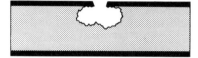

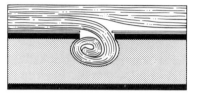

FIG. 148. Filling of bone cavity by coiled muscle flap.

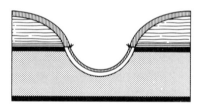

FIG. 149. Saucerisation of cavity and application of split-skin graft direct upon the raw surface.

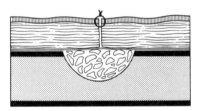

FIG. 150. Delayed filling of cavity with bone slivers and reconstitution of muscle and skin over it.

When the flap has been fashioned it is coiled into a ball and held in this form by one or two transfixion sutures. The coiled flap is then pushed firmly into the cavity in the bone and should fill it completely (Fig. 148). Soft tissues are then closed over the mouth of the cavity with sutures that transfix the base of the flap, thus preventing its being displaced from the cavity. Finally, a solution of the appropriate antibiotic drug is instilled into the cavity and about the muscle flap, and the wound is closed, usually without drainage.

Exteriorisation of cavity by direct skin grafting. If it is impracticable to fill the cavity with overlying soft tissues or with a muscle flap it is often advisable to apply split skin grafts directly to the walls of the cavity. For this purpose the cavity must be well saucerised—that is, it must be shallow in relation to its surface area (Fig. 149). To achieve this state it may be necessary to cut away overhanging edges of the cavity.

Skin grafting of the surface of the cavity may be done by cutting strips of split skin—rather thin— each about 2 centimetres wide and laying them on a base of *tulle gras*. A series of such strips is laid in the cavity and pressed against the walls so that they are in intimate contact with bone over the entire area. Each strip may overlap the preceding strip by a few millimetres to ensure complete coverage by skin. The skin is held against the walls of the cavity by fluffed cotton soaked in paraffin and flavine emulsion, and the cavity is then packed with soft gauze or a sponge to ensure moderate but not excessive pressure. Further dressings are applied on the surface and held in place by one or two crepe bandages, firmly applied. The site should be left undisturbed for seven days, after which the dressings are changed. Subsequently, daily saline irrigations and packing with soft gauze are continued until the skin is stable.

Delayed obliteration of cavity by cancellous sliver grafts. In some centres chronic osteomyelitic cavities are filled with cancellous bone grafts at the primary clearance operation. This plan is often successful but there is considerable risk of reinfection of the haematoma in which the grafts are embedded and of consequent failure of the grafts

to be revascularised and incorporated. It is better, therefore, to defer any attempt to fill the cavity by bone until the chronic infection has been overcome by one of the methods described above, and until time has been allowed for the tissues to settle down. At that stage—perhaps three to six months after the primary operation—it is justifiable to refreshen the walls of the cavity after removal of the contents or skin lining, and to pack it with bone slivers obtained from the ilium (Fig. 150). The chances of success will be greater if the bone grafts can be covered on the outer aspect by a good layer of healthy muscle.

The same principle may be applied when excision of diseased bone has left a complete gap in one of the long bones. Once the infection has been overcome and full skin healing obtained, the gap may be bridged by a cancellous bone graft from the iliac crest. In this case a solid piece of bone may be preferred to slivers or chips (Nicoll 1956), and it may be held in place by an intramedullary nail driven down the host bone and penetrating the graft throughout its length.

Comment

The requirements for success in the treatment of chronic purulent osteomyelitis are: 1) removal of all sequestra and foreign material; and 2) total elimination of dead space. The most reliable method of obliterating a cavity is by filling it with a flap of muscle. This is often a permanent solution to the problem, and it is by no means always desirable to replace the muscle at a later stage by bone grafts. Bone grafting is needed only when the strength or continuity of the bone is impaired, or to fill in a skin-filled cavity for cosmetic reasons. Even when strength is impaired sufficiently to demand some reinforcement of the bone, grafting of the cavity itself by bone may not always be the best solution to the problem. The alternative that is sometimes to be preferred is to reinforce the intact normal part of the bone by an onlay bone graft applied to the side of the bone opposite to the cavity.

EPIPHYSIODESIS

The operation of epiphysiodesis implies permanent arrest of growth at an epiphysial plate. It is achieved by a combination of bone grafting by cortico-cancellous grafts bridging the growth plate, and partial destruction of the growth cartilage itself. Arrest of epiphysial growth for correction of inequality of limb length is applicable mainly to the lower femoral epiphysis or to the

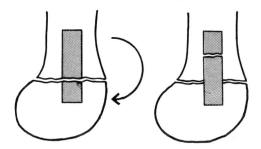

FIGS 151–152. Epiphysiodesis. Figure 151—A rectangle of cortex including part of the epiphysial growth plate is cut free. Figure 152—The excised piece of bone has been reversed and reinserted in the slot as a bone graft to bridge the epiphysial plate.

upper tibial and upper fibular epiphyses, or to both levels together. Rarely, it may be applied to other sites, such as the lower end of the tibia or the lower end of the fibula, when growth of these bones is uneven. There is little place, if any, for epiphysiodesis in the upper limb.

PRELIMINARY STUDIES

Before epiphysiodesis is undertaken it is essential that accurate measurement of the length of each limb be made, preferably by the radiological technique of scanography. From tables of expected future growth, based on skeletal age rather than on chronological age (Anderson and Green 1947), the correct timing of the operation is then worked out; or the alternative simple technique of Menelaus (Menelaus 1966; Westh and Menelaus 1981) may be used.

TECHNIQUE

Medial and lateral vertical incisions about 5 centimetres long are made over the selected epiphysial plate. One-third of each incision is over the epiphysis and two-thirds over the diaphysis. Each incision is deepened to the periosteum, which is incised vertically. The edge of the epiphysial plate is identified as a whitish line crossing the line of incision more or less transversely. For further identification it may be prodded with a straight needle: whereas this does not sink into bone, it sinks readily into the cartilage of the epiphysial plate.

On each side of the bone a rectangular area is marked out by lightly scratching the surface with an osteotome. The rectangle should measure about 3 centimetres in vertical length by about 1.5 centimetres in width (Fig. 151). Two-thirds of the rectangle should be over the diaphysis and one-third over the metaphysis. With a thin sharp osteotome about a centimetre wide this rectangular piece of bone, crossed near one end by the epiphysial plate, is cut out: it consists mainly of cortical bone, with some underlying cancellous bone adherent to it. Before the grafts are reinserted in their beds as much of the epiphysial cartilage as is accessible from within the slots that have been cut out is scooped away with a small gouge or awl in order to help to promote fusion.

The excised strips of bone, which will form the bridging bone grafts, are now reversed by turning them through 180 degrees as shown in Figure 152. Each graft after reversal is put back into the rectangular slot from which it was taken. Reversal of the graft causes the longer metaphysial piece of cortex to bridge the epiphysial plate whereas the former epiphysial part of the graft, together with the fragment of epiphysial plate, is transposed to the metaphysial area. After the graft has been impacted into its bed the periosteum is sutured over it and the skin wound is closed.

POST-OPERATIVE MANAGEMENT

A plaster splint to immobilise the joint is worn for three weeks. Thereafter exercises are encouraged in order to restore full joint movement.

Comment

The cortico-cancellous bone graft bridging the epiphysial plate on each side of the bone soon becomes incorporated and locks the epiphysis to the metaphysis. Further longitudinal growth is thus prevented. Observation for several months after the operation is desirable because it is just possible, though exceptional, that arrest of growth may fail on one or other side, thus leading to deformity. It is important that such a complication be recognised early so that corrective measures may be taken.

EXCISION OF OSTEOID OSTEOMA FROM A LONG BONE

A typical osteoid osteoma grows in the cortex of a long bone—often the femur or the tibia. It is surrounded by a dense mass of new bone which forms a fusiform swelling as seen in the radiograph. The swelling may or may not be palpable clinically, depending upon its site. Operation entails removal of the central core or so-called nidus which is the essential lesion, together with a reasonable margin of surrounding bone. The bone should be excised as a block rather than piecemeal.

PRELIMINARY STUDIES

It is important before operation to identify the central nidus and to locate its position accurately. The nidus cannot always be seen clearly in plain radiographs because it may be obscured by the dense surrounding bone. The lesion will show as a local "hot" area in a radioisotope (technetium) scan, but tomographs may be required to identify the nidus. Usually it will be found to occupy the centre of the fusiform mass of dense new bone (Fig. 153). Accurate localisation before operation is important because it is desirable to remove the lesion in a single block with the surrounding bone, rather than to attempt to reveal the actual lesion at the time of operation.

TECHNIQUE

The basic technique is the same no matter which long bone is affected or which part of the cortex.

Exposure. According to the localisation of the lesion as revealed by radiographs, the affected bone is exposed by the most convenient route. The periosteum is incised and muscles are stripped from the affected part of the bone over a small length above and below the swelling, and held aside by two pairs of bone levers.

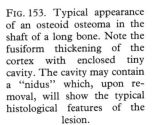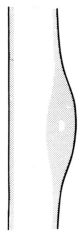

Fig. 153. Typical appearance of an osteoid osteoma in the shaft of a long bone. Note the fusiform thickening of the cortex with enclosed tiny cavity. The cavity may contain a "nidus" which, upon removal, will show the typical histological features of the lesion.

Marking out the area to be excised. In most cases the extent of the fusiform bony swelling will be clearly revealed when the bone is exposed, and it is easy with the help of the pre-operative radiographs to define the area of bone that needs to be removed. If in an unusual case there is still doubt about the site of the lesion in relation to the bone mass, new radiographs should be taken in the operation theatre after opaque markers have been placed approximately where the lesion is expected to be found. It should thus be possible to confirm the site of the lesion and to ensure that the wrong part of the bone is not removed.

Removal of block of bone containing the lesion. It is recommended that the block of bone, the extent of which has already been outlined, be removed by making appropriate cuts through the entire thickness of the cortex with a rotating or oscillating power-driven bone saw. The technique is the same as that for cutting a cortical bone graft (p. 72). When the four sides of the block have been cut right through to the medulla, the block should be already loose and may be levered out with a slender chisel or elevator. If the block of bone is still adherent, as it may be at one or more of the corners, it may be freed either by further cuts with the bone saw or by completing the cut with a thin osteotome.

Examination of specimen. It is useful to radiograph the specimen immediately after its removal in order to confirm that it does in fact contain the central nidus of the osteoid osteoma itself. If this is not shown to be present in the specimen the wrong piece of bone may have been removed inadvertently. Further radiographs should then be taken of the affected bone to see if the central nidus is still present in the remaining cortex; if so, the appropriate further piece of bone must be removed. An alternative method is to scan the excised fragment with a gamma camera; but this presupposes that ^{99m}technetium has been injected before the operation so that it will be taken up selectively in the region of the osteoid osteoma.

Closure. It is impracticable to close the periosteum, and all that is necessary is to suture muscles over the defect and to close the skin with or without suction drainage as may seem appropriate.

POST-OPERATIVE MANAGEMENT

Usually splintage is not required and the affected limb may be left free after the application of a snug crepe bandage over copious gauze dressings. In the case of the lower limb weight bearing may usually be resumed as soon as the skin is healed.

Comment

This operation is almost exactly comparable to the taking of a cortical bone graft, for instance from the medial surface of the tibia. To cut the block of bone out cleanly with a motor saw is far preferable to piecemeal removal of the lesion and the surrounding bone with chisels and osteotomes in an attempt to find the central lesion. This is not easily identified under such circumstances, and in any case the surrounding bone is often so dense that chipping it away with a chisel is unnecessarily laborious. It seems better to remove the lesion encased in its surrounding block of bone, which should then be radiographed or scanned before being sent for histological examination.

BIOPSY OF MUSCULO-SKELETAL TUMOURS

Biopsy of suspected tumours of bone or soft tissue always requires careful planning, and must never be undertaken casually. A badly sited or poorly executed biopsy may prejudice the successful eradication of a malignant tumour. A survey in the United States of America (Mankin *et al.* 1982) showed that complications arose in the skin, soft tissue or bone of the biopsy area in more than 17 per cent of the patients. The plan of treatment had to be altered on account of problems related to the biopsy in 18 per cent, an otherwise unnecessary amputation had to be carried out in 4.5 per cent, and in 8.5 per cent the prognosis and outcome were judged to have been adversely affected. Especially significant was the finding that these biopsy-related problems occurred very much more frequently when the biopsy was performed at a referring centre rather than at a treating centre, where presumably surgeons have greater experience and skill in the correct siting and execution of a biopsy operation.

It is therefore incumbent upon every surgeon who undertakes biopsy for a suspected tumour to be fully conversant with all the requirements, the problems and the techniques, so that a representative piece of tissue will be obtained without compromising in any way the technical success of a subsequent operation for excision of the tumour.

Furthermore, it is generally to be advised that the surgeon who is to undertake the definitive excision of the tumour should himself be responsible for the biopsy. Thus if the patient is to be referred to another centre for the definitive treatment it is better that the transfer be made before rather than after the biopsy.

Pre-biopsy studies. Since biopsy usually is—or should be—the penultimate step in the management of a tumour, it is important that any other diagnostic studies that are relevant and contemplated should have been completed before the biopsy is undertaken. Biopsy is only one event—albeit often a crucial one—in the staging of a tumour, and the results of previous investigations may have a bearing on the planning of the biopsy. These preliminary investigations may include haematological and biochemical studies of the blood, ^{99m}technetium and ^{67}gallium citrate radioisotope scanning, plain radiography and CT scanning of the primary lesion and of the lungs, and peripheral angiography; and there should be full consultation with the radiologist and with the other specialists concerned.

Open or closed biopsy? In general, open biopsy is preferred to biopsy by needle or trephine, except in certain anatomical situations and when certain types of tumour are suspected. Despite the greater risk of spillage of tumour cells and of complications such as haematoma or infection, open biopsy has the advantage that a relatively large and representative specimen of the tumour is likely to be obtained, thus permitting a more certain histological diagnosis and more accurate grading of the tumour. On the other hand, the use of closed biopsy is widely accepted for suspected tumours

in inaccessible situations such as the spine. It is also often acceptable when the tumour material is expected to be of a homogeneous kind such as a round cell tumour, a metastasis or a local recurrence. In these instances a needle biopsy is likely to yield representative tissue. The use of closed biopsy, however, clearly demands the availability of a co-operative pathologist skilled in the interpretation of such limited samples.

Excision biopsy. Excision biopsy is justifiable only in certain well defined circumstances—for instance, when the tumour is almost certainly benign, or when a small lesion is confined within an expendable bone such as the fibula, the clavicle or a rib. Except in these and a few other rare instances, incisional biopsy is to be preferred.

Tourniquet. Whether or not a tourniquet should be used is a matter of controversy. But the advantages gained from the use of a tourniquet seem to outweigh the theoretical objections—for instance, that tumour cells may be flushed out into the general circulation when the tourniquet is released. Two precautions in the use of the tourniquet should, however, be observed. These are: 1) that an exsanguinating Esmarch bandage should not be applied over the site of the tumour (lest tumour cells be disseminated); and 2) that the tourniquet should be removed and all bleeding points secured before the biopsy wound is closed. Of course, if on the basis of immediate histological studies the surgeon decides to proceed with excision of the tumour under the same anaesthetic, this second precaution would not apply.

Siting of biopsy wound. The placement of the biopsy wound is crucial: whereas it must afford reasonable access, it is paramount that it must not jeopardise the technical success of a subsequent excision operation. The cardinal rule is that the biopsy site must be capable of being excised entire with a malignant tumour, whether at local resection or at amputation. A misplaced biopsy incision may lead to the necessity for amputation when local excision might otherwise have been feasible. Correct planning of the biopsy thus demands that the surgeon must have a thorough knowledge of limb-conserving resection procedures as well as a familiarity with standard and non-standard amputation flaps.

Transverse incisions for biopsy are to be avoided, especially in the limbs, because they cannot readily be excised *en bloc* with longitudinally directed segments of bone or musculo-aponeurotic compartments (Simon 1982). For similar reasons, the incision should be kept away from the major neuro-vascular bundles. Thirdly, the biopsy route should not traverse any musculoskeletal compartment that is not involved with the tumour to reach one that is involved. In the pelvic region, incision through the buttock should be avoided, especially if subsequent local pelvic resection or limb-conserving hemipelvectomy is envisaged (Simon 1982).

In selecting the particular part of the tumour from which to take the biopsy specimen, the surgeon should bear in mind that the periphery of the tumour, close to the pseudocapsule, is usually the most representative part: tissue taken from the centre of the mass may be necrotic.

It is not always necessary to take a specimen of bone in the case of a bone tumour: soft parts of the tumour will often have penetrated the bone, and these may be sampled instead of the bone itself. If a bone has to be windowed to obtain tumour material this should be done with extreme care lest the bone be weakened to the point of pathological fracture. The opening should be as small as is practicable, and it should be round or oval: angular openings are much more prone to set up a weak spot that may lead to fracture.

Frozen section and immediate definitive operation. When facilities permit, examination of frozen sections of soft tissue specimens at the time of biopsy is to be advised. Even if immediate definitive operation is not envisaged, frozen sections may indicate whether or not a representative piece of tissue has been obtained, so that if this is not the case a further specimen may be taken.

When the circumstances are appropriate, there is much to be said for proceeding to immediate definitive eradication of the tumour on the evidence of the frozen sections, provided that the diagnosis is positively established by full accord between radiological and other investigations and the histological features. It is imperative, however, that definitive excisional operation be deferred if there is any doubt whatever about the diagnosis.

Examination of the specimen. Tissue that is to be studied by light microscopy after appropriate staining should be preserved in formaldehyde. A separate specimen should be set aside for bacteriological culture. If electron microscopy studies are envisaged, a specimen should be stored in glutaraldehyde rather than in formaldehyde.

CHAPTER THREE

Neck and Cervical Spine

The cervical spine is a borderland between the fields of orthopaedic surgery and neurosurgery. In most orthopaedic centres operations in this region are undertaken infrequently, especially if the surgeon—like the authors—adopts a conservative attitude to degenerative lesions of the cervical spine and to disc protrusions without involvement of the spinal cord. Probably the commonest reasons for surgical intervention in the cervical spine are fractures with displacement, and rheumatoid arthritis.

There are serious potential hazards in all operations upon the neck, and the surgeon should have filled a considerable apprenticeship before he embarks upon such procedures without the assistance of his senior.

CONTENTS OF CHAPTER

RELEASE OF CONTRACTED STERNOCLEIDOMASTOID MUSCLE FOR INFANTILE TORTICOLLIS

In torticollis from contracture of the sternocleidomastoid muscle on one side, the muscle may be released either at the lower end or at the upper end. Release at the lower end is the usual method and is the method to be described here. Often the child is aged from three to five years at the time of operation.

TECHNIQUE

Position of patient. The patient lies supine with a small pad between the scapulae to throw the base of the neck forwards. The head is rotated slightly away from the side affected.

Incision. The incision is placed about a centimetre above the medial quarter of the clavicle and

the lateral half of the manubrium of the sternum. Before making the incision the surgeon should draw the skin downwards so that the line of incision is over the clavicle. He may then cut straight through the skin and platysma in the knowledge that deeper structures will not be endangered.

Exposure and division of the muscle. With the skin and platysma retracted the tight sternal and clavicular heads of the sternocleidomastoid muscle come into view with the covering layer of fascia. The fascia is divided at the medial and lateral margins of the muscle and teased away from it. A blunt-pointed curved haemostat is then insinuated behind the heads of the muscle, and working both from the medial and from the lateral side the surgeon frees the muscle heads from the deeper tissues. With a director or haemostat still in place behind the muscle as a protection for the underlying tissues the muscle is then divided cleanly with a knife. Some surgeons crush the muscle between the blades of a haemostat before dividing it, in order to reduce bleeding.

Correction of deformity. The patient's head is now manipulated into a position of over-correction, so that the affected sternocleidomastoid muscle is put on the stretch. This is done by rotating the chin towards the side of the operation and approximating the opposite ear to the adjacent shoulder. If during this manoeuvre it is seen that resistance to full correction is still offered by the strong deep cervical fascia, which lies immediately behind the muscle, this may be judiciously divided with extreme care to avoid injury to the internal jugular vein and the subclavian artery and vein, which all lie close to the operation area.

Closure. When full haemostasis has been secured the platysma is repaired with fine absorbable sutures. The skin may be closed with a subcuticular stitch to ensure that the scar is unobtrusive.

POST-OPERATIVE MANAGEMENT

The child should lie as much as possible with the head in the corrected position—that is, with the ear of the opposite side approximated to the adjacent shoulder. This position may be maintained by a wide gauze head band held in place upon the pillow by sand-bags. After removal of the suture at seven days an over-corrected position may be maintained by a light collar of moulded plastic foam. This is worn for three weeks and thereafter corrective exercises are supervised by a physiotherapist for two to three months.

Comment

This simple operation demands careful execution because of the proximity of major vessels to the deep aspect of the muscle. Because of the hazard presented by these vessels it is surprising that surgeons for many years continued to release the tight muscle blindly by subcutaneous tenotomy. What is not surprising is that this often failed to give full correction of the deformity, for the natural tendency would be for the cautious surgeon to keep the tenotome on a too superficial plane for fear of damaging the deeper structures, so that in many cases the division of the posterior fibres of the muscle was almost certainly incomplete.

APPLICATION OF SKULL CALIPERS FOR NECK TRACTION

Skull traction is used mainly to aid reduction of acute subluxation or dislocation of the cervical spine, or to maintain reduction; and occasionally to help to stabilise the spine during and after operations such as intervertebral fusion.

THE CONE (CONE-BARTON) CALIPER

The Cone (Cone-Barton) caliper (Fig. 154) (Cone and Turner 1937) is convenient and easy to apply. It has screw-operated points that enter the outer table of the parietal bones without the need for preliminary drilling, and the shoulder on each pin automatically prevents over-penetration.

TECHNIQUE

Position of patient. The patient lies supine, preferably with the head supported upon the special head rest provided on most operation tables. Alternatively, he may rest upon a flat trolley.

Determining correct position for insertion of pins. A narrow tape is used to mark a line commencing at the tip of the mastoid process on one side and crossing the vertex of the skull at right angles to the sagittal line to extend down the opposite side of the skull to the mastoid process. While the tape is held in position the caliper is opened slightly wider than the skull and placed in position over the tape. A suitable point for insertion of the pin on each side is thus easily found: usually it will be 2 or 3 centimetres above the top of the ear (Fig. 154).

FURTHER MANAGEMENT

The head end of the bed should be elevated so that the slope provides counter-traction. As a general rule traction should be applied with the head and neck in the neutral or slightly extended position.

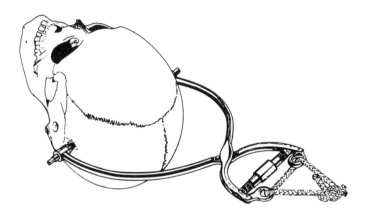

FIG. 154. Cone (Cone-Barton) skull caliper. The drawing shows the position of the pins in the parietal bones.

A small area of the scalp above the ear on each side should first be shaved. If local anaesthesia is to be used anaesthetic solution is infiltrated in an area 1.5 centimetres in diameter with its centre at the site selected for insertion of the pin. The caliper is then brought back into position and the special steel pin is introduced into the conical end of the caliper on each side. The exact point where the pin will pass through the skin may be penetrated by a fine (No. 15) scalpel blade to reduce contamination of the pin as it passes through the skin layer. The caliper is now closed down upon the scalp so that the point of each pin enters the tiny skin incision. With the square-ended key, each pin is screwed home so that the point enters the bone and automatically penetrates the correct distance. It is best to tighten each screw alternately so that the pressure is equal on the two sides. A few turns of sterile gauze may be wrapped around the conical ends of the caliper, but no further dressing is required. Suitable cord is attached to the two lugs of the caliper and the desired weight is attached with the cord suspended over a pulley.

The caliper should be inspected twice daily to ensure that a satisfactory grip is maintained, and it may be tightened as necessary. Close watch must be kept for any sign of infection about the pins.

THE CRUTCHFIELD CALIPER

The Crutchfield skull traction caliper (Fig. 155) is fixed into the upper part of the skull. Its successful placement and retention need careful planning. The pins designed to penetrate the outer table of the skull have protective shoulders to prevent their penetrating too deeply at the time of insertion or tightening. Their diameter corresponds to that of special drills used to prepare the holes in the skull.

TECHNIQUE

The patient lies supine upon a completely flat trolley or operation table. The tongs are offered to the head directly above the external auditory meatus. A small area of hair is shaved around the proposed site of each pin, and the exposed scalp is cleaned.

To decide the exact point for insertion of the pins requires much care. When in place, the pins must enter the skull exactly at right angles. Allowance must be made for the thickness of the scalp and for the depth of insertion if the correct angle of pin entry is to be achieved. The points of insertion must also be exactly level on either side of the vertex. If there is any angling of the line of traction the upper pin is liable to pull out, with sudden loss of traction.

The area of the scalp selected for the insertion of each pin is infiltrated with local anaesthetic. When the anaesthetic has taken effect the scalp is incised with a small cruciform incision. The drill bit, attached to the brace, is inserted through the incision and rested gently upon the skull. Any sudden movement is painful for the patient and should be avoided. The alignment of the drill is now checked in two planes to ensure that it is at right angles to the bone. The drill is then rotated slowly so that the bit enters as far as its protective shoulder allows. The procedure is repeated on the other side.

The tongs are now inserted. The locking nut (Fig. 155) is freed so that it cannot interfere with

tightening of the tongs. The compressing screw is then tightened and the locking nut is screwed home, but not too tightly.

Daily tightening of the caliper is necessary to maintain a good hold. First the locking nut is

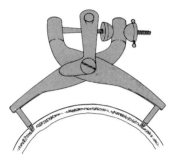

Fig. 155. Crutchfield skull caliper. The pins are shouldered to prevent penetration beyond the outer table of the skull.

undone three or four turns. The compressing screw is then gently tightened, and the locking nut is screwed home again.

For the patient's comfort it is important to remember that anything knocking against the tongs transmits the vibration directly to the skull because of the tight fit. This is very uncomfortable and disturbing.

FUSION OF ATLANTO-AXIAL JOINT

Atlanto-axial fusion is effected by wiring the posterior arch of the atlas to the spinous process of the axis and incorporating in the wire loop a cortico-cancellous bone graft after rawing of the recipient bone of the atlas and axis. This is not an operation that should be undertaken by the occasional operator or novice. There are potentially serious hazards, especially if full reduction of any atlanto-axial displacement has not been gained. The technique to be described is basically that of McGraw and Rusch (1973).

PRELIMINARY STUDIES AND PREPARATIONS

It is necessary to determine from radiographs before operation to what extent the atlanto-axial joint is unstable, and in which position there is the

greatest stability: usually this is in moderate extension. In a case of severe instability it is advisable to apply skull calipers to facilitate longitudinal traction during and after the operation. If necessary, the calipers may be inserted under local anaesthesia before the induction of the general anaesthetic. In cases of long-standing disability without severe displacement skull caliper traction may be omitted.

TECHNIQUE

Position of patient. Although it is common practice to undertake this operation with the patient prone, the authors prefer to have the patient in the lateral position with the head suitably supported on a firm pad or rest so that there is no lateral inclination. The head should be in a position of slight extension. If skull calipers have been applied for the purpose of maintaining traction, the line of pull of the weight is so adjusted that the head is held in the optimal position.

by 3 centimetres wide is cut from the wing of the ilium. It should consist of the outer cortex together with the cancellous layer (see p. 76). The graft is trimmed and shaped to fit the prepared bed. It should be just long enough to extend from

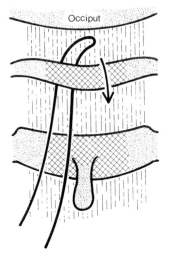 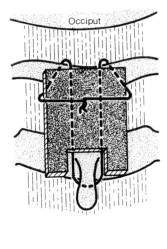

FIGS 156–157. Technique of wiring bone graft to posterior arches of atlas and axis (after McGraw and Rusch 1973). Figure 156—Looped wire being inserted deep to arch of atlas from below, ready to be brought down over spinous process of axis. Rawed areas of the atlas and axis are shown cross-hatched. Figure 157—Graft in position; wire twisted superficial to graft to hold it in place.

Exposure. A midline incision is made from the lower margin of the occiput to the spinous process of the third cervical vertebra—that is, the second palpable spinous process. The muscles are stripped from the underlying posterior arch of the atlas and from the spinous process and laminae of the axis vertebra. The muscles are held aside by self-retaining retractors. In stripping the muscles from the back of the atlas the surgeon must take care to avoid injuring the vertebral artery, which lies only about 1.5 centimetres from the midline.

Preparation of bed for graft. A flat raw surface is prepared on the back of the posterior arch of the atlas and on the laminae of the axis by cutting away the cortex finely with a small chisel. Care must be taken not to remove more than a very thin layer of cortex, lest the remaining bone be rendered unduly fragile (Fig. 156).

Preparation of bone graft. A rectangular piece of bone measuring approximately 4 centimetres long

the upper margin of the posterior arch of the atlas to the lower margin of the spinous process of the axis. A deep notch should be cut in the lower end of the graft to accommodate the spinous process of the axis (Fig. 157).

Wiring the graft in position. A length of strong (gauge 20) stainless steel wire is formed into a loop and passed deep to the posterior arch of the atlas in a proximal direction after separation of the posterior occipito-atlantoid membrane from the bone (Fig. 156). The loop of wire is then turned downwards over the posterior arch of the atlas and hooked below the spinous process of the axis. This loop of wire is drawn tight by steady traction upon the ends of the wire: excessive force must not be used for fear of fracturing the bone. The bone graft is now laid in position in close contact with the rawed bed, and the ends of the wire are folded round the sides of the graft, in which small notches should be cut to accommodate the wire, and tied or twisted near the midline (Fig. 157).

Any projecting end of the wire should be turned over and buried in the tissues.

Closure. The muscles are sutured together in the midline over the graft, and the skin is closed with interrupted eversion sutures without drainage.

POST-OPERATIVE MANAGEMENT

If skull calipers are in position weight traction may be maintained for four to seven days, after which a cervical brace is applied. This should be worn for ten to twelve weeks according to the progress of union.

Comment

The lateral posture as described offers advantages to the anaesthetist and also to the surgeon. In particular, the position of the head is easily adjusted. A further advantage is that the risk of harmful pressure upon the eyes, which has on occasions led to serious complications including blindness, is eliminated.

OCCIPITO-CERVICAL FUSION

Occipito-cervical fusion may extend from the occiput to the atlas or, more usually, to the axis vertebra. Exceptionally an even greater number of segments may be included. The operation entails exposure of the base of the occiput and of the posterior aspect of the upper segments of the cervical column. After rawing of the bones they are then bridged by abundant slivers of cancellous bone. This operation should not be undertaken by the inexperienced surgeon.

TECHNIQUE

Position of patient. The patient is positioned in the lateral posture as for atlanto-axial fusion. It is usual to apply skull calipers at the beginning of the operation and to maintain traction during the operation.

Exposure. The exposure is the same as for atlanto-axial fusion (page 116) except that it extends upwards over the base of the occiput. The bones are exposed by stripping aside the muscles from the base of the occiput and from the posterior elements of the relevant vertebrae. Great care must be taken to avoid injuring the vertebral arteries (Fig. 158) or their branches by keeping the deep dissection within 15 millimetres of the midline and by separating the tissues by blunt dissection. Alternatively, the arteries may be located where they wind round the articular masses of the atlas and suitably protected.

Preparation of bed for grafts. The backs of the relevant vertebrae are rawed in the same way as for atlanto-axial fusion. The occiput is rawed over an area of 3 or 4 centimetres which extends proximally (backwards) from the margin of the foramen magnum.

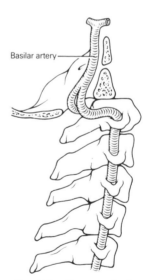

Fig. 158. Course of the right (and higher up of the left) vertebral artery. The two arteries join to form the basilar artery.

Application of grafts. Cancellous grafts are obtained from the ilium and laid in the prepared bed. Generally, bone chips or long slivers are preferred to a solid sheet of cortico-cancellous bone because it is impracticable to anchor such a graft to the occiput by wire in the manner recommended for atlanto-axial fusion. The bone grafts are held in place by firmly suturing the muscles over them in the midline.

POST-OPERATIVE MANAGEMENT

If there is no marked instability of the affected region of the spine a Minerva-type plaster jacket may be applied either immediately or within a few days of the operation. If there has been marked instability it is better to maintain traction through skull calipers for the first four weeks and' thereafter to apply a Minerva jacket. An alternative method of external fixation is to apply a "halo" to the skull and to incorporate the bars in a plaster jacket.

POSTERIOR FUSION OF CERVICAL SPINE

Posterior cervical fusion may be confined to one intervertebral joint or it may extend over several segments, depending upon the nature and extent of the pathology. Basically the method consists in rawing the posterior elements (laminae and spinous processes) and laying in cancellous bone grafts from the ilium. Grafting is usually combined with wire fixation of the spinous processes in order to maintain a stable position while the grafts become incorporated.

TECHNIQUE

The technique is basically similar to that of atlanto-axial fusion (p. 116). Either a solid sheet of cortico-cancellous iliac bone is used or, more usually, large cancellous slivers. In either case the graft material should be abundant. Heavy gauge wire should be used to anchor the spinous processes.

POST-OPERATIVE MANAGEMENT

If the fusion is designed to bridge only one intervertebral space and if good fixation by wire has been secured, it is sufficient to rely upon a cervical brace to support the neck until the grafts are consolidated. If the fusion extends over several segments it may be wise to provide more efficient immobilisation by means of a Minerva-type plaster jacket. It may be well to defer the application of the plaster until the patient is able to cooperate—usually a week or two after the operation—and in the meantime to rely upon a brace.

ANTERIOR CERVICAL FUSION

An intervertebral joint in the cervical spine may be fused by removal of the intervertebral disc from the front and insertion of a cancellous bone graft in the resulting cavity. Any joint from the third cervical vertebra to the first thoracic may be fused in this way. The operation may be confined to a single intervertebral space, or two or more joints may be fused at the same operation. This operation should not be undertaken by the inexperienced operator.

PRELIMINARY STUDIES

The precise level of the lesion for which fusion is to be undertaken is not always easily established. The level is determined from a combination of clinical observation with particular reference to neurological signs in the upper limbs, plain radiographs, and if necessary cineradiography or discography.

TECHNIQUE

Position of patient. The patient lies supine. A small pad is placed between the scapulae to allow the neck to rest in a slightly extended position. The head is rotated 10 degrees to the right.

Incision. The approach is on the left side of the neck between the midline structures (trachea, oesophagus and thyroid gland) and the carotid sheath. (Some surgeons make the approach on the right side.) For fusion of a single joint a transverse incision in a skin crease at the approximate level of the affected joint is appropriate. If multiple joints are to be fused an oblique incision along the anterior margin of the sternocleidomastoid muscle is to be preferred.

important structures and it may be exposed by retracting the carotid sheath laterally and the midline structures in the opposite direction. Access is limited proximally by the superior thyroid artery and distally by the inferior thyroid artery. If necessary, one or other of these vessels may be divided. The pretracheal fascia is incised just medial to the carotid artery. The plane deep to the pretracheal fascia is opened up by blunt dissection towards the midline (Fig. 159). The thyroid gland, trachea and oesophagus are retracted further across. To expose the prevertebral muscles and the anterior longitudinal ligament behind the oesophagus the prevertebral fascia, which is semi-transparent, is divided vertically near the midline. The cervical sympathetic chain lying over the longus colli muscle just lateral to

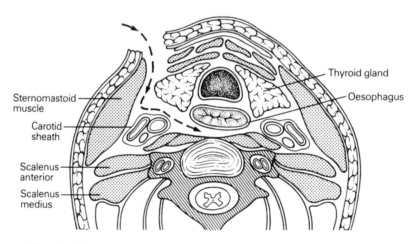

FIG. 159. Transverse section through neck indicating the route of approach to the vertebral bodies.

Exposure of spinal column. First the fascia along the medial border of the sternocleidomastoid muscle is incised vertically and the muscle is mobilised and retracted laterally. The sternohyoid, sternothyroid and omohyoid muscles are retracted medially and inferiorly. The carotid sheath is thus exposed and the common carotid artery is identified by feeling its pulsation. Between the medial border of the carotid sheath and the lateral margin of the anterior midline structures (thyroid gland, trachea and oesophagus) the pretracheal fascia is not overlaid by

the vertebral bodies is identified and preserved. Close to the midline the glistening anterior longitudinal ligament covers the fronts of the vertebral bodies and the intervening discs.

Identification of level. Unless the level chosen for fusion is clearly identifiable by large osteophytes or other structural features shown in the radiographs it is wise to identify the joints to be fused radiographically. To this end a radio-opaque marker is placed over the disc at the supposed correct level and a lateral radiograph is taken.

Preparation of bed for graft. A rectangular flap of anterior longitudinal ligament with its base medially is raised and turned over to expose the selected disc. Disc material is removed and the opposing vertebral end plates above and below are cut away with a fine chisel, with care to preserve the anterior margin to restrain the graft. The resection of the vertebral end plates should be sufficient to expose cancellous bone.

Preparation of bone graft. The dimensions of the space between the rawed vertebrae are measured and a cortico-cancellous bone graft removed from the crest of the ilium is trimmed to size, the graft being orientated so that its rounded cortical margin—that is, the upper margin of the crest—is directed anteriorly.

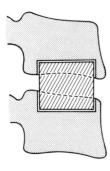

FIG. 160. Diagram showing method of locking the graft by recessing the vertebral bodies behind the anterior cortex.

Insertion of graft. The neck is extended to widen the space between the vertebral bodies, which may be further spread apart by judicious retraction with blunt hooks. This enables the graft to be inserted in the prepared space, and when the extension and traction force is released the graft is locked in place by the overhanging anterior margins of the vertebral bodies (Fig. 160). It is thus stable without further fixation.

Closure. The structures fall naturally into place and light repair of the fascial planes and of the platysma suffices. The skin wound may be closed with a subcuticular suture.

POST-OPERATIVE MANAGEMENT

When a single cervical joint has been fused it is sufficient to support the neck in a well moulded brace for eight to ten weeks. If fusion has been carried out at more than one level, more rigid support from a Minerva-type plaster jacket may be advisable. This is best applied two weeks after the operation when the wound is well healed and the patient fit enough to sit upon a stool.

Comment

Although anterior fusion is nowadays often advised in preference to posterior fusion, it is important that the hazards be borne in mind and avoided by a meticulous technique. Possible hazards during the exposure include perforation of the pharynx or oesophagus, injury to the recurrent laryngeal nerve, and injury to the sympathetic chain with consequent Horner's syndrome. The left recurrent laryngeal nerve is probably less vulnerable than the right: hence the common choice of approach through the left side of the neck (Robinson *et al.* 1962). To avoid damage to important structures the surgeon must have a detailed knowledge of the anatomy of the neck, and unless he undertakes the operation regularly he should freshen his knowledge by dissection in a cadaver.

The need for extreme caution in the removal of disc material hardly needs to be emphasised. The spinal cord is very close to the back of the intervertebral disc, and careless or hasty avulsion of disc material or injudicious use of the chisel in removing the vertebral end plates may easily cause irreversible damage to the cord, as is testified by a number of court actions that have been reported.

CHAPTER FOUR

Thoracic and Lumbar Spine

The range of orthopaedic operations that are carried out routinely upon the spine is small: two operations—removal of extruded disc material and intervertebral fusion—together make up the great bulk of the spinal work undertaken at most orthopaedic centres.

In conditions affecting this region careful selection of patients for operation is especially important. Indifferent results are all too frequent, and before advising operation the surgeon must be satisfied that a remediable organic lesion is indeed present: there is no room here for a hit-or-miss approach.

It is important also that the first operation be made effective: revision operations necessitated by technical faults at the initial procedure are notoriously prone to fail— perhaps from extensive scarring or perhaps partly because the patient has become demoralised. Most orthopaedic surgeons have encountered those tragic cases in which the patient seems to become worse after each successive operation and ends up a chronic spinal invalid. If there is any way in which such depressing cases can be made less frequent it is by precision in diagnosis and precision in operative technique.

CONTENTS OF CHAPTER

COSTOTRANSVERSECTOMY FOR DRAINAGE OF PARASPINAL ABSCESS

Costotransversectomy entails removal of the transverse process of a thoracic vertebra and of the proximal part of the related rib in order to gain access to the side of the vertebral body for drainage of an abscess. The operation is now seldom required except in countries where spinal tuberculosis is still common.

PRELIMINARY STUDIES

Good antero-posterior radiographs are essential to outline clearly the soft-tissue shadow thrown by the abscess (Fig. 161). Often the bulge is apparent on both sides of the midline, but the shadow is usually larger on one or other side: this side should be selected for the decompression. In order to ensure that the operation is carried out at the correct level it is wise to obtain a radiograph the skin incision, and with a periosteal elevator the medial part of the muscle mass is stripped from the lamina of the vertebra and, a little more later-

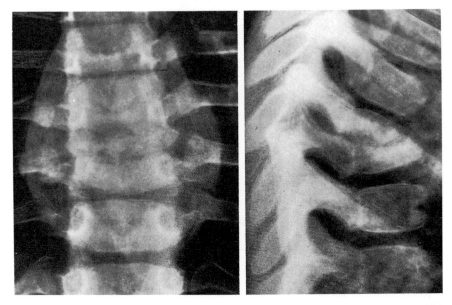

FIG. 161. Paraspinal abscess from tuberculosis of the lower part of the thoracic spine in a child. The abscess is seen as a fusiform shadow on either side of the spinal column.

before operation with an opaque marker placed over the rib that has been selected for removal. The opaque marker will show whether in fact the rib has been correctly chosen. As a general rule the rib to be removed should be that which lies over the most prominent part of the paraspinal abscess shadow.

TECHNIQUE

Position of patient. The patient lies in the lateral position with the side to be operated upon uppermost.

Incision. The incision begins close to the midline and extends laterally and slightly downwards in the line of the rib that is to be resected (Fig. 162). The skin edges are spread apart with a self-retaining retractor to allow incision of the fascia overlying the posterior spinal muscles.

Exposure and removal of transverse process. The posterior spinal muscles are divided in the line of

ally, from the back of the transverse process. When the whole of the transverse process has been cleared it is divided at its base with a sharp osteotome and cut free with blunt-pointed scissors (Fig. 163).

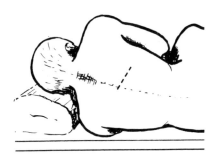

FIG. 162. Costo-transversectomy. The skin incision.

Excision of medial part of rib. Deep to the transverse process is found the related rib, the medial end of which is inclined steeply forwards towards the articulation of the rib with the postero-lateral part of the vertebral body. When the rib has been cleared of muscle as far laterally as about 8 centimetres from the midline the periosteum is incised along the back of the rib and stripped from the bone with a suitable curved elevator. In this manoeuvre care should be taken to ensure that the pleura and the medial wall by the vertebral body. In cases of chronic abscess the pleura is thickened. In most cases the abscess is easily opened by passing a blunt, well curved bone lever anteriorly along the side of the vertebral body. The surgeon

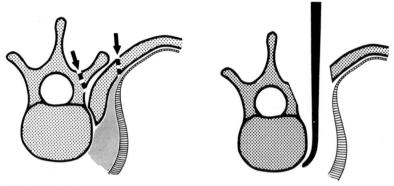

FIGS 163–164. Costo-transversectomy. Figure 163—Diagram showing site of division of transverse process and rib. Pus has distended the space between the pleura and the vertebral body. Figure 164—After excision of the transverse process and of the head and neck of the rib, the cavity is widened by careful insertion of a blunt-ended, well curved bone lever and evacuated by suction.

instrument remains close to bone and does not transgress the periosteal layer. The next stage is to divide the rib at the lateral extremity of the incision, 7 or 8 centimetres from the midline. The outer end of the rib is then grasped with sequestrum forceps, and with curved blunt-pointed scissors aided by gentle twisting of the rib its medial attachments are severed and the whole of the exposed part of the rib, including the head, is removed (Figs 163–164).

Location of abscess. In the depth of the wound the lateral wall of the cavity is now formed by

should make sure that he feels the blunt point of the instrument to be in contact with bone throughout. The instrument enters the abscess cavity and pus gushes forth from the wound. Evacuation of the abscess may be aided by passing a curved suction tube towards the front of the vertebral body (Fig. 164).

Closure. In cases of chronic abscess—almost always tuberculous—the wound may be closed in layers once all the pus has been evacuated. The skin is closed with interrupted eversion sutures.

ANTERO-LATERAL DECOMPRESSION OF SPINAL CANAL

This operation—not very aptly named because the opening into the spinal canal is lateral rather than antero-lateral—may be regarded as a radical extension of costotransversectomy, being designed to give access to the lateral aspect of the pedicles of three or four contiguous vertebrae. Then by removal of the pedicles the spinal canal is opened from the side.

Like costotransversectomy, the operation is done with the patient in the lateral position. A curved incision outlines a flap based at the midline. Its length depends upon the extent of the exposure required: usually three or more ribs are exposed according to the extent of the underlying lesion.

After stripping of the muscles the transverse processes and the medial ends of the ribs are excised, as in costotransversectomy. Next the intercostal nerves are identified and traced medially. They lead the surgeon to the intervertebral foramina and thus to the pedicles of the vertebrae. When the pedicles have been cleared they are removed piecemeal with nibbling forceps.

For further details of this operation the reader is referred to the papers by Alexander (1946) and Capener (1954) and to the monograph by Griffiths, Seddon and Roaf (1956).

SPONDYLOTOMY FOR REMOVAL OF PROLAPSED INTERVERTEBRAL DISC

This operation, often referred to as laminectomy—a term that may be inappropriate because sometimes little or none of the lamina is removed—was reported by Mixter and Barr in 1934. The operation entails removal of part of the posterior wall of the spinal canal in order to expose the dural sac with the contained cauda equina, and displacement of the lateral edge of the sac medially to reveal deep to it the bulging disc material that has escaped; this is removed together with other accessible parts of the nucleus pulposus.

TECHNIQUE

Position of patient. The patient is placed prone on a special supporting frame or mattress (Fig. 165). An unsupported area is left in front so that there is no pressure on the abdomen. This prevents any impairment of ventilated respiration, which would cause venous dilation and increased bleeding. The patient's head is supported on a special horseshoe-shaped support which allows full choice to the anaesthetist of the head and neck position. Great care is taken to place the

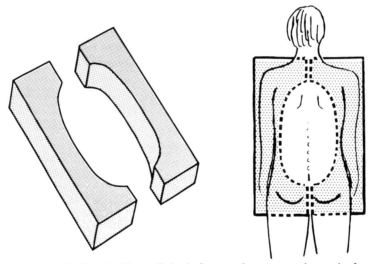

FIGS 165–166. Shaped pillows of plastic foam used to support the trunk of a patient in the prone position for removal of prolapsed lumbar disc. The shoulders, sternum and pelvis rest upon the pillows, but the lower chest and the abdomen are free from the pressure of body weight.

The description that follows refers to the exploration of a single intervertebral joint, but it must be appreciated that in many cases, if not in most, the surgeon will wish to explore two intervertebral levels and in exceptional cases three. Nevertheless the basic technique at each level is the same, and it is simply repeated at the second or third level.

patient's arms on well-padded supports on either side of the head. Care must be taken when moving the arms into position that the brachial plexus is not strained. The padding of the arm supports prevents any pressure damage to the nerves in the arms.

Incision. A gently curved skin incision about 12

centimetres long is made from the spinous process above the suspected level of the prolapse down to the sacrum (Fig. 166). An indication of the spinous process level is obtained by noting that the spinous process of the fourth lumbar vertebra is level with the iliac crest.

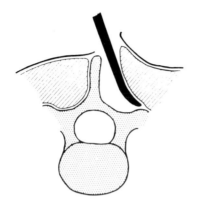

FIG. 167. Stripping of posterior spinal muscles from spinous processes and laminae.

The deep exposure. Before the incision is deepened the plain antero-posterior radiograph is checked to ensure that there is no spina bifida. If a spina bifida is present the lack of the lamina means that the spinal theca is exposed to any forceful deep incision. If the anatomy is normal the supraspinous ligament is preserved. Incisions are made on either side of the spinous processes at the definitive level and above and below. These are deepened on each side to the lamina. Distally the deep incision is extended down to the sacrum on the side of the lesion. With a Cobb's periosteal elevator the paraspinal muscles on each side are separated laterally from the spinous processes (Fig. 167). This elevator is broad enough to avoid any danger of slipping between adjacent laminae and penetrating to the spinal theca. A large self-retaining retractor such as the Harvey Jackson is inserted to separate the muscles.

Identifying the required level of exploration. The anatomical level is next to be confirmed. The sacrum has a posterior wall formed of a continuous sheet of bone and is therefore easily identified.

The lateral radiograph of the sacrum is checked to identify any mobile first sacral segment. Tapping on the sacral bone with the Cobb's periosteal elevator produces a hollow sound which is different from that obtained by tapping a lamina. Counting from the sacrum, the correct level of operation is identified. If there is any doubt concerning the level, a bone-holding forceps is clamped on the probable spinous process above the surgical site and a lateral radiograph is taken on the table.

Exploration of site of prolapse. The interspinous ligament is incised with a number 12 blade on a 3L handle. The hooked shape of this blade prevents any chance of the blade's slipping and penetrating

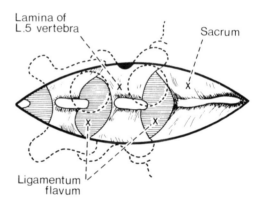

FIG. 168. Removal of prolapsed disc at two levels. Diagram showing outline of circular windows to be cut through laminae and ligamenta flava for access to the spinal canal. In many cases sufficient access can be gained without removal of bone from the lamina.

the spinal canal. A bone spreader is then inserted between the spinous processes and deep to the supraspinous ligament, which remains intact. The spreader is opened and a greatly improved view of the ligamentum flavum is obtained, bridging the space between the laminae. The adjacent laminae are cleared of all soft tissue remnants by a small periosteal elevator (Fig. 168).

The next stage is to enter the spinal canal. This must be done very delicately because the disc prolapse may be pressing the dura tightly against the deep surface of the ligamentum flavum. A 15 blade on a 5 or 7 handle is used. The ligamentum flavum is incised longitudinally as close to the median line as possible. The blunt end of a Watson-Cheyne probe is used to test for the breach in the ligamentum flavum. When the opening has been shown, a wet neuro-pattie soaked in saline is passed through to separate the dura from the deep surface of the ligamentum flavum. With this in position it is safe to incise the ligamentum flavum laterally from the initial longitudinal incision. The opened corner of ligamentum flavum is raised, being gripped by long fine-toothed forceps such as Waugh's tonsil dissecting forceps. A small area of the ligamentum is then excised. Further removal of ligamentum is achieved by the use of bone cutting punch forceps (for instance, Kerrison pattern). These cut upwards away from the dura and are therefore safer than down-cutting forceps which would cut towards the dura.

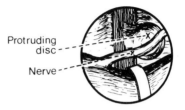

FIG. 170. Enlarged view through the circular window showing protruded globule of disc material with nerve stretched over it.

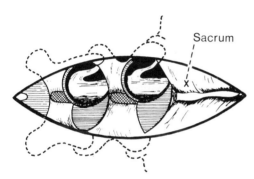

FIG. 169. The circular windows have been cut out. The spinal theca and the issuing nerve are seen through each opening.

Access to the space between the laminae is improved by widening the arc of the bone spreader. It is often unnecessary to excise any bone from the margins of the laminae, but a small fringe may be nibbled away if necessary (Fig. 169).

Identification and removal of prolapsed disc material. The field is now clear for inspection of the issuing nerve and the posterior aspect of the intervertebral disc (Fig. 170).

First, excess dural fat is teased away to expose the bluish surface of the dura, which forms the tough outer wall of the spinal theca. An O'Connell nerve root retractor or an equivalent fine, blunt

instrument is used to press gently on the theca to check its tension. If there is a large underlying bulging disc the theca will be very tense.

The recurved end of the nerve root retractor is faced laterally and it is gently passed lateral to the theca and advanced until it reaches the posterior surface of the vertebral body. It is then gently rotated so that the recurved end is anterior to the theca. The dura can then be displaced medially, exposing the underlying disc bulge. The relevant nerve root may have been displaced medially, anterior to the dura, or laterally, with the bulging disc occupying the axilla of the nerve root.

Any bleeding is cleared by an Adson or equivalent sucker. It is noted that these suckers have a hole made in their shaft. This is usually left uncovered as the degree of suction is sufficient to clear blood from the spinal canal. If it is closed the suction is so powerful that tissue is sucked into the sucker end and it is thereby blocked.

If no bulging disc is seen this may be because of the patient's position on the table or the action of the bone spreader in flattening a bulging disc by spreading the posterior longitudinal ligament. If the disc cannot be identified by vision it can be sought by probing with the sharp end of a Watson-Cheyne probe. This is then inserted into the disc space. With the disc certainly identified, the theca and nerve are protected by the nerve root retractor. The disc is incised with the fine-bladed scalpel. In a florid case this allows disc material almost to extrude spontaneously.

The disc space is then explored by a fine pituitary rongeur, such as a Beck's rongeur with a 2 millimetre bite. If there is a large prolapse it may be possible to remove a large part of the disc in one piece. If not, the disc removal is performed piecemeal. The disc material resembles white crab meat.

Further disc material is removed by the use of larger and angled rongeurs. They must be passed gently into the disc space. Many angled rongeurs cannot easily be passed into the disc space because of the sharpness of their angle. They must not be forced in. No rongeur should be inserted more than 2 centimetres into a disc space, for fear of its penetrating the anterior longitudinal ligament and damaging the great vessels.

At the conclusion of this stage of the operation the nerve which was previously stretched or displaced is shown to be free of all obstruction and mobile. Some small portion of disc material may have been displaced down along the nerve root canal. The patency of the canal can be checked by passing a fine soft catheter along the root canal. An endobronchial catheter number 6 is suitable for this.

Closure. The erector spinae muscle is allowed to fall back into place and held by suture of the overlying aponeurosis. Skin is repaired by tension sutures and interrupted eversion sutures. Drainage is not required.

POST-OPERATIVE MANAGEMENT

A programme of early activity is recommended. After one to three days in bed the patient is allowed up and is encouraged to walk. At that stage gentle spine flexion and extension exercises are begun on the bed, the patient assisting flexion by pulling himself forward with a rope attached to the foot of the bed.

Comment

The standard operation as described above is straightforward and not unduly difficult in a clear-cut case of disc prolapse in the lower lumbar region. The main essential is a delicate surgical technique whereby unnecessary damage to the spinal canal, and particularly to the theca and the issuing nerves, is avoided.

Removal of the initial window in the posterior wall of the spinal canal, through which to approach the theca and the disc, must be undertaken with particular care: a too hasty incision through the ligamentum flavum may lacerate the theca, which lies close under the deep surface of the ligament. Once the initial opening has been made it can be enlarged with relative safety, for the plane between the ligament and the theca is then easily defined.

When the exploration reaches a deeper plane, display of the issuing nerve and of the back of the intervertebral disc may be hindered by bleeding from small veins that form a network upon the posterior surface of the spinal column. Such bleeding may have to be controlled by neuropatties moistened in saline. These have radio-opaque markers and an attached thread which is led to the surface of the wound to aid their identification and retrieval. Several can be packed proximally and distally to control bleeding at the site for incision into the disc space. A slender sucker tube with a single perforation to control the suction is also indispensable.

The posterior surface of the disc is best exposed by teasing away the overlying areolar and fatty tissue with fine non-toothed forceps while the dural sac is held medially by the sucker tube or by a suitable fine retractor. The surface of a bulging disc has a characteristic white glistening appearance, and once it is exposed to view there is no difficulty in incising it safely with a fine-bladed knife.

One of the difficulties in lumbar disc operations is to be sure from inspection and palpation of a disc whether it is normal or abnormal. The major prolapse or the sequestrated disc is unmistakable: these are the lesions that the surgeon likes to find, and removal of such a disc is always attended by dramatic relief of pain. Doubt arises in cases of slight bulging, when the variation from normal may be ill defined. When such a disc is encountered it is usually advisable to explore adjacent levels before a decision is made to incise the posterior wall of the disc and to tease out the disc material. In a doubtful case it may also be wise to extend the exposure by removal of laminae in order to be sure that the exploration has been comprehensive and that a hidden lesion such as a displaced disc sequestrum is not overlooked.

The need to avoid over-penetration of the disc with pituitary forceps has already been emphasised. Many cases are on record in which the anterior longitudinal ligament has been perforated and damage has been inflicted upon the great vessels lying in front of the spinal column (Birkeland and Taylor 1969). It is only necessary to remove relatively loose pieces of disc material from the interior of the disc: nothing is gained by over-zealous efforts to remove the entire disc.

VARIATIONS OF TECHNIQUE

There is some difference of opinion among surgeons as to the position of the patient and as to the extent of the exposure. Some surgeons find over-riding advantages in the lateral posture of the patient, particularly in the greater comfort that it provides for the anaesthetist and for the surgeon (Fig. 195). It also allows full flexion of the lumbar spine with widening of the interlaminar spaces achieved without the need for a bone spreader.

The knee-chest (tuck) position has also been used but it is not recommended because it imposes an unnecessary risk of renal complications secondary to compression of major vessels in the lower limbs (Keim and Weinstein 1970).

With regard to the exposure of the theca and nerves, some surgeons prefer to use a much wider exposure than that described, by removing the entire lamina on one side as well as the ligamentum flavum. Some surgeons go so far as to remove spinous processes and to undertake complete laminectomy in order to deroof the whole width of the spinal canal. This certainly allows a comprehensive view of the spinal theca and of the issuing nerves. In a clear-cut case such a wide exposure seems unnecessary, but if the findings prove indefinite as viewed through a small window it is a simple matter to enlarge the opening secondarily to obtain a wider view.

MIDLINE PROTRUSIONS

Disc protrusions extending towards the midline may usually be suspected before operation, from impairment of cauda equina function. Their removal may entail a transdural approach. The posterior wall of the dura is incised vertically and the edges are retracted with fine holding sutures. The nerves of the cauda equina are separated and retracted away from the midline, to reveal the bulging disc in the depth of the wound. The extruded disc material is removed in the usual way after incision of the anterior wall of the theca and of the posterior longitudinal ligament. When the disc has been dealt with the incision in the dura is closed with fine interrupted absorbable sutures.

POSTERIOR FUSION OF THORACIC SPINE

Posterior fusion of the thoracic spine is seldom required except in cases of severe scoliosis, when it is used to stabilise the spine after correction has been gained by Harrington rods, by Luque rods, or by some other means. In these cases the patient is usually an adolescent girl. Occasionally it may be found necessary to carry out the operation with the patient in traction or in a plaster jacket, when a suitable window must be cut to allow access.

The technique usually employed is that recommended by Moe (1958), which consists essentially in denuding each of the postero-lateral (facet) joints of articular cartilage, roughening the subchondral bone, and driving in a cancellous sliver graft between the joint surfaces. At the same time the backs of the laminae are roughened in petal fashion and the whole series of laminae in the area to be fused is bridged by sliver grafts obtained from the spinous processes and from the ilium.

The number of segments to be fused depends upon the length of the curve. Often almost the whole length of the thoracic spine is involved and indeed the fusion may have to be extended to the upper lumbar region.

TECHNIQUE

Position of patient. The position may be dictated to some extent by a retentive apparatus attached to the patient. The lateral posture is often the most practicable.

Incision. A posterior midline incision is made, corresponding in length to the number of segments to be fused. A separate incision is made over the wing of the ilium on one or both sides for removal of bone grafts.

Exposure of laminae and posterior (facet) joints. The deep fascia is incised in the midline and separated from the spinous processes on each side. With a broad rounded elevator the erector spinae muscles are stripped from the spinous processes and then from the backs of the laminae as far laterally as the facet joints. The muscles are spread apart by self-retaining retractors. Remnants of adherent muscle are cleared from the bones, and the facet joints are opened and thoroughly exposed by removal of ligamentous tissue.

Preparation of surfaces for grafting. With fine sharp chisels the surface of each lamina is roughened by raising small flakes of the surface bone in such a way that each flake remains attached at its base in the manner of a petal of a flower (hence the term "petalling" for this technique). Each facet joint in turn is then denuded of articular cartilage from each surface, and the subchondral bone is roughened by multiple small chisel cuts.

Preparation of bone grafts. As much bone as can readily be obtained is taken from the wing of the ilium on one or both sides (see p. 75). The grafts are cut up into small elongated slivers, sized appropriately to fit between the rawed surfaces of the facet joints.

Application of grafts. Cancellous sliver grafts are impacted securely into each of the facet joints in turn. Attention is then turned to the laminae, which must be bridged together through the whole length of the fusion area. To a slight extent this can be done by turning over some of the "petals" that have been raised from the backs of the laminae, but main reliance is placed upon bridging the spaces with slivers obtained from the spinous processes, which are cut off where they join the laminae. The fusion area may be further reinforced by iliac grafts if sufficient bone is available.

Closure. The grafts are held in place by suturing the erector spinae muscles over them. The fascia and skin are closed with interrupted sutures.

POST-OPERATIVE MANAGEMENT

The fusion operation is usually only part of a long programme of treatment of scoliosis, details of which are beyond the scope of this book.

ANTERIOR FUSION OF THORACIC SPINE

Anterior fusion of the thoracic spine through a transpleural approach is undertaken mainly for destructive lesions in tuberculosis. Owing to the steep decline in the incidence of tuberculosis the operation is now seldom required in Western countries. It is still used commonly, however, in countries where florid spinal tuberculosis is still prevalent. For details of the operation the reader is referred to the paper of Hodgson and Stock (1960).

POSTERIOR LUMBAR INTERVERTEBRAL FUSION WITH SCREW FIXATION

Posterior fusion with screw fixation is applicable mainly to the lowest two lumbar intervertebral joints. A prerequisite is that the neural arches must be intact. The technique to be described is that of Boucher (1959), as modified by Kirwan (1977). Internal fixation is by a pair of screws at each level. At the lumbo-sacral joint the screws traverse the outer part of the lamina and pass downwards and outwards into the ala of the sacrum. At the L.4–5 joint each screw traverses the outer part of the lamina of the fourth lumbar vertebra and is directed downwards and slightly outwards to engage the body of the fifth lumbar vertebra. This fixation is combined with posterior bone-grafting with cortico-cancellous slivers from the ilium.

of L.4–5 fusion, however, the L.5–S.1 joint is also abnormal and should then be fused at the same time.

Position of patient. It is more convenient to undertake this operation with the patient in the prone position rather than in the lateral position. Nevertheless, there are many surgeons who prefer to do the operation with the patient on the side. If the prone position is used special care must be taken that the abdomen is free from pressure from the body weight, which might restrict respiration. Long pillows of plastic foam (Fig. 171) extending longitudinally on each side to support the shoulders and manubrium sterni above and the pelvis below, but allowing the lower part of the

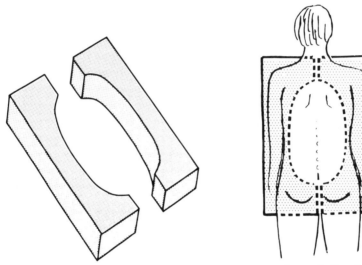

FIGS 171–172. Shaped pillows of plastic foam used to support the trunk of a patient in the prone position for posterior spinal fusion. The shoulders, sternum and pelvis rest upon the pillows, but the lower chest and the abdomen are free from the pressure of body weight.

TECHNIQUE

The description that follows relates to fusion of the lowest two lumbar joints—that is, the L.4–5 joint and the L.5–S.1 joint, the neural arches at each level being intact. In appropriate cases the L.5–S.1 joint alone may be fused, and very occasionally the L.4–5 joint may be fused without fusion of the L.5–S.1 joint, provided that the latter has been proved to be normal: in most cases

thorax and the whole abdomen to be unencumbered (Fig. 172), offer a solution to this problem.

Incision. In its upper half the incision is a vertical one in the midline extending from the spinous process of the third lumbar vertebra to the lower edge of the spinous process of the fifth lumbar vertebra. Thence the incision curves in a gentle sweep to the left to cross the posterior superior spine of the ilium in an oblique direction downwards and outwards (Fig. 173). In the first part of the operation—that devoted to fixation of the vertebrae by screws—only the proximal (vertical) part of the incision is developed.

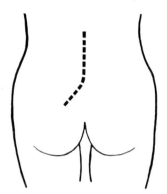

FIG. 173. Posterior fusion of lumbar spine. The skin incision.

Exposure of spinous processes and laminae. The spinal aponeurosis is incised in the midline over the tips of the spinous processes of the fourth and fifth lumbar vertebrae and over the proximal part of the spine of the sacrum. The muscles are stripped from the sides of the spinous processes and from the interspinous ligaments with a large blunt curved elevator (Fig. 174), and in like manner the small deep muscles are cleared from the backs of the laminae and posterior cortex of sacrum and from the intervening ligamenta flava. The muscles can then be spread widely apart with a deep self-retaining retractor so that the whole width of each lamina is cleanly exposed right down to the facet joints. These joints need not be opened except in so far as it may be desirable to remove large osteophytes.

Exploration of nerves in spinal canal and foramina. Depending upon the nature of the case, it may be desirable to open the spinal canal by removal of ligamentum flavum in the manner described in the section on laminectomy for prolapsed intervertebral disc (page 125). In the absence of neurological features, however, it is usually unnecessary to open the spinal canal.

Fixation of L.5 to S.1 with screws. The point at which the screw is to be entered through the

lamina on each side of the midline is marked with an awl. This point should be midway between the upper and lower margins of the lamina and should

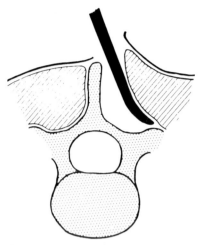

FIG. 174. Stripping of posterior spinal muscles from spinous processes and laminae.

be just medial to the capsule of the facet joint (Fig. 175). In most cases the point of entrance is about 1.75 centimetres from the midline; so the two entrance holes will be approximately 3.5 cen-

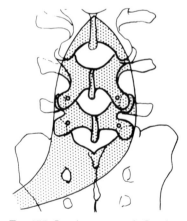

FIG. 175. Laminae exposed. Starting points for the drill holes for the screws are indicated: each lies just medial to the capsule of the facet joint, midway between the upper and lower margins of the lamina.

timetres apart. (The distance varies according to the width of the lamina, which is not constant even in patients of comparable build.)

The track for each screw is prepared with a hand drill. The drilling bit should be 3 millimetres in diameter, and the length projecting from the chuck should be known so that the penetration at any given time may be calculated by measuring the length still visible.

measured on the probe and a Sherman screw of appropriate length is driven home on each side. It will be noted that since each screw deviates 30 degrees laterally from the parasagittal plane the two screws diverge from each other at an angle of 60 degrees (Fig. 176).

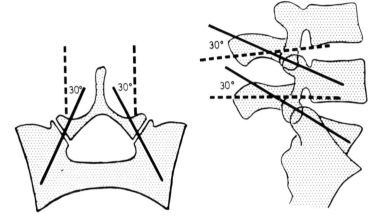

FIGS 176–177. Figure 176—Fixation of fifth lumbar vertebra to sacrum. The drills used to prepare tracks for the screws are inclined laterally at an angle of 30 degrees from the sagittal plane, as shown here, and distally at an angle of 30 degrees from an axis perpendicular to the posterior surface of the spinal column (see Fig. 177). Figure 177—For fixation both of the lumbo-sacral joint and of the L4-5 joint, the drill for the screws is directed 30 degrees downwards (distally) from an axis perpendicular to the back of the spinal column.

When the drill has entered the posterior cortex of the lamina it is tilted in the required direction, downwards and laterally. The correct direction is determined by first orientating the drill at right angles to the posterior bony wall of the spinal canal. The handle of the drill is then tilted so that the direction of travel will be 30 degrees downwards and 30 degrees laterally (Figs 176 and 177). As the drill is operated the surgeon will feel it penetrate very resistant bone in the first 2 centimetres or so of its progress—this being the cortical bone of the articular facets. The drill is then felt to drive on easily: this stage represents penetration of the soft bone of the ala of the sacrum. Penetration should not exceed 4.25 centimetres lest the anterior cortex of the sacrum be penetrated. If the drill is withdrawn and a probe substituted the anterior cortex can be readily palpated provided the drill has not been driven too far. The distance to the anterior cortex can thus be

Screw fixation of L.4—5 joint. The technique is similar to that of inserting screws across the lumbo-sacral joint except that the screws must be directed much less markedly laterally—10 or 15 degrees instead of 30 degrees. The entrance point for the drill on each side is marked as before with an awl, on a corresponding position of the lamina (Fig. 175).

After the drill has been started and has penetrated the posterior cortex of the lamina it is directed at a definitive angle which should be 30 degrees downwards relative to an axis perpendicular to the posterior wall of the spinal canal, but only 10 to 15 degrees laterally (Figs 177 and 178). A drill driven in this direction will first engage hard resistant bone (the margins of the articular facets), but after a distance of 2 centimetres or so has been traversed soft bone is reached and the drill penetrates more rapidly. The depth of the drill hole should be a little less at the L.4—5 joint than at the lumbo-sacral joint—usually 3.5 centimetres. A probe passed into the hole after withdrawal of the drill should be able to palpate the anterior cortex of the fifth lumbar vertebral body, which will receive approximately half the length of the screw.

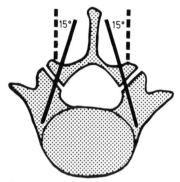

FIG. 178. Fixation of fourth lumbar vertebra to the fifth. The drills are inclined laterally only 10 to 15 degrees from the sagittal plane, as shown here. They are inclined downwards at an angle of 30 degrees (see Fig. 177).

On each side a screw corresponding to the measured depth of the hole is now driven in and tightened snugly, though with care to avoid stripping the thread in the bone.

Taking the cancellous bone grafts. Attention is now turned to the lower half of the wound, where the lower part of the incision passes obliquely downwards and laterally over the region of the posterior superior spine of the ilium. The incision is deepened through the subcutaneous fat to expose the gluteal aponeurosis—the tough fibrous layer covering the gluteus maximus and bounded medially by the crest and medial edge of the wing of the ilium where it forms the posterior superior spine. The incision through this aponeurosis is made obliquely from above downwards and medially, thus crossing the line of the skin incision almost at a right angle (Fig. 179).

Deep to the aponeurosis are the muscle fibres of the gluteus maximus arising from the wing of the ilium close up against its crest and posterior superior spine. The muscle, together with the periosteum to which it is attached, is stripped downwards and outwards with a periosteal elev-

ator to expose the raw bone of the ilium over an area of approximately 5 centimetres square (Fig. 179).

With an osteotome the crest of the ilium and the posterior superior spine are entered midway between the posterior and the anterior cortices,

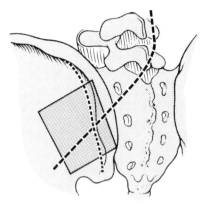

FIG. 179. Oblique diagram from half left showing the line of incision in the gluteal aponeurosis, almost at right angles to the skin incision (indicated by bold interrupted line). The extent of the rectangular iliac bone graft—to include posterior cortex and underlying cancellous bone—is indicated.

and with the same osteotome a "window" measuring about 5 centimetres long by 4 centimetres wide is outlined upon the posterior cortex of the ilium (Fig. 179), which is penetrated with the osteotome down to but not through the anterior (deep) cortex. The "lid" thus outlined is lifted free together with some of the underlying cancellous bone and placed in a tray for use as a graft. Numerous further substantial slivers of cancellous bone are taken from the part of the ilium thus opened, and particularly from the region of the posterior superior spine where the bone is relatively thick.

Preparation of recipient bed and application of grafts. Attention is now turned again to the upper half of the wound, where the laminae of the fourth and fifth lumbar vertebrae and posterior cortex of the upper part of the sacrum are rawed with a gouge. (The instrument devised by Capener is often ideal for this purpose.) Only a thin layer of cortex is to be removed—just enough to expose raw subcortical bone. This decortication may extend also along the sides of the spinous processes, especially near their bases. Here again only a very thin layer of bone must be removed; otherwise the processes may be weakened to the point of fracture.

The slivers of cancellous graft bone are laid upon the raw area on each side of the spinous processes, extending from the upper margin of the lamina of the fourth lumbar vertebra above to the posterior cortex of the sacrum below. Finally, the substantial cortical "lid" obtained from the posterior wall of the ilium is fashioned with a nibbling forceps into the shape of an H, the horizontal bar of which is driven between the spinous processes of the fourth and fifth vertebrae as shown in Figure 180. This cortical lid serves to hold the cancellous slivers in place and also to promote a strong plate of bone on the posterior face of the fusion area.

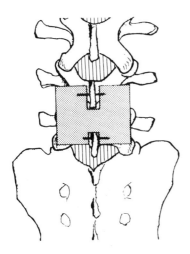

FIG. 180. The H-shaped graft applied between the spinous processes of the fourth and fifth lumbar vertebrae, covering the cancellous sliver grafts (not shown). The H-graft has been locked in position by cross pins.

If the spinous processes are of good length the H-graft may conveniently be secured in position by small cross pins (cut from Kirschner wire) driven transversely through the spinous processes superficial to the graft (Fig. 180).

Closure. The erector spinae muscles are brought together and the overlying aponeurosis is sutured in the midline to hold them in place. Likewise, the gluteal aponeurosis and the underlying fibres of the gluteus maximus are replaced in position and repaired with absorbable sutures. There is inevitably dead space in the donor area, and consequently suction drainage from this region and also from the subcutaneous area of the midline incision is recommended. The skin is closed with deep tension sutures and interrupted skin edge sutures.

POST-OPERATIVE MANAGEMENT

At the conclusion of the operation gauze dressings are secured by adhesive strapping, and if desired a further layer of surgical gauze may be held in place by a many-tail bandage.

The patient should lie flat on the back for the first twelve hours in order to minimise the risk of haematoma formation. Thereafter, there need be no special restrictions and the patient may turn freely in bed or recline propped up on pillows.

Exercises for the lower limbs and static exercises for the posterior spinal muscles are carried out under the supervision of a physiotherapist. Walking is permitted after three to seven days according to progress: sticks or elbow crutches may be provided at first. After discharge from hospital two or three weeks from the time of operation, muscle exercises may be continued and ordinary daily activities are resumed progressively as strength is regained.

Comment

It must be emphasised that the operation described is not applicable in cases of spondylolisthesis with defect of the pars interarticularis, for rigid fixation depends largely upon an intact neural arch.

Provided the steps of the operation are carried out as outlined above, no special technical difficulty is to be expected. Care must be taken, of course (as with any lower lumbar fusion), to identify with certainty the vertebrae concerned in the operation, for cases are known in which fusion has been carried out at the wrong level. The key to the identification is the sacrum. Provided exposure is adequate the sacrum is easily identified positively by the broad sheet of continuous bone that forms its posterior surface. It also gives a characteristic hollow sound when tapped with a forceps. From this starting point the laminae of the fifth and of the fourth vertebrae are easily identified. Nevertheless, if there should be any doubt at all about the identification of level, a radiograph should be obtained after an opaque marker has been placed on the bone concerned.

Drilling the holes for the screws demands care but does not present undue difficulty provided the landmarks and the angles noted above are used. It is to be emphasised that the drill holes do not traverse the facet joints but lie just medial to them, fixing lamina to ala of sacrum in the case of the lumbo-sacral joint and lamina to fifth lumbar vertebral body in the case of the L.4–5 joint. In making the drill holes care should be taken not to overpenetrate the bone: the drill should stop short of the anterior cortex of the sacrum and of the anterior margin of the vertebral body of the fifth vertebra. The anterior cortex in each case can be identified by palpation with a probe.

If the screws have been inserted correctly, the fixity obtained is very striking. Before insertion of the screws the affected vertebra is often unstable and can be moved freely by grasping the spinous process. After fixation with screws no movement at all can be demonstrated between the two vertebrae.

The screws are well away from the midline and consequently there is no risk of damage to the spinal theca. It is possible for a screw to lie in contact with an issuing nerve where it lies close to the pedicle of the vertebra. The nerve slides away from the screw, however, and any ill-effect is confined to sciatic pain in the distribution of the nerve. If this should occur it may be advisable to remove the offending screw or to re-insert it in a slightly different location.

It is important that the bone grafts should not project beyond the limits of the laminae concerned in the fusion; nor should muscle be stripped unnecessarily beyond the proposed site of fusion. Such disturbance even of soft tissues can lead to later trouble in the joints concerned.

Support for the spine in either a plaster jacket or plaster bed has sometimes been recommended, but with the remarkable fixity afforded by the screws it is safe to omit any external support. Any movement imparted to the spine during ordinary activities is absorbed by the freely mobile joint above the fusion area and distally by the hip joints. Thus the joints concerned in the fusion are not subjected to any significant moving force.

LATERAL (INTERTRANSVERSE) FUSION OF LUMBAR SPINE

This operation entails the placing of precisely fashioned grafts between the transverse processes or, in the case of fusion to the sacrum, between transverse processes and the alae of the sacrum. The transverse processes are deeply placed, especially in the lower lumbar region, and the correct fashioning and placing of the grafts demand a meticulous technique. The operation should not be attempted by inexperienced surgeons except with close supervision. The technique to be described is basically that of Adkins (1955).

TECHNIQUE

Position of patient. The authors prefer the patient to be placed in the lateral posture, but if preferred, the operation may be done with the patient prone (see previous section for details of positioning). It is immaterial whether he lies on the left side or on the right: in the authors' practice this is governed by the leg from which the graft is to be taken; usually the patient lies on the left side and the graft is taken from the left tibia. In positioning the patient the assistants should flex the lowermost hip and knee 90 degrees so that the shin lies parallel with the edge of the operation table. The uppermost limb rests upon a platform, with the hip and knee fully extended (Fig. 181).

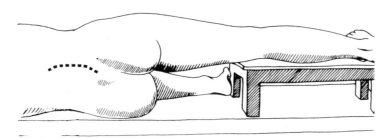

FIG. 181. Lateral fusion of lumbar spine. Position of patient. Resting the upper leg upon a platform helps to ensure that the spine is straight. The slightly curved line of incision is shown.

Incision. The main part of the incision is a vertical one placed about a centimetre away from the spinous processes. At each end it curves across the midline. Its length depends upon the number of segments to be fused.

Exposure of transverse processes. On each side of the midline the muscle mass lying upon the spinous processes and laminae is pushed aside by an elevator as far as the postero-lateral (facet) joints (Fig. 182). To gain further access in a lateral

far laterally and a centimetre or so deeper than the plane of the laminae.

The transverse processes are best identified by feel, the surgeon using blunt scissors. As each transverse process is identified it is stripped of muscle and aponeurosis by blunt dissection with scissors until the tip of the transverse process is reached. The tip likewise is isolated by blunt dissection and a cup-ended retractor (a long-handled spoon-gouge can serve the purpose well) is slid over the tip of the transverse process to lever the lateral muscles out of the way (Fig. 183). This enables the transverse processes to be clearly seen and thoroughly stripped of soft tissue down

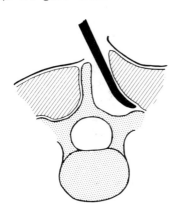

FIG. 182. Stripping the posterior spinal muscles from the spinous processes and laminae with a blunt lever.

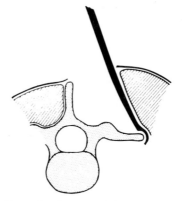

FIG. 183. A cup-ended retractor placed over the tip of the transverse process is used to lever the muscles out of the way, thus exposing the transverse process to full view.

direction the erector spinae mass is divided transversely a little above its attachment to the sacrum. This allows the dissection on each side to proceed

to raw bone. If the sacrum is to be included in the fusion the ala is likewise identified on each side and stripped of soft tissue.

Preparation of beds for grafts. The bed for each graft is prepared by first cutting a shallow notch in the uppermost transverse process to be fused (Fig. 184). If the graft is to be between transverse processes a similar notch is then cut in the upper margin of the lowermost transverse process; but if the fusion is to extend to the sacrum a deep slot proportionate in size to the proposed graft is cut into the ala. The slot should penetrate almost as far as the anterior cortex and should be about 2 centimetres long (Figs 184 and 187).

The length of the required graft is determined by measuring the gap to be bridged with the aid of a caliper: the graft should be a centimetre longer than the gap to be bridged, to allow for deep notching of its ends (Figs 184–187).

graft on each side is fashioned as shown in Figures 185 and 186, with a deep notch at each end to receive the transverse process. If the fusion is to be extended to the sacrum, the lower end of the graft is not notched but is bevelled at one corner to facilitate its insertion into the slot in the sacrum in a jam fit (Fig. 187).

Insertion of grafts. If the graft is to be fitted between transverse processes it is held in a sequestrum forceps and one end is fitted to the corresponding notch at the base of the upper transverse process, the other end sloping outwards to allow the notch to engage the tip of the lower transverse process (Fig. 185). This end of the graft is then forced medially so that it lies vertically between the transverse processes in a jam fit (Fig. 186).

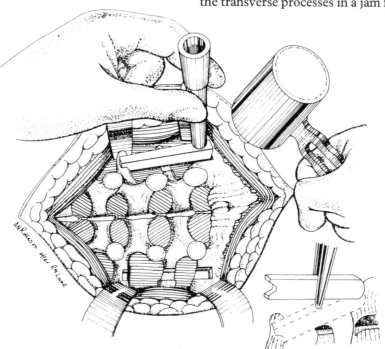

FIG. 184. Lateral (transverse process to ala of sacrum) lumbar fusion. On the right side (upper half of picture) a tibial graft, notched into the transverse process of the fourth lumbar vertebra, is being impacted into a deep slot cut in the ala of the sacrum. On the left side (lower half of picture) the bed is seen prepared for a graft. Inset shows method of inserting the graft.

Preparation of grafts. The authors use tibial grafts 1.5 centimetres wide and of a length commensurate with the distance to be bridged. In the case of fusion between transverse processes the

If the graft is to enter the sacrum its upper end is first engaged in the notch in the transverse process of the uppermost vertebra and the lower end is then impacted into the slot in the sacrum as shown in Figure 188. Any extra chips of cancellous bone that have been obtained may be placed around the fusion area.

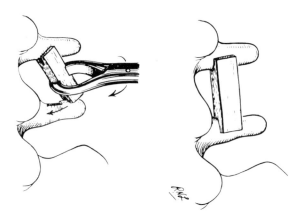

FIGS 185–186. Shape and fitting of cortical intertransverse process graft. It is important to secure a jam fit.

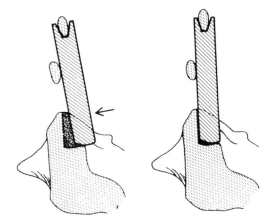

FIGS 187–188. Shape and fitting of transverse process to ala graft. An intermediate transverse process (that of the fifth lumbar vertebra) is displaced forwards after being divided at its base.

Internal fixation by spinous process clamp. By means of a special dual plate or clamp that grips the spinous processes rigidly it is possible to provide internal fixation of the affected joint or joints while incorporation of the bone grafts is occurring. The clamp* (Fig. 189) is appropriate to all cases in which grafts are inserted between transverse processes. It is applicable to lumbo-sacral fusion (grafts between fifth lumbar transverse

* Supplied by Howmedica Ltd, London, England.

process and ala of sacrum) only when the sacrum possesses a spinous process large enough to be gripped by the clamp.

Application of the clamp is simple. The spinous processes to be gripped are thoroughly cleared, and the angle between spinous process and lamina on each side may be deepened a little with a fine chisel to gain a greater usable expanse of spinous process. The device consists of two plates which are clamped together by the tightening of only two nuts. Each plate has teeth incorporated on its inner surface, and when the two plates are clamped together the teeth bite into the bone and grip it securely (Fig. 190). Two lengths of plate are available, and the choice depends upon the number of segments to be bridged.

The clamp is applied as follows. The female plate (Fig. 189) is placed in position and the two perforations mark the location of holes to be made through spinous process or interspinous ligament. When these holes have been drilled (a leather punch is ideal for the purpose) the studs incorporated in the male component are passed through the holes and through the female component. It remains then to apply and tighten the nuts with the special box spanner that is available. Tightening should proceed only to the point when the teeth on the plates bite into the bone: excessive tightening may crush the bone so completely that all rigidity is lost.

Closure. The wound is closed in layers, usually without drainage.

POST-OPERATIVE MANAGEMENT

Formerly, it was the authors' practice routinely to apply a plaster jacket incorporating one thigh, to give partial support to the lumbar spine during incorporation of the grafts. The patient remained in bed for only a few days before resuming walking in the plaster, which was usually changed two weeks after the operation. Support in a plaster spica-jacket may still be wise if internal metallic fixation is omitted, but when rigid fixation of the spinous processes by the special clamp described has been achieved it has been thought unnecessary to use a plaster jacket, and accordingly the patient has been allowed to lie free in bed for the first few days and thereafter gradually to resume walking, at first with the aid of elbow crutches.

wise to rely upon the use of a plaster spica-jacket, even though it is clear that no form of external splint can immobilise the lumbar spine fully.

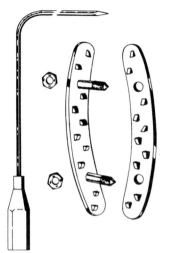
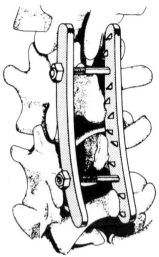

FIGS 189–190. Figure 189—The Crawford Adams spinal plate or clamp, designed for easy application to the spinous processes. The projecting teeth penetrate the spinous processes to give secure fixation when the male and female plates are clamped together. The special box-spanner has a trocar-point handle designed to transfix muscle and skin at the site of each nut and thus to give direct access for tightening. Figure 190—The plates in position before tightening of the nuts.

As in all cases of operation upon the spine, the use of a turning bed (for instance the Stryker Circ-o-Lectric vertical turning bed) offers great advantages in the first few days after operation.

Comment

In this technique the precision of a cabinet-making job is required. The essence of the operation is to lock the strut grafts rigidly in place to promote their speedy incorporation. This is made difficult by the fact that the transverse processes are often very fragile. They need to be handled carefully; otherwise they may break off at the base. It is therefore particularly important that any notch that is cut in the edge of the transverse process to receive the end of the graft should be very shallow, lest the bone be unduly weakened.

Internal fixation by the special clamp described has proved valuable. Its limitation is that it cannot be used in every case of lumbo-sacral fusion because the spinous process of the sacrum may be of inadequate size. In such an event, it is probably

ALTERNATIVE TECHNIQUE

A variety of methods of lateral and postero-lateral fusion have been reported (Rombold 1966, Scott 1967, Watkins 1953). Differences lie mainly in the approach, in the source of the donor bone, and in the placing of the grafts. Many surgeons use twin incisions, one on each side of the midline over the outer ends of the transverse processes. These give a more direct approach to the transverse processes, though the exposure is still deep.

Another alternative is the use of cancellous bone from the iliac crest in preference to tibial bone. Iliac bone is so soft that it is difficult to fashion it with precision to ensure a jam fit of the grafts. Those who use cancellous bone therefore tend to abandon the principle of a jam fit and rely on the placing of multiple cancellous slivers about the transverse processes and along the lateral aspect of the facet joints and adjacent parts of the laminae.

ANTERIOR LUMBAR INTERVERTEBRAL FUSION

Anterior fusion of a lumbar intervertebral joint is effected by placing blocks of cancellous bone between the adjacent vertebral bodies after clearance of the disc from the front and removal of the vertebral end plates to expose vascular spongy bone. The operation may be carried out by a transperitoneal or by a retroperitoneal approach.

TRANSPERITONEAL INTERVERTEBRAL FUSION

Transperitoneal intervertebral fusion is applicable particularly to the lumbo-sacral joint and to that between the fourth and fifth lumbar vertebrae in cases of degenerative disc disease or spondylolisthesis. The technique of Freebody (1964, 1971) is recommended, and for a detailed account of the procedure the original papers should be consulted.

TECHNIQUE

It is convenient to take bone from the wing of the ilium for grafting before the main part of the operation is begun. For this preliminary stage the patient is placed in the left or right lateral position.

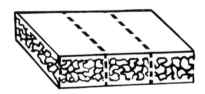

FIG. 191. Anterior intervertebral fusion. Block graft from ilium, to be divided into three parts as indicated.

A rectangular block of bone (Fig. 191) measuring 7.5 centimetres by 4 centimetres and comprising both cortices is cut from a thick part of the ilium as described on page 76. The abdominal area is then re-draped for the main part of the operation.

Position of patient. For the main part of the operation the patient lies supine. Provision must be made for Trendelenburg tilt.

Exposure. Through a left paramedian incision the intestines are packed off proximally, with the patient in the 30 degrees Trendelenburg position. The posterior peritoneum is infiltrated with adrenalin and saline solution (1 part in 200 000). The peritoneum is then incised vertically. The infiltration facilitates dissection and preservation of the presacral nerves. Vessels crossing the sacral promontory in a longitudinal direction are clamped and ligated. The tissues are then retracted to expose the front of the fifth lumbar vertebra and the sacral promontory. Steinmann pins are driven into the fifth lumbar vertebral body to hold the great vessels proximally out of harm's way.

For exposure of the joint between the fourth and fifth lumbar vertebrae it is necessary to approach the area from the left side of the great vessels, above the aortic bifurcation. The aorta and the vena cava are then displaced to the right after ligature of the left lumbar vessels.

Preparation of bed for graft. In degenerative disc disease it is necessary first to excise the intervertebral disc as completely as possible, with due regard to the safety of the spinal theca, and then to chisel away the vertebral end plates, leaving plain parallel surfaces of spongy bone. In doing this it is well to leave the anterior wall of the vertebral body intact, so that the grafts will be slightly recessed and consequently not liable to displacement (Fig. 192). In spondylolisthesis the adjacent ends of the vertebral bodies are recessed more deeply to allow the fitting of a long oblique graft.

Preparation and insertion of grafts. In cases of degenerative disc disease the bone graft is cut into three pieces, each so proportioned that when placed in the intervertebral space in the sagittal plane, with the edges directed proximally and distally (Fig. 192), the graft makes a jam fit between the vertebral bodies. In antero-posterior depth each graft should be wide enough to penetrate to within 5 millimetres of the posterior longitudinal ligament. The three grafts are jammed in side by side to fill virtually the whole width of the intervertebral disc space.

In cases of spondylolisthesis with considerable shift of the upper vertebra upon the lower, it is necessary to place the graft obliquely. In these cases the long axis of the graft will correspond in direction with the oblique line joining the centres of the two vertebral bodies. Deep excavations are

and fitting of the grafts that alone can provide inherent stability. It should not be undertaken by the occasional operator in this field unless he has gained a good apprenticeship at the hands of an expert. Nor should it be embarked upon by one who is unfamiliar with abdominal surgery.

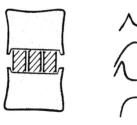

FIG. 192. *Left*—The three grafts in position as seen from the front. *Right*—Side view to show method of locking the grafts.

made in the opposing aspects of the vertebral bodies and the graft is so shaped that it can be forced into position by opening up the front of the disc space and firmly locked in place when the distraction is released. The remaining spaces between the vertebrae at each side of the main graft are filled with cancellous sliver grafts.

Closure. The posterior peritoneum is repaired by a fine absorbable suture and the anterior abdominal wall is closed in layers.

POST-OPERATIVE MANAGEMENT

If rigid fixation of the grafts has been achieved the patient may lie free in bed for four to six weeks and then gradually resume walking. If less stable impaction of the grafts has been secured—as may be the case in spondylolisthesis or in fusion of two levels simultaneously—it may be wise to enforce a greater degree of immobilisation by resting the patient in a plaster bed for the first four weeks.

Comment

This operation is attended by its best results in the hands of surgeons who practise it regularly and become proficient in the precise fashioning

In men, a hazard that requires mention is that of causing disturbance of sexual function—loss of ejaculation due to retrograde flow of semen into the bladder—by inadvertent damage to nerves of the pre-sacral plexus. Even though the risk is small when the operation is carried out with the precautions mentioned here, nevertheless instances of such damage do occur from time to time. When posterior fusion or lateral fusion is appropriate, therefore, it is probably to be preferred to anterior fusion.

EXTRAPERITONEAL INTERVERTEBRAL FUSION

In tuberculous disease involving an intervertebral joint and in cases of degenerative disease or spondylolisthesis affecting the lumbar spine proximal to the lumbar 4–5 joint, the extra-peritoneal approach is to be preferred. The patient should lie in the right lateral position to allow the vertebral column to be approached from the left—that is, from the side of the aorta rather than of the more fragile inferior vena cava. The exposure is the same as that used in operations upon the kidney and ureter. The peritoneum having been displaced forwards with the ureter, the affected intervertebral joint is reached from the antero-lateral aspect, either in front of the psoas muscle or through its anterior fibres. Preparation of the space for the bone graft and fitting of the graft are along the lines already described. For further details of this approach to the spine the reader is referred to the description of Hodgson and Wong (1968).

DECOMPRESSION OF SPINAL CANAL FOR SPINAL STENOSIS

This operation is usually carried out in the lumbar region, though occasions arise when it is necessary at other levels. It should be preceded by plain radiography, with oblique films as well as the normal antero-posterior films and lateral films in flexion and in extension, and by myelography. In this way the likely extent of the stenosis—whether from primary congenital narrowing of the canal or from encroachment upon it of acquired derangements such as osteophyte formation or vertebral displacement—may be determined. The actual dimensions of the canal may be measured by CT scanning.

extradural fat. Pulsation of the theca is an indication that it is not deprived of adequate space, but the converse is not necessarily true, for pulsation may not always be visible even when the spinal cord, the issuing nerves and the thecal space are unimpaired.

TECHNIQUE

The operation consists in deroofing of the bony spinal canal by removal of laminae and intervening ligamenta flava and, in most cases, decortication of the lateral walls of the canal (Fig. 194).

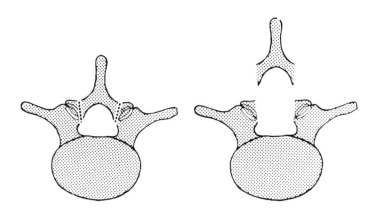

FIGS 193–194. Decompression of spinal canal for spinal stenosis.
Figure 193—Cross-sectional diagrams showing the amount of bone to be removed. Figure 194—The canal de-roofed.

In the usual type of case spinal stenosis is secondary to degenerative changes with hypertrophic bone formation, and decompression corresponding in extent to two or three vertebral segments is all that is required. The principle must be, however, that decompression is extended as far as is necessary, as judged from the degree to which the spinal theca seems visibly constricted by surrounding bone, with disappearance of the normal

Position of patient. If the patient is to be operated upon in the prone position it is important that support be provided under the shoulders and pelvis so that the body weight does not rest upon the chest and abdomen, with consequent embarrassment of respiration (see p. 131). There are some advantages to be gained from having the patient in the lateral posture, particularly from the point of view of the anaesthetist (Fig. 195). This position also allows the surgeon to be seated comfortably during what is often a fairly lengthy operation.

Incision. For the purpose of this description it will be assumed that the decompression is to extend from the second to the fifth lumbar verteb-

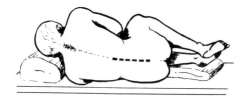

FIG. 195. Decompression for spinal stenosis. Position of patient and line of incision.

rae inclusive. The incision is a vertical one in the midline, extending from the tip of the spinous process of the first lumbar vertebra to the spine of the sacrum (Fig. 195). (It may be taken as a general rule, though not an invariable one, that the proximal limit of the crest of the ilium is at the level of the space between the spinous processes of the third and fourth lumbar vertebrae.)

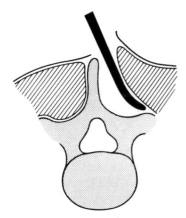

FIG. 196. Stripping of posterior spinal muscles from spinous processes and laminae.

Separation of erector spinae muscles. The deep fascia is incised in the midline and a space is opened on each side by sharp dissection between the spinous processes medially and the erector spinae muscle mass laterally. Stripping of the

muscles from the spinous processes and laminae is continued with a blunt rounded elevator (Fig. 196). The instrument must be kept close to the bone, in order to strip the muscles away cleanly without damaging them.

In this way the whole of the muscle mass on each side of the midline is reflected laterally throughout the length of the incision. The muscles are held widely apart by a deep robust self-retaining retractor. This leaves exposed the spinous processes, the posterior aspects of the laminae and, further laterally, the facet joints which at this stage need not be disturbed further.

Confirmation of level. It is essential that the vertebral level of the various structures exposed be known with certainty. Short of having a radiograph taken with an opaque marker placed over one of the bones, there is only one certain way of determining vertebral level—namely by demonstration of the sacrum. It is easy to identify the back of the sacrum because it presents a continuous sheet of bone in contradistinction to the laminae of the lumbar vertebrae, which are each separated by an interlaminar space bridged by ligamentum flavum. Moreover, the sacrum emits a characteristic hollow sound when it is tapped with a forceps. When the sacrum has thus been positively identified it is easy to establish the vertebral level of the other exposed bones by counting up from below.

In operations carried out at a higher level—for instance in the thoracic region—it is impracticable to count up from the sacrum as described, and it is best then to establish the level by radiography after an opaque marker has been placed on one of the bones.

Removal of spinous processes. It is convenient next to remove the spinous processes in the area to be decompressed—in this case from L.2 to L.5 inclusive. The processes should be removed near, but not quite at, their bases: they may be severed either with an angled bone-cutting forceps or by large nibbling forceps.

Meticulous cleaning of posterior elements. Before the actual decompression of the spinal canal is begun it is well worth while to spend time in thoroughly cleaning all the relevant laminae and interlaminar spaces. This is best done with a rounded periosteal elevator—as for instance the Robert Jones elevator. For those with little experience it is helpful to have at hand a dried specimen of the spinal column, so that the conformation of the various bony elements may be the more easily noted.

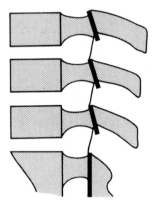

FIG. 197. Diagrammatic sagittal section showing the upward and forward inclination of the vertebral laminae in the lumbar region.

In cleaning the bones it should be remembered that the plane of the posterior surfaces of the laminae is not parallel to the plane of the body surface, for each laminae is tilted forwards through about 20 degrees, so that, in series, the laminae appear almost to be imbricated, like the tiles of a roof (Fig. 197). Between them, however, are the interlaminar spaces bridged by ligamentum flavum, which is attached not to the inferior border of each lamina but more to its antero-inferior aspect, so that the inferior border of the lamina overhangs the ligament (Fig. 197). By careful scraping with the elevator the bone surfaces and the intervening ligaments are cleared of all shreds of muscle, fat and periosteum. This is done throughout the length of spine to be decompressed.

Making the initial exposure of the dura mater. It is convenient to make the initial opening through the posterior wall of the spinal canal at the lower end of the area to be decompressed—in this case at the fifth lumbar level. Great care must be exercised in making the initial exposure of the dura mater: it is all too easy for the injudicious surgeon to cut too boldly and to break through the posterior wall of the spinal canal in a careless manner, with consequent risk of inadvertently opening the dura and even of damaging nerves of the cauda equina before he realises that he has reached the danger zone. In this connection it should be remembered that the spinal theca, which above the level of the fourth lumbar vertebra is roughly parallel with the posterior body surface, tends to sweep backwards—that is, superficially—rather sharply as it enters the fifth lumbar vertebra and sacrum. This is thus the level at which injury can most easily occur. The surgeon should also be wary of the possibility of congenital anomalies such as dural cysts, or even of congenital deficiency of the theca. Many surgeons elect to enter the spinal canal by nibbling away the base of the relevant spinous process, taking a little time so that the exposure is gradually deepened towards the spinal canal. Alternatively the bone may be cut away carefully with a rotating burr. Extreme patience should be exercised at this delicate stage of the operation, and it will be rewarded quite soon by the first glimpse of extradural fat or of the dura itself through a tiny initial opening in the bony wall of the canal.

Enlargement of initial opening and decompression of the whole area. Once the dura has been exposed through the small initial opening in the posterior bony wall of the spinal canal at the fifth lumbar level, the fenestration is easily extended proximally and laterally (Fig. 198). Bone is most easily removed with punch forceps—as for instance those of Kerrison pattern. As the opening is enlarged great care must be taken to ensure that the dura is free, as shown by the easy passage of a blunt dissector between dura and posterior wall of the spinal canal. As each bite is made with the punch forceps it is essential to observe that the blade enters this plane between dura and bone, and when the punch forceps has been closed it must not be snatched away from the site but should be withdrawn cautiously lest by mischance the dura has been nipped. Where ligamentum flavum intervenes between the laminae it may best be removed by curved blunt-nosed scissors or even by a fine knife manipulated with special caution and with the cutting edge directed away from the dura.

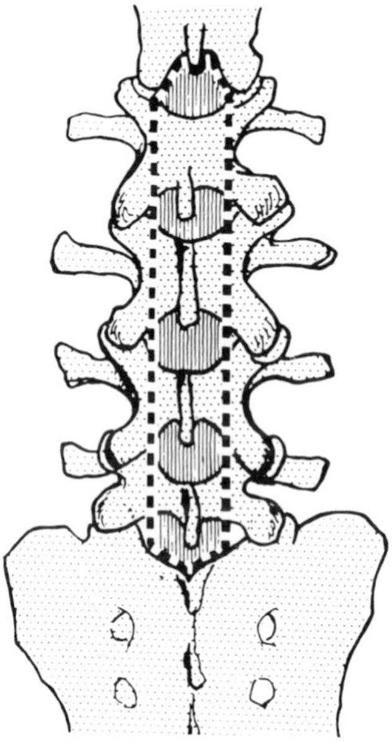

Investigation of issuing nerves and related intervertebral discs. In a classical case of spinal stenosis there is usually no impairment of nerve function with the patient at rest, and one does not expect to find evidence of direct local pressure upon a nerve. Thus straight leg raising is usually through

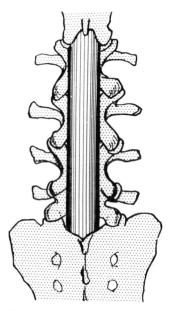

FIG. 198. Outline shows area of posterior spinal canal to be decompressed in the type of case described.

FIG. 199. The decompression completed. The spinal theca is exposed in the depth of the wound.

Once the posterior wall of the spinal canal has been removed over the planned number of segments attention must be directed towards the lateral walls of the canal. As a general rule it is wise to leave the facet articulations undisturbed, but it is permissible and usually advisable to widen the canal laterally at the expense of bone and ligament. This may be done partly with nibbling forceps and partly with a fine chisel and light hammer, care being taken to control the chisel minutely by resting the hand that holds it upon the patient's body.

When the decompression has been completed the spinal theca with its outer covering of dura mater should lie totally exposed from side to side in a cleanly outlined opening extending in the case described from the second to the fifth lumbar vertebrae inclusive (Fig. 199).

a normal range, and the tendon reflexes in the lower limb are normal. In such a case it seems unnecessary to make a formal exploration of each nerve root and of the related intervertebral disc. Nevertheless, if there is any suspicion of local mechanical embarrassment of a particular nerve then it should be explored and the nerve canal enlarged appropriately.

Dural pulsation. Visible pulsation of the dural sac is reassuring—especially so when a lack of pulsation has been observed distally and when it has returned as the decompression has been extended proximally. Nevertheless dural pulsation is not always evident in the lumbar region, and provided the decompression has been extended over the area shown to be constricted, lack of pulsation is not necessarily significant.

Closure. When the self-retaining retractor is removed the erector spinae muscles fall back into place and can be approximated in the midline and united with deep interrupted absorbable sutures. A further line of sutures is used to coapt the superficial aponeurotic layer. If desired, a tube for suction drainage may be inserted between this layer and the subcutaneous tissues and brought out in the flank before the skin edges are united.

POST-OPERATIVE MANAGEMENT

Copious gauze dressings are held in place with adhesive strips over which a many-tailed bandage may be applied if desired. The patient should lie flat on the back for the first twelve hours because this minimises the risk of formation of a haematoma. Thereafter the patient may turn and move freely in the bed. There is no need for prolonged recumbency. Usually the patient may be allowed out of bed after two or three days or even earlier. After the wound has healed exercises are encouraged both to rehabilitate the spinal muscles and to restore mobility of the spine.

Comment

In a well-established case of spinal stenosis decompression is a satisfying operation because of the often total relief of symptoms that it affords. Nevertheless it is a somewhat demanding operation, to be carried out with meticulous patience. The essentials are to gain adequate decompression over the required extent while avoiding damage to the dura. A hurried and careless technique can all too easily lead to perforation of the dura and—more important—damage to the contained nerves.

The need to enlarge the spinal canal laterally as well as posteriorly has already been mentioned. This point was emphasised by Naylor (1979), who advised special care to ensure that the emerging spinal nerves are free from constriction in the lateral recesses of the canal.

CHAPTER FIVE

Shoulder Region

Operations upon the shoulder are generally necessitated by the effects of trauma rather than of congenital anomalies or degenerative disease. Fractures, dislocations and tendon ruptures present the bulk of the problems. Advances in the surgery of the shoulder have not been spectacular in recent decades. Nevertheless much thought has been devoted to the problems of devising a reliable technique of total replacement arthroplasty, for which there is a need particularly in rheumatoid arthritis. A number of techniques are at present on trial, of which one example will be given in this chapter.

CONTENTS OF CHAPTER

SCREW FIXATION OF CLAVICLE TO CORACOID PROCESS FOR DISLOCATION OF ACROMIO-CLAVICULAR JOINT

This operation is undertaken for complete dislocation (conoid and trapezoid ligaments ruptured) rather than for subluxation (conoid and trapezoid ligaments intact), which seldom demands active treatment.

TECHNIQUE

Position of patient. The patient lies supine, with the affected shoulder raised forwards by means of a sand-bag under the scapular region and the head inclined towards the opposite side.

Exposure. The tip of the coracoid process is palpated. An incision starting over this point is extended upwards in the line of a shoulder strap as far as the posterior border of the clavicle (Fig. 200). When the deep fascia has been incised in the same line the groove between the deltoid muscle and the pectoralis major is identified. The muscles are separated over a distance of about 5 centimetres and held apart with a self-retaining retractor. To increase the exposure the deltoid may be detached from its origin from the clavicle over a distance of 2.5 centimetres.

Superiorly the upper surface of the clavicle is cleared of soft tissue close to its outer end and vertically above the coracoid process. Inferiorly the upper surface of the coracoid process is identified and cleared of soft tissue.

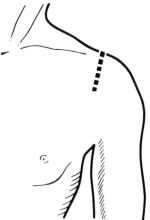

Fig. 200. Stabilisation of acromio-clavicular joint. The skin incision.

Drilling the clavicle and the coracoid process. At a point on the upper surface of the clavicle vertically above the coracoid process a small notch is made in the bone with an awl to serve as the starting point for a drill hole. On the basis that a 4.5 millimetre lag screw is to be used, the hole is made with a 3.2 millimetre drill directed vertically downwards towards the upper surface of the coracoid process mid-way between its base and tip. Under direct vision the drill is driven on through the whole thickness of the coracoid process, to emerge at its inferior surface.

Insertion of screw. The drill having been withdrawn, threads are cut in the bones with a suitable tap. The depth of the track between the upper surface of the clavicle and the deep surface of the coracoid process is measured with a depth gauge while the acromio-clavicular dislocation is held reduced by firm downward pressure upon the clavicle. A lag screw 4 millimetres in diameter and of the appropriate length is passed through the hole in the clavicle, guided into the hole in the coracoid process and driven home firmly (Fig. 201), though with care to avoid stripping the thread in the coracoid.

If a fully threaded screw is used instead of a lag screw it is important that the drill hole through the clavicle be enlarged to provide a clearance fit for the screw, so that when the screw is tightened

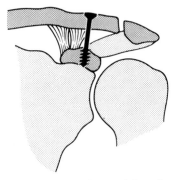

Fig. 201. The screw is passed through a drill hole in the clavicle to engage the coracoid process.

the clavicle will be drawn down towards the coracoid process, thus ensuring full reduction of the displacement.

Closure. The wound is closed in layers, without drainage.

POST-OPERATIVE MANAGEMENT

Dressings are held in place by an elastic adhesive bandage, and a sling is worn for the first week. Thereafter gentle shoulder and elbow exercises are encouraged, though with avoidance of full elevation. It is recommended that the screw be removed two months after its insertion, when it may be assumed that the soft tissues are sufficiently healed.

Comment

The main essential in this operation is to gain a clear view of the coracoid process, so that the drill hole may be made and the screw inserted under direct vision. It is a mistake to attempt to insert the screw blindly, as has sometimes been advised.

If preferred, a self-tapping screw may be used, thus avoiding the need to tap the threads. But the holding power of the screw is likely to be enhanced if the threads are pre-tapped.

EXCISION OF OUTER END OF CLAVICLE

When the outer end of the clavicle is to be excised for degenerative or post-traumatic arthritis of the acromio-clavicular joint it is important to preserve the conoid and trapezoid ligaments, which anchor the outer end of the clavicle to the coracoid process. The bone must therefore be divided lateral to these ligaments. This limits the length of bone to be removed to little more than 1.5 centimetres. In contrast, when the outer end of the clavicle is to be removed for long-standing upward displacement of the clavicle at its outer end, due to dislocation of the acromio-clavicular joint with disruption of the conoid and trapezoid ligaments, it is wise to remove a greater length of bone—up to 5 centimetres.

EXCISION WITH PRESERVATION OF CONOID AND TRAPEZOID LIGAMENTS

TECHNIQUE

Position of patient. The patient lies supine, with a rather flat sand-bag placed behind the scapula on the affected side to throw the shoulder forwards.

Incision. An incision in the sagittal plane (Fig. 202) is recommended. It begins anteriorly,

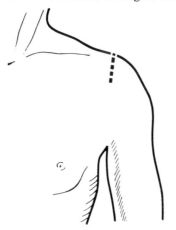

FIG. 202. Excision of distal end of clavicle. The skin incision.

immediately lateral to the coracoid process, and arches backwards over the lateral end of the clavicle to end close to the posterior margin of the acromion process. The incision is thus about 5 or 6 centimetres long.

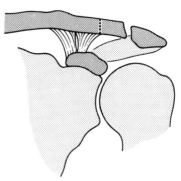

FIG. 203. Interrupted line shows site of division of the clavicle, immediately lateral to the coraco-clavicular ligaments.

Exposure of acromio-clavicular joint and lateral end of clavicle. It should be remembered that the acromio-clavicular joint lies in the sagittal plane. In the normal subject, the joint can be palpated about 3 centimetres medial to the tip of the acromion. To expose the joint the skin edges are retracted medially and laterally, the platysma is split in the direction of its fibres, and the underlying clavicle is reached by blunt dissection. Then the exposure is pursued laterally until the outer articular margin of the clavicle and the acromio-clavicular joint are identified. The antero-superior ligaments of the joint and the capsule may be divided at this stage to open the joint.

Division of clavicle and removal of lateral fragment. The point at which the clavicle is to be divided should be marked upon the surface with an osteotome. In an adult this point should usually be 1.5 centimetres medial to the acromio-clavicular joint (Fig. 203). It is necessary to check that the site selected is lateral to the conoid and trapezoid ligaments; their position is easily noted from the position of the coracoid process, which forms their inferior attachment.

Before the bone is divided it is wise to clean its outer end by sharp dissection, all the ligamentous and muscular tissue being separated with a small knife blade held always close to the bone. This stripping of musculo-ligamentous tissue should extend as far round the bone to its deep aspect as is possible. At the projected point of division it should be possible to pass a curved spike or dissector from front to back deep to the bone to display the full thickness that is to be divided. The clavicle may be divided either by hand instruments such as a slender osteotome or a nibbling forceps, or by a powered instrument such as a high-speed dental-type burr.

When the division is complete the medial cut end of the isolated lateral fragment of the clavicle is levered upwards by an elevator (for example, Bristow's) so that a sharp bone hook may be thrust into the cut surface (Fig. 204). While a steady

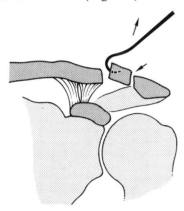

FIG. 204. Lifting the lateral fragment with a bone hook thrust into the cut surface, to allow division of the deeper structures close to the bone.

upward pull is exerted on the hook, remaining deep attachments of the outer end of the clavicle are divided close to the bone with a fine-bladed knife, and finally the deep ligaments and remaining part of the capsule of the acromio-clavicular joint are severed to free the bone fragment.

Before closure, the cut surface of the main (medial) fragment of the clavicle should be inspected to make sure that no sharp edge or bone spicule remains. Likewise, the articular surface of the acromion should be cleared of any exuberant osteophytes.

Closure. The fibres of the deltoid muscle are allowed to fall together and may be approximated

with one or two fine absorbable sutures. The skin wound is closed without drainage.

POST-OPERATIVE MANAGEMENT

The wound is covered with dry gauze and elastic adhesive strapping, or by a proprietary dressing of similar type. The arm may be rested in a sling for greater comfort, but after a few days active or assisted shoulder abduction exercises should be begun under the supervision of a physiotherapist. After removal of the sutures at 10 days exercises are intensified until a normal range of shoulder movement is restored.

EXCISION FOR LONG-STANDING UNREDUCED UPWARD DISLOCATION OF CLAVICLE AT ACROMIO-CLAVICULAR JOINT

In these cases the outer end of the clavicle is considerably elevated and projects under the skin. Trimming of the bone is undertaken largely for cosmetic reasons as well as for discomfort where the displaced lateral extremity of the bone projects. Since the conoid and trapezoid ligaments are disrupted, excision need not be restricted to the part of the clavicle that lies lateral to them, and accordingly sufficient bone should be removed to eliminate the visible deformity. This may entail removal of as much as 3 to 5 centimetres of the clavicle.

TECHNIQUE

Incision. A longitudinal incision in the line of the clavicle, and placed over its anterior border, is appropriate (Fig. 205).

Exposure and removal of appropriate length of bone. In the type of case under consideration the outer extremity of the clavicle has lost its muscle attachments and lies unanchored in the subcutaneous tissue. This part of the bone is therefore best exposed first, by a knife cut straight down upon it, and the whole circumference of the bone is easily cleared by sharp dissection with a fine knife held close to the bone surface. The outer end of the clavicle being now grasped with a seques-trum forceps or similar instrument, dissection is carried medially along all aspects of the bone.

muscle, by bringing together the edges of trape-zius above and deltoid below. The subcutaneous tissue should also be closed as a separate layer before the skin edges are approximated.

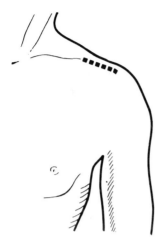

FIG. 205. Excision of widely dis-placed outer end of clavicle proximal to coraco-clavicular ligaments. The skin incision.

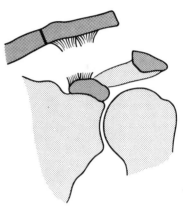

FIG. 206. Diagram showing the site of division of the clavicle and the amount of bone to be removed. The stump of the clavicle should be rounded off.

This part of the dissection is most easily carried out with slender blunt-nosed scissors curved on the flat, the instrument being kept close to the bone at all times.

When the required length of bone has been displayed and cleared (Fig. 206) a pack or a mal-leable retractor is laid beneath it to protect the deeper tissues while the bone is divided. The division is perhaps most easily accomplished with bone nibblers, and after the lateral fragment has been discarded care should be taken to ensure that the medial stump of the clavicle is rounded, any sharp edge or bone spicules being removed.

Closure. It is best to try to bury the outer cut end of the remaining fragment of the clavicle with

POST-OPERATIVE MANAGEMENT

This is the same as for excision distal to the coraco-clavicular ligaments, as described above.

Comment

When a large part of the clavicle or even the whole of it is to be removed particular care is required in order to avoid damage to the dome of the pleura and, further medially, the external jugular vein and the great vessels. In these circumstances the need to keep the dissection very close to the bone is obvious. The hazards mentioned do not apply, however, when the length of clavicle to be removed is less than 3 centimetres.

REPAIR OF RUPTURE OF TENDINOUS CUFF OF SHOULDER

The tendinous cuff of the shoulder—often termed the rotator cuff—comprises the tendons of supra-spinatus, infraspinatus and teres minor in that order from before backwards. Rupture—either a

sudden traumatic event or a quiet disintegration of a degenerate tendon—may be confined to the supraspinatus component (Fig. 207), or the tear may widen with the lapse of time so that eventually a large defect exists. The head of the humerus is then separated from the acromion process only by the subacromial bursa.

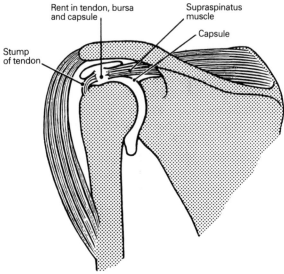

FIG. 207. Tear of supraspinatus shown diagrammatically. Note that the subacromial bursa communicates with the shoulder joint through the rent.

PRE-OPERATIVE STUDIES

It is wise to investigate the pathology by arthrography of the shoulder before operation is decided upon. A short-bevelled spinal needle is entered a centimetre below the anterior margin of the acromion process and thrust backwards to enter the articular cartilage of the humeral head. The needle is then withdrawn from the cartilage to allow injection of about 20 millilitres of contrast medium into the joint. Radiographs are taken immediately. Flow of the fluid from the joint into the subacromial bursa, as shown in the radiograph, indicates a rupture of the tendinous cuff.

TECHNIQUE

No matter whether the tear is thought to be small or large, it is best approached through an acromion-splitting incision approximately in the coronal plane. A small tear may be repaired by direct suture of the tendon to the bone. A large tear cannot be closed in this way and satisfactory repair can be accomplished best by lateral advan-

cement of the whole of the supraspinatus muscle in its fossa, in the manner described by Debeyre *et al.* (1965).

Position of patient. The patient lies in the lateral posture with the affected shoulder uppermost. The whole upper arm is draped in a sterile stockingette tube to permit adjustment of the position of the shoulder during the course of the operation. In the early stages of the operation it is convenient to apply light longitudinal traction on the limb. This may be arranged by tying a sterile bandage around the wrist, over suitable padding: a weight is then applied to the end of the bandage and suspended over the foot of the table.

Incision. The medial half of the incision lies a centimetre above and parallel with the upper margin of the spine of the scapula. Laterally it curves slightly backwards to cross the acromion process: thence it extends downwards over the outer aspect of the deltoid muscle for a distance of 4 centimetres beyond the margin of the acromion (Figs 208 and 209).

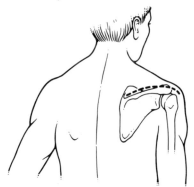

FIG. 208. Acromion-splitting exposure of supraspinatus muscle and tendinous cuff. The skin incision.

Exposure of supraspinatus muscle. The trapezius muscle is divided transversely parallel with the spine of the scapula and about a centimetre proximal to it—that is, in the line of the skin incision. The main part of the belly of the supraspinatus is then exposed simply by division and reflection of the overlying fascia.

Further laterally, the acromion process is split with an osteotome in the direction of the skin incision. The anterior half of the acromion, to which is attached the clavicle, may then be swung forwards, the space between the two parts of the bone being held open with a self-retaining retractor.

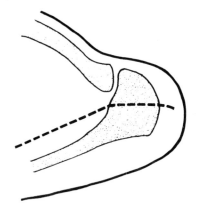

FIG. 209. The line of incision through muscle and bone.

Beyond the margin of the acromion the deltoid muscle is split and its edges are retracted, with care not to injure the axillary nerve. Deep to the acromion the subacromial bursa is opened. In this way the whole of the supraspinatus muscle is uncovered. The extent of the rupture of the tendinous cuff is clearly revealed: through the rent the humeral head is visible to a degree that depends upon the extent of the rupture.

Direct re-attachment of ruptured tendon to bone. If the rent in the tendon is small—involving the supraspinatus component alone—direct re-attachment of the tendon to the bone of the greater tuberosity may be feasible.

The repair is best made with the arm held abducted 90 degrees by an assistant. First a notch or groove is cut with a chisel along the upper margin of the greater tuberosity, close to the natural sulcus that exists between the tuberosity and the articular surface of the humeral head. Four drill holes, each about 1.5 millimetres in diameter, are then made from the depth of the groove through the thickness of the greater tuberosity to emerge at its lateral surface (Fig. 210). Mattress sutures of strong absorbable material or—perhaps better—stainless steel wire, looped through the ruptured tendon, are then passed

through the drill holes and tied at the outer aspect of the tuberosity in such a way as to draw the tendon down into the groove in the bone.

Repair by advancement of supraspinatus muscle. In the case of an extensive rupture of the tendinous cuff it is not practicable to close the gap by direct suture to the bone as described. The most satisfactory way of effecting repair is then to detach the belly of the supraspinatus from the supraspinatus fossa of the scapula and to slide the muscle bodily in a lateral direction, to enable the gap in the tendon to be closed.

In detaching the muscle from its bony sulcus the surgeon must make every effort to preserve the suprascapular nerve and the adjacent arteries and veins, which enter the belly of the muscle on its deep aspect. With care, a neurovascular pedicle may be mobilised to allow the muscle to be shifted laterally about 2 centimetres. Thus advanced, the tendon may be attached without difficulty to the

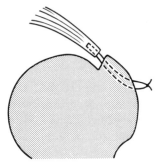

FIG. 210. Method of attaching supraspinatus tendon to greater tuberosity.

greater tuberosity of the humerus in the manner described (Fig. 210). The sides of the advanced tendon are then sutured to the adjacent components of the tendinous cuff by interrupted absorbable sutures.

Closure. The split fibres of the deltoid muscle are approximated with interrupted sutures. Close to the margin of the acromion these sutures serve to hold the two parts of the split acromion process together. The trapezius muscle is repaired along the line of its detachment from the spine of the scapula. Before skin closure a tube may be placed in the supraspinatus fossa for suction drainage.

POST-OPERATIVE MANAGEMENT

To ensure the best chance of healing of the tendon at its junction with the bone the limb should be supported in right-angled abduction and moderate flexion and medial rotation in a plaster-of-Paris shoulder spica. After four weeks the lid of the spica is removed to allow abduction exercises from the plaster. When good deltoid function has been regained one or two weeks later the plaster may be discarded. Thereafter intensive exercises must be continued with the aim of restoring active shoulder abduction from the resting position.

Comment

In general, the results of repair of ruptures of the tendinous cuff of the shoulder have been disappointing. Many of these patients are elderly and the tendon tissue is degenerate. It tends to heal poorly after suture, and the rent is prone to recur. Despite an unhealed rupture many patients have eventually regained active power of abduction by deltoid action alone, a new fulcrum presumably developing beneath the acromion process. These factors have often deterred surgeons from attempting repair in an elderly subject. Certainly attempted repair should be considered with caution in the elderly: probably it is worth waiting 3 to 6 months or so before operation in the expectation that reasonable function may be regained by physiotherapy alone.

Before the technique of muscle advancement was advocated by Debeyre et al. (1965) suture of a wide rent was technically so unsatisfactory that success was always unlikely. Lateral advancement of the muscle makes the repair simple, though it must be suspected that in a proportion of cases the viability of the muscle is prejudiced by its total separation from the bony fossa, with inevitable damage at least to the smaller vessels. It is indeed possible that in some cases the reported success of the muscle advancement technique depends upon the provision of a bulky pad between the head of the humerus and the under surface of the acromion rather than upon effective restoration of supraspinatus power.

EVACUATION OF CALCIFIED DEPOSIT FROM SUPRASPINATUS TENDON

This operation entails splitting of the thin tendinous sheet superficial to the calcified deposit and curettage of the small cavity within the substance of the tendon.

PRE-OPERATIVE STUDIES

It is essential that good quality radiographs be available at the time of operation in order to aid localisation of the deposit, should it not be immediately seen. The series of radiographs should include a true antero-lateral film with the forearm directed forwards, an axial projection and, if necessary, antero-oblique and postero-oblique tangential projections.

TECHNIQUE

Position of patient. It is convenient to place the patient in the lateral posture with the affected shoulder uppermost. The arm should be fully draped in sterile stockingette. It is a good plan to arrange slight distal traction upon the limb by gripping the wrist with a soft bandage, to the other end of which is attached a weight of half a kilogram, which is suspended over the foot of the table. The surgeon stands behind the patient.

Incision. The incision is a vertical one extending distally from the lateral margin of the acromion process at its anterior corner for 3 or 4 centimetres.

Exposure of tendinous cuff. After incision of the deep fascia the fibres of the deltoid muscle are split through the whole thickness of the muscle and the edges are drawn apart with a self-retaining retractor. Deep to the muscle will be found the flimsy walls of the sub-deltoid bursa. Some areolar tissue has to be removed in order to clean the superficial aspect of the tendinous cuff, which is composed at this level of muscle fibres, becoming tendinous, and with a mesh of fine blood vessels upon its surface.

Location and evacuation of calcified deposit. Often the site of the calcified deposit is immediately apparent where it forms a prominence upon the surface of the tendinous cuff, the white material showing through the superficial fibres, surrounded by a zone of redness. In other cases— especially in those that are chronic—it is difficult to find the deposit. A thorough search of the area is made by rotating the limb to and fro, so that all parts of the tendinous cuff come into view through the deltoid-splitting incision. A point suspected of being the site of the deposit may be investigated by making a tiny cut through the tendon in the direction of its fibres with a number 15 blade. When the blade enters the deposit there can be no doubt about its identification because white chalky material immediately begins to exude. When the deposit has been thus located, the tendon fibres are split sufficiently to allow complete emptying of the small calcium-containing cavity.

Closure. The small incision in the supraspinatus tendon is closed with fine absorbable sutures. The deltoid fibres fall together and may be coapted with one or two fine sutures. The skin is closed with interrupted non-absorbable sutures.

POST-OPERATIVE MANAGEMENT

A simple gauze dressing held in place by adhesive tissue is all that is required. The arm may be rested in a sling for a few days, but active mobilising exercises should be practised from an early

stage and intensified as pain lessens, and increasingly so after removal of the sutures 10 to 12 days after the operation.

Comment

The operation presents no special problem except that the calcified deposit may not be obvious when the surface of the supraspinatus tendon complex is inspected. It is usually immediately obvious in the acute case with intense local pain, but it may not be obvious in a chronic case. It is in these cases that careful pre-operative radiography is essential. Provided that the position of the arm at radiography is known, and that this position is reproduced during the operation, the radiographs give a useful guide to the position of the calcified deposit. The axial view taken with the hand directed forwards, as in the anatomical position, will often show the deposit to be on a line that continues the anterior outline of the clavicle and acromion process distally into the arm, and if this is the case the incision should be placed accordingly. The antero-posterior radiograph is also a useful guide: if it shows the deposit in clear profile lateral to the greater tuberosity of the humerus, and not overlying the tuberosity (the hand being directed forwards in the anatomical position), the deposit must clearly lie approximately in the mid-lateral plane. If the deposit is seen overlying the tuberosity, further tangential projections should be made to show whether it is anterior or posterior to the mid-lateral line.

In the event that the deposit cannot be seen from the superficial aspect of the tendon it is necessary to make tiny exploratory stab incisions with a very fine knife in the area defined radiographically until the cavity is opened and white material begins to exude.

PUTTI-PLATT OPERATION FOR RECURRENT ANTERIOR DISLOCATION OF SHOULDER

This operation was devised independently by Putti (quoted by Valtancoli 1925) of Italy and by Platt (quoted by Osmond-Clarke 1948) of Manchester, England. The aims of the operation are two-fold. Firstly it is designed to obliterate the

anterior recess of capsule which is created by stripping of capsule and periosteum from the front of the neck of the scapula at the time of the first dislocation and which is a characteristic feature of most cases of recurrent dislocation of the shoulder. This pocket-like recess is obliterated by suturing into it the tendinous stump of the divided subscapularis muscle.

Secondly, the operation aims to create a check ligament to limit lateral rotation of the humerus, and thus to prevent the dent or groove in the postero-lateral aspect of the head of the humerus from rotating forwards to the anterior margin of the glenoid, where it is liable to slip over the edge with consequent subluxation. This check ligament is formed partly by attachment of the subscapularis tendon to the front of the scapular neck and partly by overlapping of the divided ends of the subscapularis, thus shortening the muscle.

TECHNIQUE

Position of patient. The patient lies supine, with the affected shoulder thrust forward by a firm sand-bag under the scapula.

Exposure. The routine anterior exposure of the shoulder (p. 10) is convenient, but in women especially—in whom a prominent scar may be embarrassing—the axillary approach (see p. 13) (Fig. 212) should be preferred. The subsequent steps in the operation are the same no matter which incision is used.

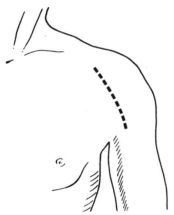

FIG. 211. Putti-Platt repair for recurrent anterior dislocation of shoulder. The skin incision.

In the standard exposure the skin incision extends 10 centimetres downwards and laterally from the coracoid process over the delto-pectoral groove (Fig. 211). When the deep fascia has been divided the cephalic vein is seen in the delto-pectoral groove: it is retracted medially. The interval between the deltoid and the pectoralis major is opened up as far proximally as the clavicle (Fig. 213).

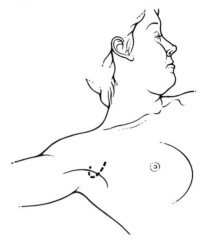

FIG. 212. Axillary incision. This is often to be preferred—especially in women—because the scar is much less conspicuous.

The coracoid process, with the attached conjoined biceps (short head) and coracobrachialis muscles, is thus revealed: it is cleared and the borders of the muscles are defined (Fig. 213). The coracoid process is divided with an osteotome a centimetre from its tip and reflected distally with the coracobrachialis and short head of biceps (Fig. 214). At this stage special care must be taken to avoid injury to the large musculocutaneous nerve, which enters the deep surface of the coracobrachialis 7 or 8 centimetres below the coracoid process.

An assistant now applies a steady lateral rotation force to the arm in order to stretch the subscapularis muscle, which comes clearly into view when the coracobrachialis and biceps have been reflected distally. The borders of the subscapularis are defined, and a blunt curved lever is passed from above downwards deep to its tendon, about 2.5 centimetres from its attachment to the humerus. Stay sutures are inserted into the belly of the muscle near the musculo-tendinous junction to prevent excessive retraction when the muscle has been divided.

The subscapularis is then divided close to the musculo-tendinous junction, about 2.5 centimetres from the insertion into the humerus.

Identification of pathological anatomy. The edges of the opening in the capsule are held apart with stay sutures to allow inspection of the inter-

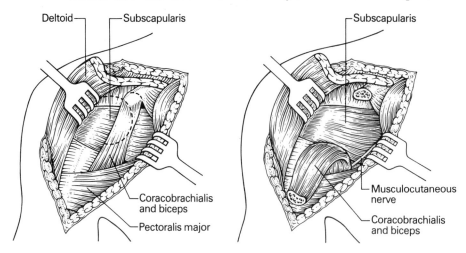

FIGS 213–214. Putti-Platt repair. Figure 213—After separation of the deltoid and pectoralis major muscles, the conjoined coracobrachialis and biceps muscles are seen attached near the tip of the coracoid process. Deep to them lies the subscapularis, the fibres of which, running horizontally, become tendinous as they approach their insertion into the humerus. The broken line shows the position of the head of the humerus. Figure 214—The coracoid process has been divided and the coracobrachialis and biceps have been reflected distally. Note the musculocutaneous nerve, which may be hazarded by injudicious retraction.

Sometimes the tendon is blended with the underlying capsule and the two structures are divided together. At other times the capsule is distinct

ior of the joint. Looking towards the front of the glenoid, the surgeon will now see clearly whether or not the capsule and the glenoid labrum have

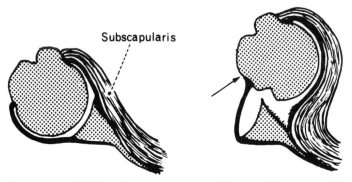

FIGS 215–216. Pathology of recurrent anterior dislocation. Figure 215—The normal state. Figure 216—Diagram showing how the capsule and periosteum are stripped from the front of the neck of the scapula, creating a deep pocket between periosteum and bone. The postero-lateral dent in the humeral head is also shown.

from the tendon and remains intact when the tendon is divided. In that event the capsule is now opened separately in the same line as the subscapularis tendon.

been detached from the rim of the glenoid, as is nearly always the case. In that event the rent where the capsule and labrum are separated from the glenoid margin leads to a small pocket in front of the neck of the scapula, where bare bone is exposed (Fig. 215). If the arm is now abducted, laterally rotated and extended the head of the

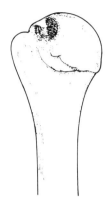

FIG. 217. Typical defect (dent) in the head of the humerus in recurrent dislocation of the shoulder. In a case of anterior dislocation the defect is postero-lateral.

humerus will be readily dislocated or subluxated from the glenoid. By rotating the humerus laterally to its fullest extent it is often possible just to display the groove or dent in the postero-lateral aspect of the humeral head which is a nearly constant feature of recurrent dislocation (Fig. 217) and should have been looked for before operation by radiographs taken with the arm in medial rotation (Fig. 218). Even if the groove cannot be seen it may be palpated with a curved spike or probe.

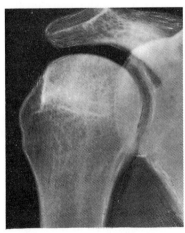

FIG. 218. Postero-lateral defect of humeral head shown radiographically by an antero-posterior projection with the shoulder held in 70 degrees of medial rotation.

Repair. When it has been confirmed that there is separation of the capsule from the anterior margin

of the glenoid, stabilisation is effected in the following way. First the bare area of the bone at the front of the scapular neck is scarified by multiple shallow cuts with an osteotome in order to promote bleeding and thus to facilitate adhesion of the soft tissues to the bone.

The next step is to suture the distal stump—that is, the tendinous stump—of the subscapularis into the pocket that lies between the front of the neck of the scapula and the stripped-up capsule and periosteum (Fig. 219). In order to secure the

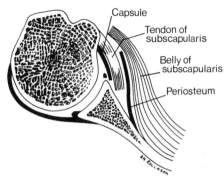

FIG. 219. Horizontal section showing anatomy of Putti-Platt repair. The tendon of subscapularis lies in the osteo-periosteal pocket and the belly of the muscle overlaps it.

stump of the subscapularis in the depth of this pocket it is necessary to place the humerus in full medial rotation, but before this is done it is easier to insert the three sutures that will hold it in position. The insertion of these sutures is one of the key parts of the operation. The sutures are of strong (Number 3) catgut or other absorbable material and are inserted as mattress sutures with a needle threaded on at each end.

To insert the sutures the flap of capsule and periosteum is pulled forwards with a Kocher's forceps or with a stay suture so that the point of the needle can be inserted from without inwards from the space between the subscapularis muscle and the stripped-up periosteum. The needle enters the periosteum and should emerge at the very depth of the pocket, where it is gripped and withdrawn (Fig. 220). Each end of the suture is brought through in this way and is then passed through the tendinous stump of the subscapularis nearly a centimetre from its cut edge.

When three separate sutures have been inserted

in this fashion the arm is rotated medially to its full extent in order to allow the stump of the subscapularis to be drawn down by the sutures into the capsulo-periosteal pocket (Fig. 220). The sutures are best tied by hand with only moderate tension. From this point onwards the arm must be held by an assistant in medial rotation to prevent disruption of the sutures.

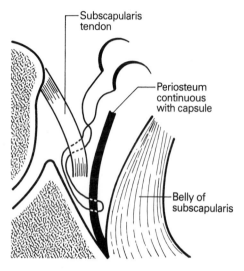

FIG. 220. Enlarged diagram showing method of inserting the deep sutures to hold the tendon of subscapularis in the osteo-periosteal pocket.

The next step in the repair is to bring the proximal flap of capsule forwards and laterally so that it overlaps the subscapularis tendon and to suture it here with three or four absorbable sutures. The belly of the subscapularis is then stretched forwards and laterally over the capsule by means of the stay sutures previously inserted, and sutured to the soft tissues in the region of the lesser tuberosity of the humerus. In other words the divided ends of the subscapularis are overlapped like a double-breasted jacket (Figs 219 and 220).

Closure. It remains only to re-attach the coracoid process with two sutures through the soft tissues, to repair the deltoid muscle if it has been partly detached from the clavicle, and to suture the skin without drainage.

POST-OPERATIVE MANAGEMENT

It is important that the arm be held in medial rotation for the first three weeks after operation. At the conclusion of the operation copious folds of absorbent gauze are placed in the axilla and between the arm and the trunk, and the arm is bandaged to the trunk with the forearm across the chest by several wide crepe bandages reinforced with elastic adhesive bandage. In order to apply these bandages satisfactorily at the conclusion of the operation the patient should be placed in a sitting position while still anaesthetised, the back being supported on a narrow smooth board. The bandages are placed around the trunk and board together, and after completion of the bandaging the board is withdrawn.

The patient is allowed up immediately and should practise wrist and finger exercises and, to a limited extent, elbow flexion and extension so far as the bandages permit. Three weeks from the time of operation the bandages are removed and a simple sling is applied. After a further week active mobilising exercises for the shoulder are begun, but attempted lateral rotation is avoided.

Comment

This operation is straightforward and provides the opportunity for a clean anatomical dissection of the structures at the front of the shoulder. There are only two points of special importance; the first one of caution and the other one of difficulty. Special caution is needed to avoid damaging the musculocutaneous nerve during retraction downwards of the coracobrachialis and biceps muscles. The nerve enters the deep surface of the muscles obliquely. As the muscles are reflected downwards it may be seen coming in from the medial aspect. It is in danger of being stretched by too vigorous retraction or even of being accidentally divided if it is not identified and protected.

The main point of difficulty in the operation is in the insertion of the key sutures which hold the stump of the subscapularis tendon deeply in the pocket in front of the neck of the scapula. The difficulty is to get these sutures deeply enough between the belly of the subscapularis and the neck of the scapula. Inserting the sutures is made easier by the use of very small but thick and strong needles such as the Mayo trocar-pointed needle. As already noted, twin needles should be used on each strand of suture material, and each needle is passed from the outside of the periosteum (between periosteum and subscapularis muscle) in such a way that the point enters the capsulo-periosteal pocket at its very depth. The needle is then gripped by the point and pulled through into the pocket and thence through the stump of the subscapularis in mattress fashion (Fig. 220).

Of the many operations that have been devised for the stabilisation of the shoulder in cases of recurrent dislocation, most—whether or not by deliberate intent—lead to fibrous buttressing of the anterior capsular pocket into which the humeral head was wont to subluxate, and many of them cause restriction of the extreme range of lateral rotation. This is beneficial, for full lateral rotation allows the defect in the humeral head to come forward to the anterior glenoid margin and to subluxate over it. The Putti-Platt operation, in its design, is intended to achieve both anterior fibrous buttressing and restriction of lateral rotation, and it is nearly always effective while still permitting virtually normal function. The Magnuson and Stack (1943) operation, in which the subscapularis muscle is advanced laterally to a new insertion on the upper end of the humerus, similarly restricts lateral rotation but without deliberately buttressing the front of the joint.

GLENOPLASTY BY ANTERIOR BONE BLOCK FOR RECURRENT ANTERIOR DISLOCATION OF SHOULDER

This operation is designed to extend the bearing surface of the glenoid fossa anteriorly by screwing a suitably shaped piece of iliac bone to the front of the neck of the scapula. The bone graft is placed outside the capsule so that the synovial lining will provide a gliding membrane over the raw bone.

TECHNIQUE

Position of patient. This is the same as for the Putti-Platt operation (p. 157).

Exposure. The shoulder is exposed anteriorly in the manner described for the Putti-Platt operation. The steps of that operation are followed as far as the point at which the joint capsule is opened to allow inspection of the interior of the joint.

Preparation of bed for graft. It is necessary to raw the anterior surface of the neck of the scapula to promote bony fusion of the graft to the host. The area to be rawed is about 2 centimetres wide and it should extend backwards towards the body of the scapula for at least 2.5 to 3 centimetres. In this area periosteum is stripped and the cortical bone is deeply scarified or flaked off with a sharp chisel or rasp, or with a dental burr.

Preparation of bone graft. Selection of the appropriate piece of bone from which to shape the graft demands much care. The graft is taken from the wing of the ilium, and it is usually best to include with it part of the iliac crest. The piece of bone required will measure approximately 2 centimetres wide by 3 centimetres long: it is wise to take rather more bone than will be needed in order to allow scope for shaping the graft.

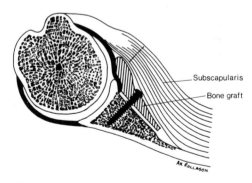

Subscapularis
Bone graft

FIG. 221. Anterior bone block for recurrent anterior dislocation of shoulder. Horizontal section showing shape and position of the bone graft. Dotted line shows site of division of the subscapularis.

The final product should be thick at the end that will border the glenoid fossa, and from there it should gradually taper to thinner bone where it will lie upon the body of the scapula (Fig. 221). The glenoid end should thus be represented by the thick crest of the ilium, and this should be carefully shaped so that when the graft is screwed in position it will present a concave surface that continues the general contour of the glenoid fossa. It will thus provide a bearing surface for the head of the humerus, with only the synovial membrane and capsule interposed between them.

The deep surface of the graft must be rawed by shaving away the cortex, and the raw surface should match accurately the surface of the bed already prepared for the graft.

Application and fixation of graft. The graft is laid in position with care to ensure that the margins of the joint capsule and synovial membrane are trapped between the graft and the rawed anterior surface of the glenoid (Fig. 221). While the graft is held in position by an assistant a suitable hole is drilled through graft and body of glenoid to receive a screw. A screw of appropriate length is then inserted and driven home. Care must be taken not to tighten the screw too forcibly for fear that the screw head may crush the soft cancellous bone of the graft.

Soft-tissue repair. If desired, the application of a bone graft as described may be combined with reefing of the subscapularis muscle in the manner of the Putti-Platt operation. The remaining steps are the same as those already described in the previous section.

POST-OPERATIVE MANAGEMENT
This is the same as for the Putti-Platt operation (p. 160).

Comment
This operation is useful for the small group of patients with recurrent anterior dislocation of the shoulder in whom the joint is so unstable in consequence of ligamentous laxity that the Putti-Platt operation alone may be inadequate.

The main difficulties of the operation are, firstly, to shape the bone graft accurately so that it will in effect form a prolongation forwards of the articular surface of the glenoid fossa; and secondly, to fix the graft securely to the body of the glenoid through the somewhat limited access that is available. It is an operation that demands precision, but one in which patience and meticulous technique are well rewarded.

GLENOPLASTY BY POSTERIOR BONE BLOCK FOR RECURRENT POSTERIOR DISLOCATION OF SHOULDER

This operation is analagous to the anterior bone block operation just described. It should probably be regarded as the standard operation for recurrent posterior dislocation of the shoulder, because a soft-tissue reinforcement operation alone, on the lines of the Putti-Platt operation but at the back of the joint, tends to be unreliable on account of the large size of the defect, or dent, that is nearly always present at the antero-medial part of the head of the humerus.

TECHNIQUE

Position of patient. The patient lies in the lateral posture with the affected shoulder uppermost.

Exposure. An incision 12 centimetres long is made over the lower border of the spine of the scapula, extending laterally as far as the tip of the acromion process (Fig. 222). The deltoid origin is detached from the spine of the scapula and outer aspect of the acromion, and the deltoid cuff is retracted downwards and laterally to expose the infraspinatus and teres minor muscles. These are separated by blunt dissection and the teres minor is retracted downwards.

The infraspinatus is divided 2 centimetres from its insertion into the middle facet of the greater tuberosity of the humerus (Fig. 223). An adequate exposure of the posterior aspect of the joint is thereby obtained. The joint capsule is incised vertically about 2 centimetres from the glenoid margin to enable the interior of the joint to be inspected and the pathological features to be confirmed.

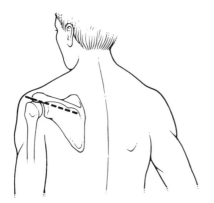

FIG. 222. Posterior exposure of shoulder. The skin incision.

Preparation and fitting of bone block. Preparation of the bed for the graft, taking of the graft from the iliac crest, shaping of the graft and its application

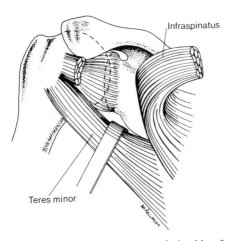

FIG. 223. Posterior exposure of shoulder for stabilisation against recurrent posterior dislocation.

to the back of the neck of the scapula with a screw (Fig. 224) are basically similar to the corresponding steps described in the previous section.

Closure. The operation is completed by repair of the infraspinatus muscle over the graft, and closure of the wound in layers.

POST-OPERATIVE MANAGEMENT

This is the same as for the anterior bone block operation.

Comment

As in the anterior bone block operation, the essentials for success are careful shaping of the iliac bone graft and secure fixation of the graft to the neck of the scapula after thorough rawing of the bed that is to receive it. A hazard of the operation

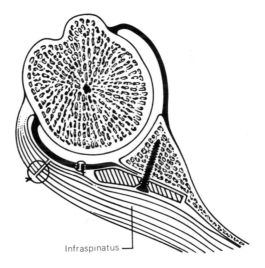

FIG. 224. Posterior bone block for recurrent or persistent posterior dislocation of the shoulder. Horizontal section showing shape and position of the bone graft.

relates to the terminal part of the suprascapular nerve, which penetrates the deep aspect of the infraspinatus muscle after entering the infraspinatus fossa at the lateral border of the spine of the scapula. If proper care is not exercised the nerve may be damaged as the infraspinatus is retracted medially to gain access to the neck of the scapula.

ARTHRODESIS OF SHOULDER

The technique to be described entails rawing of the articular surfaces of the glenoid fossa and of the humeral head, transfixion of the joint with a three-flanged nail or screw, and deflection of the acromion process downwards into a notch cut in the upper end of the humerus. This operation should not be attempted by the inexperienced surgeon, and the orthopaedic surgeon in training should always have the assistance and guidance of his chief.

POSITION FOR ARTHRODESIS

It is essential that the shoulder be fixed in the best position for function—that is, in moderate abduction and with enough medial rotation to enable the hand to be brought to the mouth. The recommended position is: abduction 40 degrees, forward flexion 20 degrees, medial rotation 25 degrees.

TECHNIQUE

Position of patient. The patient lies supine with sand-bags under the shoulder and buttock to roll the patient slightly towards the opposite side.

Incision. The anterior approach to the shoulder is used (see page 10), but the incision over the delto-pectoral groove and coracoid process is prolonged proximally and arched backwards over the shoulder, in the line of the shoulder strap, to end at the posterior margin of the acromion process near its junction with the spine of the scapula (Fig. 225).

Exposure of joint. When the joint capsule has been exposed together with the overlying tendon of subscapularis the long tendon of biceps is identified in the upper part of the bicipital groove of the humerus. The tendon is freed from its tunnel and drawn forwards. The joint is then opened widely by a vertical cut through the medial part of the capsule and the blended tendons (subscapularis below and supraspinatus above).

Rawing of articular surface. The articular cartilage of the glenoid fossa and of the head of the

humerus is removed with gouges and chisels to expose raw bleeding bone. So far as possible the opposing articular surfaces are shaped in such a way that they are in intimate contact when the shoulder is placed in the optimal position for fusion.

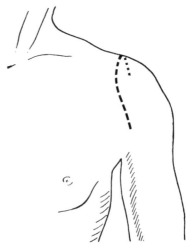

FIG. 225. Arthrodesis of shoulder. The skin incision.

Internal fixation. The arm is now carefully adjusted so that the shoulder rests in the correct position for fusion, as described above. The position is held carefully by an assistant while a guide wire is driven across the joint from the outer aspect of the neck of the humerus. The guide wire should enter the glenoid fossa near its centre, and should be so directed as to engage the thickest part of the scapula. (It is useful to have a dried skeleton of the shoulder at hand for reference.) A three-flanged nail or a heavy duty cannulated bone screw of appropriate length is then driven home over the guide wire, with care to ensure that the rawed articular surfaces of the humerus and glenoid are not distracted from one another (Fig. 226).

Deflection of acromion into humerus. To facilitate downward deflection of the acromion process the spine of the scapula is partly divided close to the base of the acromion. Likewise the clavicle is cut partly through so that the whole acromion may be readily turned downwards to engage in a notch that should be cut in the upper end of the humerus to receive it (Fig. 226). It may be possible to fix the acromion to the upper end of the humerus with a screw directed downwards and slightly medially.

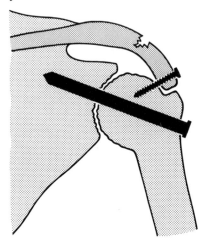

FIG. 226. Arthrodesis of shoulder. After rawing of the articular surfaces, the humeral head and the glenoid are transfixed by a three-flanged nail or screw in the optimal position. Then the acromion process is deflected downwards after partial osteotomy at its base, and secured in a slot in the humeral head.

POST-OPERATIVE MANAGEMENT

For the first two weeks the arm is rested upon an abduction shoulder splint which has been prepared and fitted for a trial period before the operation. After two weeks, when the sutures are removed, a plaster-of-Paris shoulder spica is applied with the patient in the sitting position, care being taken to ensure that the shoulder remains in the ideal position for fusion.

Comment

The need to arthrodese the shoulder arises very seldom, especially now that the incidence of tuberculosis and of poliomyelitis has been enormously reduced. The operation is a difficult one, partly because the correct angle for fusion—which is critical—is not easily judged in the anaesthetised patient, and partly because the rather soft humerus and the very small socket do not lend themselves well to rigid internal fixation. The operation should therefore be undertaken only by experienced orthopaedic surgeons.

Caution. One point needs special emphasis: that is, that in a case of totally paralysed and flail shoulder muscles with intact hand function, the greatest care must be taken not to pull heavily on the limb during the positioning of the patient. In the relaxed anaesthetised patient it is all too easy for an assistant, helping to roll the patient over in order to insert a sand-bag behind the scapula, to cause a traction lesion of the brachial plexus. The senior author has seen this happen in his own operation theatre, with disastrous consequences to the function of the limb.

TOTAL REPLACEMENT ARTHROPLASTY OF SHOULDER

Arthroplasty of the shoulder—undertaken mostly for severe rheumatoid arthritis and occasionally for degenerative arthritis—is still in a stage of development, and it is not possible to predict how it will evolve in the future. Prominent among the several methods that have been devised are those of Neer *et al.* (1982), Lettin *et al.* (1982) and Bayley and Kessel (1982). All except that of Kessel entail the fitting of a high-density polyethylene socket in the region of the glenoid and a ball-shaped stemmed metal head in the humerus after removal of the natural head: in Kessel's technique the arrangement is reversed, so that the ball is fitted to the glenoid and the socket to the humerus.

In general, the technique of insertion of these devices is similar in all. The basic steps are exemplified in the following description of the arthroplasty devised by Mr M. Laurence (1991) of Guy's Hospital in London. For details of the alternative techniques mentioned above the reader is referred to the original papers. Arthroplasty of the shoulder should not be attempted by the inexperienced surgeon, and the orthopaedic surgeon in training should always have the guidance of an expert in the technique.

THE LAURENCE TECHNIQUE

The technique to be described has the merit of simplicity and the technical advantage that the socket of the ball-and-socket joint is cemented not only to the glenoid fossa—too small in itself to provide adequate anchorage—but also to the acromion process and the coracoid process. Only one size of prosthesis* is available and this may be used for either the right or the left shoulder. The humeral prosthesis, of cobalt-chrome alloy, resembles a miniature femoral head prosthesis

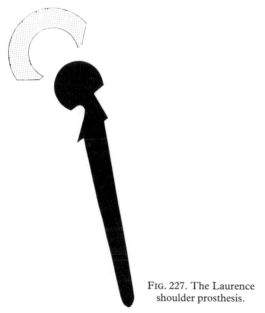

FIG. 227. The Laurence shoulder prosthesis.

(Fig. 227): the head diameter is 25 millimetres. The hemispherical glenoid prosthesis is of high density polyethylene, with an outside diameter of 50 millimetres (Fig. 227).

TECHNIQUE

Position of patient. The patient lies supine, with the affected shoulder thrown forwards by a sandbag placed under the scapular region. In the pre-

* Supplied by Corin Ltd, London, England.

parations for operation, the affected limb is draped separately and enclosed in a sterile stockingette tube to permit easy handling by the surgeon or his assistant during the operation.

Incision. The incision, 9 or 10 centimetres long, extends distally from a point just below the clavicle in the line of the delto-pectoral groove

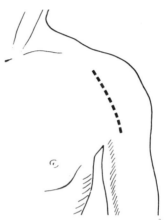

FIG. 228. Laurence arthroplasty of shoulder. The skin incision.

(Fig. 228). A useful surface marking for this is the coracoid process: the delto-pectoral groove lies immediately lateral to it. Distally, the incision follows a line which if projected downwards would cross the middle of the antecubital fossa midway between the medial and the lateral epicondyle of the humerus.

Exposure of shoulder joint. The exposure is basically the standard anterior exposure of the shoulder (see p. 10). The sulcus between the deltoid and the pectoralis major is identified. (If there is any difficulty in this the cephalic vein, which lies in the groove, is a useful landmark.) The cephalic vein is retracted medially to allow the interval between the deltoid and the pectoralis major to be opened up by dissection with blunt-nosed scissors. A few tributaries crossing the sulcus to enter the cephalic vein require division.

The dissection is deepened lateral to the coracoid process, where the fibres of the subscapularis muscle, running transversely, are easily identified: laterally they blend with the capsule of the shoulder joint.

Next the tendon of the long head of the biceps is identified in the bicipital groove of the humerus, which is easily palpated about 2.5 centimetres lateral to the tip of the coracoid process. The aponeurosis that converts the bicipital groove into a tunnel is divided longitudinally, exposing the tendon in the groove. The tendon will shortly be divided, but in order to prevent downward retraction of the distal stump the tendon is first anchored in its groove by two or three absorbable sutures transfixing the tendon and the overlying aponeurosis. The tendon is then divided proximal to the point of suture.

Attention is now turned to the tendon of the subscapularis muscle, already identified. This is incised close to the joint, where the tendon is already blended with the joint capsule. Tendon and capsule are incised together, opening the gleno-humeral joint. The exposure of the joint is widened by excision of the anterior part of the capsule and synovial membrane.

Removal of humeral head. An assistant should now grasp the upper arm and deliver the upper end of the humerus forwards to give a clear view of the whole of the head and neck. At this stage the limb is maintained in the neutral (anatomical)

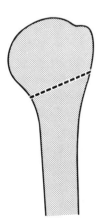

FIG. 229. Line of division of the neck of the humerus.

position. The neck of the humerus is divided with an osteotome or powered saw to allow removal of the head. The line of the bone section, commencing at the medial angle of the neck, slopes upwards and laterally (Fig. 229).

The head is removed either entire or, if more convenient, piecemeal. The proximal stump of the

tendon of the long head of biceps is divided proximally and removed. By working upwards and laterally under the acromion process and deltoid, the remains of the subacromial bursa are removed.

Preparation of bed for socket. When the humeral head and greater tuberosity, together with most of the anterior part of the capsule, have been removed, three bony components will be seen ranged round the medial and superior aspects of the cavity that remains (Fig. 230). (In the cases for

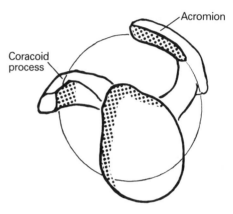

FIG. 230. The circle encloses the three bony parts to which the socket is anchored—namely the greater (upper) part of the glenoid fossa, the coracoid process and the acromion process.

which shoulder arthroplasty is usually required—namely severely destructive rheumatoid arthritis or osteoarthritis—the supraspinatus tendon complex will almost always have been disrupted, so that the cavity of the shoulder joint proper and of the subacromial bursa have become one.) These three bony components are: postero-medially, the glenoid fossa; superiorly, the under surface of the acromion process; antero-medially, the coracoid process.* Together they form the outline of a cavity which, suitably prepared, will accept the high density polyethylene socket that forms the female part of the prosthetic joint.

To prepare the bed for the socket the three bony

* In some cases of advanced degenerative disease with long-standing disruption of the supraspinatus tendon complex, the glenoid fossa and the under surface of the acromion process are more or less confluent due to the formation of osteophytic bone outgrowths above the glenoid which meet up with the medial border of the acromion.

surfaces are roughened by removal of the surface bone. This is conveniently done with a powered burr. In the case of the glenoid fossa remains of articular cartilage are removed, usually only from the upper two-thirds of the cavity, and the subchondral bone is made rough by multiple small cuts with a fine chisel. Holes are then drilled in all three bony prominences in order to key in the cement that will hold the prosthetic socket. The holes may be 6 to 8 millimetres in diameter: one or two may be drilled in the glenoid, at least two in the acromion process, and one in the coracoid process. A trial fit is made of the socket that is to be used or of a template of the same diameter, and if necessary further bone may be removed to allow correct seating of the prosthesis.

mouth of the socket is: 35 degrees of forward inclination from the lateral axis, and 30 degrees of lateral angulation from the vertical axis (Figs 231 and 232). With the cup thus correctly orientated it is held pressed in position until the cement sets.

Trial fit of humeral prosthesis. It is a simple matter to scoop out the cancellous bone of the upper third of the humeral shaft to accommodate the stem of the humeral head prosthesis. Before this is cemented in, it is well to insert the prosthesis without cement and to articulate the two parts to assess the freedom of movement. It is important to ensure that enough capsule at the inferior aspect of the joint has been removed to allow passive abduction through 90 degrees.

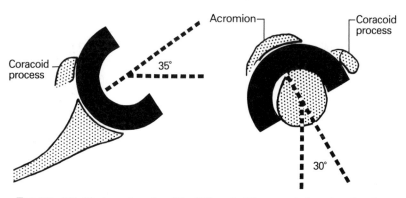

FIGS 231–232. Horizontal section (Fig. 231) and oblique vertical section showing correct orientation of the socket: its axis is inclined forwards 35 degrees from the coronal plane (Fig. 231) and 30 degrees outwards from the vertical plane (Fig. 232). Note that the socket abuts on the coracoid process and the acromion process.

Fixation of plastic socket by cement. Acrylic cement is prepared in the normal way, and when it is ready for insertion it is divided into three parts, one for the glenoid fossa, one for the acromion process, and one for the coracoid process. Each lump of cement is pressed firmly about the respective bony prominence, with care to ensure that cement enters the drill holes. Although separate lumps of cement are used to invest each bone, they may become confluent, especially in the case of the glenoid fossa and the acromion process.

When all is ready the polyethylene cup is pressed into the cement-lined bed and its orientation is adjusted. The recommended axis of the

If all is well, the prosthesis is removed and reinserted after the medullary cavity has been filled with cement. At this point it is necessary to check that the orientation of the humeral head is correct: with the arm in the anatomically neutral position—this can be maintained most easily by flexing the elbow through 90 degrees and ensuring that the forearm is directed forwards—the humeral head should face directly medially.

Assembly and closure. When the cement has set, the humeral head is pressed into the socket. With this particular prosthesis the two parts engage with a snap fit, which helps to prevent subluxation when the arm is relaxed and dependent. Considerable pressure is needed to force the head into the socket through the slightly crimped opening.

In closure, the deltoid is approximated to the pectoralis major with a few absorbable sutures after a suction drainage tube has been placed deep to this muscle layer. The skin is closed in the normal way and the limb is supported in a sling.

POST-OPERATIVE MANAGEMENT

Immobilisation is not required. For the first few days the arm should be rested comfortably upon a pillow on the bed. After three or four days the patient is encouraged to be up and about, the limb being supported in a sling. At about this time passive shoulder movements are begun. A week or so later, active movements are attempted and are assisted by the physiotherapist, who may use slings or, preferably, a pool to lessen the force of gravity.

Comment

Like shoulder arthroplasty in general, the main purpose of this operation is to relieve pain. Restoration of active movement, though obviously desirable, is less important than comfort. With this operation, as with most other types of shoulder arthroplasty, ability to lift the arm against gravity beyond the range that can be achieved by scapular rotation is a bonus rather than an expectation. Some flexion/extension movement is usually regained, and with assistance or with gravity eliminated the range of abduction may be 90 degrees but seldom more.

As already noted, the technique gives wider fixation of the socket than do those methods in which the socket is fixed solely to the glenoid fossa. It is important that full advantage be taken of this by meticulous exposure and roughening of the three bony points to which attachment is made, with careful siting of the keying-in holes. It is also important to apply the cement not too dry, so that it thoroughly invests the three bony points and penetrates deeply into the drill holes.

It may be questioned whether it would not be advisable to make provision for attachment of the short superior tendons—supraspinatus and infraspinatus—to the prosthesis; or alternatively, to so design the prosthesis that the greater tuberosity could be left intact. In the type of case that lends itself to shoulder arthroplasty, however, the tendinous cuff is almost invariably disintegrated and its repair is impracticable.

AMPUTATIONS ABOUT THE SHOULDER

In amputations at the shoulder the head of the humerus should be retained whenever possible in order to preserve the normal contour of the shoulder.

AMPUTATION THROUGH THE NECK OF THE HUMERUS

TECHNIQUE

Position of patient. The patient lies supine but the upper part of the trunk is rolled into the semi-lateral position with the affected shoulder uppermost, this position being maintained by a large sand-bag beneath the scapular region.

Marking out the skin incisions. It is convenient to mark out on the skin surface the outline of the incisions before the operation is begun. The outline is designed to form a lateral flap corresponding broadly to the deltoid muscle. The outline begins anteriorly at the coracoid process and follows the anterior border of the deltoid as far as its insertion. The outline then curves backwards and proximally along the posterior border of the deltoid as far as the posterior axillary fold. The two ends of this outline are joined in a line passing under the axilla (Fig. 233).

Dissection and division of major vessels and nerves. When incisions have been made through skin and fascia in the outlines already drawn, attention is first directed to the anterior part of the wound, where the interval between the deltoid muscle and the pectoralis major is developed. The site of this interval is marked by the cephalic vein, which should be ligated and divided high in the

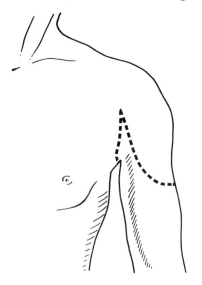

FIG. 233. Amputation through neck of humerus. The skin incision.

wound. When the two muscles have been separated the pectoralis major is traced distally as far as its insertion into the humerus. The muscle is divided there and reflected medially.

Dissection now in the angle between the pectoralis minor and the coracobrachialis reveals the neurovascular bundle traversing the axilla. The axillary artery and vein are doubly ligated by transfixion ligatures and divided immediately below the pectoralis minor. The four major nerves—the median, the ulnar, the radial and the musculocutaneous—are then individually pulled distally and divided cleanly as high up as possible and allowed to retract.

Division of remaining muscles and of neck of humerus. The deltoid muscle is traced to its insertion into the humerus, divided there and reflected proximally together with the overlying skin flap. The latissimus dorsi and teres major are severed close to their insertions at the bicipital groove of the humerus.

The level of bone section, which should be through the surgical neck of the humerus, is marked upon the surface. About 2 centimetres distal to this the triceps muscle, the two heads of the biceps and the coracobrachialis are divided transversely. The humerus is divided with a hand saw and the limb discarded.

Closure. The triceps muscle, the two heads of the biceps and the coracobrachialis are sutured together over the end of the divided bone. Likewise the pectoralis major is swung outwards and attached in the region of the cut bone end. The lateral flap, comprising skin and underlying deltoid muscle, is trimmed as necessary to allow the edges to be sutured smoothly to the periphery of the wound. Suction drainage should be provided deep to this flap.

POST-OPERATIVE MANAGEMENT

Copious gauze dressings are held in place by crepe bandages carried round the trunk and reinforced by an elastic adhesive bandage. The drainage tube should be removed after 48 hours.

DISARTICULATION OF THE SHOULDER

TECHNIQUE

The technique of disarticulation of the shoulder is broadly similar to that of amputation through the neck of the humerus. The incision, the treatment of vessels and nerves, and the raising of the skin flap with the deltoid muscle are the same as described in the previous section.

After division of the latissimus dorsi and the teres major the arm is rotated strongly medially to expose the short lateral rotator muscles—supraspinatus, infraspinatus and teres minor—which are divided close to the bone together with the posterior part of the joint capsule. Next the arm is rotated laterally to allow division of the subscapularis muscle and the remainder of the capsule. Division of the triceps muscle then frees the limb, which is discarded.

In closure of the wound the divided ends of the pectoralis major, triceps, biceps and coracobrachialis are drawn towards the glenoid fossa and sutured there to fill the conspicuous hollow. The area is further covered by the flap of deltoid muscle, which is sutured below the glenoid fossa. Any undue prominence of the acromion process is then trimmed away to give a more even contour to the shoulder.

Finally the edges of the skin flap are trimmed appropriately so that it fits accurately to the periphery of the wound. The skin edges are united with interrupted eversion sutures after provision has been made for suction drainage deep to the deltoid layer.

POST-OPERATIVE MANAGEMENT

This is the same as for amputation through the neck of the humerus.

FORE-QUARTER AMPUTATION

Fore-quarter or interscapulothoracic amputation ablates the whole upper limb together with the corresponding half of the shoulder girdle (clavicle and scapula) and the related muscles. A detailed description of the operation is not required here: it is performed very infrequently, almost always for malignant tumour in the proximal part of the extremity, and generally it is undertaken only by those with wide experience in the field of orthopaedic surgery or of cancer surgery.

TECHNIQUE

The operation is most conveniently performed with the patient in the lateral position, with the affected limb uppermost. The surgeon works first and mainly from the back, and makes a secondary incision anteriorly in the later stages.

The first incision begins at the medial end of the clavicle and follows the bone laterally as far as the acromion process, where it turns backwards over the shoulder and then follows the axillary border of the scapula down as far as the inferior angle;

there it turns medially onto the chest wall, ending close to the mid-line (Fig. 234).

The various muscles holding the scapula and humerus to the back of the trunk are divided well clear of the scapula and the clavicle is divided close to its medial end. Thus separated from its posterior attachments, the scapula falls forwards so that the subclavian vessels and the brachial plexus come into view in the upper part of the wound. The trunks of the brachial plexus are divided near the spinal column and the vessels are ligated and divided.

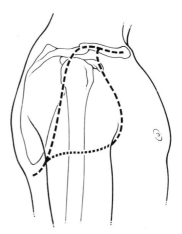

FIG. 234. Forequarter amputation (Littlewood technique). The skin incisions.

From the front a second incision is made: this begins over the middle of the clavicle and extends downwards close to the delto-pectoral groove. Thence it extends across the anterior fold of the axilla and downwards and backwards on the upper part of the lateral chest wall to join the first incision near the lower end of the axillary border of the scapula (Fig. 234). This allows division of the remaining muscles and separation of the whole limb with the scapula and clavicle.

Comment

Those seeking a detailed description of the operation should consult the original paper of Littlewood (1922).

CHAPTER SIX

Upper Arm and Elbow

Arm and elbow injuries figure prominently in fracture surgery. Indeed injury accounts for a high proportion of the operations that are undertaken in this region. It is a region where a precise knowledge of the anatomy pays dividends, for on every aspect there are nerves or major blood vessels that are liable to be damaged, not only as a consequence of fracture or dislocation but also by injudicious surgery.

CONTENTS OF CHAPTER

INTRAMEDULLARY NAILING OF FRACTURED HUMERUS

This section should be read in conjunction with the general description of intramedullary nailing in Chapter 2 (p. 84). As with other long bones, nailing may be "closed" if an acceptable position of the bone fragments can be secured without exposing them; or open, when exposure of the fragments is required in order to gain adequate reduction.

CLOSED NAILING

Closed nailing is applicable only when the fragments are in acceptable position or when adequate reduction can be gained by closed methods.

TECHNIQUE

Position of patient. The patient is placed in the lateral position with the affected arm uppermost and the elbow flexed to a right angle. It is advantageous to have the arm resting upon a platform over the body: an easily constructed platform used by the authors is shown in Figure 235: alternatively, a large Mayo table may be adapted for the purpose. Provision should be made if necessary for the application of longitudinal traction on the humerus through a Kirschner wire which may be inserted through the olecranon process. Provision should also be made for use of the image intensifier or for radiographic films during the operation. It is not practicable to use a tourniquet.

Reduction of fracture. An attempt is made to reduce the fracture by closed manipulation supplemented if necessary by skeletal traction. The

dow" allows the introduction of a Steinmann pin which, held in a hand chuck, is thrust proximally along the medullary canal for 8 to 10 centimetres

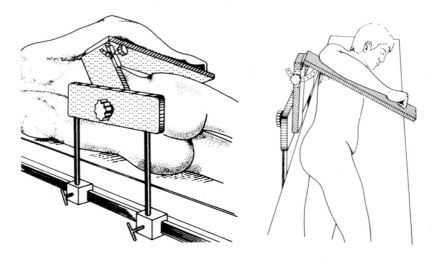

FIG. 235. Adjustable platform to support the upper arm, elbow and forearm for operations upon the posterior aspect of the humerus.

position is checked radiographically, preferably by the image intensifier, and if an acceptable position has been gained the operation proceeds in the following stages. If an acceptable reduction is not achieved, closed nailing is abandoned in favour of the open technique (p. 175).

Incision. It is best always to introduce the nail at the distal end of the humerus, never at the upper end. The incision for the introduction of the nail is therefore made in the midline of the posterior aspect of the arm: it extends from the tip of the olecranon process proximally for about 6 centimetres. The lower end of the triceps aponeurosis and muscle is split to expose the olecranon fossa of the humerus and the posterior cortex of the humeral shaft immediately proximal to the fossa.

Preparation of entrance point for guide wire. With a 4-millimetre drill or a narrow gouge the cortex of the olecranon fossa is penetrated and the instrument is driven proximally into the medullary canal of the humerus. This initial opening is enlarged proximally with fine bone-nibbling forceps to extend 1 or 2 centimetres up the shaft of the humerus (Fig. 236). This elongated "win-

to form a starting track that will direct the guide wire along the correct course.

Introduction of guide wire. A guide wire, preferably of the olive-tipped type, is thrust along the

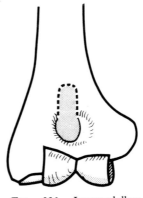

FIG. 236. Intramedullary nailing of humerus. The floor of the olecranon fossa has been perforated and the opening has been extended upwards about a centimetre to allow access for the reamer and nail.

track prepared for it and is advanced across the site of fracture into the proximal fragment of the humerus. It should penetrate almost to the sub-chondral bone of the humeral head: this point is easily felt because the advance of the guide wire comes to an abrupt halt. The position of the wire is checked by the image intensifier.

Reaming of medullary canal. The canal is reamed in the usual way by flexible reamers passed in turn over the guide wire. Depending upon the size of the bone, the initial reamer may be 6 or 7 millimetres in diameter. Reaming is continued until the canal is large enough to receive a fairly stout nail, usually about 9 or 10 millimetres in diameter.

Alternative method: drilling out the canal. If in a case of old ununited fracture sclerotic bone blocks the medullary canal it may be difficult to pass a guide wire across the site of fracture. In that event it is easier to drill out the canal with long twist drills driven by a hand brace. The initial drill should be about 4 millimetres in diameter. When a suitable track has been drilled it may be enlarged appropriately by further twist drills, or a guide wire may be passed to allow further enlargement of the canal with flexible reamers.

Insertion of nail. Before the nail is driven in, the olive-tipped guide wire should be changed for a plain one or, if the fracture is stable, it may be discarded.

The correct length of nail is determined from the calculated length of guide wire within the bone, the position of the tip of the wire having been observed radiographically. The length of nail should be so chosen that the tip of the nail penetrates into the head of the humerus almost to the subchondral bone. Distally, the base of the nail should be just within the opening in the posterior cortex of the lower end of the humeral shaft, so that it does not abut on the olecranon fossa.

When a nail of the correct length and diameter has been selected it is inserted through the distal opening, preferably with the removal slot orien-tated posteriorly. It is then driven on with light blows of the hammer, its position being checked periodically with the image intensifier.

Insertion of cross screw. It is essential in the case of the humerus, unlike the other long bones, to place a screw transversely in the lower end of the humerus, either immediately distal to the nail or through a drill hole in the nail, to prevent the nail from sliding distally—a common complication if the screw is omitted. The screw, preferably of narrow gauge, is easily placed through an appro-priate drill hole which may be antero-posterior if the screw is to penetrate a hole in the nail, or in the coronal plane if the screw is placed distal to the end of the nail.

POST-OPERATIVE MANAGEMENT

Provided a firm grip of the fragments has been secured with the nail, external protection by a plaster or splint is unnecessary. The arm may simply be supported in a sling. Early finger and elbow exercises are encouraged, and within a few days active and assisted shoulder exercises may be begun.

Comment

Closed nailing of the humeral shaft does not present any special difficulty, except sometimes that of gaining adequate reduction. It must be emphasised again that the nail should always be introduced from below, rather than through the tuberosity of the humerus as has sometimes been recommended. Introduction through the tubero-sity is liable to interfere with the restoration of shoulder function, whereas a nail introduced in the olecranon fossa does not significantly affect elbow movement once the tissues have healed.

In contradistinction to nails required for the femur and the tibia, a nail inserted into the humerus need not be of very wide diameter: since the humerus is not a weight-bearing bone, strains upon it are relatively small, and usually a nail of, say, 10 millimetres will suffice provided it is tight enough in the medullary canal to prevent rotation of the fragments.

Another point worthy of note is the need to prevent the nail from sliding distally by means of a cross screw. The authors have several times seen cases in which the nail slid downwards into the olecranon fossa, necessitating re-operation within a few days of the primary procedure, through neglect of this precaution.

OPEN NAILING

When adequate reduction of the fracture cannot be achieved by closed methods open nailing is required.

TECHNIQUE

Position of patient. This is the same as for closed nailing.

Incision. The fracture site is exposed through the posterior approach, made through a midline posterior incision as described on page 16. The long head and the lateral head of the triceps are separated, and the medial or deep head is incised vertically, with care to protect the radial nerve.

Reduction of fracture. If the fracture site is not immediately obvious it is approached from above and from below, normal bone away from the fracture being first exposed. The fracture surfaces are cleared of blood clot, fibrin and—in late cases—fibrous tissue and callus, so that they may be fitted together in exact apposition. The fragments are held reduced by bone-holding forceps or by a bone clamp during the subsequent stages of the operation.

Medullary nailing. The remaining stages of the operation, namely the preparation of the opening for the guide wire, the introduction of the guide wire, reaming of the canal and the driving of the nail are the same as in closed nailing.

POST-OPERATIVE MANAGEMENT

This is the same as for closed nailing.

Comment

Open nailing of the humeral shaft does not present special problems. Special care is needed to avoid injury to the radial nerve or its branches. In high fractures of the shaft the ulnar nerve and the brachial artery are also vulnerable.

USE OF THE HUCKSTEP NAIL

In a difficult case of non-union of a fracture of the shaft of the humerus the use of the Huckstep perforated intramedullary nail, supplemented by transfixion screws, should be considered. The technique of inserting this device, which is used mainly for difficult fractures of the femoral shaft, is described on page 335. This account should be consulted.

NAILING FOR FRACTURE OF NECK OF HUMERUS

Even though the proximal fragment is very short after fracture of the neck of the humerus, nevertheless intramedullary nailing is often the method of choice when internal fixation is required. For these very high fractures the exposure of the fracture itself should be through the anterior route (p. 10). In other respects the operation follows the same lines as those described in the previous section. It is of course particularly important that the nail should penetrate right up to the subchondral bone of the humeral head, in order that the best possible grip be obtained. As in the case of fracture of the shaft of the humerus, a Huckstep nail may be used, to allow the introduction of multiple cross screws.

PLATE FIXATION FOR FRACTURE OF SHAFT OF HUMERUS

The technique of internal fixation of fractures by plating was described in Chapter 2 (p. 82). Plating is applicable to most fractures of the humeral shaft as an alternative to medullary nailing.

When function of the radial nerve is unimpaired the approach to the humeral shaft may be through the anterior incision (p. 14) with splitting of the brachialis muscle in the direction of its fibres. If, however, there is evidence of damage to the radial nerve the posterior approach (p. 16) is to be preferred because it allows direct examination of the nerve at the same time that the fracture is dealt with.

Most fractures of the humeral shaft unite readily, and simple plating is usually adequate. Nevertheless there is probably some advantage in using a plate of the dynamic compression type: this plate has slotted holes so shaped that as the screws are driven in the fragments are pressed together (see page 70).

POST-OPERATIVE MANAGEMENT

Unless fixation by a plate is exceptionally rigid it is wise to support the limb in a full length arm plaster from axilla to metacarpal heads, with the elbow held at a right angle. If this is deemed unnecessary a simple cuff of plaster round the upper arm may suffice. The initial plaster should be changed at two weeks when the sutures are removed, and thereafter protection is continued until union of the fracture, as shown radiographically, is well advanced. It is important to encourage shoulder exercises from an early stage. Later, when the plaster has been removed, elbow exercises must be practised assiduously.

Comment

Although plate fixation of humeral fractures usually gives good results, fixation by an intramedullary nail is generally to be preferred for fractures near the middle of the shaft, because of its greater rigidity. On the other hand, in fractures near the lower end of the humerus plating, combined if necessary with screw fixation of isolated condylar fragments, offers better fixation than an intramedullary nail.

BONE GRAFTING FOR DELAYED UNION OR NON-UNION OF FRACTURE OF HUMERAL SHAFT

The techniques of bone grafting were described in Chapter 2 (p. 78). These techniques apply to fractures of the humerus as to most other long bones, and further detailed description is not required here.

As in fractures of the other major long bones, bone grafting may be either by the technique of applying cancellous sliver grafts about the site of fracture (Phemister 1947) or by cortical onlay grafting, in which a cortical bone graft is screwed across the fracture in the manner of a metal plate. Generally, cancellous sliver grafting is to be preferred to cortical onlay grafting, though in most cases it is advisable to supplement the technique by securing rigid fixation of the bone fragments by a stout intramedullary nail driven in from below (see p. 172) or by a Huckstep perforated nail with transfixion screws (p. 335).

Onlay cortical bone grafting is a reasonable alternative, but it entails disturbance of a tibia as the donor site for a graft, as compared with the lesser hazard of taking sliver grafts from the iliac crest; and the incidence of union is not greater after cortical grafting than after cancellous grafting combined with nail fixation.

The anterior exposure of the humerus (p. 10) is appropriate for cancellous sliver grafting or for onlay cortical grafting, but if grafting is to be combined with intramedullary nailing, which entails a midline posterior incision just above the olecranon process for the introduction of the nail, the posterior approach to the humeral shaft (p. 16) may be found more convenient.

POST-OPERATIVE MANAGEMENT

Whether or not the limb should be protected in a plaster-of-Paris splint after the operation depends upon the rigidity of any internal fixation device that may have been used. If fixation has been achieved by an intramedullary nail, external support may be dispensed with and soft dressings only applied. A sling should be worn for the first few weeks, but early mobilising exercises for shoulder and elbow may be encouraged.

If rigid fixation has not been provided, support for the limb in a plaster-of-Paris splint from axilla to metacarpal heads should be provided, the elbow being held at a right angle. Splintage should be continued until radiographs show union of the fracture to be well advanced, and thereafter intensive mobilising exercises for the elbow are begun.

FIXATION OF FRACTURE OF OLECRANON PROCESS

FIXATION BY INTRAMEDULLARY SCREW

Many different types of screw have been used to secure a separated olecranon fragment to the main body of the ulna. The screw that is recommended is the Venable hip screw, which has an overall diameter of 6 millimetres and a core diameter of 4 millimetres. The screw is used for intramedullary fixation: it is of just the right calibre to pass down the medullary canal and yet to grip its walls securely; thus there is no need to attempt to pass the screw through the cortex of the ulnar shaft.

TECHNIQUE

Position of patient. The patient lies supine with the affected arm across the chest. It is convenient to attach a weight of about 0.5 kilogram (a mallet serves the purpose well) to the wrist with a sterile bandage (applied over padding) and to suspend the weight over the side of the table, in order to stabilise the limb. If a tourniquet is used it should be placed high on the upper arm.

Incision. The incision is an almost vertical one, but curved a little towards the lateral side in order to be well clear of the ulnar nerve. It begins about 3 centimetres proximal to the tip of the olecranon process, and after crossing the olecranon it extends about 5 centimetres downwards over the back of the ulna (Fig. 237).

Exposure of fracture surfaces. The fibres of the triceps muscle are split strictly in the midline: where they are aponeurotic over the olecranon they are separated by sharp dissection to expose the fracture. In this dissection care should be taken to preserve as fully as possible the soft-tissue attachments to the olecranon fragment lest

the blood supply to the bone be imperilled: the main or distal fragment on the other hand may be stripped to expose a wide area of its posterior surface. The fracture surfaces are then inspected in order to confirm that the fragments are suitable for internal fixation by a screw: if comminution is considerably more severe than was expected from examination of the radiographs (as is not infrequently the case), consideration should be given to fixation by a tension band wire (p. 178) or, in the worst cases, to excision of the olecranon.

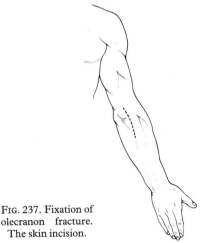

FIG. 237. Fixation of olecranon fracture. The skin incision.

If there is little or no comminution, so that the olecranon fragment is virtually in one piece, preparation for screw fixation should proceed. First the fracture gap is opened by retraction of the proximal fragment with a bone hook. This allows the fracture surfaces to be cleared of blood clot and fibrin, and at the same time the joint cavity may be inspected through the fracture gap and any small loose bone fragments or clots removed. Accurate fitting of the fracture surfaces together is essential, in order to preserve a smooth articular surface without any "step". The fragments should be coapted under direct vision to ensure a perfect fit: nothing short of this should be accepted.

Insertion of screw. It is important that hairline reduction be maintained while a suitable drill hole is made and a screw inserted. Undoubtedly the most satisfactory instrument for holding the frag-

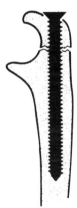

FIG. 238. Screw fixation for fracture of olecranon process. The Venable screw obtains a rigid hold within the medullary canal.

ments at this critical juncture is the Charnley bone clamp. To apply this a drill hole is first made in the shaft of the ulna about 3 centimetres distal to the fracture line to receive the peg of the Charnley device. The other jaw of the clamp is fitted with the double hook device which grips the superior surface of the olecranon: thus when the clamp is closed the fragments are held immovably.

A hole for the screw is now prepared by drilling down from the superior surface of the olecranon into the medullary canal of the ulna with a drill 4 millimetres in diameter. Next the olecranon fragment alone is drilled out to allow a sliding fit of the screw, which demands a drill 6 millimetres in diameter. Finally a Venable hip screw of appropriate length—usually 7.5 centimetres—is driven securely home (Fig. 238).

Checking the position. Before the wound is closed the position of the screw and the state of the fracture should be checked by the image intensifier or by radiographic films. If the position is in any way unsatisfactory the screw must be removed and the appropriate adjustments made.

Closure. The fibres of the triceps muscle and of the aponeurosis are united with fine absorbable sutures and the skin is closed without drainage.

POST-OPERATIVE MANAGEMENT

It is usually advisable to support the limb in a plaster from upper arm to metacarpal heads with the elbow at a right angle. Splintage is maintained for three to four weeks. Mobilising exercises may then be commenced.

Comment

The first point to note about this operation is that it is possible to damage the ulnar nerve in the exposure. The nerve lies surprisingly close to the olecranon, and great care must be taken in the dissection to divide the triceps strictly in the midline of the arm. Likewise, care must be taken not to injure the nerve by over-vigorous retraction of the medial edge of the wound.

The second important point is that replacement of the olecranon fragment must be anatomically perfect; otherwise there will be a step on the articular surface which in the course of time may lead to wear-and-tear degeneration of the joint. To ensure a perfect fit of the fragments the entire area of the fracture surfaces must be clearly exposed to view and thoroughly cleared of interposed tissue. Great care is needed in drilling the proximal fragment for the screw, to avoid splitting the bone.

FIXATION BY TENSION BAND WIRE

Fixation by a tension band wire looped over twin Kirschner wires is appropriate when the olecranon fragment is split or comminuted to an extent that precludes the use of an intramedullary screw (as described in the previous section), but when the articular surface is not so damaged that excision of the olecranon is demanded.

Position of patient. The positioning of the patient and the application of a tourniquet are the same as described in the previous section.

Incision. This is the same as described in the previous section (Fig. 237).

Insertion of Kirschner wires. When the fracture has been fully reduced in the manner previously described, two 1.5 millimetre Kirschner wires 7.5 centimetres long are driven, side by side and parallel to one another, from the superior aspect of the olecranon process, through the olecranon, into the shaft of the ulna. The wires should be spaced about one centimetre apart and should penetrate a distance equal to about three-quarters of their length, leaving one quarter protruding (Fig. 239).

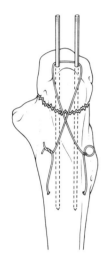

FIG. 239. Fixation of olecranon fracture by tension band wire. The wire, passed through a drill hole in the ulna, is looped over Kirschner wires that penetrate the olecranon, and tightened posteriorly.

Insertion of wire through drill hole, and assembly. With a 2 millimetre drill, a transverse hole is drilled through the shaft of the ulna from side to side, about 4 or 5 centimetres distal to the level of the fracture. Through this hole a length of stainless steel wire (gauge 26) is passed, and the two ends of the wire are turned up proximally to lie over the fracture site. These protruding ends of the wire should be of unequal length. In the longer wire a loop is formed and twisted two or three turns: this loop should lie about 2 centimetres proximal to the drill hole in the ulna. This same end of the wire is then looped over the protruding Kirschner wires, as shown in Figure 239, so that a figure-of-eight is formed. Moderate tension is applied and the two wires are twisted together.

It only remains now to tighten this twisted junction equally with the looped part of the wire, which may be tightened as necessary, to give equal tension on the two sides. Excess wire is cut away, as is the loop, and the twisted wire junctions are turned over and buried either in the bone or in adjacent muscle, to avoid any prominence under the skin.

Attention is now turned again to the Kirschner wires protruding proximally from the upper surface of the olecranon. These are shortened appropriately and turned over posteriorly so that the ends may be punched into the bone to avoid any subcutaneous prominence.

Closure. The split aponeurosis of the triceps is repaired with absorbable sutures. After a further check that there is no undue prominence of the wires the skin is closed in the normal way.

Comment

As in the case of fixation of the olecranon by a screw (see previous section) it is important to ensure that the articular surface of the olecranon is smooth and not stepped. It is a mistake to leave any gross irregularity of this articular surface. Indeed, if a congruous fit of the ulna with the humerus cannot be restored it is probably better to excise the olecranon process and to suture the triceps to the remaining stump of the ulna.

The purpose of looping and twisting the longer end of the tension wire is to allow for even tightening of the two sides of the figure-of-eight tension band. It would be equally appropriate to tighten the two ends of the wire over the olecranon itself, except that it would be more difficult to bury the cut ends of the wire and to avoid prominence under the skin.

The essential principle of this technique is that the two Kirschner wires are used to provide purchase for the tension band on the olecranon fragment. Tensioning of the wires then draws the olecranon into close apposition with the shaft fragment. The extension force theoretically exerted by the tension band is counteracted by the flexion force exerted by the triceps.

EXCISION OF OLECRANON PROCESS FOR COMMINUTED FRACTURE

When extensive comminution of an olecranon fracture precludes the restoration of a perfectly smooth articular surface, excision of the fragmented olecranon may be preferable to attempted reconstruction. After excision of the fragments it is important that the triceps be attached securely to the remaining stump of the olecranon.

TECHNIQUE

Position of patient and exposure of fracture surfaces. These are the same as for screw fixation of fractured olecranon (see p. 177).

Excision of fragments. It is important that the aponeurosis of the triceps that extends over the back and sides of the olecranon should be preserved: comminuted fragments must be excised by sharp dissection, with the knife kept close to the bone.

Reconstruction of triceps mechanism. When the olecranon fragments have been removed there will be found to be a gap of about 2 centimetres between the distal end of the triceps muscle where

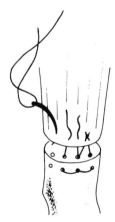

FIG. 240. Method of suturing triceps to ulna after excision of fractured olecranon process.

it has been cut from the bone, and the remaining stump of olecranon. It is not practicable to pull the muscle down to reach the bone; nor would this be advisable because excessive tightness of the triceps would prevent the restoration of a full range of elbow flexion.

In many cases there is some remaining continuity of aponeurotic fibres at each side of the olecranon, but it is nevertheless desirable that the gap between the muscle and bone be bridged. An effective way of doing this is to turn down a flap of triceps muscle consisting of perhaps half its width, the flap being based laterally or anteriorly. Before the muscle flap is turned down, the aponeurosis over it should be split in the midline and reflected towards each side.

With the elbow flexed 90 degrees, the rotated muscle flap is sutured to the stump of the olecranon by mattress sutures of stainless steel wire (gauge 32) inserted through 1-millimetre holes drilled through the cortex of the ulna posteriorly, medially and laterally, the holes emerging on the fracture surface (Fig. 240). When the muscle has been thus reattached to bone, the overlying aponeurosis is sutured back over the muscle to reinforce the repair.

POST-OPERATIVE MANAGEMENT

The limb is supported in a plaster splint extending from the upper arm to the metacarpal heads with the elbow at a right angle. The plaster is retained for three weeks and thereafter active mobilising exercises are encouraged.

Comment

It is important that the repair of the triceps mechanism be made without tension. It is a mistake to suture the triceps to the bone with the elbow fully extended: there may be too much tension on the muscle, so that when the elbow is flexed to the right angle the sutures may tear out. It is better to make the repair with the elbow at a right angle or extended only a few degrees beyond the right angle.

After operation it is unwise to immobilise the elbow in a position of extension beyond the right angle. Immobilisation in extension or near full extension favours oedema of the hand and fingers and may prejudice the restoration of full elbow flexion.

It might seem likely that excision of the olecra-non would leave the elbow unstable and liable to subluxate, but this has not proved to be so in practice. Indeed, provided that not less than half of the articular surface remains, a strong and serviceable elbow is restored.

EXCISION OF HEAD OF RADIUS

The following description applies only to adults. Excision of the head of the radius is not recommended in children because of the risk of proximal migration of the radius.

TECHNIQUE

Position of patient. The patient lies supine with the affected forearm laid across the chest, the elbow being flexed about 80 degrees. It is convenient to attach a weight (a small mallet may serve) to the wrist by a soft bandage applied over padding, and to suspend it over the side of the table in order to keep the limb steady. A tourniquet may be used on the upper arm.

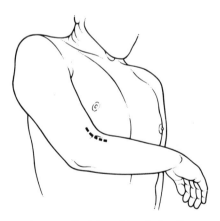

FIG. 241. Excision of head of radius. The skin incision. Note that the fore-arm should be held fully pronated.

Incision. Before the incision is made the forearm should be fully pronated. This brings the posterior interosseous nerve forwards and reduces its vulnerability to injury in the lower part of the wound. The incision begins over the lateral supracondylar ridge of the humerus 2.5 centimetres above the lateral epicondyle. It extends vertically downwards across the humero-radial joint and for 2.5 centimetres distal to it (Fig. 241).

Exposure and removal of radial head. Sharp dissection immediately in front of the supracondylar ridge and lateral epicondyle, with the knife kept

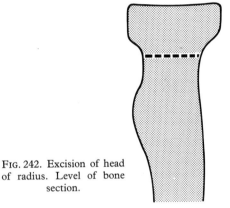

FIG. 242. Excision of head of radius. Level of bone section.

close to the bone, divides the capsule and synovial membrane, thus opening the elbow joint. The incision through the joint membranes is continued distally with scissors to expose the head of the radius. Retraction of the wound edges must be done lightly: heavy leverage with bone spikes may damage the posterior interosseous nerve, which lies in the supinator muscle a little in front of the wound. It is useful and permissible, however, to insert slender, well curved bone levers or Macdonald dissectors round the neck of the radius so long as they are held lightly.

With the bone thus exposed it is a simple matter to divide the neck of the radius transversely just below the head (Fig. 242). Fine-pointed bone-cutting forceps are suitable for this purpose but a thin osteotome may be used if preferred. It is important that the bone be divided cleanly and that the remaining cut surface should be smooth and flat: small spurs or projections must be smoothed away with bone nibblers. If the operation is being done for fracture of the head of the radius it is necessary to be sure that no fragment of bone is left behind in the joint or in the neighbouring soft tissues.

Closure. The incision in the capsule is closed with fine absorbable sutures. The skin is closed with interrupted eversion sutures.

POST-OPERATIVE MANAGEMENT

A crepe bandage is applied snugly over copious gauze dressings. A plaster-of-Paris splint extending from the upper arm to the metacarpal heads with the elbow at a right angle is worn for two weeks. Thereafter active mobilising exercises are begun.

Comment

The potential hazard to the posterior interosseous nerve should always be borne in mind in any operation upon the outer side of the elbow. The hazard and the safeguards against it were discussed by Strachan and Ellis in 1971. Important points are that the forearm should be pronated while the incision is made, and that the incision should not extend more than 2.5 centimetres distal to the joint line.

Many surgeons prefer soft dressings and a sling rather than a plaster splint in the post-operative management. The authors employ plaster splintage because it adds to the patient's comfort and affords the best conditions for wound healing. Moreover, the hand can often be used to better advantage when the elbow is held in plaster without a sling than it can when the arm rests continuously in a sling, especially when this is of the collar-and-cuff type.

SUPRACONDYLAR OSTEOTOMY OF HUMERUS FOR CORRECTION OF VARUS DEFORMITY

This operation is used mainly in children with varus deformity from malunited supracondylar fracture of the humerus. The aim of the operation is to excise an appropriate wedge of bone from the lateral side of the lower humerus and then to angle the bone to close the wedge-shaped gap. The technique to be described applies to children, but the operation in adults is broadly similar.

PRELIMINARY STUDIES

Great accuracy is required if the deformity is to be corrected sufficiently and yet not excessively: the angulation must be exactly right. To facilitate this, comparable antero-posterior radiographs are obtained of both upper limbs with the elbows straight and the forearms in full supination. By drawing lines on the radiographs to indicate the long axis of the humerus and of the ulna on each side, the difference in the angle subtended by these lines in the normal arm and in the deformed arm is measured.

Alternatively, a tracing of the radiograph may

be made on plain paper and the outlines of the bones cut out. On the side of the deformity the paper model is cut across in the supracondylar region of the humerus and the fragments are angulated until the pattern can be superimposed accurately upon that of the normal arm. The angle of correction is then measured with a protractor: the length of the base of the wedge at the lateral cortex should also be measured. When the angle of correction has been thus determined, a template may be cut from paper or from lead sheet for use at the time of operation.

TECHNIQUE

Position of patient. The child lies supine with the affected limb on the side of the table alongside the body. A tourniquet may be applied high on the upper arm.

Incision. The correct level of the osteotomy is about 2 centimetres proximal to the lateral epicondyle of the humerus. A vertical incision 6 centimetres long is made on the lateral side of the arm with its centre at that level.

Marking out the site of osteotomy. After incision of the deep fascia the lateral aspect of the humerus is exposed between the triceps posteriorly and the brachioradialis and, lower down, the extensor carpi radialis longus anteriorly. The periosteum is incised vertically and stripped from the front and back of the bone over a length of about 4 centimetres. The periosteum at the medial side of the humerus should be left intact to serve as a hinge. Slender well curved bone levers are inserted to retract the periosteum and the muscles: retraction anteriorly should be gentle to eliminate any risk of stretching the radial nerve.

With a thin osteotome or an awl the wedge to be removed is outlined on the surface of the bone, its dimensions having been ascertained before operation in the manner described (Fig. 243).

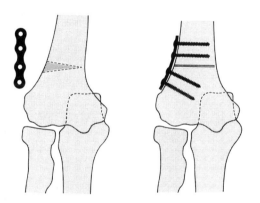

FIGS 243–244. Figure 243—Site of wedge to be cut from humerus for correction of cubitus varus. The angle of the wedge is equal to the angular correction required. Figure 244—After excision of the wedge the gap is closed and the fragments are fixed with a four-hole plate.

Division and angulation of bone. The wedge of bone is removed piecemeal, either with a sharp thin osteotome or with sharp-pointed bone cutting forceps; or with a high-speed dental burr. A slender bridge of cortex should be left intact at the medial side. By gentle force the humerus may now be angulated to close the wedge. In a young child this can be done without fracturing the medial cortex, for the bone is pliable and bends suffi-

ciently. In an older child or adult, however, the medial cortex usually breaks with a snap.

Internal fixation. At this stage it is wise to assess the shape of the arm in comparison with the normal side to make sure that the correction is exactly right. The fragments are then secured with a plate and four screws applied to the lateral aspect of the bone (Fig. 244). Care should be taken to ensure that the plate does not bridge the epiphysial growth plate.

With the osteotomy thus fixed, the final test is made to ensure that the forearm folds correctly upon the upper arm, the hand coming in line with the front of the shoulder.

Closure. The deep tissues are approximated with two or three light absorbable sutures, and the skin is closed without drainage.

POST-OPERATIVE MANAGEMENT

Gauze dressings are held in place with a crepe bandage over which a well padded arm plaster from axilla to metacarpal heads is applied, with the elbow at a right angle and the forearm midway between pronation and supination. The plaster is changed at two weeks, when the sutures are removed. A new close-fitting right-angled arm plaster is applied and retained until adequate union is shown radiographically, usually six to eight weeks from the time of operation.

Comment

The need for accuracy in determining the required angle of correction has already been emphasised. In the actual technique of operation due regard must be paid to the position of the radial nerve, which at this point lies antero-lateral to the humerus, anterior to the front wall of the incision. Excessive retraction of the soft tissues anteriorly may stretch or bruise the nerve. The risk of nerve injury is reduced if the elbow is kept flexed to relax the anterior tissues while the osteotomy is performed.

It is important that the osteotomy be well stabilised before the wound is closed; otherwise the position of the fragments may change while the limb is within the plaster. Leaving an intact medial hinge at the time of osteotomy adds greatly to the stability of the fragments. Nevertheless main reliance must be placed upon the plate and screws. The temptation to use a very short (two-hole) plate should be resisted in favour of a four-hole plate, which prevents angulation in the antero-posterior plane as well as in the coronal plane. Care must be taken to avoid any rotational displacement at the site of osteotomy, which may lead to incorrect folding of the forearm upon the arm.

ALTERNATIVE TECHNIQUE

A two-stage procedure designed to preserve stability of the fragments was described under the title "osteotomy-osteoclasis" by Moore in 1947. At the first stage a wedge of bone is excised but a substantial bridge of cortex is left at the medial side. The excised bone is finely fragmented and replaced in the osteotomy gap.

Two weeks later, with the child anaesthetised, the humerus is forcibly angulated to correct the deformity, the previously intact medial bridge of cortex being fractured deliberately. It is assumed that at this stage granulation tissue and early callus between the bone fragments are sufficiently "sticky" to prevent major displacement, while still allowing angulation sufficient to correct the deformity. Success depends upon removing just the right amount of bone at the first stage of the procedure.

For further details Moore's original paper should be consulted.

REMOVAL OF LOOSE BODY FROM ELBOW JOINT

Commonly, loose bodies in the elbow originate from an area of osteochondritis dissecans of the capitulum of the humerus. The loose body may be solitary, and there are seldom more than two or three bodies except in synovial chondromatosis. Generally the loose body is in the anterior compartment of the joint and is best removed through a lateral incision.

TECHNIQUE

Position of patient. It is convenient to rest the affected forearm upon the upper abdomen, the wrist being held by an assistant or by a small weight attached to the wrist by a bandage and suspended over the opposite side of the table. A tourniquet should be used on the upper arm. The surgeon stands on the affected side.

Exposure of joint. A vertical incision is made over the lateral supracondylar ridge of the humerus (Fig. 245). The muscles attached to the front of the supracondylar ridge are stripped away by dissection close to the bone. As the dissection proceeds medially, the knife soon enters the joint

through the synovial membrane, and the opening is easily enlarged with scissors. Usually it is unnecessary to divide capsule and synovial membrane distal to the joint level.

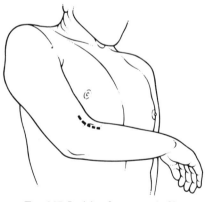

FIG. 245. Incision for removal of loose body from elbow. This incision permits exposure of either the anterior or the posterior compartment of the joint.

Location and removal of loose body. With the elbow held flexed the anterior part of the synovial membrane is easily retracted forwards so that a clear view is obtained of the interior of the anterior compartment of the joint; the loose body is nearly always found without difficulty. It may be grasped with a toothed dissecting forceps and removed.

Closure. The detached extensor muscles are sutured back in position and the skin is closed with interrupted sutures.

POST-OPERATIVE MANAGEMENT

The elbow is supported by crepe bandages over liberal gauze dressings. Unless there has been extensive exploration of the joint, splintage is not required. Mobilising exercises should be begun as soon as the skin is healed.

EXTRACTION OF LOOSE BODY FROM POSTERIOR COMPARTMENT

Very occasionally, a loose body may be found in the posterior compartment of the elbow joint. It may be removed through a similar skin incision to that just described, but the posterior instead of the anterior surface of the lateral supracondylar ridge of the humerus is stripped. With the knife kept close to the bone the synovial cavity is easily entered. The loose body is usually found easily and removed: often it lies in the olecranon fossa.

An alternative approach to the posterior compartment is through a vertical triceps-splitting incision.

RELEASE OF TRAPPED MEDIAL EPICONDYLE FROM ELBOW JOINT

Entrapment of the avulsed medial epicondyle within the elbow joint (Fig. 246) occurs almost joint by the negative pressure created as the joint surfaces are opened apart.

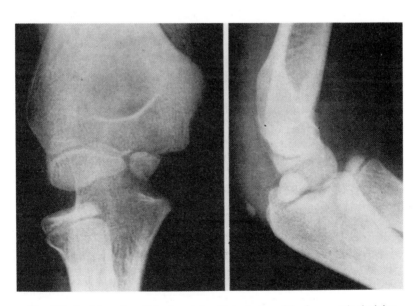

FIG. 246. Avulsion of medial epicondyle with inclusion of the fragment in the joint.

exclusively in children. It is thought that there is momentary subluxation of the joint, and that the medial epicondyle, avulsed by the pull of the attached forearm flexor muscles, is sucked into the

RELEASE BY MANIPULATION

It is worth while making an attempt to extract the bony fragment (to which the flexor muscles are still attached) by manipulation. If the attempt fails the surgeon may then proceed immediately to open operation.

TECHNIQUE

The principle is to reverse the negative pressure within the joint by the introduction of a medium-sized hollow needle and then to cause tension on the flexor muscles of the forearm while at the same time the forearm is abducted upon the humerus in order to open up the medial side of the joint (Fig. 247).

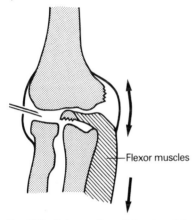

-Flexor muscles

FIG. 247. Release of medial epicondyle trapped in elbow joint. A hollow needle has been introduced into the joint from the lateral side. The joint is about to be manipulated into valgus (upper arrow) and at the same time the flexor muscles are to be made taut by extension of the wrist and fingers or by electrical stimulation.

The manipulation is carried out with the patient anaesthetised and supine. First a suitable hypodermic needle is introduced into the joint from the lateral side. The needle enters immediately in front of the lateral epicondyle of the humerus and is directed medially and slightly backwards along the front of the condyle to enter the joint cavity (Fig. 247). With the needle still in position, an assistant now grasps the upper arm firmly to fix it, and the surgeon takes hold of the hand and forearm. With the elbow straight and the forearm fully supinated an abduction force is applied to the forearm and at the same time the wrist and fingers are fully dorsiflexed.

This manoeuvre causes the forearm flexor muscles to be tensed and thus to exert a pull upon the displaced medial epicondyle which may be sufficient to dislodge it from the joint. It has been suggested that a more effective pull upon the muscles may be promoted by electrical stimulation at the motor point. Release of the fragment is checked radiographically.

If the bone fragment is successfully released by closed manipulation in the manner described it is necessary only to rest the elbow in the right-angled position by means of a plaster splint retained for two weeks or so, and thereafter to encourage active mobilising exercises but without any passive forcing.

RELEASE BY OPEN OPERATION

If manipulation fails to release the fragment the surgeon should proceed immediately to operative extraction.

TECHNIQUE

Position of patient. The patient lies in the semi-lateral position, the trunk being rolled towards the affected side so that the arm may rest upon its lateral border on the arm platform. A tourniquet may be used high on the upper arm.

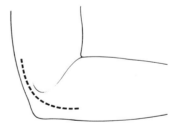

FIG. 248. Release of trapped medial epicondyle by operation. The skin incision, shown passing behind the medial epicondyle.

Incision. The incision, initially 4 or 5 centimetres long, is a longitudinal one placed just behind the medial axis of the limb, beginning over the medial condyle of the humerus (Fig. 248). Half the incision should be proximal to the level of the elbow joint and half distal. Since in these cases there is often considerable swelling, with some distortion of the bony landmarks due to avulsion of the medial epicondyle, there may be some difficulty in placing the incision accurately. It may be necessary to use the landmarks at the lateral side of the joint—the lateral epicondyle and the head of the radius—to determine precisely the level of the joint. It is particularly important that the proximity of the ulnar nerve should be borne in mind. The nerve is superficial at this level, and it may easily be damaged by a too deep skin incision that is injudiciously placed.

Identification of ulnar nerve. As a first step in the operation the ulnar nerve should be identified so that it may be protected from harm. This is best done by blunt dissection with dissecting scissors. There should be no difficulty in identifying the nerve where it lies behind the medial condyle and the medial supracondylar ridge of the humerus, and from here it may be followed down into the upper part of the forearm. The nerve should be kept under view to prevent its being injured.

Identification of flexor muscles and extraction of bone fragment. Next the upper part of the flexor mass of the forearm close to its origin is sought at the medial side of the joint. If necessary the incision may be extended distally for this purpose. Although there may often be considerable swelling and bruising of the tissues the muscle mass, partly tendinous, is found without difficulty as it turns laterally in its upper part to enter the joint (Fig. 247). By abduction of the forearm upon the upper arm the joint may be opened up sufficiently at the inner side to allow the muscle origin with the attached bone fragment to be easily withdrawn from the joint.

Testing the joint for stability. In these cases the elbow has usually been momentarily subluxated or even dislocated, and consequently it is necessary to ensure by inspection that the articular surfaces are correctly apposed and that there is no obstruction to a good range of flexion and extension and of rotation. The degree to which the joint is unstable on abduction and adduction stress with the joint extended should also be ascertained.

Re-attachment of medial epicondyle. The site on the medial condyle from which the epicondyle has been avulsed will be easily identified. It is not necessary to do more than to re-attach the epicondyle close to this point by means of absorbable sutures through the adjacent soft tissues (Fig. 249).

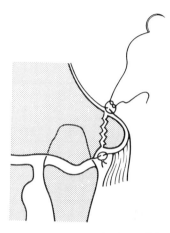

FIG. 249. The avulsed medial epicondyle is re-attached in its normal position by sutures through the soft tissues.

Closure. The tourniquet having been released and any bleeding points secured, there is little need for deep sutures and usually the skin alone need be closed. Before closure, however, it is important to ensure that the ulnar nerve lies secure and intact in its groove and that it is well away from any sharp edge of bone.

POST-OPERATIVE MANAGEMENT

It is wise to protect the elbow for two weeks in a right-angled plaster extending from the upper arm to the metacarpal heads. This is applied over a lightly applied crepe bandage and a generous layer of cellulose padding. After removal of the plaster active elbow exercises are encouraged, but any forcible movement should be prohibited.

Comment

The incidence of successful extraction of the bone fragment by manipulation is probably less than 50 per cent: nevertheless it is worth a trial before operation is resorted to.

It is important to establish before manipulation or operation whether or not the ulnar nerve is intact: it may have suffered contusion from the initial injury. Great care must be taken during operation to ensure that the nerve is not damaged, particularly during incision of the skin.

Extraction of the bone fragment with attached

muscles by operation does not present difficulty, but it is important to ensure, after its release, that the joint surfaces are congruous and that there is no other associated injury. It has to be appreciated that inclusion of the bone fragment in the joint is only a part of a rather more extensive disruption at the medial side, with subluxation or even dislocation that may be only momentary.

ARTHRODESIS OF ELBOW

Arthrodesis of the elbow is nowadays carried out only exceptionally, and a detailed description is not required here. For a fuller account the reader is referred to the paper by Van Gorder and Chen (1959).

POSITION FOR ARTHRODESIS

If one elbow is to be fused, the other being mobile, a position close to the right angle or just below the right angle (perhaps 80 degrees of flexion) with the forearm pronated 15 or 20 degrees is recommended. If both elbows are to be stiff, one should be fixed in flexion of about 100 degrees (to enable the hand to reach the mouth) and the other flexed no more than 75 degrees. By the use of trial plaster splints in different positions of flexion the patient will be helped to determine for himself which is the most useful position of the elbow in his particular circumstances.

TECHNIQUE

The technique is not standardised. Often, by the time an elbow comes to arthrodesis the anatomy is grossly distorted from the normal, and the technique has to be adjusted to suit the pathological anatomy. In general, the approach should be made from the medial side with the arm abducted upon a side table and rotated laterally at the shoulder. In some cases a lateral incision may also be required.

Exposure and clearance of joint. Through the medial incision, which follows the line of the ulnar nerve, the first step is to identify the nerve and to

lift it from its bed behind the medial epicondyle out of harm's way. The medial epicondyle is then detached from the humerus with a chisel so that the attached mass of flexor muscles may be retracted forwards.

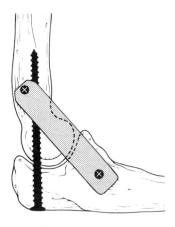

FIG. 250. Arthrodesis of elbow. The joint has been exposed from the medial side after transposition of the ulnar nerve. Fixation has been achieved by a heavy screw transfixing the ulna to the humerus, and by a strut graft.

The joint is now opened widely from the medial side by excision of ligaments and joint capsule. This allows the forearm to be abducted upon the humerus to give access to the interior of the joint. In this manoeuvre care must be taken to avoid injury to the brachial artery and the median nerve.

Remains of articular cartilage and synovial membrane are excised down to raw bone, both on the humeral and on the ulnar side of the joint. Depending upon the nature of the pathology, it may be necessary also to raw the surfaces of the humero-radial joint or, in cases of disability resulting from old injury rather than from infection or rheumatic disease, it may be appropriate to excise the head of the radius with the aim of preserving forearm rotation.

Fixation. When the articular ends of the humerus and of the ulna have been rawed and reshaped to fit together as snugly as possible it may be practicable to transfix the joint by a wide diameter screw (for instance a Venable hip screw) inserted from the back of the olecranon process and driven longitudinally along the medullary canal of the humerus. To reinforce the fixation the elbow should be buttressed by a cortical graft cut from the tibia or, if more appropriate, a cortico-cancellous graft from the iliac crest. A flat raw bed should be prepared for the graft by chiselling

away the medial aspect of the medial condyle of the humerus and the adjacent medial surface of the ulna, the ulnar nerve being held well forwards out of harm's way. The graft is then fixed in place across the angle by one screw at each end (Fig. 250). Supplementary cancellous grafts may be added as required. The ulnar nerve is laid in a new bed in front of the elbow (see below) and the wound is closed.

POST-OPERATIVE MANAGEMENT

Post-operative treatment depends upon the rigidity of the internal fixation secured at operation. If fixation is rigid a closely fitting plaster from axilla to metacarpal heads may be sufficient, but if the rigidity of the fixation leaves something to be desired it may be advisable to apply a full plaster-of-Paris shoulder spica.

ANTERIOR TRANSPOSITION OF ULNAR NERVE

This operation entails freeing the ulnar nerve from its groove at the back of the medial epicondyle of the humerus and bringing it forward in front of the condyle. In a patient with a reasonably thick layer of subcutaneous fat it is permissible to lay the nerve superficial to the common flexor muscle origin. Transposition deep to the muscles is nevertheless to be preferred, and this is the technique to be described.

TECHNIQUE

Position of patient. The patient lies supine with the shoulder abducted and the arm resting upon a side table in full lateral rotation, with the elbow semi-flexed. A tourniquet may be used high on the upper arm.

Incision. The incision follows the line of the ulnar nerve. It begins at the mid-point of the upper arm, skirts the medial epicondyle posteriorly, and ends at the junction of the upper and middle thirds of the forearm. Caution is required in order to avoid damage to the nerve.

Isolation of ulnar nerve. Behind the medial epicondyle the nerve is easily identified through its covering of deep fascia. The fascia is carefully divided with blunt-pointed scissors, first in a proximal direction and then distally. In the distal dissection the humeral fibres of the flexor carpi ulnaris muscle, which cross the nerve anteriorly, should be divided. The nerve is then traced along its course between the flexor carpi ulnaris medially and the flexor digitorum superficialis laterally. The nerve is lifted from its bed and drawn anteriorly without tension and without undue stripping of surrounding vascular tissue.

Below the level of the epicondyle the nerve may be found partly tethered by branches destined for the flexor carpi ulnaris muscle. With care, these branches can be dissected proximally and separated from the main body of the nerve for a sufficient distance to allow the nerve to lie in a straight course.

Division of flexor muscle origin. Blunt-pointed scissors are passed deep to the flexor muscle origin about a centimetre distal to the medial epicondyle.

By opening the scissors the muscles are freed from the deeper structures. The muscle mass is divided about a centimetre from its origin.

Division of medial intermuscular septum. In the proximal part of the incision the sharp-edged tough medial intermuscular septum is identified where it extends proximally from the medial condyle of the humerus. The lower third of the septum is excised in order to allow the ulnar nerve to take a straight course from the postero-medial aspect of the upper arm to the anterior aspect of the elbow.

Re-siting of nerve. The nerve is laid upon the surface of the brachialis muscle, where it is not far separated from the median nerve. It is placed deep to the flexor muscle origin, which is then sutured over it. It is important to ensure that the nerve lies in a straight course without any kinking.

Closure. Fascia and skin are closed with interrupted sutures.

POST-OPERATIVE MANAGEMENT

After operation the elbow should be rested in a right-angled plaster with the forearm in semi-pronation for three weeks. Thereafter mobilising and muscle strengthening exercises are encouraged.

Comment

Although this is seemingly a straightforward operation it must be carried out very carefully if serious consequences to the ulnar nerve are to be avoided. Cases are on record of paralysis of the nerve after its transposition.

It is important that the nerve be handled with great gentleness and that so far as possible its vascular supply be preserved.

It is also important that the nerve be transposed entirely deep to the flexor muscle origin: if it is embedded in the muscle it is liable to become strangled in scar tissue. Transposition to a superficial position—just deep to the subcutaneous fat—has often been carried out but it cannot be recommended except in obese patients.

Equally important is the need to cut away the lower part of the medial intermuscular septum; otherwise the sharp medial edge of the septum may damage the nerve as it passes forwards over it. Likewise any tendency to kinking in the lower part of the wound must be overcome by division of any constricting tissue.

EXCISION OF OLECRANON BURSA

Excision of a bursa overlying the olecranon process is not often required because in a high proportion of cases bursitis is relieved by aspiration, instillation of hydrocortisone, firm bandaging and avoidance of local pressure. Gouty bursitis also may often be relieved by conservative measures. When excision is required the bursa has usually been present for a considerable time, with mild inflammation leading to marked thickening of the wall of the bursa.

TECHNIQUE

Position of patient. The patient lies supine. The affected arm is laid across the chest so that the olecranon region is uppermost. It may be convenient to tie a soft sterile bandage around the wrist and to attach a weight of half a kilogram: the weight, suspended over the opposite side of the table, maintains the limb in the required position and obviates the need for an assistant to steady it. A tourniquet may be used high on the upper arm.

Incision. A vertical incision centred over the convexity formed by the bursa is recommended (Fig. 251). Its length must depend upon the size of the bursa, but in most cases it will be about 5 to 7 centimetres long. A transverse incision is permissible, but if this is used great care must be taken to avoid injury to the ulnar nerve at the medial end of the incision—an accident that can happen surprisingly easily.

Dissection of bursa. With skin edges and subcutaneous fat retracted medially and laterally the thick wall of the bursa is encountered. There is no difficulty in separating the wall of the bursa from the overlying tissues as far as its peripheral margins. This dissection is accomplished most easily by blunt-nosed scissors curved on the flat.

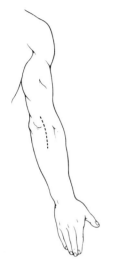

FIG. 251. Excision of olecranon bursa. The skin incision.

When the posterior aspect of the bursa has thus been exposed and cleaned, it is permissible to make an opening into it so that its full extent can be ascertained by palpation from within the cavity. The edge of the sac may then be grasped with an artery forceps so that the sac can be easily manoeuvred during dissection on its deep aspect (Fig. 252). This blunt dissection proceeds as before, with care to keep closely to the plane between the wall of the bursa and the surrounding tissues—mainly fatty tissue peripherally but periosteum overlying the upper end of the ulna on the deep aspect.

Even though the deep wall may be adherent to periosteum the bursal wall is continuous all round and it may be separated from periosteum and expanded aponeurosis of the triceps by sharp dissection. The aim should be to remove the bursal wall in its entirety.

Closure. Any defect created in the triceps expansion and periosteum may be closed by fine absorbable sutures, as may the subcutaneous tissue. In closure of the skin it is recommended

that interrupted mattress sutures be used and that two or three of the sutures should be placed deeply to transfix the triceps expansion and periosteum (Fig. 253). In this way the skin is held

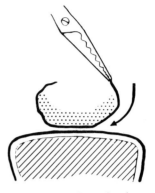

FIG. 252. The bursa has been opened after exposure of its posterior (superficial) wall. The cut edge of the bursal wall is gripped by an artery forceps to allow light traction to be exerted while the deep aspect of the bursa is dissected out.

down to the bone; so the risk of haematoma beneath the skin is reduced. With the same objective in mind it is a wise precaution to release the tourniquet before the wound is closed, so that all bleeding points may be sealed.

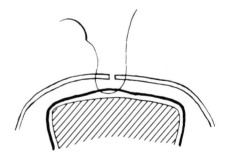

FIG. 253. During closure some of the skin sutures are passed through the periosteum to prevent raising of the skin flaps by haematoma.

POST-OPERATIVE MANAGEMENT

At the conclusion of the operation a firm crepe bandage 15 centimetres wide is applied snugly over layers of gauze and surgical cotton. The elbow is rested in a sling in a position of 90 degrees of flexion for the first few days, though gentle active flexion and extension exercises may be practised from the beginning.

Comment

This seemingly simple operation has occasionally been marred by complications. The risk of damage to the ulnar nerve during injudicious exposure and dissection of the bursa has already been mentioned. It is easily avoided by employing a vertical rather than a transverse skin incision and by keeping the dissection close to the wall of the bursa throughout.

Another common complication is the formation of a haematoma in the area of the dissection, giving a new swelling in place of the old one. This is best avoided by painstaking attention to all bleeding points after removal of the tourniquet before closure, by passing some of the skin sutures deeply to grip the underlying triceps expansion and by snug, though not over-tight, bandaging with a wide crepe bandage over gauze or cotton.

STRIPPING OF EXTENSOR ORIGIN FOR TENNIS ELBOW

Although the exact pathological lesion in tennis elbow is still unknown it seems clear that it is related to the site of origin of the extensor muscles of the forearm from the lateral supracondylar ridge of the humerus and from the front of the lateral epicondyle. Elevation of the tendinous attachment of these muscles from the bone and adjacent ligaments is a reliable method of treatment for resistant tennis elbow with marked tenderness localised to this region.

TECHNIQUE

Position of patient. The patient lies supine. It is convenient to place the affected arm across the chest. A useful refinement is to tie a soft bandage round the wrist and to suspend upon the bandage a suitable weight on the opposite side of the table—a steel mallet serves the purpose well. The arm is thus steadied in position so that the assistant is freed from the task of supporting it. A tourniquet may be used high on the upper arm.

Incision. The incision is centred on the lateral epicondyle (Fig. 254). The upper limb of the incision, 3 or 4 centimetres long, extends proximally from the epicondyle over the lateral supracondylar ridge of the humerus. The lower limb of the incision, of similar length, extends vertically downwards from the epicondyle. The forearm is held in full pronation while the incision is made.

This helps to ensure the safety of the posterior interosseous nerve by displacing it forwards away from the line of the incision.

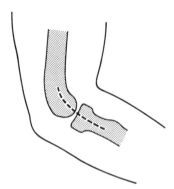

Fig. 254. Stripping of extensor origin for tennis elbow. The skin incision. Deep landmarks are shown.

Exposure and reflection of extensor origin. The dissection begins in the proximal half of the wound, where a vertical cut is made straight down to the bone of the supracondylar ridge of the humerus, which is easily palpated in the lateral axis of the limb. With a fine knife and a periosteal elevator tendinous tissue together with the blended periosteum is stripped from the anterior and posterior aspects of the supracondylar ridge over a width of a centimetre or more.

Attention is now directed towards the middle and lower part of the wound, where the lateral epicondyle and the bone immediately in front of it will be seen to be covered by a broad sheet of tendinous aponeurosis. Further distally the proximal apex of the extensor muscle mass will be seen giving place to tendon fibres. These tendons, though partly blended, are arranged in three groups (Fig. 255): the brachioradialis, extensor carpi radialis longus and extensor carpi radialis brevis in front; the extensor origin proper (comprising extensor digitorum communis, extensor digiti minimi and extensor carpi ulnaris) in the middle; and the anconeus behind.

A broad strip of the tendinous aponeurosis where it covers the lateral epicondyle and the adjacent bone anteriorly and superiorly is marked out and incised (Fig. 255) to allow its reflection distally together with the central part of the fan-shaped musculo-tendinous origin. Reflection is carried out by grasping the proximal cut end of the aponeurosis in a forceps and lifting it laterally away from the bone (Fig. 256), and as the reflection proceeds the tendon fibres are divided with a fine knife at the point of their attachment to the bone. It is convenient to peel the aponeurosis

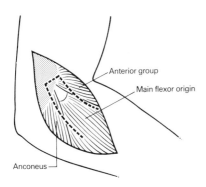

FIG. 255. Exposure of lateral epicondyle and of the three adjoining groups of muscles. Interrupted line marks out the flap of tissue to be reflected downwards.

distally over a distance of 3 or 4 centimetres—that is, as far as the lower margin of the head of the radius, which is easily identified by palpation. (There is no need to open the synovial cavity of the elbow joint.)

Thinning of aponeurosis and shaving of bone surface. Although elevation of the musculotendinous

origin alone is probably sufficient, it is nevertheless to be recommended that the thick tendinous aponeurosis be thinned down by shaving off the deep surface with a fresh knife-blade. The surface of the lateral epicondyle and of the adjacent bone anteriorly and superiorly is then shaved off as a thin flake with a fine chisel.

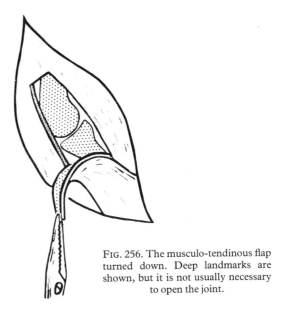

FIG. 256. The musculo-tendinous flap turned down. Deep landmarks are shown, but it is not usually necessary to open the joint.

Reattachment of extensor aponeurosis. The reflected sheet of aponeurosis is laid back in position, a fraction more distally than in the natural state—that is, with slight lengthening—and it is anchored by a few fine absorbable sutures to the adjacent soft tissue anteriorly and superiorly.

Closure. After removal of the tourniquet and sealing of any bleeding points, the skin is closed with interrupted mattress sutures.

POST-OPERATIVE MANAGEMENT

First, a dressing of dry gauze and crepe bandage is applied. A light plaster-of-Paris cast extending from the upper arm to the metacarpal heads is then applied with the elbow flexed 90 degrees and the forearm in neutral rotation. The plaster is retained for two weeks, after which the sutures are removed and elbow exercises are encouraged.

Comment

As in all operations upon the lateral aspect of the elbow, the position of the posterior interosseous nerve should be borne constantly in mind. The nerve is vulnerable if the incision is extended distally into the forearm beyond the level of the neck of the radius, and especially if it inclines forwards too much below the lateral epicondyle. In this operation the nerve is not endangered provided the operation is carried out as described. Even so, it is a wise precaution to pronate the forearm fully before making the skin and fascial incisions.

The operation is entirely extra-articular, and it is unnecessary to open the cavity of the elbow joint.

Some surgeons avoid applying a plaster splint after the operation, but the use of a plaster is to be recommended because it helps to reduce post-operative pain and it maintains the comfortable right-angled position of the elbow which allows reasonably active use of the hand.

Many other operations have been described for tennis elbow. Bosworth (1955) advised excision of the annular ligament, with or without division of the common extensor origin. Kaplan (1959) sought to denervate the humero-radial joint. Garden (1961) relied upon elongation of the tendon of extensor carpi radialis brevis just proximal to the wrist, believing that tension upon the origin of this muscle alone at the lateral epicondyle was responsible for the pain. Roles and Maudsley (1972) incriminated entrapment of the radial nerve, and released the nerve at the front of the elbow.

Admittedly there are cases in which the cause of pain at the outer side of the elbow may be other than the "tendonitis" that has been assumed here (Capener 1966), and thus there may be occasions when one or other of the operations mentioned may be appropriate. Nevertheless it does seem that in the great majority of cases the pathology—whatever its nature—is localised to the epicondylar region and tendinous origin, and that therefore it is logical to counter it by a direct rather than a remote intervention.

AMPUTATION THROUGH UPPER ARM
(ABOVE-ELBOW AMPUTATION)

LEVEL OF AMPUTATION

In general, as much length as possible should be preserved. To allow room for the mechanism of a prosthetic elbow, however, the level of section through the humerus should be not less than 4 centimetres proximal to the articular surface. Amputations above the level of the axillary fold do not leave a stump long enough to move a prosthetic limb, and such amputations must be fitted as for a disarticulation of the shoulder. Nevertheless it is important if possible to preserve the head of the humerus, which cosmetically is of value in giving a normal contour to the shoulder.

TECHNIQUE

Position of patient. The patient lies supine. It is not practicable to use a tourniquet.

Marking out the skin flaps. It is well to mark out with ink the outlines of the skin flaps before the incisions are made. When the required level of bone section has been determined the level is marked upon the skin surface.

Equal anterior and posterior flaps are designed starting from this level. Each flap is equal in length to slightly more than half the diameter of the limb at the level of proposed bone section. The anterior flap begins in the mid-medial line of the arm and sweeps distally and laterally to cross the front of the arm, and then to curve proximally again to the mid-lateral line of the arm level with the starting point. The outline of the posterior flap is of corresponding dimensions.

Reflection of flaps and division of vessels and nerves. After the skin flaps have been fashioned, each is reflected together with the subcutaneous tissue and deep fascia as far as the level of proposed bone section. The first step in the subsequent dissection is to identify and ligate the brachial artery with double ligatures. The vessel is then divided. The main veins are treated similarly. Next the median, ulnar and radial nerves are identified, pulled distally, divided cleanly with a fresh knife blade and allowed to retract proximally.

Division of muscles. The anterior muscles are divided transversely 1 centimetre distal to the planned level of bone section. The muscles retract slightly so that their cut surfaces will be flush with the cut surface of the humerus. Posteriorly, the triceps muscle is not divided at the same level but is dissected free for a length of 5 or 6 centimetres distal to the level of bone section. The triceps is then divided at this distal level, later to be turned proximally as a muscle flap to cover the end of the stump.

Division of humerus. At the level of bone section the periosteum of the humerus is incised circumferentially and stripped proximally. The humerus is sawn through with a hand saw and the lower part of the limb is discarded. The cut edges of the bone are smoothed with a rasp.

Myoplasty. The flap fashioned from the triceps muscle is trimmed to a thickness of about half a centimetre and is then brought forward to cover the sawn surface of the humerus. If the muscle flap is too long it is trimmed appropriately and the cut edge is then sutured to the brachialis and biceps muscles.

Closure. The skin and fascia are trimmed if necessary so that the flaps lie smoothly in place to cover the end of the stump, without tension and yet without undue laxity. The edges of the fascia are united with fine absorbable sutures and the skin flaps with interrupted eversion sutures. Before final closure it is advisable to insert a polythene tube for suction drainage.

POST-OPERATIVE MANAGEMENT

Copious gauze dressings are held in place with wide crepe bandages, snugly applied to give even support over the circumference and end of the stump. It may be wise to change the dressings after two days, when the drainage tube should be removed. The skin sutures should remain for two weeks. Exercises to preserve shoulder movement should be practised from an early stage.

AMPUTATION THROUGH ELBOW JOINT

Disarticulation through the elbow has the important advantage over above-elbow amputation that rotation of the humerus can be transmitted to the prosthesis, for the flared and flattened lower end of the humerus can be gripped securely by the socket.

TECHNIQUE

Position of patient. The patient lies supine with the arm resting upon a side table. A tourniquet may be used but care must be taken to ensure that it is placed as high as possible on the upper arm, well clear of the operation area.

Marking out the skin flaps. It is advisable to mark the outline of the flaps upon the skin before the incisions are made. Equal anterior and posterior flaps are recommended. They should be slightly over-generous, to ensure that the stump will be covered without tension. The outline of the anterior flap begins at the medial epicondyle of the humerus and curves across the front of the upper forearm in a convex sweep, finally curving proximally again to end at the lateral epicondyle (Fig. 257). The lowest point of the flap should be about 2 centimetres distal to the insertion of the biceps tendon. The outline of the posterior flap follows a similar course upon the back of the upper forearm, its lowest point extending 4 centimetres distal to the tip of the olecranon process.

Reflection of flaps and division of anterior structures. The anterior and posterior skin flaps are fashioned and reflected proximally. The deep dissection is begun on the medial side, where the forearm flexor muscles are detached from the

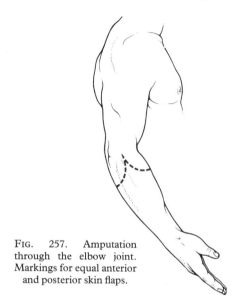

FIG. 257. Amputation through the elbow joint. Markings for equal anterior and posterior skin flaps.

medial epicondyle of the humerus and turned distally. The median nerve and the accompanying main vessels are next identified where they lie just medial to the tendon of the biceps muscle. The brachial artery is ligated and divided just proximal to the level of the joint: likewise the accompanying veins. The median nerve is drawn distally, divided as high as possible and allowed to retract. The ulnar nerve is treated similarly where it lies behind the medial epicondyle. The tendon of the biceps is divided and the brachialis muscle is detached from the coronoid process of the ulna. Next the radial nerve is identified where it lies between the brachialis muscle and the brachioradialis, divided and allowed to retract.

Attention is next directed to the extensor muscles of the forearm which arise from the lateral epicondyle and from the adjacent part of the humerus. These muscles should be exposed and divided about 8 centimetres distal to the lateral epicondyle and turned up proximally as a flap which will be used later to cover the end of the stump.

Completion of disarticulation. It remains only to divide the tendon of the triceps muscle just above the olecranon and then to cut the joint capsule anteriorly and at the sides to sever the forearm.

Myodesis and myoplasty. It is not necessary to trim the lower articular surface of the humerus, which forms the end of the stump. The articular cartilage is left intact. The triceps tendon is pulled distally and anteriorly and sutured to the distal ends of the brachialis and biceps muscles. The flap of forearm muscles formed from the extensor group, which remains attached to the lateral epicondyle of the humerus, is used to cover the under surface of the humeral condyles. The fleshy flap of muscle is unnecessarily bulky and should be trimmed to a thin pad before being folded across the condyles and united at the medial side of the joint to the severed origins of the flexor muscles. The edges of the flap are drawn out to widen it and to ensure complete coverage of the bone. The edges are sutured to periosteum or muscle remnants in front of and behind the humeral condyles.

Closure. The skin flaps and fascia are approximated in the coronal plane, and any excess of skin is trimmed away to ensure smooth coverage of the end of the stump without undue tension yet without too much laxity. As there is no oozing from the bone, drainage of the wound may usually be avoided, provided haemostasis has been made complete after removal of the tourniquet.

POST-OPERATIVE MANAGEMENT

Wide crepe bandages are applied smoothly over copious gauze dressings to ensure even pressure over the sides and end of the stump. In the absence of complications the initial dressings may be left until the end of the second week, when the sutures are removed.

CHAPTER SEVEN

Forearm, Wrist and Hand

The hand is a borderland between the fields of orthopaedic surgery and plastic surgery. Indeed hand surgery is tending to become a distinct speciality served by surgeons skilled in both these disciplines, to which an increasing number of surgeons are devoting their whole careers.

In this chapter only those standard operations that are likely to be within the compass of the general orthopaedic surgeon have been included. The higher flights of hand surgery, which include such operations as pollicisation of the index finger, transfer of innervated island pedicle flaps and major reconstructive procedures are beyond the scope of this book.

CONTENTS OF CHAPTER

INTRAMEDULLARY NAILING OF ULNA

This section should be read in conjunction with the general description of medullary nailing in Chapter 2 (p. 84). The ulna lends itself well to intramedullary nailing because there is easy access to the medullary canal through the olecranon process. Nailing is appropriate either to a fresh fracture or to a fracture that shows delayed union or non-union. Nailing is usually carried out by the open technique, but closed nailing may be appropriate occasionally for a fresh fracture without significant displacement. The following description refers to open nailing.

TECHNIQUE

Position of patient. The patient lies supine with the arm resting upon a side platform. The limb and the body should be so draped that during part of the operation the forearm may be placed across the chest to facilitate access to the medullary canal through the olecranon process. A tourniquet may be used on the upper arm.

Exposure. The incision for exposure of the fracture surfaces is over the medial (subcutaneous) margin of the ulna between the flexor and the extensor muscle groups. The incision for insertion of the nail is in the midline of the back of the elbow, centred over the tip of the olecranon process.

If the upper end of the radius is to be exposed at the same operation—for instance to reduce a dislocation of the head of the radius in a Monteggia fracture-dislocation—the posterior incision described on page 19 may be used as an alternative.

Exposure and reduction of fracture. The fracture surfaces are displayed after exposure of a short length of normal bone above and below the fracture site. The surfaces are cleared of blood clot, fibrin or fibrous tissue to allow precisely accurate coaptation of the fragments.

Particular care should be taken to ensure that there is no rotational deformity. This is automatically corrected in a fresh fracture if the spikes and crevices of one fragment can be made to fit

their counterparts on the opposite fragment. It is less easily achieved in a case of long-standing fracture with non-union. In such a case it is necessary to rely upon matching the contours of the ulnar shaft on the proximal and the distal fragments.

When the fracture has been reduced the position is held temporarily by clamping the fragments with a suitable bone-holding forceps.

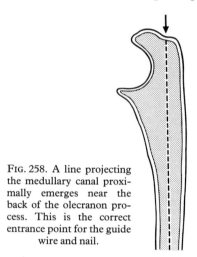

FIG. 258. A line projecting the medullary canal proximally emerges near the back of the olecranon process. This is the correct entrance point for the guide wire and nail.

Preparation of track for nail. The forearm now being placed across the patient's chest, the olecranon process is exposed. An opening is made in the superior surface of the olecranon by a small gouge or awl. The opening should be close to the posterior margin of the bone, in line with the upward prolongation of the medullary canal (Fig. 258): intrusion upon the coronoid notch is thereby avoided.

When the cortex has been breached the line of the medullary canal is identified by passing into it a strong awl or a Steinmann pin. This is withdrawn and a suitable guide wire is introduced into the medullary canal and driven distally across the fracture, through almost the full length of the bone. The medullary canal is then reamed out with flexible power-driven reamers inserted over the guide wire. A diameter of 6 or 7 millimetres is usually adequate.

As an alternative to this method of reaming, the

medullary canal may be prepared by drilling out the medulla direct with a long 6-millimetre drill on a hand brace. Often this is the simpler method, particularly if the medullary canal is markedly narrowed by sclerotic bone. Sometimes it is practicable, and easier, to drill proximally and distally from the fracture site.

Insertion of nail. If a guide wire has been used it should now be removed: the nail may usually be driven in directly, without a guide. A nail of the correct length and diameter is selected after measuring the length of the ulna with a ruler on the surface. The nail should be long enough to penetrate distally almost as far as the head of the ulna; proximally the end of the nail should be sunk a few millimetres deep to the superior cortex of the olecranon process. The nail is inserted through the opening in the olecranon and driven down by light blows with the hammer: close observation of the fracture site is required lest distraction or rotational deformity occur. As the point of the nail nears the distal end of the ulna its position should be checked repeatedly with the image intensifier.

POST-OPERATIVE MANAGEMENT

The after-care depends upon the rigidity of the fixation achieved by the nail, which in turn will depend to some extent upon the site of the fracture, and secondly upon the condition of the radius.

If the radius is intact and the ulna has been securely fixed, external support may not be required. On the other hand, if the radius has also been fractured and immobilised by internal fixation at the same operation, or if fixation of the ulna is not completely rigid, then support for the limb in a full-length plaster splint with the elbow flexed 90 degrees is recommended.

Comment

Intramedullary nailing of the ulna usually presents little difficulty because the bone is easily exposed and introduction of the nail through the olecranon process is straightforward. To some extent the technique may be varied according to the circumstances of each individual case.

For instance, it may sometimes be easiest to drill out the medullary canal to the required size by introducing a drill into each fragment in turn from the site of fracture, the proximal fragment thus being drilled in a proximal direction and the distal fragment in a distal direction. If this is done it may be easier also to pass the selected nail proximally along the proximal fragment from the fracture site by the retrograde technique (see p. 91), leaving only 2 or 3 millimetres of nail protruding at the fracture site to engage the medullary canal of the distal fragment as the fracture is reduced. The nail is then driven down from above into the distal fragment. This retrograde technique of drilling and nailing is usually practicable only if both bones of the forearm are fractured: if the ulna alone is fractured or if the radius has already united it may not be possible easily to disengage the ulnar fragments sufficiently to allow the drill or the nail to be introduced through the site of fracture. Drilling the canal and driving the nail must then be carried out from above, as described.

Care should be taken not to over-ream the medullary canal. The cortex of the ulna is often thin, especially towards the lower end, and if the canal is reamed or drilled too widely the cortex may be reduced to egg-shell thinness and may disintegrate.

INTRAMEDULLARY NAILING OF RADIUS

This section should be read in conjunction with the general description of intramedullary nailing in Chapter 2 (p. 84).

The radius does not lend itself so well as the ulna to nailing because there is no easy access to the medullary canal. Access can be gained at the dorsal surface of the extreme lower end of the bone, but at best it is rather restricted, and to some extent the preparation of the track and the insertion of a nail may encroach upon the lower articular surface of the radius. When both the radius and the ulna are fractured, however, it is possible to introduce the nail at the fracture site and to shunt it into position without disturbing either end of the bone.

TECHNIQUE

Position of patient. The patient lies supine, with the affected limb resting upon the arm platform and with the elbow semi-flexed. A tourniquet may be used on the upper arm.

Exposure. If the fracture is in the lower half of the radius the bone may be approached directly from in front, between the flexor carpi radialis medially and the brachioradialis laterally. If the fracture is in the upper half of the radius the anterior exposure reported by Henry (1945) may be used. This was described on page 17.

Exposure and reduction of fracture. Normal bone should be exposed a little distance above and below the site of fracture and each fragment should then be cleared towards the fracture. All blood clot, fibrin and fibrous tissue must be removed from the fracture surfaces to allow accurate coaptation. Care must be taken to avoid any rotational deformity.

Preparation of medullary canal. The medullary canal must be reamed or drilled out to a uniform diameter—usually 6 or 7 millimetres—to receive the intramedullary nail. There are two methods of preparing the track, and the method used will depend upon the circumstances of each case.

The first method is to make an opening into the medullary canal from the extreme lower end of the radius at the dorsal aspect, where the cortex curves forwards to join the articular surface (Fig. 259). The initial opening may be made with an awl or small gouge, and a pilot track may be made upwards from this point with a rigid instrument such as a Steinmann pin held in a hand chuck. A guide wire may then be passed through this opening and driven on towards the proximal end of the radius. Over the guide wire flexible reamers are used to enlarge the medullary canal to

the desired diameter. The guide wire is then removed ready for the insertion of the nail.

The second method, which may not be appropriate if the ulna is intact because of the difficulty

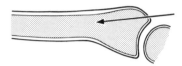

FIG. 259. Diagram showing a possible site at the lower end of the radius for the insertion of a nail. Because of the rather inadequate access nailing of the radius is usually reserved for cases in which no other method will satisfactorily serve the purpose.

of delivering each fragment separately into the wound, is to drill out the medullary canal of each fragment in turn from the fracture site, using a solid drill operated by a hand brace (Fig. 260) instead of a guide wire and cannulated reamer. Each fragment should be drilled to within about a centimetre of the end of the bone: no attempt should be made to bring the drill point out through the lower cortex of the radius.

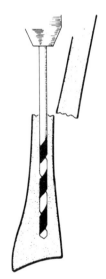

FIG. 260. Intramedullary nailing of radius. Preparing a track for the nail by drilling from the site of fracture.

It should be noted that when the bone is drilled from the fracture site the nail must also be introduced at that site, as described below.

Insertion of nail. The correct length for the nail is easily determined by measuring the length of the radius externally. If the nail is to be introduced through the lower dorsal cortex the length should be about 2 centimetres less than the total length of the bone. If the nail is to be introduced at the fracture site and shunted into position it must be considerably shorter, usually about half or two-thirds of the length of the bone, depending upon the site of the fracture. The diameter of the nail should equal the diameter of the drill or reamer used for preparing the medullary canal.

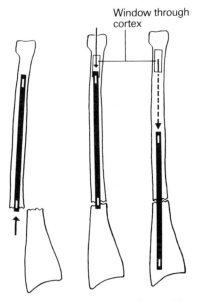

FIGS 261–263. Intramedullary nailing of radius. Technique of shunting the nail into position after its introduction at the site of fracture. Figure 261—Nail inserted at fracture site and driven into longer fragment. Figure 262—Fracture reduced. Window cut in bone just clear of nail. Figure 263—Nail punched down into shorter fragment through the window. An angled punch is used.

If the nail is to be introduced from below through an opening in the cortex of the lower end of the radius, no special problem is presented. It is best to remove the guide wire before the nail is hammered in. In this situation there is no particular advantage in driving the nail over a guide wire.

If the nail is to be introduced through the fracture site it is driven first into the longer of the two fragments until only 2 or 3 millimetres of the point of the nail still protrude from the fracture surface (Fig. 261). The fragments are then reduced accurately so that the small protruding part of the nail engages the medullary canal of the other fragment. (Care must be taken at this stage to ensure that the fragments are in the correct rotational position.) To drive the nail down into the other (shorter) fragment a window must now be cut through the cortex of the longer fragment over the end of the nail (Fig. 262). With an angled punch inserted through this window the nail is then driven down into the shorter fragment (Fig. 263).

POST-OPERATIVE MANAGEMENT

This is the same as for intramedullary nailing of the ulna (p. 199).

Comment

Intramedullary nailing of the radius has been little used because of the difficulty of gaining access to the medullary canal. The access afforded at the lower dorsal cortex, as described above, is far from ideal because the cortical opening is liable to encroach to some extent on the articular surface of the distal end of the radius. For this reason many surgeons reserve intramedullary nailing of the radius for cases of special difficulty—for instance in old fractures with non-union and perhaps some loss of healthy bone due to infection and sequestrum formation. In such a case nailing may be combined with the insertion of a cancellous block graft after removal of infected bone (see p. 204).

The retrograde method of driving the nail into the longer fragment from the fracture site, and then driving it down into the shorter fragment through a window in the cortex (Figs 261–263), is often a satisfactory method of getting the nail in position across the fracture, but only when a concomitant fracture of the ulna creates sufficient mobility of the fragments to allow access at the fracture site. The method is applicable mainly when the fracture site is situated towards one end of the bone so that the fragments are of unequal length. Because of the shunting that must take place in the longer fragment it is clear that with this technique the nail can never occupy more than about two-thirds of the length of the medullary canal. Nevertheless it is a very useful technique to have at one's command.

INTRAMEDULLARY NAILING OF RADIUS AND ULNA TOGETHER

Both bones of the forearm may be nailed at the same operation, or alternatively one bone may be plated or bone-grafted while the other is nailed.

Often, the presence of a fracture of both bones makes preparation of the medullary canal for nailing rather easier than it is when one bone is intact, because of the much greater mobility of the fragments and the consequent ease with which they may be delivered from the wound for drilling from the fracture site. As a rule it is preferable to use a separate incision for each bone.

PLATE FIXATION OF FRACTURES OF THE FOREARM BONES

The technique of internal fixation of fractures by metal plates and screws was described in Chapter 2 (page 82). Fixation by plates is used frequently in fractures of the shafts of the radius and ulna, which must unite with perfect apposition and alignment if normal function is to be restored. Plating is appropriate either to fractures of the radius or ulna alone, or to fractures of both bones.

The authors prefer to use a simple four-hole plate, which is regarded as no more than a bone suture to maintain normal apposition and alignment: it is used in conjunction with external support from a plaster-of-Paris splint. It is recognised, however, that many surgeons prefer to use heavier plates, with six or even eight screws, aiming to gain such secure fixation that supplementary support from a plaster splint is not required. The principle of applying compression across the fracture by the use of slotted-hole plates (see p. 70) may also be adopted.

For plating of the ulna, a direct approach to the bone through an incision over the medial (subcutaneous) surface is used. The plate may be applied either to the anterior or to the posterior aspect of the ulnar shaft.

For plating of the radius in its lower half, the direct anterior approach may be used; the incision lies between the flexor carpi radialis and the brachioradialis, just lateral to the radial artery. For fractures of the middle of the shaft or in the proximal half of the radius this exposure should be extended proximally in the manner described by Henry (1945) (p. 17). If both bones of the forearm are to be plated, separate incisions should be used for each bone.

In the plating of forearm fractures it is especially important that rotational deformity be avoided. Since plating is undertaken mostly for fresh fractures, preservation of correct rotational alignment does not usually present difficulty because the interdigitating spikes of cortex can be locked together accurately after removal of blood clot and granulation tissue. It is also important to preserve normal length in each bone; otherwise the correct relationship of the two bones at the inferior radio-ulnar joint is likely to be disturbed.

POST-OPERATIVE MANAGEMENT

If rigid fixation by strong plates has been achieved it may be appropriate to avoid external support, but in other cases it is safer to advise splintage in a plaster-of-Paris case until radiological evidence of union is present—often a matter of ten to twelve weeks. In the immediate post-operative period, however, a complete encircling plaster is best avoided because of the risk of swelling. Instead, crepe bandages are applied over copious gauze dressings and the limb may be left without further external support, or a posterior plaster gutter splint may be applied, the anterior aspect of the arm and forearm being left uncovered by plaster.

The peripheral circulation must be watched closely in the first three days, and if there is any doubt about the integrity of the circulation there should be no hesitation in splitting the bandages and dressings right through to the skin and opening up the gutter splint as far as is necessary.

After two weeks, when the sutures are removed, a complete plaster may be applied over a thin layer of cellulose wool, with the elbow at 90 degrees and the forearm mid-way between pronation and supination.

Comment

In many cases plate fixation of the forearm bones is an alternative to intramedullary nailing, though nailing is favoured much less in the case of the forearm bones—particularly the radius—than in the other major long bones. In general, plating of the radius and ulna is a simple procedure and in the great majority of cases union of the fractures occurs without difficulty.

Although it may be possible by the use of special rigid plates to eliminate the need for external support by plaster-of-Paris (Hicks 1961), the authors nevertheless often prefer to have the additional safeguard of a plaster splint because without it there is a risk that rotational forces at the fracture site may eventually lead to loosening before union has occurred, with the possible consequence of delayed union or non-union.

BONE GRAFTING FOR DELAYED UNION AND NON-UNION OF FRACTURES OF FOREARM BONES

The techniques of bone grafting were described in Chapter 2 (p. 78). Both cancellous sliver grafting by the technique of Phemister (1947) and onlay cortical grafting are used for the forearm bones. Either the radius or the ulna may be grafted alone, or grafts may be applied to both bones at the same operation. The exposure of the radius and ulna is the same as for plate fixation (p. 202).

Cancellous bone grafting. Cancellous sliver grafting is often combined with rigid internal fixation of the bone by an intramedullary nail.

First the fracture is exposed and any necessary adjustment is made to the position and alignment of the fragments. If necessary the fracture surfaces are freshened. Care is required to ensure that there is no rotational deformity. This may present difficulty because these fractures are usually old and the original digitations of the cortex are likely to have been effaced by local resorption. Reliance must therefore be placed on matching up the surface contours of the two fragments. When this has been achieved medullary nailing is carried out by the technique described on page 198.

Finally thin flakes or slivers of soft cortical bone from the ilium are laid about the freshened bone ends, bridging the fracture and extending partly round the circumference of the bone. The muscles are sewn together over the slivers to hold them in place and the skin wound is closed.

Onlay cortical grafting. Onlay cortical bone grafting still has an important place in the treatment of old ununited fractures of the forearm bones. Such grafts have the advantage of providing rigidity as well as promoting new bone formation about the site of fracture.

Grafts are best taken from the medial cortex of the tibia as described on page 72. Usually a graft for a forearm bone is about 7 or 8 centimetres long and is drilled for four screws, two to be inserted in each fragment. The graft is applied in the same manner as a metal plate, as described in the previous section, the surface of the recipient cortex having been shaved into a flat surface with a chisel.

After the graft has been screwed into position the corners and edges of the graft may be bevelled off to provide a smoother surface for the overlying muscles. The screw heads should also be well countersunk, and care should be taken to ensure that the points do not penetrate too far through the bone into the soft tissues.

Onlay cancellous/cortical grafts. Onlay grafts of cancellous iliac bone, with one cortex preserved intact on the graft, also have a place in the management of non-union. They may be fixed in place with screws, as described above. Such grafts, however, are not strong enough in themselves to provide rigid fixation of the fracture; so they are usually combined with internal fixation by an intramedullary nail.

Block grafting for bone defect. When non-union is associated with actual loss of bone—whether from destruction at the time of injury or from deliberate excision of infected bone or sequestrum—the method of filling the defect described by Nicoll (1956) is to be recommended (Fig. 264).

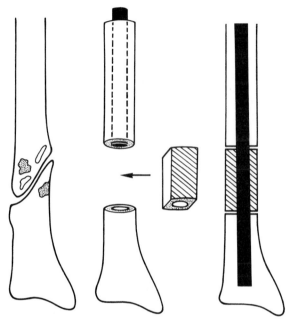

FIG. 264. Excision of infected bone adjacent to ununited fracture and substitution by a block of cancellous (iliac) bone (Nicoll 1956). *Left*—The ununited infected fracture. *Centre*—the infected pseudarthrosis has been excised and a graft from the ilium prepared. An intramedullary nail has been driven down as far as the gap. *Right*—Bone graft inserted and nail driven on through graft into distal fragment.

The recipient bone ends are trimmed appropriately to remove all dead or infected bone, and squared off to leave a neat regular gap. This prepared gap is then filled with a single block of cancellous bone taken from a thick part of the ilium (see p. 76). Finally the bone fragments and the graft are secured either by a plate, as recommended by Nicoll, or, preferably, by an intramedullary nail (Fig. 264). If a nail is to be used, it is convenient to drill the graft longitudinally to receive the nail before it is removed from the ilium (Fig. 103, p. 76).

POST-OPERATIVE MANAGEMENT

After bone-grafting of the forearm bones, whether by cancellous sliver grafts or by onlay cortical grafts, it is wise to support the limb in a plaster-of-Paris splint extending from upper arm to metacarpal heads, with the elbow at a right angle and the forearm mid-way between pronation and supination.

The initial plaster should be no more than a slab or gutter splint, the anterior aspect of the arm and forearm being left uncovered by plaster lest post-operative swelling impede the circulation. Even the gauze dressings and crepe bandages may obstruct the circulation, especially is they become soaked in blood which subsequently dries hard. The surgeon must therefore be prepared to split the dressings and bandages right through to the skin if there should be any embarrassment of the circulation in the first two or three days after operation.

After two weeks, when the sutures are removed, a snugly fitting encircling plaster may be applied and retained until there is good radiological evidence of incorporation of the grafts.

Comment

The choice between cancellous sliver grafting and onlay cortical grafting is often a matter of individual preference. Each method can give good results in the ordinary case of delayed union or non-union. If there has been previous infection, however, the use of soft cancellous bone is to be preferred because it entails less risk of recrudescence of the infection.

If part of the shaft of a bone has been lost through sequestration or has had to be excised to clear up infection, the Nicoll technique of block grafting as described above can give gratifying results.

EXCISION OF LOWER END OF ULNA

The lower end of the ulna is excised mainly on account of loss of the normal relationship between the ulna and the radius at their lower ends. Often there is proximal displacement of the radial component of the joint relative to the head of the ulna. A common cause is a fracture of the lower end of the radius with shortening due to compaction of the bone (Fig. 265). The head of the ulna is then

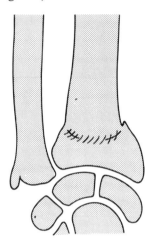

FIG. 265. Old fracture of lower end of radius united with shortening and consequent subluxation of inferior radio-ulnar joint.

unduly prominent and its distal extremity is level with or even distal to the styloid process of the radius, whereas in the normal wrist the tip of the radial styloid is lower by about a centimetre. Forearm rotation is impaired and often painful at the extremes of the range.

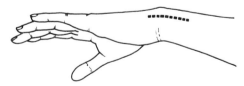

FIG. 266. Excision of lower end of ulna. The skin incision.

In excision of the lower end of the ulna about 2 or 2.5 centimetres of the bone should be removed, together with the investing periosteum.

TECHNIQUE

Position of patient. The patient lies supine, with the forearm and hand resting upon an arm platform or side table. A tourniquet may be used on the upper arm.

Incision. A vertical dorso-medial incision is made over the subcutaneous aspect of the ulna (Fig. 266). It is about 5 centimetres long, with its lower limit immediately distal to the styloid process of the ulna.

Exposure and removal of head of ulna. The incision is deepened directly on to the bone. So far as is possible dissection should then be made between the outer aspect of the periosteum of the ulna and the surrounding soft tissues. It is not practicable, however, to isolate the whole of the

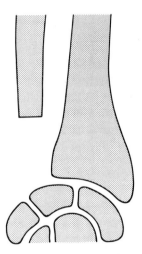

FIG. 267. After excision of lower end of ulna. Note the amount of bone removed.

lower end of the ulna extraperiosteally, and accordingly, when the dissection reaches a deeper plane, the periosteal cuff may be opened and periosteum stripped from the bone. Distally, periosteum and ligaments are firmly attached to the end of the bone and these attachments are better left intact at this stage.

The next step is to divide the ulna 2 to 2.5 centimetres proximal to the styloid process (Fig. 267). The bone section may be made with nibbling forceps, with fine-pointed bone-cutting forceps, or with a high-speed powered dental-type burr, according to preference. The division must be clean and in the transverse plane.

With the bone thus divided, a sharp bone hook may be inserted in the cut surface of the distal fragment, and with this the fragment may be drawn towards the operator and twisted as necessary to enable the firm ligamentous attachments at its distal end to be divided cleanly with a small-bladed (number 15) knife, which should be kept close to the bone. The bone fragment is thus cut free and discarded.

Attention is finally directed to the remaining cuff of periosteum from which the bone fragment has been shelled out. Part of the cuff will have already been mobilised and this should now be removed together with those parts of it that lie deep to the bone, which are still adherent to fibro-fatty tissue and must be freed by sharp dissection. Distally the triangular fibrocartilage and capsule of the wrist joint are both left undisturbed.

Closure. After release of the tourniquet and securing of any persistent bleeding points, subcutaneous fibro-fatty tissue is approximated with two or three sutures of fine absorbable material and the skin is closed with non-absorbable sutures.

POST-OPERATIVE MANAGEMENT

Rigid splintage is not required. It is usually sufficient to bandage the area firmly with a crepe bandage 10 centimetres wide over copious gauze dressings. The patient is encouraged to be up and about within a few hours of the operation. Early attention should be paid to the restoration of full movement of the fingers, elbow and shoulder, preferably under the supervision of a physiotherapist. After the first week wrist mobilising exercises are begun, and at this stage particular attention should be paid to rotation exercises to promote full supination and pronation.

Comment

This simple operation gives almost uniformly good results. Caution is to be enjoined, however, on the risks of excising too great a length of the ulna. There is a moderate margin of safety, but if a length greater than 5 centimetres of the lower end of the ulna is removed, there is a risk of disturbance of smooth rotation of the forearm, especially in patients with rheumatoid arthritis. Rotation is not necessarily restricted, but the normal smooth movement is marred by subluxation of the superior radio-ulnar joint at a certain point in the arc.

Another worthwhile precaution has already been noted—namely to remove as much of the periosteum that surrounds the excised bone fragment as possible, in order to prevent the possible re-formation of a spur of bone.

OPEN REDUCTION AND FIXATION OF SMITH'S FRACTURE BY BUTTRESS PLATE

This operation was described by Ellis (1965), who devised a special plate to give anterior support to the lower end of the radius after reduction of the displacement. The lower end of the plate is flared out to give a broad area of contact with the small lower fragment (Fig. 268). An ordinary plate may be used in the same way as the buttress plate. In either case it may be necessary to bend the lower end of the plate to match the normal curve of the anterior cortex of the lower end of the radius.

TECHNIQUE

Position of limb. The limb rests upon a side table with the forearm supinated. The fingers and thumb may be controlled by a "lead hand". A tourniquet may be used on the upper arm.

Incision. The incision is a vertical one over the front of the lower end of the radius. It lies just lateral to the radial artery.

Reduction of fracture. It is best to expose first the normal bone of the radial shaft 5 or 6 centimetres proximal to the styloid process. The radius is then followed down to the site of fracture. If the

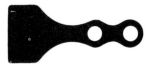

FIG. 268. Ellis's buttress plate. Note the flared lower end, designed to support the lower fragment of the radius.

lower fragment of the radius has been shifted forwards (Fig. 269) the fractured cortex of this fragment will be immediately encountered.

The fracture is now opened up by a suitable lever such as a Macdonald's dissector, to allow complete clearance of all blood clot and fibrin, so that there is nothing to prevent interlocking of the fragments. Then by a combination of leverage and backward pressure upon the lower fragment by a

in contact with the lower fragment almost down to the level of the wrist joint. The plate is screwed to the proximal fragment by two screws after suitable drill holes have been made (Fig. 270).

Closure. The skin alone is sutured.

POST-OPERATIVE MANAGEMENT

Additional support to the wrist by a plaster-of-Paris splint is recommended. The initial plaster should be no more than an anterior shell held in position by crepe bandages. After two weeks, when the sutures are removed, a light encircling plaster from upper forearm to metacarpal heads is applied, the plaster being well moulded about the site of fracture and in the palm.

The plaster should be retained until union is well advanced—usually about eight weeks from the time of operation. It is by no means always necessary to remove the plate, but its removal should be advised if it causes any local discomfort.

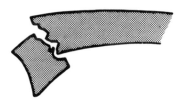 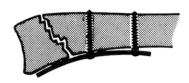

FIGS 269–270. Smith's fracture. Figure 269—Typical anterior displacement of the distal fragment of the radius. Figure 270—Fracture stabilised by buttress plate screwed to the anterior surface of the proximal fragment.

thumb placed over a swab the fragment is reduced to its normal position.

Reduction presents more difficulty when the lower fragment is comminuted than when it is in one piece: if it is not possible to gain exact apposition the surgeon should ensure at least that the articular surface is directed downwards and only slightly forwards, as in the normal wrist.

Application of buttress plate. If necessary the Ellis buttress plate may be bent into a curve by plate benders to fit the concavity of the anterior surface of the lower end of the radius. The plate is then placed in position, with the flared lower end

Comment

The Ellis buttress plate is more satisfactory than an ordinary plate screwed to both fragments because its flared lower end gives better support to the lower fragment. In any case it is often not practicable to use a screw in the lower fragment because the bone is fragmented and fails to afford a satisfactory grip to a screw.

The main essential of the operation is to ensure that reduction is complete, as judged from the restoration of a perfectly smooth contour to the anterior surface of the radius, without any step. The surgeon should also be sure that the articular surface of the lower end of the radius is directed downwards and only slightly forwards as in the normal wrist, and that any distortion of the joint surface due to comminution of the lower fragment is corrected. If there is doubt about this the position should be checked by a radiograph or by the image intensifier before the wound is closed.

SCREW FIXATION OF OBLIQUE FRACTURE OF BASE OF FIRST METACARPAL

The type of case for which internal fixation is described in this section is that in which an oblique fracture involves the articular surface of the base of the first metacarpal. The main fragment is displaced dorsally and proximally, leaving a small triangular volar fragment articulating with the trapezium (Bennett's fracture-subluxation) (Fig. 271). The aim of the operation is to reduce the displacement under direct vision and to fix the two fragments with a transverse screw so accurately that the articular surface is smooth, without any step (Fig. 273).

of the trapezium is exposed, care being taken to retract the radial artery dorsally out of the field of operation.

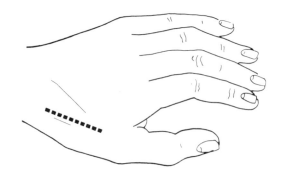

FIG. 272. Operative reduction of Bennett's fracture-subluxation. The skin incision.

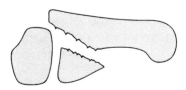

FIG. 271. Oblique fracture through base of first metacarpal with proximal displacement of the major fragment (Bennett's fracture-subluxation).

TECHNIQUE

Position of hand. The hand rests upon a side table with the thumb uppermost. It should be supported by a "lead hand". A tourniquet may be used on the upper arm.

Exposure. The skin incision is a longitudinal one, parallel with and just behind the extensor pollicis brevis tendon (Fig. 272). It is about 4 centimetres long with its centre over the trapezio-metacarpal joint.

The skin edges are retracted and the dorsal surface of the base of the displaced first metacarpal is exposed by reflection of the periosteum by sharp dissection, the knife being kept close to the bone. More proximally, the dorso-lateral surface

Discovery of the small volar fragment and reduction of fracture. To ensure accurate reduction it is necessary to secure a full end-on view of the articular surface of the base of the first metacarpal. To allow this full exposure of the articular surface, the whole base of the first metacarpal must be subluxated from the trapezium by freeing the collateral attachments of the capsule and ligaments at each side of the joint and then placing the metacarpal in a position of forced opposition.

In freeing the capsule from the margins of the articular surface of the metacarpal the knife should be kept close to the bone throughout. In the dissection on the radial side the tendons of extensor pollicis brevis and abductor pollicis longus are pushed forwards with the capsule, off the dorsal aspect of the bone.

When the metacarpal is now placed in full opposition and rotated a little medially or laterally, the articular surface of its base is clearly exposed and the fracture line comes into view.

Nearly always there is a considerable step between the small volar fragment and the main dorsal fragment, which is displaced proximally.

The fracture line is opened up from the articular surface to allow clearance of any blood clot or fibrin that may have congealed between the fracture surfaces. Reduction is then easily obtained by strong traction on the thumb, which is still held in the position of opposition, combined with countertraction in a proximal direction on the small triangular volar fragment by means of small nerve hooks gripping the adjacent soft tissues.

Insertion of fixation screw. When the fracture has been thus reduced and when it has been confirmed by palpation with a probe that there is no remaining step on the articular surface, a suitable drill hole is prepared to receive the selected screw. The drill track should be made horizontally—that is, parallel to the articular surface of the metacarpal and about 5 millimetres distal to it. The drill is entered at the dorsal surface of the main fragment and is driven through into the small volar fragment.

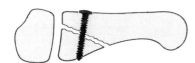

Fig. 273. Fixation of Bennett's fracture-subluxation by transfixion screw.

The initial drill hole should be equal to the core diameter of the screw, but the hole in the dorsal (main) fragment should subsequently be drilled out wider to allow a sliding fit. This ensures that when the screw is driven home into the lesser fragment the fracture surfaces are drawn together (Fig. 273). Because of the small size of the volar fragment a fine-gauge screw should be selected: its overall diameter should preferably be not more than 3 millimetres.

Closure. With the two fragments thus securely fixed together the trapezio-metacarpal joint is reasonably stable when the subluxation is reduced by extending the metacarpal. Nevertheless it is important to close the marginal incision in the capsule at the base of the metacarpal by fine interrupted sutures gripping the periosteum. When the capsular ligaments have thus been reconstructed it remains to close the skin with interrupted sutures.

POST-OPERATIVE MANAGEMENT

A light plaster-of-Paris splint enclosing the forearm and metacarpals and well moulded round the base of the thumb is worn for four weeks. By that time healing is sufficiently well established to allow gentle use of the hand without further rigid support.

Comment

It may not seem easy at first to demonstrate the small triangular volar fragment from this approach. The secret is to gain a thorough exposure of the whole area of the articular surface by sufficient separation of the capsule and ligaments from the articular margin of the base of the first metacarpal.

Even then, the view is not adequate until the metacarpal is strongly opposed into the palm or rotated so that its base is subluxated dorsally into the wound. With the articular aspect of the fracture line thus exposed there is no special difficulty in clearing the fracture surfaces and then gaining good reduction by strong longitudinal traction upon the metacarpal and a proximal counter-pull upon the smaller fragment.

Even if the triangular volar fragment is very small it is usually possible to secure it adequately if a screw of small diameter is used. Provided the screw is inserted accurately, fixation is quite rigid, so that little reliance need be placed upon external splintage.

This technique of fixation ensures more certain reduction than alternative methods in which the fragments are secured semi-blindly by a Kirschner wire.

STABILISATION OF OBLIQUE FRACTURE OF METACARPAL WITH RECESSION OF KNUCKLE

Oblique fracture of the shaft of a metacarpal may lead to significant shortening with consequent ugly recession of the knuckle. Although such fractures will unite readily without special treatment and do not lead to any loss of function, the cosmetic blemish from the recessed knuckle may be distressing, especially in women. Thus consideration may have to be given at the initial stage of management to stabilisation of the fractured bone at normal length. Open reduction, with fixation by small transverse screws or by plate and screws, is one method that may be used.

A somewhat simpler method, in that it does not involve open operation, is to draw the fractured bone out to full length by manual traction and

Correction of shortening. Provided the fracture is recent, there is no difficulty in overcoming the shortening by traction upon the finger against counter-traction upon the upper arm, the elbow being flexed 90 degrees. It is best that traction be maintained by assistants so that the surgeon has both hands free to introduce the transfixion wire.

Introduction of wire. A stiff Kirschner wire of 1.5 to 2 millimetres diameter should be selected. It is well to mark the course of the wire on the back of the hand with dots of ink to help to ensure that it is directed accurately.

In the case of a fracture of the metacarpal of the middle finger the wire should be introduced at the

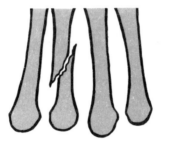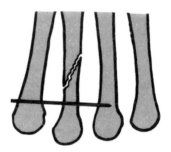

FIGS 274–275. Stabilisation of oblique fracture of a central metacarpal by transfixion of injured and adjacent bones with a stiff wire. Length is preserved and recession of the knuckle prevented.

then to anchor the distal fragment to the adjacent metacarpals by transfixing the bones with a stiff wire. This method is applicable only to the middle or ring finger because there has to be an intact metacarpal on each side of the injured one if rigid stabilisation is to be achieved (Figs 274 and 275).

TECHNIQUE

The procedure may be carried out either with general anaesthesia or with regional anaesthesia.

Position of patient. The patient lies supine with the affected hand resting upon the arm platform of the operation table.

junction of neck and head of the index metacarpal in the mid-lateral plane and directed horizontally towards the ulnar side of the hand so that it penetrates the neck of the middle metacarpal and enters the head of the ring finger metacarpal (Fig. 275). In the case of fracture of the ring finger metacarpal the wire is introduced through the head of the fifth metacarpal near its junction with the neck, and is directed transversely and slightly distally towards the head-neck junction of the middle metacarpal.

The correct length of wire should be determined before its introduction, so that the surgeon will know precisely when the wire has penetrated to the correct depth: the optimal length is easily determined by measurement upon the dorsal surface of the hand.

When all is ready and the surgeon is satisfied that the knuckle has been restored to its correct location the wire is introduced through a tiny nick made in the skin with a fine-pointed knife blade. When the wire has penetrated to the pre-determined depth it is cut off with a wire cutter, leaving about 3 or 4 millimetres protruding through the skin. Finally, the shape of the hand is assessed clinically with the fingers flexed and then extended, and by radiography. If for any reason the normal contour of the knuckles is not restored, the procedure should be abandoned in favour of open reduction and internal fixation.

POST-OPERATIVE MANAGEMENT

To reduce the discomfort entailed by transfixion of the bones and protrusion of the wire, it is advisable to apply rather voluminous gauze dressings and to envelop the protruding tip of the wire in sterilised felt or a small sponge, and then to apply a plaster-of-Paris support to hold the wrist in slight extension. The plaster is brought down just below knuckle level and across the palm of the hand in such a way that finger flexion is not impeded. Stabilisation by the wire should be maintained for two and a half to three weeks, by which time intrinsic stability will be sufficient to allow removal of the wire.

Comment
This simple method can work well, but accurate introduction of the wire calls for considerable skill because the metacarpals, especially in women, are slender and it is easy to fail to transfix all three metacarpals. There is also the disadvantage of leaving a wire protruding through the skin, with risk of pin-track infection, and it is to help to prevent this that encasement in plaster-of-Paris—which itself helps to persuade the patient to keep the hand dry—is recommended.

It is important that perfect reduction of the deformity is seen to be gained at the time of the operation, and that if perfect reduction cannot be secured and maintained, the pin should be removed immediately and a decision made on whether to accept the situation or to proceed to an alternative method.

OPEN REDUCTION AND FIXATION
BY SMALL PLATE AND SCREWS

The A.O. mini-fragment set may be used with advantage for the management of these fractures.

TECHNIQUE

Position of patient. The patient lies supine with the affected hand on an arm board at the side. A tourniquet should be used.

Exposure. Through a longitudinal incision over the affected metacarpal, any interosseous muscle is stripped away from the fracture site by a small, sharp periosteal elevator.

Procedure. Blood clot is cleared from between the fragments. The fragments are reduced and held accurately in position by the pointed bone-holding forceps or small Verbrugge forceps. A plate is chosen of such a size that it will allow two screws to fix it on each side of the fracture. Because the metacarpal head fragment (distal fragment) may be small, one of the T-shaped or offset plates may have to be selected. (The offset parts of the plate may be bent to the contour of the metacarpal by the use of the bending pliers contained in the set.) The appropriate plate is held in place across the fracture with the special plate-holding forceps provided. Screws 2 millimetres in diameter are used to hold the plates. A 1.5 millimetre drill is centred in each plate hole using the drill guide. The screw length required is determined for each screw by the miniature depth gauge. Each hole is tapped with the 2 millimetre tap and screws of the correct length are inserted.

Closure. Usually skin closure alone is needed. The tourniquet is released with the hand elevated.

POST-OPERATIVE MANAGEMENT

A non-adhesive dressing and a crepe bandage are applied. Gentle active hand movements are encouraged from the beginning, but the patient must be warned against using the hand forcefully until the fracture has united—usually after about six weeks.

INTRAMEDULLARY NAILING FOR FRACTURE OF SHAFT OF METACARPAL

Nailing is appropriate especially for displaced fractures near the middle of a metacarpal, when the fracture is transverse and when closed reduction is impracticable. This section should be read in conjunction with the general description of intramedullary nailing in Chapter 2 (p. 84).

TECHNIQUE

Position of hand. The hand rests upon a side table with the dorsal surface uppermost and the palm supported by a rolled towel. A tourniquet may be used on the upper arm.

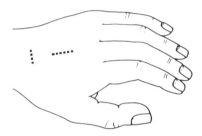

FIG. 276. Intramedullary nailing for fracture of shaft of metacarpal. The skin incisions.

Exposure. Since the metacarpals are subcutaneous the requisite exposure may be obtained by a direct vertical incision over the site of fracture (Fig. 276). A second incision or a prolongation of the first incision is required over the base of the metacarpal, where access of the nail to the medullary canal is to be gained.

Reduction of fracture. The extensor tendon overlying the fracture is retracted medially or laterally according to which is the easier. The fracture surfaces are thus exposed together with a short length of normal bone proximal and distal to the fracture. The fracture surfaces are cleared of blood clot and fibrin.

By this stage the reason why manipulative reduction was impossible will have become apparent: often there is excessive overlap of the fragments, which cannot be drawn out to length by closed methods because of the rigidity of the adjacent metacarpals. Occasionally, soft tissue is caught up and button-holed by one or other of the fragments so that it cannot be disengaged by closed manipulation. With the fragments in view it is a simple matter to free any obstruction and to gain full end-to-end reduction by a combination of traction and leverage with a blunt instrument such as a Macdonald dissector. Internal fixation as described below may not be necessary if the position of the fragments is stable after reduction.

Introduction of intramedullary nail. Pin is perhaps a better term than nail for the fixation device. Usually a stout Kirschner wire or a guide wire serves the purpose well.

The pin is introduced at the dorsal surface of the base of the metacarpal, which is made as prominent as possible by acute flexion of the wrist. The entrance hole for the pin is made with an awl from the dorsal corner of the articular surface. The awl must necessarily be introduced at an angle to the line of the medullary canal, and being straight and rigid it usually cannot be thrust along the full length of the canal. It is necessary therefore to bend the tip of the selected pin into a slight curve so that after its introduction through

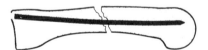

FIG. 277. Internal fixation of fracture of shaft of metacarpal by intramedullary wire.

the prepared hole it will find its way along the medullary canal. To ensure this it is desirable that the pin should be slightly flexible so that it may adapt itself to the line of the metacarpal.

When the pin has been introduced almost as far as the head of the metacarpal it is cut off close to the base of the metacarpal with a wire cutter (Fig. 277).

POST-OPERATIVE MANAGEMENT

For the first three weeks after operation it is well to protect the hand by a light dorsal plaster slab extending from forearm to metacarpal heads and held in place by a firm crepe or cotton bandage. Active finger movements are encouraged from the beginning.

Whether or not the pin should be removed when union is consolidated depends upon indi-vidual circumstances. If the base of the pin is palpable under the skin, or if the metal pin used is suspect from the point of view of total resistance to corrosion—as some Kirschner wires and guide wires are—removal of the pin should certainly be advised. If a pin that is entirely buried within a metacarpal has to be removed it may be necessary to make a small window over the point of the pin and to force the pin backwards out of the bone until the base can be gripped with pliers.

SCREW FIXATION FOR FRACTURE OF SCAPHOID BONE

Fixation of a fracture of the scaphoid bone by a screw is suitable for certain unfavourable types of fresh fracture, for delayed union and for non-union (Maudsley and Chen 1972, Leyshon *et al.* 1984, Herbert and Fisher 1984). It is not appro-priate if the proximal fragment is very small (that is, when the fracture is through the proximal pole) or when the proximal fragment is avascular.

TECHNIQUE

The technique to be described relates to the inser-tion of the special screw devised by T. J. Her-bert*; but other types of cancellous screw of suitable proportions may be used with minor modifications of the freehand technique. The special feature of the Herbert headless screw is that the leading threads are of coarse pitch where-as the trailing threads are of fine pitch (Fig. 279). Thus the two halves of the fractured bone are drawn together.

Position of patient. The patient lies supine with the forearm resting upon a side table, palm upper-most. The position of the hand may be controlled by a "lead hand". A tourniquet may be used on the upper arm.

Incision. The skin incision, about 3.5 centi-metres long, begins 2 centimetres proximal to the tuberosity of the scaphoid bone. This eminence is easily palpated at the front of the wrist at the level of the flexor crease, and immediately lateral to the

* Supplied by Messrs Zimmer Inc, Warsaw, Indiana, USA.

tendon of flexor carpi radialis. From this point the incision extends distally, curving slightly laterally over the thenar muscle mass to end 1.5 centi-metres distal to the tuberosity of the scaphoid (Fig. 278).

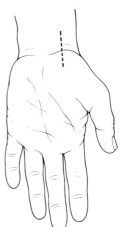

FIG. 278. Anterior ex-posure of scaphoid bone for screw fixation or bone grafting. The skin incision.

Exposure of scaphoid bone. The skin edges being retracted, a small superficial palmar branch of the radial artery is sought and protected. The flexor carpi radialis tendon is retracted medially (ulnar-wards) after incision of its sheath. The scaphoid bone now lies in the depth of the wound and is easily exposed by incision of the anterior capsule of the wrist joint. The edges of the capsule are best held aside by holding stitches. The scaphoid bone is well revealed in its entire length and the fracture is clearly visible.

It is important at this stage to examine the state of the fracture, to ascertain whether it is mobile or held to some extent by fibrous tissue, and to see whether there is any displacement and if so whether it can be reduced. Full reduction is clearly necessary, and by experiment the surgeon must ascertain whether it can be achieved by altering the position of the wrist, or perhaps by a direct pressure against the displaced fragment by a flat instrument.

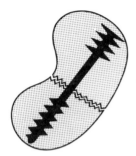

FIG. 279. Fixation of scaphoid fracture by Herbert screw. Note that the leading threads of the screw are of coarse pitch whereas the trailing threads are of fine pitch. As the screw is driven in the fragments are therefore drawn together.

Directing the drill by the Zimmer jig. A special jig and other instruments are supplied by the makers of the Herbert screw, but the use of the jig is not essential. If the jig is to be used the tiny hooked spike designed to engage over the proximal pole of the scaphoid bone is made to so engage and the drill guide is brought down into contact with the tuberosity of the scaphoid as far posteriorly as possible. Once the jig is correctly inserted, the drill hole will automatically be correctly sited.

The first drill, 2.4 millimetres in diameter, is equal to the core diameter of the trailing thread of the screw. The depth of penetration by this drill is stopped automatically by a shoulder at about 7 millimetres. This drill is followed by the longer drill, 1.9 millimetres in diameter, which is passed down the drill guide and should penetrate into the proximal pole of the scaphoid. Threads are then cut in the proximal pole by means of a special tap provided. Finally the screw is driven in with a special hexagonal screwdriver. As the trailing thread sinks into the distal fragment increasing resistance is felt, and the two fragments of the scaphoid are drawn tightly together (Fig. 279).

Insertion of screw by freehand technique. It may be difficult to fit the jig to gain entrance to the bone at the optimal site, and in such a case the screw may be inserted freehand. First the 2.4 millimetre drill is inserted at the tuberosity at

such a point that the drill can be directed accurately towards the proximal pole. The drill is inserted to the appropriate depth, penetrating only the distal fragment. The 1.9 millimetre drill follows, and is driven right on into the proximal pole of the scaphoid. The hole is then tapped all the way with the special tap provided. Finally the screw is inserted and tightened.

Bone grafting. If it is considered advisable, a small bone graft may be inserted into the fracture gap at the time of screw fixation.

Closure. The anterior capsule is closed with fine absorbable sutures and the skin is closed without drainage.

POST-OPERATIVE MANAGEMENT

Provided good fixation has been achieved, there should be no need for external immobilisation. Nevertheless the authors prefer to give additional support to the wrist by a light plaster-of-Paris splint, retained for six weeks.

Comment

Insertion of a screw into the scaphoid bone does not present special difficulty because the whole length of the bone is under direct vision, and it is relatively easy to ensure that the drill passes correctly in the long axis of the bone, even when the drilling is done freehand. The correct length for the screw can also be ascertained accurately because the length of the bone can be measured. The Herbert screw offers advantages over an ordinary lag screw in that there is no screw head, and the trailing thread is driven inside the bone. The compression effect of this screw arises from the fact that the leading thread is of coarse pitch, whereas the trailing thread is of finer pitch, and thus the two fragments are drawn together as the screw is tightened. The screw not only provides immobility, but by drawing the fragments into very close coaptation it prevents the ingress of synovial fluid between the fracture surfaces, which may well be an important factor in preventing union.

BONE GRAFTING OF SCAPHOID BONE FOR UNUNITED FRACTURE

To a great extent, bone grafting of fractures of the scaphoid bone has given place to fixation by a screw (see p. 213), particularly since methods of screw fixation have been refined (Herbert and Fisher 1984) and may be combined with the insertion of a small graft at the time of screw fixation. Nevertheless grafting may still have an occasional place in cases of long-standing non-union, provided the fracture is not proximal to the waist of the bone and that the proximal fragment is free from avascular necrosis. The technique to be described is based on that of Russe (1960). A similar method was favoured by Mulder (1955). It employs an inlay graft cut from the crest of the ilium.

Incision. The tuberosity of the scaphoid bone is identified by palpation, and an incision 2.5 to 3 centimetres long is made vertically proximally from the tuberosity, between the flexor carpi radialis on the medial side and the radial artery (Fig. 278). These structures are retracted with the skin edges and the incision is deepened to expose the distal two-thirds of the front of the scaphoid bone. The area of bone that is exposed is almost entirely non-articular. More proximally the bone is covered with articular cartilage and this should not be disturbed.

Demonstration of fracture. It is essential to gain a clear view of the fracture line, which encircles the

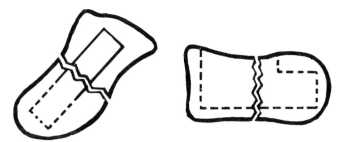

FIGS 280–281. Bone grafting of scaphoid bone. Figure 280—Orientation of slot for graft, as seen in antero-posterior view. Figure 281—The slot shown in longitudinal section. Note its boot-like shape.

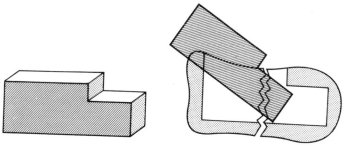

FIGS 282–283. Figure 282—The graft, shaped from iliac bone to match the cavity. Figure 283—Method of introducing the graft.

TECHNIQUE

Position of limb. The patient lies supine with the forearm, fully supinated, resting upon a side table. The fingers and thumb may be stabilised by enfolding their tips in a "lead hand". A tourniquet may be used on the upper arm.

bone usually in its middle third but sometimes closer to the proximal pole. The fracture gap may be open, simulating a joint between the fragments, or it may be bridged by fibrous tissue. So long as the fragments are in normal relationship one to the other, there is no need to disturb the fracture surfaces once the fracture line has been demonstrated. If there is difficulty in demonstrating the fracture it is wise to place a radio-opaque marker on the bone that has been exposed and to obtain a radiograph. Occasionally a surgeon has been surprised to find that he had exposed the wrong bone.

Preparation of slot for bone graft. The slot lies in the direction of the long axis of the scaphoid bone (Fig. 280) and it is cut out from the front. The slot should be so deep as to reach almost to the posterior shell of the bone. In other words it should penetrate through virtually the whole thickness of the bone (Fig. 281). The slot is open anteriorly throughout the distal two-thirds of the bone, crossing the fracture line. In the proximal pole of the scaphoid the slot is excavated from the interior without opening the surface, as shown in Figure 281; articular cartilage is thus left intact. The slot is best cut with a fine chisel about 3 millimetres wide. Its walls must be cleanly cut and strictly parallel, and the distal end wall must be cut square. Proximally, as already noted, the cavity is undercut into the proximal pole of the scaphoid. The cavity is thus boot-shaped (Fig. 281) and the graft must exactly fit the "boot".

Preparation of bone graft. A piece of bone fractionally larger than the outside dimensions of the proposed graft is cut from the crest of the ilium in the manner described on page 76. It should include one cortex of the ilium, the remainder of the graft being of firm cancellous bone. The graft is placed on a fresh sterile cloth or work board, and with a fine chisel it is cut precisely to the dimensions of the cavity that has been prepared for it (Fig. 282). The graft should be so cut that the cortical surface forms the deep surface of the graft.

Fitting and impaction of graft. The finished graft, like the cavity already prepared for it, is boot-shaped and the manner of insertion is to place the toe of the boot first into the slot so that it will occupy the cavity undercut in the proximal pole of the scaphoid (Fig. 283). With the "toe" thus in position the remainder of the graft is easily driven down into the slot and it automatically locks into position. To ensure a tight fit the graft may be punched home lightly with a rectangular punch. The wound is then closed.

POST-OPERATIVE MANAGEMENT

The wrist should be protected in a scaphoid-type plaster-of-Paris splint until union is shown to be well advanced—usually a matter of ten to twelve weeks.

Comment

This operation demands a precise technique because it depends for its success upon firm impaction of the carefully fashioned graft in both fragments of the scaphoid bone. It is particularly important that the graft be in one piece. A graft as slender as this is easily fractured during its preparation and particularly during its insertion if the slot made to receive it is even fractionally narrower than the graft.

Another important requirement is that the graft should penetrate deeply into the body of the scaphoid bone, preferably almost through to the posterior cortex. The operation is one in which painstaking care and precision are well rewarded.

SCREW FIXATION FOR OBLIQUE FRACTURES OF PHALANGES OF THE HAND

Certain phalangeal fractures with displacement of the fragments, and especially those in which the fracture line is oblique and reduction therefore unstable, may be satisfactorily treated by open reduction and fixation with a transfixion screw.

These fractures occur in almost infinite variety, and it is possible here only to suggest some general principles. These will be illustrated by the not uncommon case in which the base of the distal phalanx of the thumb is split obliquely in consequence of a sudden force applied to the tip of the straight digit.

Typically a triangular volar fragment bearing up to half of the articular surface of the phalanx is sheared away proximally and volarwards, creating a gap and step in the articular surface with subluxation of the joint (Fig. 284). Unless the articular surface can be restored to its normal contour, persistent pain and stiffness may result.

Such a fracture may often be better treated by open reduction and fixation than by conservative means. But it must be emphasised that if operation is to be undertaken, the objective must be to secure complete anatomical reduction: if this is not achieved the operation might as well not have been undertaken, as emphasised by Perkins (1958) in another but related context.

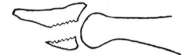

Fig. 284. Anterior marginal fracture of base of distal phalanx of thumb with subluxation of the joint.

In general plan, the operation entails exposure of the interphalangeal joint from the side and elevation of sufficient capsule, ligament and synovial membrane to expose the fracture to direct view both from the side and from within the joint. Under direct vision the displaced fragment may then be replaced and held while a suitable screw is inserted.

In this type of operation use of the A.O. mini-fragment set clearly offers great advantages.

TECHNIQUE

Position of patient. The patient lies supine, with the affected hand resting upon the arm platform. The hand itself may be supported in a "lead hand", palm uppermost. A tourniquet may be used on the upper arm.

Incision. A longitudinal incision is made in the mid-lateral line of the thumb on its radial aspect (Fig. 285). The incision extends from the middle of the proximal phalanx to the middle of the distal phalanx.

Exposure of fracture site. The dissection is deepened to the bone in the mid-lateral line of the digit. The soft tissues, including the neurovascular bundle, are mobilised forwards. By sharp

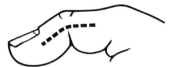

Fig. 285. Incision for exposure of interphalangeal joint and base of distal phalanx of thumb.

dissection joint capsule and periosteum are reflected anteriorly and posteriorly from the condyle of the proximal phalanx and from the base of the proximal half of the shaft of the distal phalanx. In this process the joint is opened and blood clot or fibrin is cleared away to allow direct inspection of the articular surfaces: to aid this the joint may be momentarily subluxated. The fracture line as it emerges into the joint at the base of the distal phalanx is thus brought clearly into view and the degree of displacement is ascertained.

Reposition of fragment. It is important that the displaced fragment be restored fully to its normal position. To this end the fracture line may have to be opened up to allow fibrin and bone spicules to be removed from the fracture surfaces: if necessary, the loose fragment may be further mobilised by elevation of the adjacent periosteum to allow its easy reposition. The blood supply of the fragment, however, must not be jeopardised by over-free dissection of the attached soft tissues.

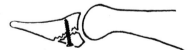

Fig. 286. Fixation of marginal phalangeal fracture by a small screw. In some cases a fine Kirschner wire may be more appropriate; or even a mattress suture of stainless-steel wire inserted through 0.5 millimetre drill holes.

Internal fixation. When the loose fragment has been accurately restored to its bed and when it has been confirmed by direct inspection that the articular surface is smooth and that no step remains, the position is held by grasping the fragment and the main part of the phalanx with dissecting forceps, while preparation is made for the insertion of a screw. In most instances, the displaced fragment of the phalanx is small and accordingly a screw of very small calibre (2 millimetres in diameter) has to be selected. A hole equal to the core diameter of the screw (1.5 millimetres) is drilled from the anterior aspect, traversing first the loose fragment and then the main part of the phalanx. The proximal part of the hole—that is, the part that traverses the loose fragment—is then drilled out by a larger drill to the overall diameter of the screw. This ensures that the fragments are drawn together when the screw is driven home (Fig. 286).

After the screw has been inserted, the articular surface of the base of the distal phalanx is again inspected to make sure that the contour is smooth.

Closure. After removal of the tourniquet the capsule and periosteum are repaired by fine absorbable sutures, and the skin is closed.

POST-OPERATIVE MANAGEMENT

It is advisable to support the injured joint by a light plaster splint, held in place by a crepe bandage, for two weeks after the operation. Thereafter, active movements are encouraged, and the hand is used progressively for light tasks and later for normal activities.

Application of Technique to Fractures of Other Digits

The technique is basically similar at other sites where an oblique fracture at the base of the pha-

lanx enters the adjacent joint. The aim should be to gain a clear exposure of the fracture and of the articular surface of the base of the phalanx, and then to mobilise the loose fragment sufficiently to

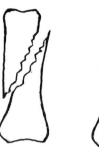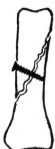

FIGS 287–288. Oblique fracture of shaft of a phalanx before and after fixation by a small-diameter oblique screw.

allow accurate reposition in its bed. A similar method of screw fixation is applicable to an oblique fracture involving the mid-shaft of a phalanx (Figs 287 and 288).

Comment

Operations of the type described require a delicate technique and gentle handling of the tissues and bone. It is all too easy to break up the small loose fragment during drilling or when the screw is driven in. This spoils the operation, for there is no second chance once the fragment has been split. It is therefore essential to ensure before the operation is undertaken that a proper range of screws of the required fineness is available. Attempts to fix the fragment with a screw that is too coarse are doomed to failure and are better not made. Equally, there is little point in undertaking the operation unless the outcome is a perfectly smooth phalangeal articular surface.

ARTHRODESIS OF WRIST

Usually the wrist should be fused in 20 degrees of dorsiflexion. The method to be described entails denuding the carpal joints of articular cartilage and applying a curved onlay graft of cortico-cancellous bone from the ilium.

TECHNIQUE

Position of patient. The patient lies supine with the forearm resting upon an arm platform. A tourniquet may be used on the upper arm.

Incision. The incision exposes the lower end of the radius, the carpal bones and the base of the middle metacarpal from behind. The incision is serpentine, like a "lazy S". It begins 2.5 centimetres proximal to the lower articular margin of the radius posteriorly, and ends over the proximal part of the shaft of the middle metacarpal (Fig. 289).

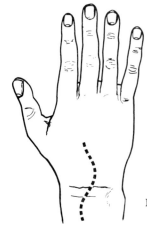

FIG. 289. Arthrodesis of wrist. The skin incision.

Skin flaps are raised and turned aside to expose the extensor tendons of the digits and wrist. These tendons are separated and retracted out of the way, medially or laterally as is found most convenient for each tendon. The extensor carpi radialis tendons, longus and brevis, may be divided from their insertions and reflected proximally.

Excision of articular cartilage. It is important that the radio-carpal joint and the intercarpal joints should be denuded of articular cartilage so far as this is accessible, in order to promote fusion between the individual bones. Cartilage is most easily removed with a fine chisel manipulated by hand, or by a dental burr. As each joint is denuded the subchondral bone is broken up or roughened, to help to promote vascularisation across the joint.

Preparation of bed for graft. The proposed graft will be placed upon the dorsum of the carpus and screwed to the lower end of the radius and to the base of the third metacarpal. To receive the graft, flat slightly sunken surfaces should be prepared with a chisel at each of these end points.

With the wrist placed in 20 degrees of dorsi-flexion and with no adduction or abduction, the length of graft required to bridge the third metacarpal to the radius, allowing 2 centimetres of overlap at each end, is measured.

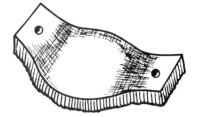

FIG. 290. Arthrodesis of wrist. Diagram showing the shape and curvature of the graft.

Taking and preparation of graft. The bone graft is obtained from the wing of the ilium. It is important that the site should be so chosen as to provide a curved graft to fit into the dorsal hollow of the wrist when it is extended 20 degrees. Such a curved graft is easily obtained from the appropriate part of the ilium: if necessary, a dried specimen of a pelvis may be studied in advance.

The graft is best cut as a rectangle, usually about 7 or 8 centimetres long and 2.5 centimetres wide: this is somewhat larger than required, but allows a margin for trimming. It should be cut out from the wing of the ilium with both cortices, so that a window is left in the iliac wing; but the iliac crest should be left intact (see p. 76).

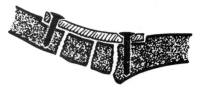

FIG. 291. Sectional diagram showing the graft seated in position and fixed with screws. Note that the inter-carpal joints have been rawed.

Once removed, the graft is further prepared by chiselling off the cortex on the convex side to leave a raw surface of cancellous bone: the cortex is left intact on the concave side (Fig. 290). The edges are then trued up to match the carpal bed in which the graft will lie, and the ends are trimmed to exactly the right length to fit the flat recesses prepared in the lower end of the radius and the base of the middle metacarpal.

Fitting of graft. Before the graft is finally fitted and screwed home, mashed cancellous bone (surplus shavings from the graft usually suffice) is laid freely within the rawed carpal joints to aid fusion. The graft is then secured in position with the wrist dorsiflexed 20 degrees. One drill hole is made through each end of the graft, to engage the radius proximally and the third metacarpal distally: then suitable screws are driven home to secure the graft (Fig. 291).

Finally any prominent corners of the onlay graft are bevelled away to leave a smooth rounded surface.

Closure. The various extensor tendons are allowed to fall back into their natural position and the wound is closed without drainage.

POST-OPERATIVE MANAGEMENT

The wrist should be supported in a plaster case until fusion is sound, usually ten to twelve weeks after operation. The first plaster should be well padded to allow room for swelling, and it is a wise precaution to split it down the back immediately after its application. The definitive plaster is applied two weeks after operation, when the sutures are removed.

Comment

This is perhaps an elaborate method of fusing the wrist but it is reliable in promoting bony fusion. Provided the graft is carefully chosen with the correct curve, it ensures fixation of the wrist in the position of function—namely in slight dorsiflexion. The ulnar-carpal joint is left undisturbed; so rotation of the forearm is preserved.

During the operation care should be taken to ensure that the surfaces of the exposed extensor tendons do not become dry: it is well to moisten the field from time to time with saline.

The cutting of the graft is a vital part of this operation. A good strong piece of bone is required, and delicate work is necessary to ensure that it is removed from the ilium cleanly without any cracks in the cortical surface. Care is also necessary when drilling the screw holes in this rather soft bone: it is all too easy to fragment the ends of the graft during drilling or by over-tight driving of the screws.

After the operation there may be considerable swelling, and it is necessary to watch the circulation carefully and to open up the plaster and dressings as necessary. The hand should be kept well elevated for the first few days after the operation.

ALTERNATIVE METHODS OF WRIST FUSION

Two other methods of arthrodesing the wrist require mention: they may be appropriate in special circumstances. These are the techniques of Smith-Petersen (1940) and of Brockman (reported by Evans 1955).

Smith-Petersen's technique. The wrist is approached from the medial (ulnar) side after excision of 3 centimetres of the lower end of the ulna. The excised bone is used as a graft, driven into a slot cut between the lower end of the radius and the carpus.

The operation has a place particularly in rheumatoid arthritis when the bones are very soft and the wrist joint is disorganised. For further details of technique Smith-Petersen's original paper should be consulted.

Brockman's technique. In this method the lower end of the radius is tapered down into the shape of a thin wedge, which is driven into a cleft created by splitting the carpal bones into equal anterior and posterior halves.

The shortening entailed in this operation makes it suitable for certain cases of cerebral palsy and of Volkmann's ischaemic contracture. For details of the technique Evans's paper should be consulted.

EXCISION OF TRAPEZIUM

In patients requiring excision of the trapezium, usually for severe osteoarthritis of the trapezio-metacarpal joint, the bone may be already deformed and the joint surface articulating with the first metacarpal may be worn away.

TECHNIQUE

Position of limb. The forearm rests on a side table on its ulnar border, with the thumb uppermost. A tourniquet may be used on the upper arm.

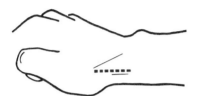

FIG. 292. Excision of trapezium. The skin incision.

Incision. The incision is vertical. It lies parallel to the extensor pollicis brevis tendon and just posterior to it (Fig. 292). Proximally, it reaches nearly to the styloid process of the radius, and distally it extends just over the base of the first metacarpal, which is easily palpated. The skin edges are retracted and the subcutaneous tissue is cleared. It is important at this stage to identify and protect the radial artery, which crosses the base of the anatomical snuff box in a downward and posterior direction.

Isolation and removal of trapezium. The first step is to identify the base of the first metacarpal bone and to open the joint between this and the trapezium. The surface of the trapezium is then cleaned by sharp dissection in a proximal direction until the joint between the trapezium and the scaphoid is entered. By means of a small elevator placed in this joint the radial artery may be held posteriorly, away from the field of operation. Then, working round the bone with a fine-bladed knife, the surgeon divides the ligaments that link the trapezium to the trapezoid bone and to the second metacarpal.

Even when seemingly isolated, the trapezium does not come away easily: patient dissection is required. As the bone begins to come free it may be grasped with a Kocher's forceps and rotated appropriately to allow the deep ligaments to be severed. On the deep aspect the knife must be kept close to the bone in order to avoid damage to the flexor carpi radialis tendon, which crosses the front of the trapezium. This tendon should be seen intact at the end of the operation.

If possible the bone should be removed entire, but occasionally small fragments break off and care must be taken to retrieve them. Excision must always be complete.

Closure. After control of bleeding points subsequent to release of the tourniquet, one or two light absorbable sutures may be used to approximate the subcutaneous tissues. If some soft tissue can be inverted into the gap between scaphoid and first metacarpal to reduce the amount of dead space, so much the better. The skin is closed with interrupted eversion sutures.

POST-OPERATIVE MANAGEMENT

A rather voluminous gauze and crepe bandage dressing is applied, holding the thumb metacarpal partly opposed. The hand should be elevated on pillows for the first two days because swelling of hand and fingers is often considerable. Active finger exercises should be practised from the beginning, and thumb movements should be encouraged as soon as pain allows.

Comment

Excision of the trapezium is a satisfactory operation for osteoarthritis of the trapezio-metacarpal joint, but the patient should be warned that the full benefit of the operation may not be gained for up to four or six months from operation. In the dissection of the bone from its neighbours a gentle technique is required. The use of too much force tends to be followed by marked post-operative pain and swelling.

ARTHRODESIS OF TRAPEZIO-METACARPAL JOINT

The technique to be described involves rawing of the opposed joint surfaces of the trapezium and the first metacarpal, and inlay of a cortico-cancellous graft from the iliac crest.

TECHNIQUE

Position of limb. The patient lies supine with the affected limb on a side table. The forearm rests on its ulnar border, the thumb being uppermost. A tourniquet may be used on the upper arm.

Incision. This is the same as for excision of the trapezium (p. 221), except that a slightly greater length of the first metacarpal is exposed.

Rawing of articular surfaces. When the trapezio-metacarpal joint has been opened the surfaces are prised apart by small hooks or by a lever in the joint, so that access may be gained to the articular surfaces. In patients selected for this operation the articular cartilage is nearly always worn away, often down to eburnated bone. The remains of the cartilage and the surface of the sclerotic bone are cut away with a fine chisel so that raw bleeding bone is exposed. When both opposing surfaces have been thus treated they are fitted together, with care to ensure that apposition is close over the whole area of the raw surface.

Preparation of slot for graft. While the opposing joint surfaces are held firmly together by an assistant a deep slot is cut across the joint with a fine chisel, preferably no more than 4 millimetres wide and with a freshly sharpened edge: alternatively a dental burr may be used. The slot should be about 2 to 2.5 centimetres long, 4 or 5 millimetres wide and nearly 1 centimetre deep. It should core almost through the thickness of the trapezium and of the base of the metacarpal. Usually about a centimetre of its length can be accommodated in the trapezium and a slightly greater length in the base of the metacarpal (Fig. 293). The slot or trench should be cut with precision so that its walls are parallel and straight, and the ends should be squared up neatly.

Taking and preparation of graft. A small graft is obtained from the iliac crest in the manner described on page 76. The finished graft must be of exactly the same dimensions as the trench in the trapezium and metacarpal. It is well to cut the graft a little larger than will be needed and then to trim it with precision after careful measurements of the trench have been made. One cortex of the ilium should be preserved on the graft; the remainder—the deep aspect—is of cancellous bone.

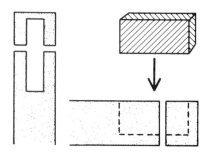

Figs 293–294. Arthrodesis of trapezio-metacarpal joint. Figure 293—Diagram showing the slot cut into the dorsal surface of the trapezium and the base of the first metacarpal. Figure 294—Side view showing the graft and the slot cut to receive it.

Insertion of graft. When the graft has been thus fashioned with the utmost care to get its size exactly right, it is inserted into the prepared slot (Fig. 294), cancellous part first, and punched home with a rectangular punch. The tourniquet is then removed and the wound closed.

POST-OPERATIVE MANAGEMENT

The joint must be supported by a plaster-of-Paris splint until union is demonstrated, usually eight or ten weeks from the time of operation. The plaster should be well moulded round the thumb metacarpal, which should be held in a position of function, moderately opposed. It is advisable to include the proximal segment of the thumb in the plaster for the first four or six weeks.

Comment

This operation does not present any special difficulty. The main essentials are, firstly, to denude the arthritic surfaces thoroughly so that raw bone is exposed; and secondly, to make sure that the slot for the graft is of adequate proportions and that the graft is a jam fit in the slot.

A technique whereby the joint surfaces are fashioned into the form of a cone and matching socket and in which a graft is not used was described by Carroll and Hill (1973). Good results have been claimed but the operation has the disadvantage that special instruments are required.

ARTHRODESIS OF METACARPO-PHALANGEAL JOINT OF FINGER

When a metacarpo-phalangeal joint of a finger is to be fused it is best placed in a position of 30 degrees of flexion. This allows good appearance and function. The method of arthrodesis is to raw the joint surfaces and then to fix the joint internally while union occurs.

TECHNIQUE

Position of hand. The hand is placed palm downwards upon a rolled towel, which allows the fingers to assume a position of semi-flexion. A tourniquet may be used on the upper arm.

Incision. A longitudinal incision is made over the back of the joint just lateral to the extensor tendon, which is retracted.

Excision of joint surfaces. The joint capsule is opened and as much of it as is accessible is removed. The collateral ligaments are divided to permit subluxation of the joint surfaces. The diseased articular cartilage is shaved away down to healthy raw bone, both from the head of the metacarpal and from the base of the proximal phalanx. The raw surfaces must be so shaped that they fit accurately together in a position of 30 degrees of flexion. This is most easily achieved if the raw surface of the head of the metacarpal is made convex and the base of the phalanx concave, as in the healthy joint.

Internal fixation. Fixation by an oblique screw or by crossed Kirschner wires is recommended. The use of a Herbert screw (see p. 213) may often

be appropriate. A screw is often satisfactory for the relatively large joints of a man, but crossed wires may be more appropriate in the slender hand of a woman, and especially for the little finger.

Fixation by screw. For insertion of a screw the lateral aspect of the shaft of the proximal phalanx is exposed about a centimetre distal to the joint surface. A notch is cut with fine nibbling forceps

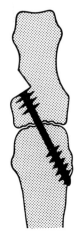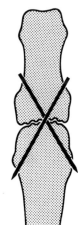

FIGS 295–296. Arthrodesis of metacarpo-phalangeal joint of a finger. Figure 295—Fixation by oblique screw after rawing of joint surfaces. It may be convenient to use a Herbert scaphoid screw, as shown here. Figure 296—An alternative method of fixation, by crossed oblique wires.

just distal to the condyle of the phalanx to allow access for the screw. The track for the screw may be prepared with an appropriate drill, or it may sometimes be simpler to use an awl or guide wire: it should be directed obliquely proximally and medially across the joint. When the initial track has been made through both bones the hole in the phalanx should be enlarged to allow a clearance fit for the screw, so that when the screw is tightened the bones are drawn together. A screw, usually about 3 centimetres long, is driven home along the prepared track, with care not to twist it too tightly lest the soft bone of the phalanx be split by the head of the screw. If a Herbert screw is to be used (Fig. 295) the track for the screw is prepared by the drills provided.

Fixation by crossed wires. Fixation by crossed Kirschner wires is effected rather more easily but it may not be quite so secure.

With the joint dislocated, a short Kirschner wire pointed at each end is driven distally and laterally from the centre of the rawed articular surface of the proximal phalanx, to emerge through the lateral cortex of the shaft: it is driven on until only a millimetre or so of the wire is left projecting at the articular surface. A second wire is then likewise inserted in the opposite diagonal. The rawed joint surfaces are then fitted together in the chosen position for fusion, and the Kirschner wires are shunted back across the joint into the head and neck of the metacarpal (Fig. 296). The wires are trimmed appropriately with wire cutters.

POST-OPERATIVE MANAGEMENT

For the first two weeks after operation the whole length of the finger is splinted with a well padded malleable metal splint laid over the dorsum of the metacarpal and finger, the splint being angulated at the level of each joint to provide fixation in semi-flexion. After two weeks the sutures are removed and a new dorsal splint is applied.

The proximal part of the definitive splint should be made from a dorsal slab of plaster-of-Paris extending from the upper forearm to the metacarpal heads. In this is embedded a malleable metal splint which extends distally over the affected finger as far as the proximal interphalangeal joint, the metal being angled appropriately over the metacarpo-phalangeal joint (Fig. 297).

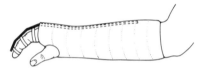

FIG. 297. Malleable aluminium splint incorporated in light forearm plaster, for immobilisation of metacarpo-phalangeal joint.

The plaster is maintained in position over the wrist with soft bandages, and the metal extension over the dorsum of the proximal segment of the finger is secured to the finger by bands of adhesive strapping, the volar surface of the finger being protected by a layer of felt.

Splintage should be maintained for six to eight weeks according to the progress of union as shown radiologically. During this time gentle active movements of the interphalangeal joints should be practised.

ARTHRODESIS OF DISTAL INTERPHALANGEAL JOINT OF FINGER

When the distal interphalangeal joint of a finger is to be fused a position of 20 degrees of flexion is usually best from the point of view both of function and of appearance. The method employed is to excise the articular surfaces and to approximate the rawed bone ends by a wire loop passed through drill holes, one in each fragment.

TECHNIQUE

Position of hand. The hand rests upon a side table with the dorsal surface uppermost. The fingers should lie semi-flexed, the palm of the hand being supported upon a rolled towel. A tourniquet may be used on the upper arm.

Incision. A broad-based U-shaped flap is outlined with its base proximally. The transverse cut should be 5 or 6 millimetres distal to the interphalangeal joint, and each vertical limb of the incision should be in the mid-lateral line of the finger, extending 5 millimetres proximal to the joint (Fig. 298). The skin flap is reflected proximally to expose the extensor expansion and the joint capsule.

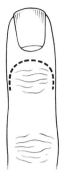

FIG. 298. Distal interphalangeal arthrodesis. The skin incision.

Excision of joint surfaces. The joint is opened from the dorsal aspect by dividing the extensor expansion, the joint capsule, and the collateral ligaments. The tip of the finger is flexed to open up the joint space, and with a fine chisel or with a dental burr the articular cartilage and the subchondral bone are removed from the head of the middle phalanx and from the base of the distal phalanx. The aim should be to leave flat surfaces of cancellous bone, and by excising a little more thickness of bone in front than behind the plane of the cut surfaces is so adjusted that when they are fitted together the joint lies in 20 degrees of flexion (Fig. 299).

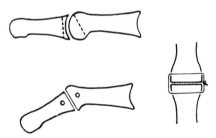

FIGS 299–301. Arthrodesis of distal interphalangeal joint of finger. Figure 299—Lines of bone section. Figure 300—The fragments drilled transversely. Figure 301—The wire loop inserted and drawn tight.

Internal fixation by wire suture. The method of fixation is to drill fine transverse holes from side to side in the head of the middle phalanx and in the base of the distal phalanx. In each case the hole should be about 4 millimetres from the freshly cut

surface (Fig. 300). The holes are best made with a drill 1 millimetre in diameter, operated either by hand or in a power-driven chuck. Through these parallel drill holes a loop of stainless steel wire (gauge 32) is passed and is tightened on the medial or lateral side to draw the two fragments together (Fig. 301). The cut edges of the wire are turned over and buried in the tissues to prevent them from forming a prominence under the skin. The skin flap is then drawn down and sutured back into position with fine interrupted sutures.

POST-OPERATIVE MANAGEMENT

It is well to splint the affected joint for about eight weeks, or until union is sound. In the first two weeks the whole finger may be supported on a malleable metal splint or in plaster, but once the wound is healed it is sufficient to use only a local splint supporting the middle and distal phalanges. The splint, carefully angulated to match the flexion of the interphalangeal joint, lies on the dorsum of the finger and is held in position by strips of adhesive strapping applied to the middle and distal segments of the finger. At an early stage exercises to restore metacarpo-phalangeal movement and proximal interphalangeal movement may be encouraged.

ALTERNATIVE TECHNIQUE

If a finger in which the distal interphalangeal joint is to be fused is small—for instance, the little finger in women—the method described above may be hardly practicable because of the small size of the phalanges. The alternative method here to be described may then be used. This entails dislocation of the joint to allow clearance of the remains of articular cartilage, and insertion of a stiff but slender wire along the medullary cavity of the distal phalanx and middle phalanx to give some rigidity while fusion is occurring. After the straight wire has been passed across the joint in the extended position the joint may be flexed to the desired position, the wire bending within the bones at the joint level.

TECHNIQUE

Position of patient. The patient lies supine with the hand resting upon the arm platform. The hand is best supported by a "lead hand" in such a way that the medial aspect of the finger to be operated upon faces the surgeon. A tourniquet may be used on the upper arm.

ior aspects of the bone. The soft tissues—extensor expansion behind and neurovascular bundle in front—are held away by slender retractors.

The medial aspect of the distal interphalangeal joint is thus presented to view, and the capsule and medial ligament are divided horizontally to open the joint. When this has been done the distal phalanx is easily angled away from the middle

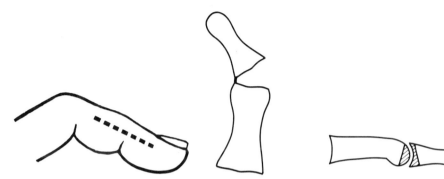

FIGS 302–304. Distal interphalangeal arthrodesis by intramedullary wire. Figure 302—The skin incision. Figure 303—Exposure of articular surfaces by angulation of joint after division of collateral ligament and capsule. Figure 304—Showing the amount of subchondral bone to be removed at the joint surfaces to ensure close contact of the opposing surfaces, with the joint slightly flexed.

Procedure. A longitudinal medial incision is made behind the position of the neurovascular bundle; that is, over the medial border of the distal

phalanx, opening up the joint and presenting the articular surfaces clearly to view (Fig. 303).

Remains of articular cartilage are removed by a

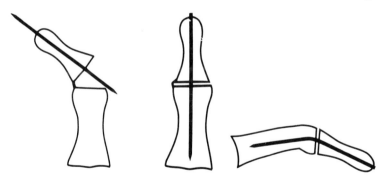

FIGS 305–307. Figure 305—Thin Kirschner wire passed from joint surface of distal phalanx to emerge through tip of finger. Figure 306—Joint surfaces apposed; wire driven proximally into middle phalanx and trimmed short at tip of finger. Figure 307—Joint forcibly flexed to desired position (usually 20 degrees of flexion), the wire being bent within the bones.

half of the middle phalanx and the proximal half of the distal phalanx (Fig. 302). While the wound edges are held apart by skin hooks dissection proceeds down to the medial surface of each phalanx and thence round to the anterior and poster-

slender bone-cutting forceps so that raw bone is exposed. The plane of the resulting raw surface should be so adjusted that the opposing sides come together cleanly when the finger is in the desired angle of flexion—usually about 20 degrees

(Fig. 304). A fine, stiff but malleable wire (0.45 millimetre diameter) is passed longitudinally down the medullary cavity of the distal phalanx from the rawed joint surface to emerge at the tip of the finger (Fig. 305), and it is pulled out until the proximal end of the wire protrudes only 2 or 3 millimetres from the raw articular surface. The opposing joint surfaces are then brought together so that the proximal part of the pin engages the medullary canal of the middle phalanx.

With the finger held straight the wire is then driven proximally throughout almost the whole length of the middle phalanx. (Penetration may be checked by holding another wire of the same length over the surface of the finger.) When the wire has been correctly inserted the excess protruding from the tip of the finger is cut off so that it lies immediately under the skin of the pulp (Fig. 306). Finally, the joint is forcibly flexed to the desired angle: this bends the wire within the bones and brings the prepared articular surfaces into close contact (Fig. 307). After removal of the tourniquet the wound is closed with fine sutures.

POST-OPERATIVE MANAGEMENT

It is wise to support the finger in a small plaster splint or alternatively by an aluminium strip splint moulded to the shape of the finger and held in place by adhesive strapping. Splintage should be changed after two weeks, when the stitches are removed. The affected joint—though not the proximal interphalangeal joint—should be supported for a total of six to eight weeks.

Removal of pin. The pin should be removed once bony fusion has occurred across the joint. The distal tip of the wire may be exposed by a horizontal incision across the pulp over the end of the phalanx. The tip of the wire is gripped by a fine needle-holder and pulled free. Although the angle created in the wire at the time of operation might be thought to impede removal of the wire, this is not the case because the wire is sufficiently flexible to find its way out if pulled firmly.

LOCAL EXCISION OF PALMAR APONEUROSIS FOR DUPUYTREN'S CONTRACTURE

Dupuytren's contracture presents in almost an infinite variety of ways, and no description can cover every case. This section will therefore be confined to a statement of principles, illustrated by the treatment of the common clinical manifestation of the disease in which a nodule beginning in the palm opposite the base of the ring finger has spread to involve the surrounding skin and has become continuous with one or two bands extending into the proximal segment of the ring finger, which is drawn into 20 or 30 degrees of flexion at the metacarpo-phalangeal joint.

PRINCIPLES OF OPERATION

The technique favoured by the authors is to excise the thickened part of the palmar aponeurosis together with any extensions into the finger, but to restrict the dissection to the abnormal tissue and not to attempt complete excision of the aponeurosis.

When the diseased tissue has been excised the main emphasis is laid on careful closure of the skin without the use of free grafts, as much flexion of the fingers being allowed as is needed to avoid tension on the suture lines until skin healing is fully consolidated, perhaps four weeks after the operation. Thereafter gradual stretching of the skin is carried out by exercises continued for two to three months or longer.

It is important to remember that in Dupuytren's contracture there is no actual loss of skin; nor is the skin abnormal except in so far as it is adherent to the underlying aponeurosis. Once the pathological tissue has been removed there is no reason why the skin should not stretch out again to normal length.

TECHNIQUE

Position of limb. The limb rests upon a side table, palm upwards. The fingers and thumb may be controlled by a "lead hand". A tourniquet should be used on the upper arm.

Incision. For the common palmar nodule extending into the base of the ring finger a serpentine incision is used. The palmar part of the incision is oblique. It begins near the ulnar border of the hand a little proximal to the proximal palmar

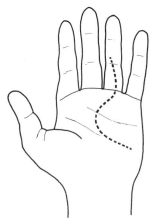

FIG. 308. Local excision of palmar aponeurosis. The skin incision.

skin crease, and extends distally and laterally to cross the proximal palmar skin crease at about its mid-point. In the mid-palm the incision turns in a wide sweep towards the base of the ring finger, where it becomes vertical and crosses into the finger mid-way between the medial and the lateral borders (Fig. 308).

An alternative incision is straight in the centre of the affected finger, lengthened in a straight line into the palm. This is less likely to damage a digital nerve, but a Z-plasty conversion of the linear incision is necessary for closure. This prevents shortening of the otherwise straight scar with time and gives greater flexibility to the skin.

Exposure and removal of thickened aponeurosis. The skin edges are reflected by gentle dissection in the plane between skin and palmar aponeurosis. Often the skin is closely adherent to the underlying thickened aponeurosis, and extreme care is needed to gain clean reflection of the skin without "button-holing" it.

When the aponeurosis has thus been displayed

the extent of the tissue that is to be removed can be assessed. So far as is possible all grossly thickened tissue should be removed, but if a wide area of the palm is affected the surgeon may have to compromise, curtailing the resection of diseased tissue in the interest of safeguarding the viability of the skin; for if the skin flaps are reflected too widely the nourishment of the skin is endangered and there may be a risk of necrosis of the edges. The aim should therefore be to excise enough tissue to release contractures and to remove prominent nodules, but to limit the area of the dissection to that permitted by strictly moderate reflection of the skin flaps.

In dissecting out thickened tissue from the palm it is often a good plan to divide the thick cord-like bands of whitish aponeurosis and to reflect them proximally and distally from the point of transection. Reflection of the distal mass may be continued right into the base of the finger.

In the dissection of the palmar aponeurosis it is of prime importance to avoid damage to the digital nerves, which run towards the interdigital clefts in close relationship with the aponeurosis. It is well to seek out the nerves and to free them from adjacent tissue before the excision of the aponeurosis is completed.

During the removal of the aponeurosis it will be found that deep extensions pass down between the flexor tendons towards the front of each metacarpal. Often these deep extensions, like the main part of the aponeurosis, are much thickened: they should be excised by sharp dissection close to the surface of the metacarpal.

In the finger a longitudinal cord-like band of diseased tissue may lie mainly on one or other side of the finger, or both sides may be affected. Dissecting the bands out demands much patience and care, for they are related very closely not only to the neurovascular bundles but also to the flexor tendon sheath.

At the conclusion of the dissection the deeper structures of the palm, namely the digital nerves, the vessels and the tendons, should be clearly displayed in the limited area of the wound, but there should be no remnant of thickened aponeurosis either in the exposed part of the palm or on the deep surface of the reflected skin.

Closure. It is important that the tourniquet be removed and all bleeding points secured before the skin is closed. It is well to spend time on securing thorough haemostasis, for a haematoma forming under the skin flaps may mar the result. In closure of the skin it is recommended that the fingers be flexed sufficiently to ensure that the edges can be sutured without the slightest tension. Everting mattress sutures of fine nylon are recommended. Drainage is not required.

POST-OPERATIVE MANAGEMENT

Before dressings are applied any residual blood that may have collected in the palm is squeezed out by firm pressure over a swab. Copious dressings of soft gauze are then applied over the palm and around the affected fingers, which are held semiflexed. More and more dressings are added until the palm and fingers are in the position used in gripping a cricket ball. The dressings are held in place by crepe bandages snugly applied, and more dressings are built up over the first turns of the bandage.

During the first few days after operation the hand is kept elevated. Finger flexion exercises within the limits imposed by the dressings are encouraged, but no attempt is made to force extension of the fingers.

On the second day the dressings should be removed to make sure that the suture line is healthy and that there has been no collection of blood beneath the skin flaps. A new dressing of similar dimensions is then applied and retained until the middle or end of the third week from operation. At that time the sutures are removed and dry dressings are continued as required.

Even at this stage no attempt should be made to force the fingers straight: wound healing is not sufficiently strong to allow any tension across the line of incision. Extension exercises are deferred until the fourth, fifth or sixth week from operation, depending upon the integrity or otherwise of the palmar skin. When this is judged to be soundly healed the patient is instructed in stretching exercises, which he may do under the supervision of the physiotherapist and also in his own home. Stretching should be gentle at first and the regaining of extension should never be hurried. The fullest recovery of extension range may not be gained in less than five or six months from the time of operation. In the later stages of rehabilitation the patient may massage the palmar skin with lanolin.

Comment

The method advocated here has the merits of simplicity and of safety. So long as the skin flaps are not reflected too far, primary skin healing can be looked for with virtual certainty. Once healing is sound—but not before—extension exercises and gentle stretching of the fingers lead to steady improvement over the months, and the final result is not inferior on the whole to that gained by more elaborate methods.

Only two further points need to be emphasised. These are, first, the need for extreme care lest a digital nerve be damaged; and second, the importance of securing full haemostasis so that all bleeding is controlled before the skin is closed. In this, more than in most operations, the outcome depends upon meticulous technique, not only in the operation itself, but also in the application of the dressings and bandages, a part of the operation that should in no circumstances be left to an unskilled assistant.

DECOMPRESSION OF SHEATH OF EXTENSOR POLLICIS BREVIS AND ABDUCTOR POLLICIS LONGUS

In de Quervain's syndrome the fibrous roof which converts the groove for the extensor pollicis brevis and abductor pollicis longus tendons on the radial styloid process into a tunnel is thickened, so that it forms a palpable and tender nodule. Simple longitudinal division of the fibrous roof may give relief of symptoms, but more certain cure follows excision of a narrow strip of the thickened fibrous sheath.

TECHNIQUE

Position of limb. The forearm and hand rest on a side table with the thumb uppermost. A tourniquet may be used on the upper arm.

Incision. Despite the general preference in the past for a transverse incision parallel to the dorsal skin crease of the wrist, a longitudinal incision

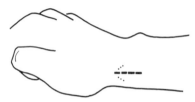

FIG. 309. Release of thickened tendon sheath in de Quervain's tenovaginitis. The skin incision. Dotted line indicates position of styloid process of radius.

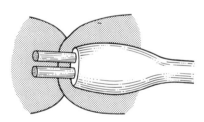

FIG. 310. The thickened part of the sheath over the radial styloid process, with the tendons of extensor pollicis brevis and abductor pollicis longus emerging.

gives easier access and obviates the risk of damage to the superficial branch of the radial nerve, which lies dorsal to the incision. The incision extends proximally from the tip of the styloid process of the radius for 2.5 centimetres (Fig. 309). It may lie directly over the affected tendon sheaths or, preferably, along the dorsal margin of the sheaths.

Exposure and division of sheath. With the skin edges retracted the thickened sheath is immediately obvious. It has a slightly glistening convex contour, and at its distal extremity the two tendons that traverse the common sheath, namely the extensor pollicis brevis and the abductor pollicis longus, are seen emerging from it. At this point the tendons are covered only by flimsy synovial tissue, which may be incised. The sheath is then traced proximally so that the full extent of its thickened roof is displayed (Fig. 310). Usually the area of thickening is about a centimetre long.

With a fine knife, two parallel longitudinal cuts are made through the thickened fibrous roof of the sheath, one at the volar and one at the dorsal margin. The cuts are separated by 2 or 3 millimetres. The intervening section of the sheath is removed. The tendons within the groove are inspected during their full excursion, produced by movements of the wrist and thumb.

Closure. The skin alone is sutured.

POST-OPERATIVE MANAGEMENT

A crepe bandage is applied over gauze dressings and retained for seven to ten days.

Comment

Like decompression of the carpal tunnel, this is a simple operation that gives almost uniformly good results. It is essential, however, to ensure that the sheath is decompressed throughout the whole extent of the thickened area. It should be noted that the sheath is sometimes a double one, with a compartment for each tendon: each should be deroofed. A full exposure is therefore required, and it is a mistake to attempt to divide the sheath semi-blindly through a small transverse incision.

DECOMPRESSION OF CARPAL TUNNEL

It is recommended that this simple operation, in which the flexor retinaculum is divided vertically, be done through a full incision under direct vision rather than semi-blindly through a short transverse incision.

TECHNIQUE

Position of hand. The patient lies supine. The forearm rests upon a side table, palm upwards. The fingers and thumb may be controlled by a "lead hand". A tourniquet may be used on the upper arm.

Incision. The incision begins at the junction of the proximal third and distal two-thirds of the thenar skin crease. It curves proximally in the line of the crease until the midline of the wrist is reached. Thence it extends vertically in a proximal direction almost up to, but not across, the

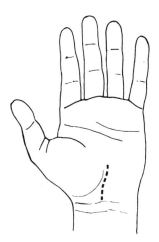

FIG. 311. Decompression of carpal tunnel. The skin incision.

transverse skin crease at the front of the wrist (Fig. 311). It is important that skin alone be cut in this initial incision, it being remembered that the median nerve lies superficially in the lower forearm and could be damaged by an injudicious incision, especially if the palmaris longus happened to be absent (Fig. 312).

Identification of median nerve and division of retinaculum. The skin edges are reflected laterally and medially, exposing aponeurotic fibres that represent the insertion of the palmaris longus into the flexor retinaculum, and more proximally the termination of the tendon of palmaris longus itself. By gentle dissection through the aponeurotic fibres in the proximal end of the wound the median nerve is now clearly identified. (It must be remembered that the palmaris longus may be absent, and that in such a case the median nerve is the most superficial structure in the wrist.)

A blunt, slightly curved director about 5 millimetres wide (a MacDonald's dissector serves well) is next passed gently down the carpal tunnel in front of the nerve. The flexor retinaculum is then

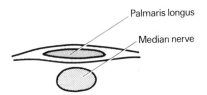

FIG. 312. Relationships of flexor retinaculum, tendon of palmaris longus, and median nerve.

carefully divided over the director with a fine knife as far as its lower limit, where the thick retinaculum gives place to thin palmar aponeurosis. In dividing the retinaculum the surgeon is wise to incline the division slightly towards the ulnar side of the midline of the hand, over the medial edge of the nerve, to ensure that the motor branch to the thenar muscles is not endangered.

Closure. After release of the tourniquet and ligature of any persistent bleeding points the skin alone is closed with interrupted sutures.

Comment

This is one of the simplest and most satisfactory operations in orthopaedic surgery. Nevertheless it demands great care, especially to avoid damaging the median nerve or its motor branch to the thenar muscles.

It should be appreciated that the nerve lies close under the skin at the front of the wrist. Only the palmaris longus and its distal aponeurotic extension lie between it and the surface, and if the palmaris longus happens to be absent the nerve is subcutaneous. In these circumstances it has sometimes been mistaken for the palmaris longus and divided—an unforgivable mistake because the nerve, with its fleshy consistency and surface blood vessels, bears no real resemblance to a tendon.

A relatively easy mistake, though one that is as easily avoided, is to damage the nerve by a too hasty and too deep initial skin incision: this accident also is more liable to occur when the palmaris longus is absent.

The small risk of damaging the motor branch to the thenar muscles is easily obviated by making the cut through the flexor retinaculum towards the ulnar side of the midline rather than directly over the nerve.

The method that is commonly used of dividing the retinaculum semi-blindly through a transverse incision close to the flexor crease of the wrist is not recommended. Mistakes will sometimes be made or the retinaculum incompletely divided if the section is not made under direct vision.

RELEASE OF CONSTRICTED FLEXOR POLLICIS LONGUS TENDON FOR TRIGGER THUMB

Trigger thumb occurs fairly frequently in infants and young children, and occasionally in adults. Operation for release of the constricted tendon by division of the thickened fibrous sheath is the same at all ages.

TECHNIQUE

The operation consists in exposure of the mouth of the fibrous flexor sheath and of the part of the flexor tendon immediately proximal to the mouth of the sheath, and excision of a strip from the thickened anterior wall of the sheath.

Position of patient. The patient lies supine with the affected arm resting upon a side table or upon the arm platform of the operation table. The forearm must be fully supinated in order to bring the volar aspect of the thumb uppermost. The hand is best held in this position by a "lead hand". A tourniquet may be used on the upper arm.

Incision. The incision is an almost transverse one on the volar surface of the base of the thumb: it lies parallel to and immediately proximal to the proximal flexor skin crease (Fig. 313). The incision in adults need be only a little more than a centimetre long, and in children correspondingly less. It is important to avoid transgressing the

antero-lateral and antero-medial margins of the digit lest the neurovascular bundle be damaged: if it is necessary to extend the incision it is better to convert it to an S-shaped one, the prolongations extending proximally from the lateral corner and distally from the medial corner in the long axis of the digit.

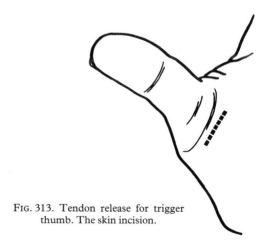

FIG. 313. Tendon release for trigger thumb. The skin incision.

Exposure and division of sheath. The skin edges being retracted proximally and distally by skin hooks, dissection is made in the subcutaneous fatty tissue in the midline of the digit by blunt-nosed curved scissors. In this way the mouth of the fibrous flexor sheath and the adjacent part of the flexor pollicis longus tendon as it enters the sheath are immediately encountered. These struc-

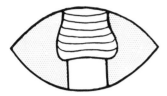

FIG. 314. The tendon is seen entering the mouth of the fibrous sheath, which is markedly thickened.

tures are cleared by further blunt dissection, and appropriate shallow blade or rake retractors are inserted to bring them fully into view (Fig. 314).

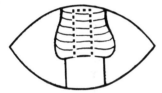

FIG. 315. The part of the anterior wall of the sheath that is to be excised is outlined.

All that now remains is to excise a strip from the anterior wall of the fibrous flexor sheath, which in these cases is considerably thickened (Fig. 315).

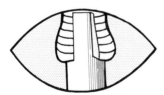

FIG. 316. The thickened section cut away, releasing the constriction of the sheath.

In adults the strip will usually be about a centimetre long (from the mouth of the sheath distally) and about 3 millimetres wide (Fig. 316). Incision of the sheath alone, without excision of a strip,

would perhaps be adequate, but it seems better to excise the thickened tissue.

When the flexor tendon has thus been decompressed, it may be observed that it is waisted in the part that was constricted beneath the mouth of the sheath, and it may seem a little swollen proximally. At this stage it is easy to confirm, by flexing and extending the thumb, that the tendon now glides freely in and out of the sheath, without any "catch".

Closure. Before closure the tourniquet should be released and any bleeding points secured. The skin incision is then closed, preferably with a subcuticular suture.

POST-OPERATIVE MANAGEMENT

The hand should be kept bandaged and dry for seven days, after which the suture is removed and full function resumed.

Comment

Sometimes in infants constricting tenovaginitis leads to fixed flexion of the thumb, which cannot be extended even with firm passive pressure. For this type of case the term trigger thumb is a misnomer, though in adults the term is apt because typical triggering or snapping is observed when the patient exerts firm active or passive force upon the thumb. Release of the thick, tight sheath is one of the more satisfying operations in orthopaedic surgery, for the cure is immediate and lasting.

The most important technical points in the operation are, firstly, to place the incision accurately so that it leads down directly to the mouth of the sheath; and secondly, to avoid extending the incision so far laterally or medially that the digital vessels and nerve are endangered: to this end the dissection in the subcutaneous plane should be confined strictly to the anterior midline of the digit, and should be carried out with fine dissecting scissors rather than with a knife.

RELEASE OF CONSTRICTED TENDON SHEATH FOR TRIGGER FINGER

Trigger finger (usually affecting the middle or ring finger) is in every way analogous to trigger thumb except that it is common in middle-aged women whereas trigger thumb occurs also in infants. Complete relief is gained by longitudinal incision of the sheath or, preferably, by excision of a narrow strip of the volar wall of the sheath at its mouth.

TECHNIQUE

The operation is carried out through a transverse incision at the base of the finger, about 5 millimetres distal to the distal palmar skin crease (Fig. 317). The incision need be little more than a centimetre long. Dissection through the subcutaneous tissue is best carried out with blunt-nosed scissors: the flexor tendons entering the fibrous sheath are encountered almost immediately. Care is needed in this dissection not to injure the digital nerves. Once the structures have been cleared of fatty tissue the thickening of the mouth of the sheath will be noted. The technique of excising a

small strip of sheath wall anteriorly is the same as described for trigger thumb (p. 232) (Fig. 315).

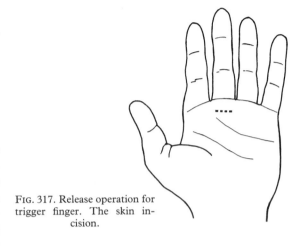

FIG. 317. Release operation for trigger finger. The skin incision.

POST-OPERATIVE MANAGEMENT

A light gauze dressing and crepe bandage are applied. The fingers may be used immediately, but the wound is best kept dry until the sutures are removed after seven to ten days.

RELEASE OF LOCKED INDEX FINGER

Locking of the index finger in about 30 degrees of flexion at the metacarpo-phalangeal joint is a clinical entity quite distinct from trigger finger from constriction of the tendon sheath. The locking is caused by a fold of the capsule of the metacarpo-phalangeal joint—particularly that part of it which is known as the accessory collateral ligament—becoming looped over the prominent volar aspect of the lateral condyle of the head of the second metacarpal. This may occur in quite young adults, especially women. In elderly patients the pathology is similar but the capsular loop may become impaled on an osteophyte in an arthritic joint rather than on the condyle as a whole.

Release is effected by incision of the accessory collateral ligament over the lateral condyle of the metacarpal head through a volar incision.

TECHNIQUE

Position of patient. The patient lies supine with the limb resting upon a side table. A tourniquet may be used on the upper arm. The hand should be supported on a "lead hand", with the palm facing upwards.

Incision. The incision is in or adjacent to the transverse palmar skin crease at the front of the metacarpo-phalangeal joint of the index finger. It is approximately 2.5 centimetres long (Fig. 318).

Procedure. The incision is deepened through the subcutaneous tissue and palmar aponeurosis, care being taken to avoid injuring the volar digital nerve which is clearly seen in a superficial plane running towards the lateral side of the index finger. The nerve is retracted laterally. Next the flexor tendons to the index finger are identified as

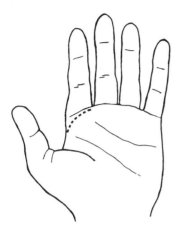

FIG. 318. Release of locked index finger. The skin incision.

they enter the mouth of the fibrous flexor sheath at the base of the finger. The incision is deepened lateral to the tendon sheath, the tendons being retracted slightly medially. On movement of the index finger it is now easy to identify the tough fibrous volar plate of the metacarpo-phalangeal joint.

At the lateral margin of the volar plate the anterior capsule of the joint is incised longitudinally with a fine knife blade and the edges of the capsular incision are retracted with fine hooks. The first glimpse will then be gained of the inferior part of the condyle of the metacarpal head and the base of the proximal phalanx: the anterior convexity of the lateral condyle is still enveloped by the thickened part of the capsule that is known as the accessory collateral ligament. The incision in the capsule is now extended proximally through this thickened condensation over the prominent anterior part of the lateral condyle, thus releasing the locking with a sudden snap.

After release of the locking the lateral condyle of the metacarpal head is inspected and any osteophyte or roughened area is smoothed off with a knife or fine chisel.

Closure. After release of the tourniquet any bleeding vessels are secured. Only the subcutaneous tissues and skin need to be sutured.

POST-OPERATIVE MANAGEMENT

A simple dry dressing is secured with a crepe bandage. It is retained until the seventh or eighth day, when the sutures are removed.

PRIMARY REPAIR OF FLEXOR TENDON IN DIGITAL SHEATH

Primary repair of a severed flexor tendon in the fibro-synovial digital sheath is a somewhat controversial subject, for whereas there are many advocates for it—in appropriate circumstances—there is nevertheless an opposing school that favours simple closure of the skin wound and secondary reconstruction at a later date. At present the advocates of primary repair seem to be in the ascendency.

Those who favour primary repair lay down strict prerequisites, of which the following would probably be an acceptable summary: 1) the wound must be clean-cut and without any contamination; 2) the phalanges and joints must be undamaged; 3) the injury must be not more than a week old in adults or two weeks in children; 4) the services of a

surgeon skilled in tendon repair work must be available, as must the requisite operation room facilities and equipment. Unless all these criteria can be satisfied primary repair should not be attempted, but the wound in the tendon sheath and the skin wound should simply be closed and the digit mobilised passively pending secondary reconstruction later.

TECHNIQUE

The operative technique is similar whether the injured tendon be in a finger or in the thumb. In the finger this description applies to repair either of the flexor digitorum profundus alone, or of the flexor digitorum profundus and flexor digitorum superficialis tendons divided together. Many would advise against attempted repair of a severed superficialis tendon if the accompanying profundus tendon were intact.

The principle of the technique is to deliver the tendon ends through the original wound in the fibro-synovial sheath and to approximate them with sutures of fine stainless-steel wire buried within the tendon tissue.

Position of patient. The patient lies supine with the affected hand resting upon a side table or arm platform. A tourniquet may be used on the upper arm, though it should be noted that some surgeons either omit the tourniquet altogether or remove it after the initial exploration, in the belief that the muscles are better relaxed and therefore the tendon ends more easily approximated in the absence of a tourniquet.

Delivering the tendon ends. The aim should be to deliver the proximal and distal ends of the divided tendon through the original wound in the fibro-synovial sheath. The skin incision may be enlarged if necessary, but the aim should be not to enlarge the incision in the tendon sheath.

As a general rule the proximal cut end of the tendon can be brought into view in the fibro-synovial incision by flexing the wrist acutely to relax the tendon, and if necessary "milking" it distally by pressure upon the palm and the base of the finger. If necessary the tendon may be exposed by a small incision in the palm, which may enable it more easily to be pushed distally. Once the tendon end is located at the site of injury, it is brought out through the wound, with care not to damage the tendon fibres: it is prevented from retracting by transfixing the fibro-synovial sheath and the contained tendon from side to side with a hypodermic needle.

The distal cut end of the divided tendon may usually be brought into view and extracted from the opening by flexing the finger.

The tendon suture. The tendon ends are laid in apposition and, if the cut surface of each fragment is not clean-cut, a tiny slice of tendon may be removed with a fresh knife blade in order to create a clean surface. The suture is carried out with 3.0 (000) braided stainless-steel wire. In order to gain a secure grip on the tendon ends the sutures should extend 8 to 10 millimetres away from the freshened surface of each stump. Two sutures are used, one for each stump. Each suture is inserted in the manner shown in Figure 319. The needle enters at one cut surface and is first directed longitudinally in the tendon substance. Emerging

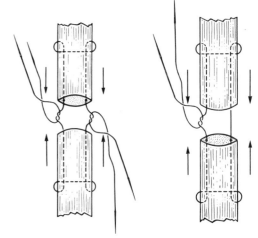

Figs 319–320. Two methods of end-to-end suture of a tendon.

at the surface 8 to 10 millimetres from the site of the tendon junction, it is then looped round to transfix the tendon transversely, as shown. With a further loop, the needle then enters the opposite lateral surface and is directed longitudinally to emerge again at the cut surface. A second identical suture is inserted in the same manner in the opposing tendon stump. As the sutures are carefully drawn together before tying, the tendon stumps are bunched together to bring the cut surfaces into close contact. The wires are then tied and the knots are concealed between the tendon ends. An alternative method of directing a single suture is shown in Figure 320.

Closure of fibro-synovial sheath. It is important that the opening in the synovial sheath be closed meticulously so that the sheath is once again a closed space within which synovial fluid is retained. This repair may be carried out with fine (5.0) sutures of nylon. The skin is likewise closed with fine non-absorbable sutures.

POST-OPERATIVE MANAGEMENT

It is recommended that the injured tendon be relaxed by immobilising the forearm and hand with the wrist in semi-flexion. In the case of a profundus tendon tension on the proximal end may be further reduced by splinting the remaining (uninjured) fingers in the straight position; since the four profundus tendons are conjoined proximally the injured tendon is thus prevented from retracting. The position is maintained by a dorsal plaster splint in which may be incorporated malleable metal splints for each individual uninjured finger. The injured finger is allowed to rest in a position of semi-flexion at the metacarpo-phalangeal and proximal interphalangeal joints.

In the early days the hand is kept elevated to reduce the risk of oedema. Splintage is discarded after three weeks, when the skin sutures are removed. Thereafter mobilising exercises are commenced.

Comment

This operation is very demanding of technical skill and should not be attempted by the occasional operator in this field. Three important principles need to be emphasised (Richards 1977). These are, firstly, that the blood supply of the tendon ends, which enters through the vincula (mesotenon), must not be jeopardised—for instance, by attempting to locate the retracted proximal end by widely incising the sheath in the palm and pulling the tendon out through the palmar wound; secondly, that the tendon tissue must not be traumatised by rough handling so that its smooth outer surface is breached and thus made liable to become adherent to the sheath; and thirdly, that the stainless-steel suture within the tendon must not strangle the tendon tissue, endangering its blood supply.

Provided the operation is carried out only when the prerequisites mentioned at the beginning of this section are met, acceptable results are to be expected in a good proportion of patients, and particularly in the young. Nevertheless, over-optimism must be cautioned against, for whereas the range of movement restored may be as high as 75 or 80 per cent of the normal range at the proximal interphalangeal joint, the range regained at the distal joint is usually less than 50 per cent of the normal, which in round figures is taken as 90 degrees both at the proximal and the distal interphalangeal joints (Richards 1977).

TENDON GRAFTING FOR SEVERED FLEXOR TENDONS IN THE DIGITAL SHEATH

When primary repair of a severed flexor profundus and flexor superficialis tendon in the digital sheath is not carried out, or fails, reconstruction is best effected by a free tendon graft provided that 1) the skin is fully healed; 2) scarring and adhesions are slight; 3) the metacarpo-phalangeal joints and interphalangeal joints are fully mobile; 4) sensibility is intact at the pulp of the finger; 5) circulation in the finger is normal; and 6) adequate surgical facilities are available.

If scarring and adhesions in and about the flexor sheath are excessive, success from free tendon grafting is unlikely and consideration should be given to the advisability of two-stage tendon reconstruction (see p. 241).

Free tendon grafting is usually undertaken only when both the profundus and superficialis tendons are divided. It entails excision of the superficialis tendon, excision of the digital sheath except at the points where fibrous pulleys should be preserved, and replacement of the profundus tendon from the point of its insertion into the distal phalanx to the upper part of the palm of the hand adjacent to the lumbrical muscle, by a free graft. The graft is obtained from the palmaris longus, from the plantaris tendon, or from one of the long toe extensors (first and fifth excluded). In certain circumstances (for instance, when there is extensive scarring in the palm) the graft may be taken up into the lower forearm, where the junction is made proximal to the volar carpal retinaculum.

TECHNIQUE

Position of patient. The patient lies supine, with the hand resting upon a side table. The remaining fingers should be held out of the way by a "lead hand", leaving the affected finger free. A tourniquet may be used on the upper arm.

Incision. For the index finger the incision is made along the mid-lateral line of the finger on the radial side, extending proximally from the level of the root of the nail to the base of the finger, where it should be prolonged in the line of the thenar crease to reach to the proximal part of the palm. A similar incision on the medial side should be made for the little finger. For the middle and ring fingers, the mid-lateral digital incision terminates at the web, and a further serpentine incision is made in the palm following loosely the distal palmar crease and more proximally the thenar crease (Fig. 321).

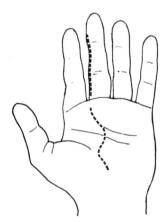

FIG. 321. Reconstruction of flexor tendon in finger. The skin incision.

Exposure of digital sheath, neurovascular bundle and palmar structures. The mid-axial incision in the finger is deepened towards the antero-lateral border of the proximal and middle phalanges so that the anterior structures, including the digital artery and nerve, are displaced forwards. By gently extending the dissection forwards from the phalanges, the digital sheath is encountered. The superficial surface of the sheath is thoroughly cleared by painstaking dissection, which may be tedious if adhesions are present. The sheath must

be exposed throughout its whole extent, across to the opposite side of the finger. During this dissection the site of severance of the tendons will be recognised.

It is important at this stage to identify the digital vessels and nerve at the base of the finger and to avoid damaging them. The palmar part of the incision is then developed, with care to avoid injury to the superficial structures (nerves, vessels), so that the superficial and deep flexor tendons are revealed and identified.

Selective excision of digital sheath. The next objective is to excise the whole of the digital sheath, except for short lengths of sheath about 6 millimetres long which should be preserved at the following points to serve as pulleys to prevent bowstringing of the tendon: 1) opposite the metacarpo-phalangeal joint; 2) at the mid-point of the proximal phalanx; 3) at the mid-point of the middle phalanx. Excised portions of the sheath are discarded. (If previous damage to the sheath precludes the formation of good pulleys, it is necessary to construct new pulleys, preferably by looping lengths of superficialis tendon round each phalanx or by Z-plasty (see below).)

Excision of tendons. The flexor superficialis tendon is removed and not replaced. It is first detached from its insertion into the base of the middle phalanx by division of the two separate slips by which the tendon gains attachment to the bone, one on either side of the profundus tendon. One of the slips should be cut as close as possible to its bony attachment, whereas the other slip should be divided about a centimetre proximal to its insertion. This short piece of tendon, attached distally to the bone, is subsequently to be laid across the interphalangeal joint deep to the tendon sheath and secured by fine sutures to the periosseous tissues, to act as a check ligament to prevent hyperextension of the joint, which is prone otherwise to occur. The superficialis tendon is next identified in the palmar part of the incision and divided cleanly in the upper part of the palm. The part of the tendon thus freed is pulled out and discarded.

Attention is next directed to the profundus tendon, which is to be removed and replaced by the tendon graft. Distally it is detached from its bony insertion at the base of the distal phalanx, and proximally it is divided opposite the mid-part of the lumbrical muscle in the upper part of the palm. The part of the tendon thus freed is pulled out and discarded.

Taking the tendon graft. According to circumstances and to the personal choice of the surgeon, the graft may be obtained from the palmaris longus, from the plantaris or from the long extensor to the second, third or fourth toe. In certain circumstances the superficialis tendon is used as a graft.

Taking the palmaris longus tendon. It is essential that this tendon be shown to be present before any exposure is made for its removal: if present the tendon stands out sharply if the wrist is actively flexed while the thumb and little finger are opposed. If the tendon is absent, it is clearly necessary to use an alternative donor site.

To harvest the tendon, when present, a short transverse incision is made immediately proximal to the proximal flexor crease of the wrist. The tendon is identified (note the importance of distinguishing it from the median nerve, which should be identified deep to the tendon) and it is lifted forwards by means of a bone lever inserted deep to it. By thus lifting it forwards and stretching the tendon its course in the forearm is clearly revealed, and a second incision may then be made over the tendon at the junction of the upper and middle thirds of the forearm. A bone lever or haemostat is passed behind the tendon through this proximal incision, and after positive identification of the tendon it is pulled out through the proximal incision and divided. It is stored temporarily in a moistened strip of gauze in a dish kept aside for the purpose.

Taking the plantaris tendon. The lower leg having been prepared (a tourniquet is not required) a longitudinal incision 3 centimetres long is made just medial to the medial border of the calcaneal tendon at a level slightly above the medial malleolus. The edges of the incision being

retracted, the medial border of the gastrocnemius where it blends with the calcaneal tendon is everted to reveal the plantaris tendon lying against the deep surface of the gastrocnemius. After division of its distal end it may be freed by a tendon stripper inserted through the lower incision and directed proximally round the tendon to the midpart of the calf, where a second short incision is made to identify the tendon and to divide it just distal to the point where the muscle belly gives rise to tendon. The tendon is protected in a moistened strip of gauze as already described.

Taking a long toe extensor tendon. The tendon for the big toe must not be disturbed: it is in any case too large. The tendon for the little toe should not be taken for fear of consequent flexion deformity due to lack of a short extensor. The tendon to the second, third or fourth toe should therefore be taken. It is perhaps best to make a full-length incision over the course of the tendon, extending proximally above the extensor retinaculum at the ankle: alternatively three short incisions may be made, leaving bridges of intact skin. The tendon is divided distally over the head of the metatarsal. It is dissected out as far as the extensor retinaculum and is then identified above the retinaculum where it is divided. The tendon may then be pulled free.

Insertion of tendon graft. Depending upon the size of the tendon to be used as a graft, the digital pulleys that have been preserved or reconstructed should be examined to make sure that they will allow free passage of the tendon. If not, the pulleys must be dilated or surgically widened.

The tendon is freed from superfluous soft tissue superficially but its surface must not be damaged or scratched. It is then laid in position after being passed through the pulleys.

Attachment of tendon to host at proximal and distal ends. At the proximal end, the junction is made at the level of the lumbrical muscle, so that part of the muscle may subsequently be used to cover the juncture. The proximal suture is made by the interlacing technique described in Chapter 2 (p. 98), the graft being threaded through two slits in the profundus tendon made at right angles to one another (Fig. 135). Fine stainless steel wire should be used for the tendon suture. If possible, part of the lumbrical muscle is then brought over as a curtain and sutured round the tendon junction with fine absorbable sutures.

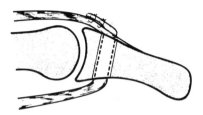

FIG. 322. A technique of attaching the tendon graft to the distal phalanx.

At the distal end a hole fractionally larger in diameter than the tendon graft is drilled antero-posteriorly through the base of the distal phalanx, well clear of the joint, to emerge on the dorsum of the finger proximal to the nail bed, where a short flap incision of the skin is made to allow its passage. The free end of the tendon graft is gripped by a mattress suture inserted by twin needles emerging from the cut surface. The needles are passed through the drill hole and through the extensor tendon to emerge at the dorsum of the finger (Fig. 322). By means of this suture the tendon graft is pulled through the hole in the phalanx in preparation for its suture to the extensor tendon near its insertion. The suture must not be made, however, until the tension on the tendon has been adjusted correctly.

Adjustment of tension. The tendon end brought through the phalanx may be locked temporarily by transfixing it with a straight skin needle just behind the point where it emerges at the dorsum of the phalanx. (The sharp point of the needle should be protected by a cork or otherwise, to protect against accidental needle stick injury.) Tension on the tendon is correct when the affected finger lies in correct relationship to the other fingers when at rest. In this normal resting position the little finger is flexed somewhat more than the index finger and the two intervening fingers are in intermediate positions of flexion. If the grafted finger does not rest in this correct position tension on the tendon graft is so adjusted that the correct posture is assumed. When this has been achieved, the tendon is anchored by three or four fine wire sutures at the point of its emergence from the dorsum of the distal phalanx.

Closure. Because of the importance of avoiding the risk of haematoma, it is essential to remove the tourniquet before closing the tissues. This allows all oozing vessels to be sealed and the field rendered perfectly dry before closure. Suture of the skin alone is required, but this should be meticulous.

POST-OPERATIVE MANAGEMENT

First the fingers of the hand are enclosed in rather voluminous gauze dressings held with a crepe bandage. Then a dorsal splint constructed from plaster-of-Paris should be applied over protective cellulose padding: the splint extends over the back of the forearm and hand and is moulded like a shell over the backs of the fingers, with the metacarpo-phalangeal and interphalangeal joints flexed about 30 degrees. The plaster splint is held on by further turns of the crepe bandage. The anterior aspects of the fingers are left uncovered by plaster so that a small range of flexion movement is allowed for.

The plaster splint is retained for three weeks. Thereafter, the sutures are removed and a new but lighter splint made from plaster or from plastic splinting material is applied as a protection, but at this stage active finger movements are encouraged within the range permitted by the splint. After a further two weeks the splint may be discarded. Carefully supervised exercises are then continued. It must be appreciated that at this early stage the tendon junctions are not fully consolidated, and flexion should not be attempted against resistance.

Comment

Tendon surgery in this difficult area of the hand is unpredictable in its outcome, depending upon a number of factors, not all of which are within the control of the surgeon. The most important requirement is a delicate surgical technique, with care not to damage the tissues by rough or unnecessary handling or by allowing the surface to become dry. The proximal and distal tendon junctions must be made with meticulous care: all raw and cut surfaces of tendon must so far as possible be oversewn and buried within the tendon substance. The degree of tension must be correct. Pulleys along the digital sheath must be adequate to prevent bow-stringing of the tendon on flexion.

Many variations of technique are practised, particularly in the manner of making the tendon junctions and also in the position of the proximal suture: some surgeons prefer to make the junction routinely above the wrist level in the lower forearm. There is good authority, however, for making the junction in the palm, so long as the tissues there are undamaged and free from adhesions (Pulvertaft 1961, 1965).

As to the choice of graft material, it is perhaps right to recommend that palmaris longus be used whenever it is present in sufficient length, and that only when this is not the case should resort be had to the use of a plantaris tendon or of one of the toe extensor tendons.

Tendon reconstruction operations in the digital sheath are sometimes impaired because of scarring

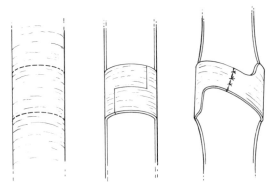

FIG. 323. Z-plasty reconstruction of narrowed flexor tendon sheath, to create a wider pulley to retain the tendon and thus to prevent bow-stringing.

and the narrowness of the sheath. It is possible to resect part of the sheath, but substantial pulley areas of the tendon sheath must remain to prevent bowstringing of the flexor tendons in action. If the pulleys are constricted they may be enlarged by serial Hegar's dilators or if necessary by Z-plasty reconstruction (Fig. 323).

TWO-STAGE RECONSTRUCTION OF FLEXOR DIGITORUM PROFUNDUS TENDON

Two-stage reconstruction of a flexor tendon divided within the digital sheath may be regarded as a last-resort operation used when simpler methods have failed. In many such cases, primary repair having been avoided or having proved unsuccessful, free tendon grafting will have been carried out unsuccessfully. Failure will often be ascribed to the formation of dense adhesions, binding the tendon in the sheath. It is in such cases as these that two-stage reconstruction may be advised, though always with a cautious prognosis.

The method to be described comprises two separate operations, with an interval between them of about eight weeks (Figs 324–327). In the first stage the damaged tendons are removed from the digital sheath, and a flexible silicone-rubber ("Silastic") rod is laid in the finger and palm to promote the formation of a new synovial sheath. Once a new sheath has been formed, the profundus tendon may be reconstructed by a free tendon graft in the manner described in the previous section. In the alternative technique to be described here, the superficialis tendon is used to replace the distal part of the profundus in the following way. At the first-stage operation, after severence of the profundus and superficialis tendons in the palm, the two proximal ends are sutured together to form a loop (Figs 328 and 329). At the second-stage operation the silicone-rubber rod is removed and the proximal part of the superficialis tendon is freed in the lower part of the forearm, turned down, and threaded through the newly formed digital sheath and secured to the distal phalanx.

The prerequisites for undertaking the operation are the same as for free tendon grafting (p. 237).

First-stage Operation

This stage comprises 1) excision of the distal parts of the flexor digitorum profundus and flexor digitorum superficialis tendons; 2) insertion of a silicone-rubber rod; and 3) suture of the stumps of the profundus and superficialis tendons in the palm to form a loop.

digital sheath throughout its length. Usually it is most convenient to identify and define the sheath at a point away from the main mass of adhesions, where the sheath and the contained tendons are healthy, and from there to work towards the scarred area. In general, the dissection proceeds in the manner described in the previous section, the objective being to expose the whole length and breadth of the sheath, from margin to margin.

When the sheath and the tendons have thus been identified in the finger attention is directed to the palm of the hand. Here it is necessary first to

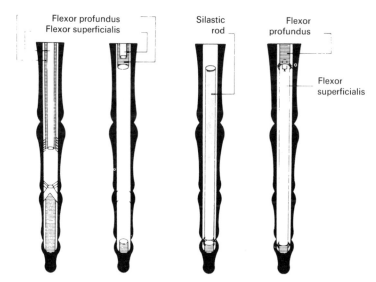

FIGS 324–327. Two-stage reconstruction of flexor tendon: the broad strategy. Figure 324—Initial state: tendons severed and adherent to sheath. Figure 325—Tendons excised. Figure 326—Silastic rod in position to promote formation of new sheath. Figure 327—Rod replaced by superficialis tendon, brought down as a graft, or by a free graft.

TECHNIQUE

Position of limb. The patient being supine, the forearm and hand rest upon a side table as described in the previous section. A tourniquet may be used on the upper arm.

Incision. The details of the incision depend upon which finger is affected, as described in the previous section.

Exposure of flexor sheath and excision of tendons. If adhesions are dense, painstaking dissection may be required in order to define and clear the fibrous

find and preserve the digital nerves and vessels as they pass from the palm to the finger. The deep and superficial flexor tendons are then traced proximally as far as the middle of the palm, where the fleshy lumbrical muscle arises from the profundus tendon. The damaged tendons are now removed in their entirety throughout the whole length of their course from the site of their insertion into the distal and middle phalanges, as far proximally as the site of origin of the lumbrical muscle in the mid-palm (Fig. 325). Where the tendons are free within the sheath their removal does not present any difficulty. Where they are adherent to the sheath they must be excised by sharp dissection. Scarred and adherent sections of the sheath must also be excised, but whenever possible an anterior bridge of healthy sheath about 7 or 8 millimetres wide should be preserved in each finger segment to help to retain the new tendon and to prevent bow-stringing.

Suturing together the divided ends of flexor profundus and flexor superficialis tendons. To facilitate the subsequent use of the superficialis tendon as a graft within the finger the cut proximal ends of the two tendons are joined by end-to-end suture after they have been freed sufficiently to allow them to be fashioned into a loop (Fig. 328). If possible this junction should be made at a point where the suture line can be covered by lumbrical muscle.

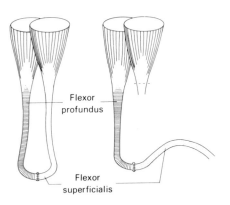

Flexor profundus

Flexor superficialis

FIGS 328–329. Method of uniting profundus and superficialis tendons in a loop, and later (Fig. 329) freeing the proximal end of the superficialis.

Insertion of silicone-rubber rod. The flexible silicone rubber (Silastic) rod, usually 4 millimetres in diameter or of comparable size in oval section, is to be placed in the remnants of the flexor tendon sheath, part of which may have had to be removed in the process of dissecting out the adherent tendons. To ensure that the remnants of the sheath will accommodate the flexible rod its track is tested for size by passing a suitable Hegar's dilator along it. Any constricted section of the sheath that holds up the dilator may be incised. When the track has been thus shown to be wide enough the selected rod is introduced along the track

(Fig. 326). It should be of such a length that it will extend from the base of the distal phalanx as far proximally as the point in the mid-palm where the union between the flexor superficialis and flexor profundus tendons has been made. The distal end of the rod should be bevelled off with a sharp knife lest the rather sharp angle formed by a clean cross section of the rod should ulcerate through the overlying skin. It is well to anchor the rod distally by one suture through soft tissue at the point of insertion of the original profundus tendon: this prevents the rod from migrating proximally. At the proximal end the cut end of the rod may be buried close to the lumbrical muscle but it should not be fixed by sutures.

Closure. No attempt need be made to close the fibrous flexor sheath where it has been incised longitudinally. It is sufficient to close the skin edges by careful suture, preferably by fine everting mattress sutures.

POST-OPERATIVE MANAGEMENT

Soft dressings only are applied: there is no need for splintage of the finger. For the first few days after operation elevation of the hand is required to control swelling. When the wound is well healed, about two weeks after the operation, passive movements of the finger joints are intensified under the supervision of a physiotherapist. It is very important that the joints be kept supple during the interval before the second-stage operation.

SECOND-STAGE OPERATION

The operation comprises: 1) removal of the silicone-rubber rod; 2) division of the flexor digitorum superficialis tendon in the forearm; and 3) redirection of the tendon through the digital sheath and attachment to the distal phalanx. The technique is applicable only if the tendons in the palm are free from major adhesions and scarring. If this is not the case, free tendon grafting should be carried out instead (see previous section, p. 237).

The second-stage operation is undertaken about eight weeks after the first stage. By this time it may be expected that the silicone-rubber rod will have promoted the formation of a new, smoothly lined sheath, and that the proximal stumps of the profundus and superficialis tendons, sutured to form a loop, will have united.

TECHNIQUE

Position of forearm. The forearm rests upon a side table as in the first-stage operation.

Incision. A limited exposure is needed at three sites: in the mid-palm to expose the joined proximal ends of the profundus and superficialis tendons; in the lower forearm to free the superficialis tendon proximally at the musculo-tendinous junction; and at the distal segment of the finger where the new tendon is to be attached to the distal phalanx. The incisions in the mid-palm and at the distal segment of the finger may coincide with those previously made in the first-stage operation: the lower forearm incision is a vertical or serpentine one extending proximally from the flexor crease of the wrist for 7 or 8 centimetres in the midline of the forearm.

Mobilisation of superficialis tendon. Through the incision in the palm the proximal stumps of the profundus and superficialis tendons, previously united to form a loop, are identified and freed from any adhesions that may have formed. Union of the two tendons where they have been sutured end to end should by this time be well advanced. Nevertheless the junction should not be submitted to unnecessary stress. If the tendons forming the loop are not healthy and free from adhesions the projected use of the flexor superficialis tendon may be abandoned and the reconstruction carried out by a free tendon graft (p. 237).

The proximal end of the silicone-rubber rod should be identified in the palmar wound, but it is left undisturbed for the moment.

Attention is next turned to the proximal incision at the front of the lower forearm. Through this opening the superficialis tendon to the finger concerned is identified by demonstrating its continuity with the loop of tendon exposed in the palm. The tendon is traced proximally until sufficient length is available to allow the tendon to reach the distal end of the finger when the loop in the palm has been unfolded. To gain adequate length the superficialis tendon must be freed up to a point at least 5 or 6 centimetres proximal to the wrist—that is, close up to the musculo-tendinous junction. At this point the tendon is divided. The tendon is then drawn down into the palm and the loop of conjoined profundus and superficialis tendons is straightened out. The superficialis tendon forms a graft continuous with the profundus tendon (Fig. 329). It remains to draw this graft through the newly formed synovial sheath and to anchor it to the base of the distal phalanx.

Removal of silicone-rubber rod and passage of tendon graft into sheath. The proximal and distal ends of the silicone-rubber rod are identified through the palmar and digital incisions. The distal anchoring suture is removed. The distal end of the tendon graft is united by a stitch to the proximal end of the rod so that as the rod is removed through the distal incision the tendon will be drawn with it into the synovial sheath to emerge at the distal end (Fig. 327).

Anchorage of distal end of tendon. It may sometimes be possible to suture the distal end of the tendon to the terminal stump of the original profundus tendon where it is attached to the base of the distal phalanx. The junction may, however, be insecure, and the authors prefer to pass the tendon through a drill hole in the base of the phalanx and to secure it with one or two sutures to the insertion of the extensor tendon at the dorsum of the finger, as described on page 239 (Fig. 322).

Closure. Before the skin is closed attention is turned to the palmar incision, where it is necessary to ensure that the junction between profundus and superficialis tendons is gliding freely and is not tethered by adhesions. Whenever possible the junction should be enveloped in a covering of lumbrical muscle. Then, after removal of the tourniquet and attention to any bleeding points, the skin wounds are closed by eversion sutures.

POST-OPERATIVE MANAGEMENT

The aim after this type of tendon reconstruction is to begin active finger movements early. In the immediate post-operative period copious gauze dressings are applied to the palm and front of the fingers and held with crepe bandages so that the fingers are in a semi-flexed grasping position. This initial dressing is retained for twelve to fourteen days. During this time finger flexion and extension exercises are encouraged within the range permitted by the bandage. When the dressings and sutures have been removed and when all the incisions are well healed, active exercises are intensified with the aim of restoring a good range of finger flexion and extension as early as possible.

Early movement after operation can be assisted by using a continuous passive motion machine. The positioning of the machine to obtain the correct arc of finger movement needs careful assessment. A machine with a variable length of travel is particularly useful in achieving this.

Comment

It must be emphasised that reconstructive tendon surgery is a highly concentrated art. Even surgeons who devote the whole of their working time to hand surgery are seriously exercised in deciding how best to tackle the more difficult problems. And even at the best level, the results are unpredictable. Such reconstructive operations, therefore, though technically well within the range of many competent orthopaedic surgeons, should never be decided upon lightly, but only after discussion with an expert in the field, or even a panel of experts.

The operation described above is included in order to illustrate, with that described in the previous section, that there is a variety of ways in which a tendon may be reconstructed, with many variations also in the details of technique. This two-stage operation, in which a new synovial lining of the sheath is promoted by the presence within it of a silicone-rubber rod, seems likely to reduce the risk of adhesions. The method relies on the assumption that the part of the tendon graft that lies within the sheath is able to gain nourishment from synovial fluid in the same way as does articular cartilage. Vascular adhesions are therefore less likely to form than they are after one-stage free tendon grafting into a freshly opened sheath.

The operation demands a high degree of technical skill. An essential point is to handle the tissues delicately, with avoidance of all unnecessary trauma. In the first stage of the operation care must be taken to ensure that the silicone-rubber rod extends distally as far as the site of insertion of the profundus tendon to the distal phalanx. It is also important that the distal end should be rounded off lest it tend to ulcerate through the skin. Proximally, the flexible rod should extend well up into the palm in order to provide a lubricated channel for almost the whole length of the tendon graft.

In the second-stage operation, which should not be undertaken sooner than eight weeks after the first stage, the important points are, firstly, to straighten out the loop formed by the junction of the profundus and superficialis tendons and to tidy up the region of the junction to ensure that it is free from adhesions and preferably clothed in a sheet of lumbrical muscle. If the tendon loop is found to be excessively matted in adhesions the superficialis tendon may still be discarded and a free graft from the palmaris longus or plantaris used instead.

Secondly, it is important to ensure that the tendon graft is attached distally with the correct degree of tension. This should be such that when the tendon has been secured to its insertion at the base of the distal phalanx the finger rests in moderate flexion, comparable to that of the adjacent fingers. Clearly, if the tendon is too slack the range of flexion is likely to be impaired, whereas if it is too tight extension will be incomplete. Thirdly, fixation of the tendon to the base of the distal phalanx should be secure enough to allow immediate active finger movements. Passing the tendon through a drill hole in the phalanx as described, and anchoring it dorsally, gives better security than suturing it to the stump of the original tendon insertion.

TENDON TRANSFER: EXTENSOR INDICIS TO EXTENSOR POLLICIS LONGUS

This tendon transfer is useful when a ruptured extensor pollicis longus tendon is frayed over a considerable distance in its groove at the back of the lower end of the radius and when in consequence direct suture is hardly practicable.

TECHNIQUE

Position of limb. The forearm rests upon a side table in semi-pronation. A tourniquet may be used on the upper arm.

Incisions. Two incisions are used. The first is a transverse one, 1.5 centimetres long, over the extensor tendons overlying the neck of the second metacarpal (Fig. 330). Its purpose is to allow the extensor indicis tendon to be divided.

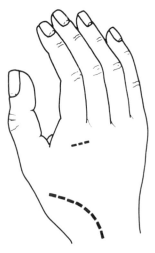

FIG. 330. Transfer of extensor indicis tendon to extensor pollicis longus. The skin incisions.

The second incision is a curved one about 6 centimetres long. It begins proximally, 2 centimetres above the dorsal crease of the wrist, just medial to the dorsal bony tuberosity of the lower end of the radius. The proximal part of the incision lies parallel to the extensor tendons of the

index finger, on their radial side. It then curves radially to cross the extensor pollicis longus tendon a centimetre distal to the base of the first metacarpal (Fig. 330).

Identification and division of extensor indicis tendon. Through the first incision over the neck of the second metacarpal the two extensor tendons of the index finger are defined. They lie side by side, the extensor indicis tendon on the ulnar side of the extensor communis tendon. When the extensor indicis tendon has been isolated it is divided about 2 centimetres proximal to the metacarpo-phalangeal joint. The proximal end of the tendon is then mobilised as far proximally as is possible through this incision.

Proximal delivery of extensor indicis tendon. After division of the fascia in the upper part of the proximal incision the tendon of extensor indicis is identified by demonstrating its continuity with the proximal stump of the tendon just divided. The tendon is then freed by blunt dissection to allow it to be pulled up and delivered through the proximal wound. Any loose attachments to areolar tissue on the ulnar side are divided up to the level of the lower end of the radius, in order to allow the tendon to be re-routed towards the base of the thumb (Fig. 331).

Preparation of extensor pollicis longus tendon to receive transfer. The lateral edge of the proximal wound is retracted to expose the tendon of extensor pollicis longus where it forms the posterior border of the anatomical snuff box. From there the tendon is traced proximally as far as the site of rupture over the lower end of the radius.

A suitable site for effecting the junction between the transferred indicis tendon and the tendon of extensor pollicis longus is chosen: this is usually midway between the lower end of the radius and the base of the first metacarpal when the thumb is fully extended. At the selected site the tendon of extensor pollicis longus is divided cleanly across with a fresh knife blade. The proximal stump is dissected free as far as the point of rupture and is discarded (Fig. 331).

The tendon suture. The tendon of extensor indicis is drawn down and laid alongside the remaining distal part of the extensor pollicis longus. The excursion of the extensor indicis should be tested by alternately pulling and relaxing the tendon. With the thumb fully extended and the first metacarpal mid-way between full flexion and full extension the extensor indicis should be held mid-way between the extremes of its excursion.

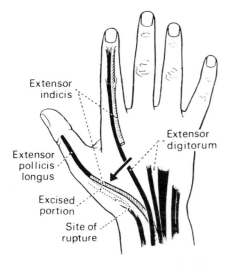

FIG. 331. Transfer of extensor indicis tendon to extensor pollicis longus. The diagram shows the tendon of extensor indicis re-routed (arrow) and sutured to the distal stump of the thumb extensor.

When these conditions have been met the tendon of extensor indicis is divided exactly level with the point of section of the extensor pollicis longus. The tendon ends are held in contact by passing straight suture needles through each tendon 1.5 centimetres from the cut end and approximating the two needles (Fig. 132, p. 97). With the two cut surfaces of the tendons thus apposed, end-to-end suture with suitable stainless steel wire is made according to the technique described on page 97. If practicable, one or two additional reinforcement sutures may be inserted. The ends of the wire sutures are buried in the tendon.

Closure. The skin alone is sutured.

POST-OPERATIVE MANAGEMENT

When suitable dressings held by a light crepe bandage have been applied a palmar plaster-of-Paris splint is constructed. It lies along the front of the forearm and the proximal half of the palm and is moulded round the volar half of the thumb to hold it in moderate though not extreme extension. The plaster should extend distally to the pulp of the thumb. It is held in position with a crepe bandage.

The plaster should be retained for three weeks, and thereafter active mobilising exercises are begun.

Comment

Transfer of extensor indicis to the extensor pollicis longus gives good results in the common type of case in which the thumb extensor is frayed and ruptured over the lower end of the radius, usually in consequence of a Colles's fracture. In other, less common circumstances in which the extensor pollicis longus tendon is severed—as for instance by a clean laceration—direct suture of the divided ends is to be preferred to tendon transfer.

The main difficulty in transfer of the extensor indicis to the extensor pollicis longus is to judge the correct tension under which the two tendon ends should be united. It is easy to suture the tendon ends under too little tension, but equally it is a mistake to attempt to join them with the thumb fully extended and the extensor indicis drawn down taut. The other obvious necessity is to effect a really firm junction between the tendon ends, so that the risk of dehiscence when the splint is removed is reduced to the minimum. Diversion of the extensor indicis from the index finger does not cause serious handicap, though it does restrict the patient's ability to point the index finger while the adjacent fingers are closed.

TENDON TRANSFERS FOR PARALYSIS OF RADIAL NERVE

When the radial nerve is irreparably damaged, active extension of wrist and digits may be restored by transfer of certain flexor muscles to activate the appropriate extensor tendons. In the original operation of Robert Jones (1921) the flexor carpi radialis was used to activate the long extensor and long abductor of the thumb and the flexor carpi ulnaris was used to activate the extensors of the fingers.

The Robert Jones operation weakened unduly the power of wrist flexion, and the preference now is to use the flexor carpi radialis to activate the extensor tendons of thumb and fingers and to use palmaris longus (when present) to activate the abductor pollicis longus (Brooks 1974). If the paralysis includes the extensors of the wrist the pronator radii teres muscle is used to activate the extensor carpi radialis brevis. The full triple transfer will be described.

TECHNIQUE

Position of patient. The patient lies supine with the arm abducted on a side table. A tourniquet may be used on the upper arm.

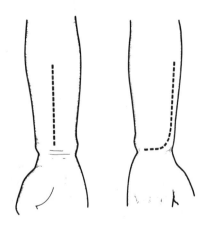

FIGS 332–333. Tendon transfers for paralysis of radial nerve. Figure 332—The anterior incision. Figure 333—The posterior incision.

Incisions. Two incisions are required, one at the front of the forearm through which to mobilise the muscles to be transferred, and one over the back of

the forearm to allow the tendon junctions to be made.

The anterior incision extends proximally in the midline of the forearm from the distal flexor crease of the wrist to the junction of the proximal and middle thirds of the forearm (Fig. 332).

The posterior incision begins immediately below the head of the ulna and crosses the back of the wrist towards the posterior margin of the

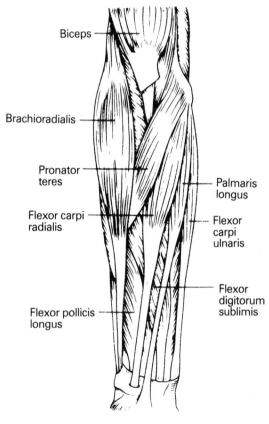

FIG. 334. The superficial flexor muscles of the forearm.

styloid process of the radius. Here it sweeps proximally (a sharp angle should be avoided) to follow the lateral border of the radius as far proximally as the junction of the upper and middle thirds of the forearm (Fig. 333).

Mobilisation of anterior muscles. The anterior incision is deepened through the fascia to expose the flexor carpi radialis tendon and, when it is present, the tendon of palmaris longus (Fig. 334). Care must be taken to avoid injuring the median nerve, which is especially vulnerable if the palmaris longus is absent. The two tendons are divided distally close to their insertions, and each tendon is transfixed by a holding stitch. This enables the tendon, and more proximally the muscle belly, to be pulled forward to allow the muscle to be freed as far proximally as the junction of the upper and middle thirds of the forearm.

Mobilisation of pronator radii teres. Through the upper part of the anterior incision the pronator radii teres muscle is identified as it passes downwards and laterally towards its insertion near the mid-point of the shaft of the radius at its lateral aspect. The tendon is detached from its insertion into the bone. It is not necessary to mobilise the muscle in a proximal direction for more than a few centimetres because the line of its pull is not to be appreciably altered.

Preparation of recipient tendons. The lower part of the posterior incision is opened up by reflection of the angled skin flap. A rectangular window is then cut in the deep fascia over the extensor tendons in the lower forearm, the distal edge of the window being at the level of the extensor retinaculum. The window should extend proximally for about 6 centimetres.

The common extensor tendons to the four fingers are now identified, as also are the tendons of extensor pollicis longus and abductor pollicis longus. The tendons of extensor indicis and extensor minimi digiti are left undisturbed. Holding stitches are inserted into each of the common finger extensors and into the long extensor and long abductor of the thumb. These stitches are useful later for controlling the tension of the tendons.

Re-routing of flexor muscles. The mobilised flexor carpi radialis muscle is withdrawn from the anterior wound and swung laterally so that its new direction may be determined. It should be laid so

that it winds round the lateral border of the forearm, with its tendon lying obliquely across the recipient extensor tendons in the direction of the little finger (Fig. 335).

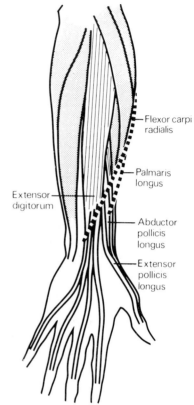

FIG. 335. Interrupted lines show new disposition of the flexor carpi radialis, which is to be attached obliquely to extensor pollicis longus and extensor digitorum tendons; and of the palmaris longus, which is to be attached to the abductor pollicis longus tendon. Recipient muscles are indicated by longitudinal hatching.

When the new line of the muscle has thus been determined a subcutaneous tunnel superficial to the deep fascia is formed by blunt dissection with scissors or with a curved haemostat. The tunnel extends from the lateral border of the anterior incision to emerge in the posterior wound. A little to the medial side a tunnel is likewise prepared to transmit the tendon of palmaris longus to its proposed point of junction with the abductor pollicis longus at the lateral border of the lower end of the radius (Fig. 335). When these tunnels have been prepared the muscles and tendons are re-routed through them to emerge in the posterior wound.

Making the tendon junctions at back of lower forearm. From this point onwards the wrist is held fully extended, with the metacarpo-phalangeal joints extended but the interphalangeal joints relaxed. The thumb is also held in extension.

By drawing taut the holding stitches already inserted in each of the common extensor tendons of the fingers and in the extensor pollicis longus tendon, any slack in the tendons is taken up. The stitches holding the four finger tendons may now be clamped together with a haemostat.

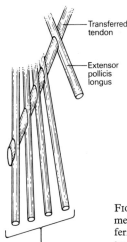

FIG. 336. Diagram showing method of attaching transferred tendon to recipient tendons of extensor digitorum and extensor pollicis longus.

(labels on figure: Transferred tendon; Extensor pollicis longus; Recipient tendons (digitorum))

With the wrist and thumb thus extended and with all slack taken up in the tendons, the tendon suture may be done with only moderate tension on the re-routed flexor carpi radialis tendon. To carry out the tendon suture the tendons of extensor pollicis longus and of each of the common extensor tendons of the fingers are button-holed in an oblique direction corresponding with the line of the transferred tendon. This line slopes distally and medially so that the slit in the tendon to the little finger is the most distal (Fig. 336). The tendon of flexor carpi radialis is then drawn through the button-holes successively from the radial to the medial side and anchored to each tendon by interrupted sutures of fine stainless steel wire. Each knot should be buried within the tendon.

The tendon of palmaris longus, which has been re-routed in the direction of abductor pollicis longus, is likewise button-holed through the recipient tendon and anchored with a wire stitch.

Suture of pronator radii teres to extensor carpi radialis brevis. Through the proximal part of the posterior incision the extensor carpi radialis brevis muscle is identified where it lies close to the detached tendon of the pronator teres. It will be recalled that the extensor carpi radialis brevis is inserted into the base of the middle metacarpal: identification may be established by pulling upon the muscle.

The pronator teres muscle, already detached from its point of insertion, is now re-routed subcutaneously round the radial side of the forearm and drawn distally with a holding stitch to emerge at the dorsal incision. The extensor carpi radialis brevis is drawn proximally to take up any slack, button-holed through the pronator teres, and sutured with fine stainless steel wire.

Closure. It is important that all bleeding points be sealed before the skin is closed in order to minimise haematoma formation and consequent adhesions. The fascial layers and the skin are closed with interrupted sutures.

POST-OPERATIVE MANAGEMENT

Plentiful gauze dressings are held snugly by a crepe bandage. For the first three weeks the wrist, fingers and thumb are held extended by a volar plaster-of-Paris splint well moulded to the forearm and palm and held in place by a further crepe bandage. In the fourth week splintage is discarded and active mobilising exercises are begun.

Comment

As with all tendon transfers there is some loss of power of the re-routed muscles. If these are to work with the greatest possible efficiency it is essential that the dissection be clean and gentle. Rough handling of the muscles or tendons is liable to lead to the formation of adhesions, with consequent impairment of free gliding. Likewise, the formation of a haematoma may lead to matting of the tissues and impaired gliding of the tendons: it is important that full haemostasis be secured before the wounds are closed.

Another important point concerns the re-routing of the transferred muscles. Care should be taken to ensure that the line of pull is as direct as possible and that there are no unnecessary kinks or bends. The subcutaneous tunnels must conform accurately to the new line of pull.

Finally, great care should be devoted to ensuring that the tendons are united with the correct tension.

A number of modifications of the original Jones's transfer have been devised. It has been quite common practice to use the flexor carpi ulnaris as the motor for extension of the fingers and thumb, the tendon being routed round the ulnar side of the lower forearm. The loss of the normal action

of flexor carpi ulnaris, however, favours radial deviation of the wrist, and it is for this reason that flexor carpi radialis is diverted instead.

To restore wrist extension many surgeons transfer the pronator teres tendon to both the extensor carpi radialis longus and the extensor carpi radialis brevis tendons. The inclusion of the long extensor, however, again tends to cause the wrist to go into radial deviation when the patient grips. A method of avoiding this tendency while still including both radial extensors of the wrist in the transfer has been described by Said (1974), who divided the tendon of extensor carpi ulnaris high in the forearm, leaving the insertion intact, and re-routed the tendon diagonally across the back of the forearm to join the pronator teres: thus the transferred pronator teres muscle is used to activate all three extensors of the wrist.

DRAINAGE INCISIONS FOR ACUTE SUPPURATING INFECTIONS OF THE FASCIAL SPACES OF THE HAND

CLASSIFICATION

If minor superficial infections are excluded there are six types of infection to be considered: 1) nail-fold infection (paronychia); 2) pulp-space infection (whitlow, felon); 3) other subcutaneous infections; 4) thenar space infection; 5) mid-palmar space infection; 6) tendon sheath infection.

SURGICAL ANATOMY

A knowledge of the anatomy of the fascial spaces of the hand is indispensable for the correct treatment of hand infections.

The nail fold and subungual space. The subcuticular plane beneath the nail fold is potentially continuous, at the base and sides of the nail, with the subungual space deep to the nail. Infection beginning in the nail fold may therefore easily spread under the nail (Fig. 337), and the resulting abscess cannot be drained effectively unless part of the nail is removed.

The pulp space. The interval between the front of the distal phalanx and the skin is traversed by

tough fibrous partitions, which subdivide the space into numerous fat-filled cells (like the cells of a honeycomb) disposed at right angles to the skin surface (Fig. 337). Infection occurring in this tough tissue is virtually within a closed compartment: tissue pressure rises rapidly and accounts for early throbbing pain.

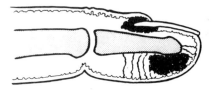

FIG. 337. Diagrammatic section showing the site of suppuration in nail-fold infection (paronychia) and in pulp-space infection (whitlow). In nail-fold infection the pus is beneath the cuticle and may extend under the nail, as shown. In pulp-space infection the pus lies in the tough fibro-fatty tissue immediately in front of the distal phalanx.

Other subcutaneous spaces. Infection may occur in the subcutaneous plane at any point in the hand. Common sites are the middle or proximal segment of a finger, and the web spaces between the digits. Less common sites are the palm of the hand and the dorsum of the hand. These superficial spaces are clearly demarcated from the deep palmar spaces next to be described, and must not be confused with them.

front. Medially it is separated from the mid-palmar space by a fibrous septum that extends deeply from the fascia on the deep surface of the flexor tendons to the fascia covering the interossei

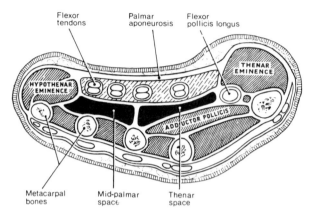

FIG. 338. The deep palmar spaces—the thenar space and the mid-palmar space—shown in diagrammatic transverse section.

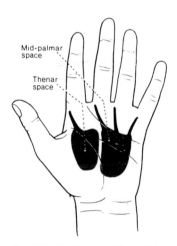

FIG. 339. Surface marking of the deep palmar spaces. The thenar space is continuous with the first lumbrical canal; the mid-palmar space with the second, third and fourth lumbrical canals. The spaces are separated by a fibrous septum.

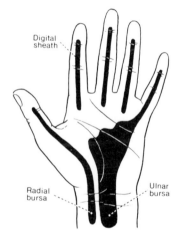

FIG. 340. The synovial flexor sheaths. The sheaths for the index, middle, and ring fingers end proximally at the bases of the fingers. Those for the thumb and little finger are continuous with the radial bursa and the ulnar bursa respectively.

The thenar space. This lies deeply under the lateral (radial) half of the hollow of the palm. It is the interval between the adductor pollicis muscle behind and the flexor tendon of the index finger and the first and second lumbrical muscles in

and adductor pollicis muscle (Figs 338 and 339). The space is prolonged forwards into the delicate sheath that surrounds the first lumbrical muscle. It sometimes communicates also with the second lumbrical canal. The lumbrical canals thus provide a potential communication between the sub-cutaneous web spaces and the thenar space: in practice, however, it is rare for infection to spread along this route.

The mid-palmar space. This lies under the me-dial (ulnar) half of the hollow of the palm. It is the interval between the interossei and metacarpal bones behind and the flexor tendons (in their sheaths) of the middle, ring, and little fingers in front (Fig. 338). Laterally, it is separated from the thenar space by the fibrous septum already de-scribed. The space is prolonged forwards into the sheaths of the second, third, and fourth lumbrical muscles. Again, despite the potential communica-tion between a web space and the mid-palmar space along the lumbrical canals, web-space infection very seldom spreads deeply to involve the palm.

The flexor tendon sheaths. Distinction must be made between the tough fibrous sheaths, which exist only in the digits, and the flimsy synovial sheaths, which line the fibrous sheaths and, in the case of the thumb and little finger, extend proxi-mally into the palm. In acute infections of the tendon sheaths (acute infective tenosynovitis) the pus is within the synovial sheath and it is confined only by the limits of the sheath. The flexor sheaths of the index, middle, and ring fingers end proxi-mally at the level of the transverse palmar skin crease (Fig. 340). The sheaths of the thumb and little finger extend proximally through the palm to end two or three centimetres above the level of the wrist. The proximal part of the sheath for the thumb is known as the radial bursa. The sheath for the little finger opens out proximally into the ulnar bursa, which encloses the grouped tendons of flexor digitorum superficialis and flexor digi-torum profundus (Fig. 340).

PRINCIPLES OF TREATMENT

When suppuration has occurred, as indicated by severe throbbing pain, intense local tenderness, pyrexia, and loss of function, the abscess should be drained surgically without further delay. After

adequate drainage has been secured the wound may be packed lightly open with vaselined gauze for two days. Thereafter, dry dressings are used and active finger exercises are encouraged.

TREATMENT OF INDIVIDUAL LESIONS

Nail-fold infection (paronychia). The subcuti-cular abscess is drained by raising the cuticle from the nail or by raising it as a short flap after incising it vertically at one or both corners (Fig. 341). If

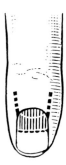

FIG. 341. Technique of drainage of paronychial abscess. For the mildest infections it is sufficient to raise the cuticle alone without incising it; but better drainage is secured by a vertical incision through the cuticle on one or both sides. When pus has extended beneath the nail it is necessary also to remove the proximal half of the nail.

pus has extended under the nail the proximal half of the nail must also be removed. This is done by cutting it across with sharp-pointed scissors and avulsing the proximal part with an artery forceps.

Pulp-space infection (whitlow). Drainage is effected by a lateral incision just in front of the plane of the terminal phalanx (Fig. 342); it is

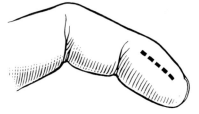

FIG. 342. Incision for drainage of pulp abscess. The incision is deepened across the pulp, in front of the phalanx, and the abscess cavity is cleared out under direct vision.

deepened transversely across the pulp of the finger but should not extend proximally beyond a point half a centimetre distal to the terminal skin crease lest the flexor tendon sheath be inadver-tently opened. An alternative method is to incise directly into the pulp over the centre of the abscess, a technique that is to be preferred if the abscess is threatening to point at the surface.

Subcutaneous infections (other than pulp-space infections). Drainage is by a short incision appropriately placed to reach the abscess without harming important structures or leaving an awkward scar. In the case of a web-space infection the incision should not divide the skin fold of the web: a short transverse incision in the palm just proximal to the skin fold is adequate (Fig. 343).

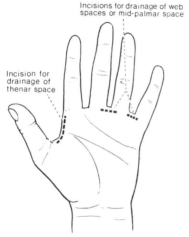

FIG. 343. Incisions for drainage through the web spaces.

Thenar space infection. Drainage is by an incision at the dorsal aspect of the first web space (Fig. 343).

Mid-palmar space infection. Drainage can be established through the web space between the middle and ring fingers or between the ring and little fingers (Fig. 343).

Tendon sheath infection. The sheath is opened at its proximal end in the palm and at its distal end (Fig. 344), and irrigated with antibiotic solution through a fine tube passed along the sheath: the tube is withdrawn and the wounds are packed lightly open. If the radial bursa or the ulnar bursa is infected it must be drained and irrigated through an additional incision in the palm (Fig. 344).

Comment

It must be emphasised first that in infections of the hand successful treatment depends first and foremost upon accurate diagnosis, without which the correct drainage incisions cannot be made. And accurate diagnosis depends in turn upon a thorough knowledge of the surgical anatomy.

There has been much discussion on the technique of surgical drainage for hand infections, and there is a tendency among some surgeons to regard only their own methods as correct. It is

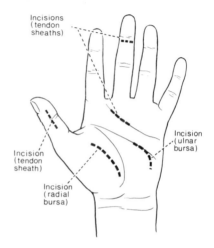

FIG. 344. Incisions for drainage and irrigation of tendon sheaths and bursae.

necessary to emphasise, therefore, that success depends largely upon the observance of certain general principles. These are as follows. Firstly, the operation must be done under favourable conditions and without undue hurry: the old method of making a hasty incision under a "whiff of gas" is indefensible. Anaesthesia may be general or regional, but it should allow time for deliberate exploration of the abscess under a tourniquet, so that its full extent can be ascertained. Secondly, the incision must be adequate to allow complete emptying of the abscess. Thirdly, the incision must not endanger important underlying structures. Fourthly, the incision must be so sited that the resulting scar is innocuous. Within the limits imposed by these principles there is often more than one way of performing the actual drainage operation.

AMPUTATION THROUGH FOREARM (BELOW-ELBOW AMPUTATION)

LEVEL OF SECTION

As much length as possible should be preserved. Useful function of the elbow is possible so long as the stump is not shorter than 5 centimetres.

TECHNIQUE

Position of patient. The patient lies supine with the affected limb resting upon a side table. A tourniquet may be used on the upper arm.

Marking out the skin flaps. The level of the proposed bone section is marked on the skin surface, measurements being taken from the tip of the olecranon. Equal anterior and posterior flaps are marked out with the base of each flap at the proposed level of bone section. Each flap should be a little longer than half the diameter of the forearm at the level of amputation.

Raising of flaps and division of muscles. The flaps outlined are cut and reflected proximally together with the subcutaneous tissue and deep fascia. All the muscles are then transected about a centimetre below the proposed level of bone section: the extra length allows for slight retraction of the muscles.

Management of vessels and nerves. The radial and ulnar arteries are clamped and ligated. The major nerves are identified, drawn distally and severed as high as possible so that the stumps retract well proximal to the level of amputation.

Division of bones. The radius and the ulna are divided transversely with a hand saw at the planned level. The cut edges are smoothed and the corners rounded with a rasp.

Closure. After removal of the tourniquet time must be spent on securing full haemostasis. The deep fascia is then closed over the end of the stump, and after any necessary trimming of skin the flaps are united with interrupted sutures. Suction drainage is recommended.

POST-OPERATIVE MANAGEMENT

Copious gauze dressings are held in place by crepe bandages evenly applied over the end of the stump with moderate tension. The drainage tube is removed after forty-eight hours, when the stump may be rebandaged. Thereafter the dressings are left in place until two weeks from operation, when the sutures are removed.

AMPUTATION THROUGH WRIST

Whenever it is practicable, amputation through the wrist is to be preferred to amputation through the forearm because the mechanism of pronation and supination can be preserved.

TECHNIQUE

Position of patient. The patient lies supine with the limb resting upon a side table. A tourniquet may be used on the upper arm.

Marking out the skin flaps. It is well to mark out the skin flaps before the incision is made. A long palmar flap and a short dorsal flap are recommended.

The anterior outline should begin at the tip of the radial styloid process; thence it extends distally towards the base of the first metacarpal but curves medially to cross the front of the palm about 4 centimetres distal to the distal flexor crease of the wrist. Thence it sweeps medially and proximally to end on the medial side of the wrist a centimetre below the styloid process of the ulna (Fig. 345).

From the original starting point a posterior flap is outlined. It extends almost horizontally across the back of the wrist from the tip of the radial styloid process, with a slight sweep distally to the level of the base of the middle metacarpal. The flaps thus outlined may prove to be over-generous and they may be trimmed appropriately during closure of the wound.

Division of tendons, blood vessels and nerves. When the skin incisions as outlined have been made the palmar and dorsal skin flaps, together

rasp. Likewise the tip of the styloid process of the ulna is removed, but the inferior radio-ulnar joint should be preserved intact.

Closure. After the tourniquet has been removed and all bleeding points secured the skin flaps are turned into position to cover the bone ends. Any excess of skin is trimmed away to ensure a smooth suture line without any tension, and the skin edges

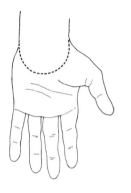
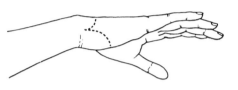

FIG. 345. Amputation through the wrist. Outline of the long anterior flap and short posterior flap.

with the fascia, are reflected proximally as far as the radio carpal joint. Next the radial and ulnar arteries are identified, ligated and divided as far proximally as possible. The median, ulnar and terminal part of the radial nerve are identified, pulled distally, divided cleanly and allowed to retract proximally. Finally all the tendons across the wrist are divided and allowed to retract.

Separation of carpus and trimming of styloid processes. The capsule of the wrist joint is divided circumferentially and the hand and carpus are discarded. The radial styloid process is trimmed off flush with the main part of the articular surface, and all sharp edges are rounded off with a

are approximated with interrupted sutures. Provided full haemostasis has been secured it should not be necessary to drain the wound.

POST-OPERATIVE MANAGEMENT

Copious gauze dressings are held snugly in place by crepe bandages which should be applied evenly to exert moderate pressure over the end of the stump. Proximally the bandage may be secured to the skin of the forearm with an elastic adhesive bandage. The bandages may be changed as required, and the skin sutures are removed two weeks after the operation.

AMPUTATIONS OF FINGERS AND THUMB

Most amputations of the digits result from trauma, and the problem is to make the most effective repair. This may entail the use of skin grafting procedures in order to preserve length; or alternatively, if some shortening can be accepted,

definitive amputation may be carried out at a more proximal level.

Sometimes a deficiency of skin in the proposed stump may be made good by the use of free skin grafts taken from the amputated member.

Split-skin Grafting for Terminal Digital Amputation

Repair by a free split thickness skin graft is appropriate mainly for amputations through the terminal pulp, especially when the bone of the terminal phalanx has not been exposed. The same technique is applicable to amputations through the distal part of the terminal phalanx, but in such a case it is necessary to cut back the bone sufficiently to allow soft tissue to enclose it, to form a base for the graft.

TECHNIQUE

A tourniquet may be used either proximally on the upper arm or, if only one finger is affected, locally round the base of the digit. The cut surface is cleaned with saline and if bone is showing it is cut back appropriately with nibbling forceps. The tourniquet may then be removed to allow adequate haemostasis to be secured. A split thickness graft is taken from the thigh or from the inner aspect of the upper arm and trimmed to size. The margins are sutured to the cut edges of the digital skin by six to eight sutures of fine non-absorbable material. The ends of the sutures may be left long and used to tie a small dressing over the grafted surface.

POST-OPERATIVE MANAGEMENT

The digit should be snugly bandaged and kept elevated so far as is practicable. The sutures are left in place for six or seven days.

Repair of Terminal Finger Amputation by Thenar Flap

Repair by a thenar flap provides full thickness skin and avoids further shortening of the finger. The inconvenience to the patient and the lack of sensibility in the graft, however, limit the application of the method.

TECHNIQUE

A tourniquet may be used on the upper arm. When the cut surface of the injured finger has been cleaned and any dead tissue removed the finger is flexed down in such a way as to lie in the most natural position upon the thenar eminence. A flap of skin with its base proximally is outlined upon the thenar eminence: its position is such that when the flap is raised it may be sutured to the cut surface of the finger without tension upon the base of the flap. It may be useful to cut a paper pattern to match the size and shape of the skin defect in order to ensure that the thenar flap is of the correct dimensions. Twenty per cent extra length should be allowed for the pedicle.

When the flap has been raised its bed and the base of the pedicle are covered with a split thickness skin graft sewn in place with six to eight fine non-absorbable sutures. The injured finger is then brought down into position and the edges of the upturned flap are sutured to the periphery of the cut surface of the finger.

POST-OPERATIVE MANAGEMENT

Small gauze dressings are applied between the donor area and the end of the finger. The finger is held flexed in position by a long strip of adhesive strapping brought round from the back of the hand and over the flexed knuckles of the finger to the base of the thumb metacarpal. Additional strips of strapping may be used to anchor the main longitudinal strip more securely. After two weeks the base of the flap is divided and both the grafted area and the donor area are tidied up as necessary.

Definitive Amputation through Finger or Thumb

LEVEL OF SECTION

In the fingers, unless the proximal phalanx and at least half of the middle phalanx can be preserved, the finger stump is of practically no functional value and amputation at the base of the finger or through the neck of the metacarpal is to be preferred. In contrast, in amputations of the thumb all possible length must be preserved, and shortening to permit formal amputation at a more proximal level is not acceptable.

TECHNIQUE

In many cases the skin flaps will have to be planned according to the extent and condition of the remaining skin. In general, anterior and posterior flaps are preferred, the anterior flap being slightly longer than the posterior. The base of each flap is at the proposed level of bone section or disarticulation. If the amputation is to be close to the nail the skin flap must be a long anterior one without any posterior flap.

When the flaps have been raised tendons, vessels and nerves are cut through at the proposed level of bone section. The bone is then divided with sharp-pointed bone-cutting forceps (care must be taken not to crush the bone) or, if the section is to be through a joint, the capsule is cut circumferentially and the terminal part of the finger discarded. After haemostasis has been secured the flaps are approximated, trimmed if necessary and united with interrupted sutures.

POST-OPERATIVE MANAGEMENT

Gauze dressings are held in place by a small crepe bandage, which in turn is anchored by strips of adhesive strapping. The hand should be elevated as much as possible during the first few days.

Amputation through Metacarpo-phalangeal Joint

TECHNIQUE

A racquet-shaped incision is appropriate. The handle of the racquet is placed dorsally, the incision beginning over the neck of the metacarpal. The periphery of the racquet encircles the base of the finger just distal to the web (Fig. 346). A generous amount of skin should be left at the first incision: the edges may be trimmed as necessary at the time of closure.

When the skin incision has been completed the extensor tendon and the joint capsule are severed through the dorsal part of the wound. This allows the base of the proximal phalanx to be pulled

forward and distally with a hook. It is then a straightforward matter to fillet out the base of the proximal phalanx from the anterior flap. Finally

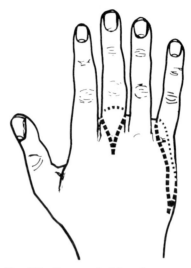

FIG. 346. Racquet incision for amputation of middle finger through the metacarpo-phalangeal joint, and extended racquet incision for amputation of little finger through the metacarpal bone.

the flexor tendons are drawn distally and severed as high as possible and the finger is discarded. The digital arteries are ligated and the nerves drawn distally and severed cleanly. The skin edges are approximated and trimmed appropriately to ensure a smooth contour. Drainage is not required.

POST-OPERATIVE MANAGEMENT

A crepe bandage is applied snugly over gauze dressings and retained until the sutures are removed a week after the operation.

Comment

Amputation through the metacarpo-phalangeal joint of a finger leaves a rather ugly gap if the middle or ring finger is the one removed, and it leaves an ugly prominence of the metacarpal head in the case of the index finger or little finger. Nevertheless it may be acceptable to a manual worker in the interests of preserving an intact metacarpus and maximum strength. If appearance rather than strength is a prime consideration, however, amputation through the metacarpal just proximal to its neck gives a more pleasing result.

Amputation through Metacarpal Bone

Amputation of a finger through the neck of the metacarpal bone is designed to eliminate the ugliness of a metacarpal stump of index or little finger,

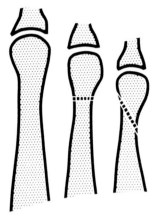

Fig. 347. Levels of bone section for amputation of ring and little fingers through the metacarpal bones.

or in the case of the middle and ring fingers to reduce the ugly gap between the remaining fingers when one finger has been removed.

Technique

The technique resembles that of amputation through the metacarpo-phalangeal joint except that the racquet incision is extended proximally as a linear cut to the junction of the middle and distal thirds of the metacarpal. The head and neck of the metacarpal are exposed and freed from the surrounding soft tissues by sharp dissection close to the bone. The bone is divided just proximal to the narrowest part of the neck (Fig. 347), and the digit is peeled distally from the investing tissues as described in the previous section.

In the case of the index finger or little finger the division of the metacarpal must be made obliquely in order to give a smooth contour without any "step" (Fig. 347). When the finger has been removed together with the metacarpal head the skin is folded into position for closure and any excess skin is trimmed away to allow a neat suture.

Post-operative Management

This is the same as for amputation through the metacarpo-phalangeal joint.

Comment

In fashioning the racquet-shaped incision it is best to err on the side of leaving too much skin rather than to run the risk of cutting away too much. It is always a simple matter to trim the edges at the time of closure.

The cosmetic benefit of amputation through the metacarpal rather than through the metacarpophalangeal joint—especially in the case of the index finger and the little finger—makes it a procedure to be recommended in preference to disarticulation when the need for strength does not outweigh the desire for good appearance.

CHAPTER EIGHT

Hip Region

The hip is a predominant field of activity for the orthopaedic surgeon, and it is a field that is especially important because painful disorders of the hip are so seriously disabling. The successful development of total replacement arthroplasty of the hip might well be acclaimed as the most important achievement of the century so far as reconstructive surgery is concerned. It has brought inestimable benefit to countless victims of degenerative and rheumatoid arthritis. It has also brought many new problems in its wake—problems of salvage after a replacement arthroplasty has come to grief. Apart from this, the hip still presents many fascinating problems, especially in relation to fracture of the femoral neck, congenital dislocation, Perthes' disease and slipped capital epiphysis. Surgical advance continues apace, and the operations described in the succeeding pages may represent but a phase in the changing scene of hip surgery.

CONTENTS OF CHAPTER

NAIL AND SCREW FIXATION FOR FRACTURE OF NECK OF FEMUR

Internal fixation of fractures of the neck of the femur was reported as long ago as 1913 by Lambotte and had been practised even earlier by Langenbeck, but it did not receive wide acceptance until the technique of fixation by a three-flanged nail was described by Smith-Petersen, Cave and

Van Gorder in 1931. Nowadays most surgeons believe that a single nail in the axis of the femoral neck may fail to provide adequate fixation, and that more rigid internal splinting is required. The following description relates to the insertion of a nail and a screw (Fig. 348). A useful alternative—fixation by compression screw—is described on page 268.

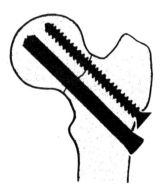

Fig. 348. Nail and screw fixation for fracture of neck of femur.

PRELIMINARY STUDIES

From good antero-posterior and lateral radiographs it should be ascertained whether the fracture is of the displaced variety or whether it is an impacted abduction fracture. The former clearly will require reduction before nailing whereas an impacted fracture, if it is nailed at all, may be nailed in the existing position. The following description relates to a displaced fracture.

TECHNIQUE

The patient must be positioned on the orthopaedic table with great care: the technical success of the operation depends to a large extent not only upon perfect reduction of the fracture but also upon the correct adjustment of the limb and of the radiographic equipment in order to facilitate accurate placing of the nail and screw. The surgeon should always supervise these initial steps in the procedure himself.

Reduction of fracture. When the patient has been laid upon the orthopaedic table an assistant holds the sound limb while the surgeon grasps the injured limb. The hip and knee are flexed 90 degrees so that the femur is directed vertically upwards towards the ceiling. Strong upward traction is then exerted upon the limb in the line of the femur while an assistant holds the pelvis. While traction is still being applied the thigh is rotated medially and the limb is then lowered to the horizontal position with medial rotation still maintained. This manoeuvre nearly always succeeds in securing anatomical reduction.

Fixation on table. Each foot is now bandaged firmly but without constricting pressure to the respective foot-piece of the orthopaedic table. The foot of the affected limb should be bandaged to the foot-piece with the limb held in slight medial rotation, so that the patella is directed about 15 degrees inwards. This ensures that the slightly anteverted femoral neck lies in the horizontal plane: in this way a true profile radiograph of the femoral neck is obtained with an x-ray beam directed horizontally. With the limb thus slightly rotated medially the prominence of the greater trochanter is directed truly laterally, and this is the chief criterion that the correct position has been attained. The sound limb is bandaged to the foot-piece in a corresponding position.

The sound limb is now abducted fully and locked in this position by clamping the appropriate swivel of the table. The injured limb is abducted about 30 degrees and locked in this position. The upright supports for the feet are next adjusted to such a height that the shafts of the femora are parallel with the floor.

Positioning the x-ray units. Two mobile x-ray units or image intensifiers are now moved into position. Positioning the vertical tube (for antero-posterior radiography) presents no special problem: the ray should be centred over the neck of the femur—that is, towards a point about 4 centimetres distal to the anterior superior spine of the ilium.

Directing the horizontal tube (for lateral radiography) calls for much care. Failure to obtain a satisfactory image is usually due to poor positioning of the patient and the x-ray units. It is usually necessary to raise the operation table a little from its lowest position to match the height of the x-ray unit: many units cannot be lowered sufficiently to allow a horizontal beam to pass through the femoral neck. It is important not only that the beam be horizontal, but that it should pass through the femoral neck at right angles to it (Fig. 349). Otherwise the image is distorted and the femoral head may not be visualised. Excessive abduction of the injured limb should be avoided because it may displace the fracture, or prevent

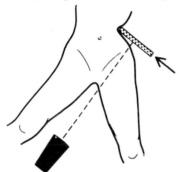

FIG. 349. For lateral radiography of the hip the film cassette must be pressed firmly into the loin as indicated by the arrow; otherwise the femoral head is not well shown. The x-ray beam (interrupted line) should be at right angles to the cassette.

the cassette or image intensifier from being brought in close enough to show the femoral head (Fig. 349). The important necessity, therefore, is that the uninjured leg be abducted fully. The machine can then be moved far enough outwards to allow the x-ray beam to be directed horizontally through the femoral neck at right angles to it. The beam passes through the leg on the shortest path, and thus allows the optimal image to be obtained, even in fat patients. This also allows the receiving medium—whether cassette or intensifier head—to be placed close in against the injured limb, clear of the main part of the table.

Skin markers and preliminary radiography. At this stage the surgeon applies radio-opaque markers to the skin to act as indicators for the insertion of the guide wire. Skin closure clips such as those of the Michel type are suitable for this purpose. A row of five clips 1 centimetre apart is

first applied over the front of the lateral part of the femoral shaft from the level of the prominence of the greater trochanter downwards (Fig. 350). Three further clips are applied just lateral to the

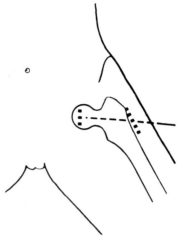

FIG. 350. Diagram to illustrate the use of skin clips as markers to aid directing of the guide wire. Five clips extend distally from the greater trochanter at centimetre intervals; then three are placed over the groin across a line joining the central one of the five lateral clips to the opposite anterior superior iliac spine. In this example a line joining the middle clips of the two rows lies over the centre of the femoral neck.

groin (over the femoral head), the centre one being on a line joining the middle one of the five vertical clips with the opposite anterior spine (Fig. 350). Antero-posterior and lateral radiographs (or image intensifier views) are now taken to check the reduction and to show the position of the opaque skin markers in relation to the femur. In the rare instances in which reduction is not adequate the drapes must be removed and the reduction manoeuvre repeated until anatomical reduction is obtained.

Incision. The incision extends vertically down the side of the thigh from the prominence of the greater trochanter for a distance of 10 to 15 centimetres, depending upon the amount of subcutaneous fat. The fascia lata, easily identified in the lower half of the wound, is split in the direction of the incision, and proximally the slit is extended upwards into the tensor fasciae latae muscle

(Fig. 351). The deeper muscle layer thus revealed is the vastus lateralis, the fibres of which run downwards and forwards. The posterior border of this muscle is sought and a curved bone lever is

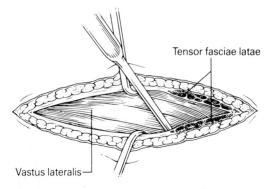

Tensor fasciae latae

Vastus lateralis

FIG. 351. Seeking the posterior edge of the vastus lateralis after incision of the fascia lata and the tensor fasciae latae muscle.

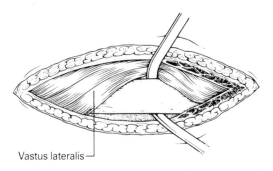

Vastus lateralis

FIG. 352. The vastus lateralis muscle has been levered forwards to expose the femur.

thrust behind the muscle and hooked over the front of the femoral shaft. The muscle is thus levered forwards and held out of the way. A second bone lever is inserted behind the femoral shaft to retract the posterior margin of the wound backwards (Fig. 352). Any remaining muscle fibres overlying the lateral aspect of the femur are now divided by a vertical cut straight onto the bone, and the periosteum is stripped over a length of about 7 to 10 centimetres from the base of the greater trochanter downwards.

Insertion of guide wires. When the bone has thus been exposed the next step is to insert guide wires along the neck of the femur from holes prepared in the lateral cortex. One guide wire will be used to

direct the nail and the other to direct the screw. That for the nail should be placed in the lower half of the femoral neck just below the central axis, and that for the screw should be in the upper half of the neck just above the central axis. Both wires should be midway between the anterior and the posterior wall of the femoral neck.

Insertion of the guide wires is facilitated by the radio-opaque skin markers that have been placed over the outer border of the femoral shaft and over the femoral head. Perusal of the radiographs taken with the skin markers in position will indicate at what point on the femoral shaft each wire should be introduced and the direction in which it should be aimed. For example, it may be found that the lower guide wire should lie in the direction of a line joining, say, the fourth of the outer row of clips to the lowest clip of the inner row. In this manner the optimal direction of each guide wire related to the antero-posterior radiograph is easily determined.

Directing the wires in relation to the lateral radiograph is also straightforward if care has been taken to ensure that the femoral neck is horizontal by directing the patella about 15 degrees medially and checking that the lateral prominence of the greater trochanter is directed truly laterally: the leg-piece of the table should also have been adjusted to ensure that the thigh lies parallel with the floor. If these criteria have been met, and if the lateral radiograph confirms that the femoral neck is horizontal by showing it to be in a line continuous with the axis of the femoral shaft, it is necessary only to be sure that the guide wires are inserted parallel with the floor. (If however the radiograph shows that the femoral neck is directed slightly forwards, as it will if the limb has not been fixed in slight medial rotation, allowance must be made for this and the guide wire must also be directed 10 or 15 degrees forwards.)

When the desired position of the guide wires has thus been established, a hole 3 or 4 millimetres in diameter is drilled through the lateral femoral cortex at the planned starting point of each wire, the drill being aimed in the direction selected for the wire: the drill should not penetrate beyond the lateral cortex. The lower guide wire, held in a hand-chuck, is then passed through the appropriate drill hole and driven along the femoral neck into the head; it should penetrate about 7 or 8 centimetres. If the wire is properly placed and directed, the surgeon is able to feel the soft cancellous bone giving way before the point of the wire. If it does not feel "right", a second guide wire and even a third may be entered through an adjacent part of the cortex and driven in a slightly divergent direction.

When the guide wire for the nail has been inserted the wire to mark the position of the screw is now driven in parallel to the first wire and about 15 millimetres above it. This wire too should penetrate about 7 or 8 centimetres. Again, a second wire for use as an alternative if the position of the first is unsatisfactory may be inserted.

When the guide wires have been inserted, their position in both the antero-posterioor and the lateral plane is checked by radiographs or by the image intensifier. If it is seen that a wire for the nail and a wire for the screw are in acceptable positions it remains only to remove any surplus wires and then to calculate the length of the nail and of the screw required, and to drive them in. If however the position of the guide wires is unsatisfactory, fresh ones must be inserted after appropriate directional corrections have been made.

Determining the length of the nail and screw. Calculation of the length of the nail and of the screw is made by first measuring the length of each guide wire that is protruding and subtracting this from the known length of the wire: this gives the length of wire within the bone. To this is added—or from it subtracted—any additional length needed to bring the tip of the screw or nail to a point 5 millimetres from the articular surface of the femoral head: the nail and the screw should come as close as this to the surface in order to provide the greatest possible fixation, but they should not come closer lest the point of the nail or the screw penetrate into the joint. In making measurements upon the radiograph the surgeon should allow for magnification of 10 per cent.

Driving the nail. The entrance hole in the cortex is enlarged in triradiate fashion with a small osteotome, or with a special trifin chisel, to allow easy entrance of the three-flanged nail. A nail of the correct length held on an introducer is then hammered in over the guide wire. Once the nail has entered the bone it is important to ensure that the guide wire is not driven on with the nail: this can happen all too easily because the point of the nail, if not exactly co-axial with the guide wire, may impinge into it and the two are driven on together. To check that this is not happening the length of wire protruding from the bone should be measured after every four or five hammer blows, the introducer or punch being removed for this purpose. If the length of wire protruding remains constant all is well, but if it becomes less between two measurements the guide wire is certainly being driven on, and it must then be immediately gripped with the hand chuck, twisted and slightly withdrawn.

As the nail nears full penetration it is well to have an assistant to apply counter-thrust against the pelvis on the opposite side of the patient. It is well also to leave the nail 3 or 4 millimetres short of full penetration at this stage, until the position of the point has been shown radiographically; thereafter the nail may be driven home further if the point is short of the optimal position.

Impaction of the fracture can also be achieved by the use of a Smith-Petersen punch over the nail. This impacts upon the femoral shaft around the nail, driving the neck fragment into the head fragment. This corrects any distraction that may have occurred as the nail was driven home. Impaction is particularly important if the screw is not used.

Driving the screw. With the nail driven home the final step in the fixation is to drive in a Venable hip screw of appropriate length—determined in the same way as the length of the nail. The core diameter of the Venable screw is 4 millimetres; so the guide wire track must be enlarged up to this bore by serial twist drills, preferably held in a power-driven chuck. The screw is then driven firmly home with a screwdriver of heavy calibre. The position and penetration of the screw are checked radiographically, and in the light of the findings any necessary adjustments are made (Fig. 348).

Closure. When haemostasis has been secured the vastus lateralis is allowed to fall back into place and its posterior margin may be anchored deeply with one or two absorbable sutures. The fascia lata and tensor fasciae latae muscle are repaired with interrupted sutures and the skin is closed without drainage.

POST-OPERATIVE MANAGEMENT

Splintage is not required: the patient may lie free in bed. Whether or not early walking is allowed depends upon the preference of the individual surgeon. Many still prohibit weight bearing for as long as three months; but an increasing proportion of surgeons—with whom the authors side—encourage immediate weight bearing with elbow crutches. The older the patient, the more important it is to get walking started at the earliest moment.

Comment

Efficient internal fixation of femoral neck fractures is not always simple and it demands considerable precision. The slogan should be: *"Get it right first time"*. All too often the operator accepts an inferior reduction, an imperfect position of the nail or screw, or incorrect length of the fixation devices. Defeat must not be accepted: perseverance is well rewarded.

Trouble is often experienced with the radiographic control. Unless the setting up of the apparatus is supervised by the surgeon himself films that are virtually useless may be produced. In particular, they often fail to show the femoral head adequately in the lateral projection. The reason for this is usually that the cassette is not pushed firmly enough into the loin, or that the beam is wrongly directed. These points must be checked every time a film is exposed. The same remarks apply to the use of the image intensifier. It is worth mentioning here that the use of an image intensifier with memory offers great advantages in that the image may be studied at leisure without adding to the radiation exposure.

If the correct rotational position of the limb is not insisted upon it often happens that the lateral radiographs show the femur semi-obliquely rather than in the true lateral projection. Acceptance of such an incorrect position makes accurate insertion of the nail and screw unnecessarily difficult.

Choosing the correct length of the nail and of the screw should not present any special problem because the length of the guide wire within the bone can be determined accurately by measuring the amount still protruding, and to this may be added or from it subtracted an amount as measured on the check radiographs. One necessary precaution needs to be mentioned, however: that is, to measure the length of the nail directly with a ruler before it is inserted, and not to rely simply on the figure engraved upon it: the length as engraved is not always the effective length that will enter the bone, for it may include the head of the nail.

A hazard that needs further mention is that of inadvertently driving the guide wire forwards with the nail. This can present a very serious difficulty if the wire is driven across the hip joint into the iliac fossa, for the guide wire may be broken off by repeated hammer blows upon the nail. In such a case the only way of retrieving the broken-off part of the guide wire is by exposing the iliac fossa and locating the tip of the wire from within the pelvis. This dilemma is, however, easily avoided if the precaution is taken of examining the guide wire repeatedly while the nail is being driven in. This entails removal of the cannulated punch and measurement of the protruding part of the guide wire to see whether it is being driven on. At the same time it is wise to grip the guide wire in a hand chuck and to rotate it to and fro: if the wire is being gripped dangerously by the point of the nail it will not rotate freely, and at this danger signal the wire should be promptly withdrawn.

All these points of detail are important: neglect of any one of them may easily lead to failure.

ALTERNATIVE TECHNIQUES

It is not universally accepted that fixation by a nail and a screw is the most effective method. The compression hip screw, the use of which is described in the section on trochanteric fractures

(p. 268), is also a satisfactory device for fracture of the neck of the femur and is preferred by many surgeons. Alternative techniques include fixation by two nails or multiple pins, the use of a triangular system of pins (Smyth 1964), the use of a single low and very oblique nail (Garden 1961), and

fixation by a specially designed nail-plate in which the nail component is telescopic so that it may shorten if some degree of absorption occurs at the fracture site (Brown and Abrami 1964, Pugh 1955). For details of these techniques the original papers should be consulted.

NAIL-PLATE FIXATION FOR TROCHANTERIC FRACTURE OF FEMUR

Internal fixation by a nail-plate is appropriate for fractures in the trochanteric region (Fig. 353). In most cases there is some displacement in the form of lateral rotation and adduction of the lower fragment: reduction is therefore required before

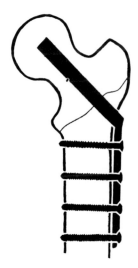

Fig. 353. Nail-plate for trochanteric fracture. A one-piece nail-plate should always be used in preference to a two-piece device. The nail should not penetrate further than shown: a margin is needed to allow for compaction of the fracture.

the fixation device is applied. Fixation by a one-piece nail-plate (for instance the Jewett type), or by a compression hip screw (described on p. 268), is recommended. The authors find no place for two-piece nail-plates, which frequently fail from loosening of the screw that joins the two pieces.

TECHNIQUE

The steps of this operation follow closely those for nail and screw fixation of femoral neck fractures (p. 260), the description of which should be read in conjunction with this section. Separate description is required here only in so far as the actual introduction of the nail-plate is concerned.

Setting up. The patient is placed on the orthopaedic table in exactly the same way as for nailing of a fracture of the femoral neck. The radiographic apparatus is also positioned in the same way.

Reduction. The displacement is nearly always reduced satisfactorily by strong manual traction on the limb, without any rotational force. Any

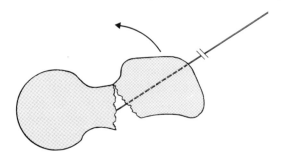

Fig. 354. The effect of excessive medial rotation of the femur in impeding the passage of the guide wire up the femoral neck. Excessive rotation opens up the fracture posteriorly, making accurate passage of the guide wire difficult.

medial rotation of the femoral shaft is liable to open up the fracture posteriorly. This angles the femoral shaft away from the femoral neck (Fig. 354). It is the commonest fault when there is difficulty in directing the guide wire into the femoral neck and head once it has been inserted through the lateral femoral cortex. After reduction of the fracture the foot is bandaged to the sole-plate of the orthopaedic table with the foot pointing directly upwards towards the ceiling. The reduction should be checked radiographically before the operation is commenced, and the opportunity should be taken to apply radio-opaque skin markers before the radiographs are taken; these serve to indicate the optimal direction of the guide wire.

The operation. The exposure is the same as described for nailing of a femoral neck fracture, except that a somewhat greater length of the femoral shaft should be exposed to accommodate the plate section of the fixation device. The first step after the bone is exposed is to insert a guide wire through a drill hole in the lateral cortex. The correct position of the wire is determined from the radio-opaque markers on the skin as shown in the post-reduction radiographs. The aim should be to pass the guide wire along the central axis of the femoral neck, though provided the wire is well within the neck a directional error of a few degrees is acceptable.

When the guide wire has been inserted (two or three may be introduced, if desired, in order to enhance the likelihood of one being in the optimal position), check radiographs are taken. If the position of the guide wire is not acceptable a fresh wire is introduced until a satisfactory placement has been made.

Selection of nail-plate. It is necessary next to calculate the appropriate angle and length of the nail-plate. The correct *angle* is selected by direct measurement on the radiograph with the guide wire in position. The appropriate *length* is determined in the same way as for nailing of the femoral neck. However, whereas in nailing the femoral neck it is necessary to drive the nail on so that its point lies quite close up to the articular surface, the nail-plate for a trochanteric fracture need not penetrate so far: an adequate grip is obtained even if the nail stops 2 centimetres short of the articular surface (Fig. 353). Indeed the length of the nail should be calculated to leave approximately this margin, for it often happens that when the nail is finally hammered home some impaction of the fracture occurs and the point of the nail penetrates further than was expected. Some "settling" may also occur after the operation, with the same consequence.

Insertion of nail-plate. The nail-plate is held on an introducer and the cannulated nail section is passed over the guide wire to bring the point into contact with the femoral cortex. If the cortex is hard it may be well to cut out notches to take the three flanges of the nail. During the introduction of the nail care must be taken to ensure that the plate section of the device lies parallel to the lateral cortex of the femoral shaft.

While the nail-plate is being hammered in over the guide wire it is necessary to make sure that the guide wire is not driven on with the nail, by measuring the length of wire protruding after each few hammer blows (see p. 264). If the guide wire is found to be penetrating the bone with the nail it must be withdrawn forthwith.

When the nail section of the nail-plate has been driven home the plate section should lie snugly against the shaft of the femur. Care must be taken to draw away any muscles that seem liable to get trapped between the plate and the bone. It is convenient then to clamp the plate firmly to the bone with a Lowman's clamp while appropriate drill holes are made through both cortices of the femur opposite the holes in the plate. Screws of appropriate length are then driven in (Fig. 353).

Closure. The reflected part of the vastus lateralis is tucked back into the posterior part of the wound and anchored with one or two light absorbable sutures. The fascia lata and the tensor fasciae latae muscle are repaired carefully with interrupted sutures. The skin is closed without drainage: deep tension sutures are useful in reducing the risk of haematoma.

POST-OPERATIVE MANAGEMENT

Splintage is not required: the patient is allowed to move freely in bed. Walking with elbow crutches is encouraged from the day after the operation. The nail-plate should be strong enough to permit virtually full weight bearing without risk of failure.

Comment

It is worth emphasising again that there is nothing to be gained from using a two-piece nail-plate. A one-piece nail-plate is applied more quickly and more easily than a two-piece one, and it does not entail the hazard of loosening at the junction of nail and plate. In fact it must be stated unequivocably that a two-piece nail-plate has virtually no place in fracture surgery.

Another important point to note is that it is a mistake to drive the nail too close to the articular surface of the femoral head. Penetration of the hip joint by the point of the nail is all too frequent, but it can be avoided if a suitable margin—perhaps 2 centimetres—is left between the point of the nail and the articular surface.

Patients with trochanteric fractures are usually old and frail, and in these cases particularly it is very important that the patient be got walking at the earliest possible moment. A patient who has

been fit enough to walk before the fracture should always be got up and encouraged to take weight on the leg on the day after operation. Nothing is to be gained by delay. But there is much to be lost because these elderly patients take progressively longer to rehabilitate with every day that is spent in bed.

For aged patients with soft bone, or indeed for any patient with a trochanteric fracture, consideration should be given to the use of a compression hip screw as an alternative to a nail-plate. This is described in the section that follows.

FIXATION OF TROCHANTERIC FRACTURE BY COMPRESSION SCREW

Sliding nail-plates—in which a three-flanged nail is free to slide telescopically in a barrel formed in one piece with a plate screwed to the lateral aspect of the femur—have been used for many years in

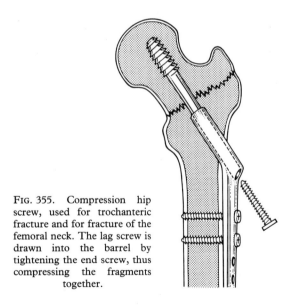

FIG. 355. Compression hip screw, used for trochanteric fracture and for fracture of the femoral neck. The lag screw is drawn into the barrel by tightening the end screw, thus compressing the fragments together.

the treatment both of fractures of the neck of the femur and of trochanteric fractures (Brown and Abrami 1964, Pugh 1955). The device that is now

used most commonly, however, is the so-called hip compression screw or "dynamic" hip screw— in reality a fracture compression screw. This comprises a lag screw designed to engage the femoral head, sliding in a barrel which, like the older devices, is directed into the base of the femoral neck and is fixed to the outer aspect of the upper femur by means of a plate integral with the barrel (Fig. 355). There is a choice of length of the lag screw and of the barrel, and also of the length of the plate. There is also a choice of angle between the plate and the barrel, though the anatomical angle of 135 degrees is commonly used. There is provision for the application of compression across the fracture by a screw device. The device may be used for fractures of the neck of the femur as well as for trochanteric fractures.

Several patterns of compression hip screw are available, including the much favoured "dynamic" screw of the A.O. system.

TECHNIQUE

Setting up of the patient on the orthopaedic table and arrangement of the radiographic equipment are the same as in the operation for fixation of a trochanteric fracture by a nail-plate as described in the previous section. The preliminary stages of the operation, up to the insertion of a guide wire, are also the same and need not be repeated here. Certain special instruments to facilitate the insertion of the device are available and should be at hand. The main steps in the operation are as follows.

Guide wire. A special ($\frac{1}{8}$-inch) guide wire is used, and a template is available to ensure that the correct angle between the guide wire and the femoral shaft (usually 135 degrees) is achieved. The aim should be to place the guide wire centrally in the neck, both in the antero-posterior and in the lateral plane. Slight deviation downwards towards the calcar and backwards towards the trochanter is acceptable. Some surgeons recommend driving the guide wire across the hip joint into the ilium, in order to obviate the tendency of the guide wire to be extruded during the later stages of the operation.

Reaming of channel for lag screw. The special cannulated reamer is slid over the guide wire and driven on through the femoral neck into the head. Penetration of the reamer should be checked radiographically: it should penetrate to within a centimetre of the articular surface, or somewhat less far in the case of a trochanteric fracture.

Reaming of channel for barrel. A reamer of wider diameter is supplied to create a channel for the barrel of the device. This also slides over the guide wire. The reamer should penetrate 2.5 to 3.5 centimetres from the lateral cortex of the femur.

Insertion of lag screw. With the special holder provided, the lag screw is passed over the guide wire through the wide channel at the base of the femoral neck to enter the cancellous bone of the upper part of the neck and the femoral head. The length of the lag screw should be such that it may be driven with certainty beyond the fracture site. For fracture of the trochanteric region a rather longer threaded portion may be used than in the case of a transcervical fracture, for which a short threaded part is required. Progress of penetration of the screw is checked radiographically.

Insertion of barrel/plate. A barrel/plate of the correct angle (determined before the operation and usually 135 degrees) and of appropriate plate length is now inserted into the prepared channel, care being taken to ensure that the plate part lies in line with the outer surface of the femur. As the device is hammered in, the plate should come in contact with the femoral cortex, to which it will be fixed by screws.

Compression of fracture by screw device. When the lag screw and the barrel have been assembled within the bone in the manner described, the compression screw is driven in to engage the stem of the lag screw and is tightened judiciously to give some degree of compression across the fracture. It is important not to over-tighten the screw, lest the threads of the lag screw pull through the bone, prejudicing the fixation.

Closure. After removal of the guide wire and fixation of the plate to the femur by screws, the wound is closed in layers in the manner already described for fracture of the femoral neck.

POST-OPERATIVE MANAGEMENT

Gauze dressings are held in place either with an adhesive pad or with a crepe bandage. The patient lies free in bed and is encouraged to carry out gentle flexion and extension exercises for the hip and knee. Within a day or two, the patient is allowed out of bed with the support of elbow crutches, a proportion of the body weight being taken on the affected limb. Subsequent management is the same as for nail-plate fixation of a trochanteric fracture, as described in the previous section.

Comment

For trochanteric fractures this method is an alternative to the well tried method of fixation by a nail-plate. The compression hip screw seems to offer certain advantages over a nail-plate, and has been adopted at most centres in preference to it. In particular, the lag screw, properly inserted, is capable of obtaining a better grip of the femoral head than does a simple three-flanged nail or nail-plate; and the sliding mechanism allows for "settling" or compaction at the fracture site, which in the case of a nail-plate may cause the nail to penetrate across the hip joint. Comparative studies (Heyse-Moore, MacEachern and Jameson Evans 1983) have tended to show that the use of the compression hip screw is attended by fewer complications than is fixation by a nail-plate.

Note on the Use of the
A.O. Dynamic Hip Screw

The setting up of the patient on the orthopaedic table is as described in the previous sections. When radiographic viewing shows that the fracture has been accurately reduced, the guide wire is inserted. The 135-degree wire guide ensures that the wire will be inserted at the correct angle to fit the barrel of the plate. Usually the guide wire enters the lateral side of the femur 5 centimetres below the tip of the greater trochanter. If the entry point of the wire is faulty the screw cannot be properly placed.

The guide wire is driven in until it is 5 millimetres from the articular surface of the femoral head. The backward-reading measure is then applied over the wire. The distance read off on the scale is the length of wire that is within the bone.

It is essential that the guide wire is central in the femoral neck both in the antero-posterior and in the lateral plane. If it is not central the screw may be so far off to one side that it penetrates the cortex. If the screw is placed too high in the femoral head the load on the head will be uneven and the head may move, allowing the screw to cut out and damage the lateral part of the acetabulum.

The reamer is now set to the distance shown on the backward-reading measure. Power reaming is used. The reamer enlarges the hole in the lateral femoral cortex to receive the barrel of the plate. The special tap is then used to cut the threads in the bone for the screw. From the measure on the tap sleeve the correct length of screw is chosen. If the bone is strikingly porotic a screw 5 millimetres longer may be substituted: this will allow a better

hold in the bone of the femoral head.

The chosen screw is inserted into the tap sleeve and screwed into the bone. The screw itself has two flats machined on its side. These fit into the tap sleeve to prevent rotation of the screw in the tap sleeve during insertion. When the screw is inserted it is important that the handle of the tap sleeve be held parallel with the femoral shaft: otherwise the flats on the side of the hip screw will not match up with the flats machined on the inner side of the barrel of the plate.

When the screw has been inserted, the plate is located over the lateral aspect of the femur and knocked home. Usually a four-hole plate is chosen to give a strong hold on the femur. Screws are driven home in the usual way after preparation of threaded tracks with the appropriate tap. Care should be taken to select a tap with long enough thread to pass right through the femur. If an unthreaded part of a tap is inserted it is liable to break at the junction of threaded and unthreaded parts, and the fragment in the bone may be very difficult to remove.

The final step in the fixation is to compress the screw into the barrel of the plate. A special compression screw with a fine thread is supplied in the instrument set for this purpose. When the screw has been tightened firmly it may be removed. In a frail and feeble patient, however, the screw may legitimately be left in place, when it acts as part of the implant.

POST-OPERATIVE MANAGEMENT

The patient may be mobilised with full weight bearing as soon as the general condition allows. If impaction occurs at the fracture site, the screw slides in the barrel of the implant and does not penetrate the femoral head as it may do in the case of a fixed appliance.

It is not usual to remove the implant. In some patients, however, there is complaint of discomfort on lying on the affected side and it is then wise to remove the metal, provided that the fracture is fully consolidated. A special extraction screw is passed down the inserter to ensure that the hip screw is withdrawn from the femoral neck.

HALF-JOINT REPLACEMENT ARTHROPLASTY OF HIP

(FEMORAL HEAD REPLACEMENT)

This operation evolved from the early arthroplasty devised by Judet and Judet (1949, 1950) in which the femoral head was replaced by a plastic (methyl methacrylate) prosthesis. Moore (1957) introduced a metal head with curved stem entering the medullary canal of the femur, as likewise

TECHNIQUE

Position of patient. The patient lies in the true lateral position with the affected hip uppermost. The limb of the affected side is supported upon a platform so that it lies in line with the trunk (Fig. 356).

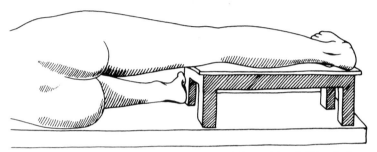

FIG. 356. Position of patient for replacement of femoral head. The platform allows the affected limb to lie in the neutral position and it facilitates exposure of the hip by the postero-lateral route.

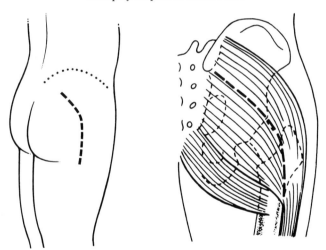

FIGS 357–358. Figure 357—Skin incision for postero-lateral exposure of hip. Figure 358—The gluteus maximus is split in the direction of its fibres. The dotted outline shows the underlying bones.

did Thompson (1952, 1954). The technique was further modified to include fixation of the prosthesis by cement (Charnley 1960). The operation is used mainly for fractures of the femoral neck that are unsuitable for nailing or in which nailing has failed, the proviso being that the articular cartilage of the acetabulum must be healthy.

Exposure. The Austin Moore or "Southern" exposure is used. This was described on page 34. The incision begins in the gluteal region 5 centimetres below and in front of the posterior superior spine of the ilium. Thence it extends to the front of the greater trochanter, where it turns vertically downwards over the line of the femur for 10 centimetres or so, depending upon the build of the patient (Fig. 357).

The gluteus maximus is split in the direction of its fibres (Fig. 358) and the margins are retracted to reveal the short transverse muscles of the hip, obturator internus and the gemelli. These muscles, and if necessary the piriformis, are divided close to their insertions and reflected backwards: they thus protect the sciatic nerve (Fig. 360). The back of the joint capsule is thus

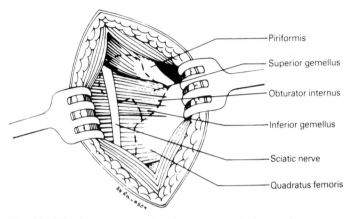

FIG. 359. The short transverse lateral rotator muscles deep to the gluteus maximus. Note that the sciatic nerve lies upon the superficial aspect of the obturator internus, gemelli, and quadratus femoris, but deep to the piriformis.

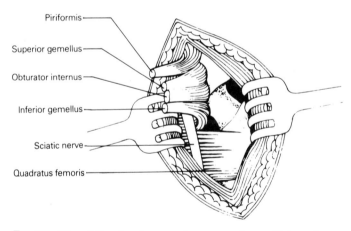

FIG. 360. The piriformis, obturator internus and gemelli have been divided close to the greater trochanter and reflected backwards, thus protecting the sciatic nerve. (In most cases sufficient access can be gained without reflecting the piriformis.) The neck of the femur is seen on a deeper plane.

namely from below upwards the quadratus femoris, the obturator internus and gemelli, and the piriformis. The sciatic nerve lies superficial to the quadratus femoris, obturator internus and gemelli but passes deep to the piriformis (Fig. 359).

Non-absorbable stay sutures are inserted in the exposed, and the capsule is opened close to the greater trochanter.

Removal of femoral head. When the capsule has been opened the fracture of the femoral neck is brought into view. If a nail has been inserted at a previous operation this is now removed. The limb is then rotated medially by an assistant to bring the stump of the femoral neck away from the head fragment, which may then be removed from the acetabulum either entire or, if more convenient, piecemeal.

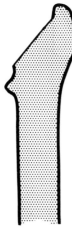

FIG. 361. The femoral head and neck have been removed after division of the bone obliquely at the base of the neck. The plane of section should match the inclination of the collar of the prosthesis, and it should allow for 20 degrees of anteversion of the prosthesis.

Selection of prosthetic head. At this stage the size of the prosthetic head required is determined either from measurement of the diameter of the original head (if it is sufficiently well preserved) or from direct measurement of the acetabulum by a caliper or by graded templates. Total reliance should not be placed on measurements alone, however: selection of the correct size of prosthetic head is so important that a trial fit must be made. A correctly sized prosthesis fits snugly into the socket without any play and yet moves freely. The fit should be so exact that a strong pull is required to overcome the vacuum when the trial prosthesis is removed.

Preparation of track in femur. The chosen prosthesis is now laid upon the surface of the medially rotated femur in a position parallel to that which it will occupy within the bone. This allows the line of section of the stump of the femoral neck to be marked out. The neck must be severed close to the intertrochanteric line, and the plane of section should conform to that of the flange or collar of the prosthesis where the stem joins the neck (Fig. 361). The bone cut is made either with a chisel or with a powered reciprocating saw. It is

important at this stage to allow for preservation of the normal angle of anteversion of the femoral neck of 15 or 20 degrees: thus the cut surface should incline a little forwards as well as medially.

When the stump of the femoral neck has thus been trimmed off at the correct level and in the correct plane, a track for the stem of the prosthesis is prepared in the upper part of the medullary canal. It may be helpful to make the initial slotted opening in the cancellous bone of the stump of the femur with a chisel. This initial slot should be carefully positioned to ensure that the femoral head will lie in the correct angle of anteversion.

Once the initial starting slot has been formed, the medullary canal is probed with a curved bone lever or similar slightly curved instrument with which the surgeon may feel the interior of the femoral shaft and may thus be sure that the cortex is not inadvertently perforated. When the medullary canal has thus been located and probed, the opening is enlarged by means of a serrated or toothed broach of the type made for this purpose. The broach has the general shape of the stem of a femoral head prosthesis; and by repeated light blows upon it with a mallet, and by reciprocal movements in the manner of a file, the track is gradually enlarged sufficiently to take the prosthesis (Fig. 407, page 302).

Making a trial fit. Before the femoral head prosthesis is cemented into the femur it is well to drive it in to its final planned position and then to reduce the artificial head into the acetabulum in order to test the assembly both for correct tension and for free mobility. If the tension is correct—that is, if the prosthesis has been driven the right distance into the femur—reduction will be accomplished without difficulty and the tip of the greater trochanter will lie approximately at the level of the centre of the femoral head as in the normal hip (Fig. 362). If this is the case the surgeon may be sure that the length of the limb will be unaltered. If the prosthesis has been inserted correctly, with due regard to the need for anteversion of 15 to 20 degrees, free mobility through a wide range of flexion, abduction, adduction and rotation should be demonstrated.

Cementing in the prosthesis. If these preliminary tests prove satisfactory the next step is to press the fully mixed acrylic cement firmly into the medullary canal of the upper femur—preferably by

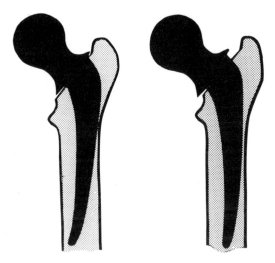

FIGS 362–363. Figure 362—Femoral head prosthesis correctly inserted. The stem has entered the cut surface of the bone high up, towards the greater trochanter, and has been seated in a valgus position, the tip of the stem resting upon the medial cortex of the femur. Note also that the centre of the femoral head is approximately level with the tip of the greater trochanter, as in the normal femur. This ensures normal length of the limb. Figure 363—Prosthesis incorrrectly inserted. It enters too low down on the cut surface of the femur and is leaning over too much into varus.

means of a ratchet-operated cement gun—and then before the cement sets to drive in the definitive prosthesis to the predetermined level.

To enable the cement to pass down the medullary canal it is well to insert a fine (size 8) polythene catheter into the canal for a distance of 10 centimetres or so in order to provide a vent for the exit of air. The catheter is removed just before the femoral head prosthesis is introduced and hammered home.

As the prosthesis is being driven in, care should again be taken to see that it takes up the desired position of anteversion. It should also be positioned in slight valgus rather than in varus—in other words the tip of the stem should be in contact with the medial wall of the femoral shaft rather than with the lateral cortex (Figs 362 and 363). Excess cement that is squeezed out of the

canal is cut away before it hardens, and care should be taken to remove any loose pieces of cement. The acetabulum having finally been wiped clean, the head is reduced into it.

Closure. If the capsule has been preserved it may be closed with two or three light absorbable sutures. The divided posterior transverse muscles (obturator internus and gemelli and sometimes piriformis) are turned back into place and sutured to the remaining soft tissues close to the posterior margin of the greater trochanter. The gluteal aponeurosis where it blends with the fascia lata is the important layer and must be sutured securely with strong interrupted sutures. The skin is closed with deep tension sutures and eversion mattress sutures, usually without drainage.

POST-OPERATIVE MANAGEMENT

At the conclusion of the operation a wedge-shaped pillow is placed between the patient's legs and attached by loosely closed Velcro straps to restrain the legs. The pillow is kept in place for two to four days while the patient is at rest in bed. It prevents excessive flexion or adduction at the hip during the early post-operative period: either of these movements may lead to dislocation of the hip. An alternative method of preventing dislocation is by means of a removable knee splint of plaster or plastic, fitted at the conclusion of the operation. By restricting knee flexion the splint also restricts hip flexion. Some patients find this less irksome than an abduction pillow.

Standing and walking (without any restraining harness) are begun on the day after operation, with the aid of elbow crutches. Hip and knee flexion exercises are encouraged under supervision, and the patient may sit out of bed for most of the day.

Comment

The three main essentials are: first, to select a prosthesis of the correct head diameter: second, to maintain correct length of the femur; and third, to preserve the normal slight anteversion of the femoral head.

It is a mistake to undertake this operation unless

a full range of prostheses of all sizes is available. Too loose a fit of the artificial head in the acetabulum leads to a localised pressure area with risk of damage to articular cartilage and eventual "wandering" of the prosthesis.

Preservation of correct femoral length is dependent upon sectioning the stump of the femoral neck close to the trochanteric line and seating the prosthesis well down. Otherwise it is easy to end up with a femur that is too long. The articulation is then unduly tight and movement may be restricted. In a femur of normal length the tip of the greater trochanter is approximately level with the centre of the femoral head. This is a useful guide, and it is well to ensure that this criterion is met when a trial fit of the prosthesis is made.

Post-operative dislocation is not to be feared if the operation is carried out as described, but the use of a triangular pillow or temporary splintage of the knee is regarded as an important precaution that should not be neglected.

Early walking may safely be encouraged with full confidence: indeed it is a mistake to confine the patient to bed, especially if she is elderly.

ALTERNATIVE PROSTHESES

A disadvantage of replacement of the femoral head by a one-piece prosthesis is that the unresilient metal head may bear unevenly against the acetabulum, with consequent progressive erosion of cartilage and bone at the point of contact—the so-called "wandering acetabulum". Erosion is particularly liable to occur if the prosthetic femoral head is not a close fit in the acetabulum—that is, if it is too small, favouring point contact. Erosion is often associated with increasing pain and disability, which may necessitate further operation, usually in the form of total replacement arthroplasty.

Attempts to eliminate this complication have centred on the development of an alternative to the one-piece metal prosthesis in the form of a two-piece articulated prosthesis incorporating semi-resilient high density polyethylene. The

device, often termed the bipolar prosthesis, consists of a relatively small metallic spherical femoral head component with stem of the usual dimensions, moving within a cup of high density polyethylene which in turn is contained in an outer metal cup (Fig. 364). The outer cup is sup-

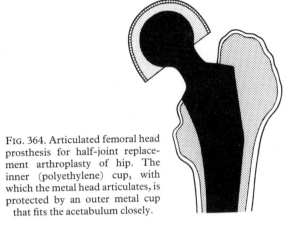

FIG. 364. Articulated femoral head prosthesis for half-joint replacement arthroplasty of hip. The inner (polyethylene) cup, with which the metal head articulates, is protected by an outer metal cup that fits the acetabulum closely.

plied in finely graduated sizes so that a very close fit in the acetabulum can be assured.

The use of a double articulation of this type offers a number of possible advantages. Firstly, movement of the femoral component within the outer cup may largely take the place of movement of the cup in the acetabulum. Secondly, the polyethylene insert, being slightly resilient, may reduce or eliminate pressure erosion of the cartilaginous lining of the true acetabulum. And thirdly, the femoral component may be constructed to such a size that, in the event of an unsuccessful outcome, it may be retained at a subsequent revision operation, and after removal of the outer cup a matching polyethylene socket may be cemented into the acetabulum to create a total replacement arthroplasty.

Various prostheses of this type, each with individual design features, have been under trial, but the conclusions are somewhat conflicting (Devas and Hinves 1983, Scales 1983, Verberne 1983).

With regard to technique of insertion, bipolar prostheses do not present any special problem: they are inserted in the manner described above for replacement by a Thompson prosthesis.

OPEN REDUCTION OF CONGENITAL DISLOCATION OF THE HIP

The description that follows applies to children of about 1 to 3 years of age. The aims of the operation are to ascertain what structure, if any, is preventing full reduction of the femoral head into the socket, and to ensure that the femoral head is placed centrally in the acetabulum by clearing away any such obstruction. At the same time the opportunity should be taken to assess the angle of anteversion of the femoral neck.

TECHNIQUE

Position of patient. The child is placed upon the table in the supine posture. The whole limb is prepared and draped with a stockingette tube so that it may be manoeuvred as required during the operation.

Exposure. Somerville's (1978) modification of the anterior (Smith-Petersen) approach to the hip is recommended. To avoid ugly scarring the skin incision is placed transversely, with its centre 1.5 or 2 centimetres below the anterior superior spine of the ilium. The skin edges are retracted proximally and distally, and the space between the sartorius muscle medially and the tensor fasciae latae muscle laterally is opened up. To improve the access the anterior 2 centimetres of the tensor fasciae latae muscle may be divided close to the crest of the ilium and the muscle displaced backwards.

The anterior margin of the iliac bone is next followed distally from the anterior superior spine to reveal the rectus muscle with its direct head arising from the anterior inferior spine and the reflected head arising more laterally from the ilium above the margin of the acetabulum. It is important to clean away fatty and areolar tissue in order that the rectus femoris muscle be clearly defined. Deep to the rectus will be found the glistening white capsule of the hip joint, and the rectus may be divided as necessary to bring the whole capsule clearly into view. At this stage a bone lever may be inserted medially between the capsule and the rectus femoris to hold the rectus and the medial structures out of the way.

Exploration of joint. The joint capsule is incised longitudinally and by cross cuts at right angles to the first incision proximally and distally, in H-pattern. The anterior and posterior flaps of capsule are retracted by holding stitches. Within, the glistening articular cartilage of the femoral head comes into view.

In most cases the head rests in either the subluxated or the fully dislocated position, and it is necessary to examine the interior of the joint carefully, firstly to locate the true acetabulum and secondly to elucidate the nature of any obstructing tissue.

In order to find the true acetabulum the femoral head must be manoeuvred out of the way: as it lies, it usually obstructs a clear view of the acetabulum. The true acetabulum is usually best revealed by flexing the hip through 90 degrees and then retracting the femoral head proximally and rotating it medially or laterally as appropriate. It is important at this stage to distinguish clearly between the shallow false acetabulum, in which the femoral head frequently lies, and the true acetabulum which is much deeper and lower. If the true acetabulum is not immediately visible even when the femoral head has been manoeuvred out of the way, it may be identified by exploration with a freshly gloved little finger. The true acetabulum can also be found by identifying the ligamentum teres and following it downwards to its origin in the floor of the true acetabulum. Once the position of the true acetabulum has been established it can be exposed to view by appropriate enlargement of the opening in the capsule or by further manoeuvring of the femur and retraction of the femoral head. The socket may then be cleared of any enclosed fat so that the articular cartilage is clearly revealed.

At this stage a thorough inspection of the cavity will reveal any obstructing agent that might prevent full reduction of the femoral head. Often the acetabular labrum—that is, the fibro-cartilaginous rim of the acetabulum often referred to as the limbus—is found to have become inturned so that it lies in contact with the articular cartilage round a considerable part of the circumference of the socket (Fig. 365). In this state the labrum is somewhat flattened against the inner wall of the socket and it has a resemblance to a meniscus of the knee joint. In some cases this inverted labrum is suffi-

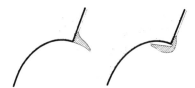

FIG. 365. Diagram to show the normal position of the acetabular labrum (limbus) (*left*) and an inturned labrum (*right*).

ciently bulky to prevent the femoral head from entering the socket to its full depth, as may be demonstrated by a trial reduction. Occasionally some other structure may be found to obstruct full reduction—for instance, an excessively bulky ligament of the femoral head (ligamentum teres).

Dealing with inturned acetabular labrum (limbus). If the labrum is found to be inturned and obstructing full reduction of the femoral head into the acetabulum it is probably best to excise it, though opinion at some centres would favour attempting to evert the labrum from the acetabulum so that it may act as a fringe round the rim of the socket, effectively deepening it as in the normal state.

Excision of the limbus does not present difficulty, provided a clear view of the components of the joint has been obtained. A small blunt hook passed into the acetabulum beyond the inturned labrum is used to lift the inturned edge of the labrum towards the operator, so that with a fine knife it may then be detached peripherally from the margin of the acetabulum, rather in the manner in which a meniscus of the knee is separated from its peripheral attachment.

Other causes of incomplete reduction. If the acetabular labrum or "limbus" does not seem to be the cause of obstruction, other possible sources of difficulty in reduction should be sought and removed. A voluminous ligament of the femoral head (ligamentum teres) may rarely be responsible. Sometimes tightness of the psoas tendon may

hinder reduction, and if so there should be no hesitation in dividing the tendon.

Determining the position of stability. Once full reduction of the femoral head deeply into the true acetabulum has been achieved it is necessary to find out in which position of the hip the reduction

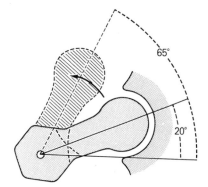

FIG. 366. Diagrammatic section of left hip, as seen from above. In normal infants the angle of anteversion is not more than 20 or 25 degrees (solid line). Excessive anteversion (interrupted line) predisposes to instability and may need to be corrected.

is most stable. Often two positions are stable: the "frog" position of abduction and full lateral rotation; and a position of abduction and medial rotation. At this stage the object is simply to ascertain which positions provide stability; other factors come into the final choice of position for immobilisation (see below).

Assessing anteversion of femoral neck. Before the wound is closed it is important to study the orientation of the femoral neck in relation to the rest of the femur, in order to note the angle of anteversion. This angle is best assessed by bending the knee to a right angle so that the tibia may be used to indicate the posterior aspect of the femur: the coronal plane is at right angles to this, and the angle of anteversion is the angle between the coronal plane and the axis of the femoral neck. In the normal hip in children the neck is directed 20 to 25 degrees anterior to the coronal plane. In congenital dislocation of the hip the angle of anteversion is often far in excess of the normal (Fig. 366), sometimes nearing 90 degrees, so that the head faces almost directly forwards. If excessive ante-version is found it may suggest the need for rotation osteotomy later.

Closure. The incision in the joint capsule is closed with fine absorbable sutures and the wound is closed in layers without drainage.

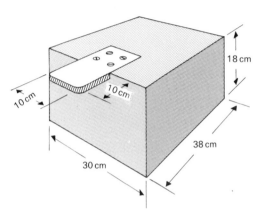

FIG. 367. Easily made support to facilitate application of plaster spica after reduction of congenital dislocation of hip.

POST-OPERATIVE MANAGEMENT

At the conclusion of the operation the lower trunk and the limbs are encased in plaster-of-Paris. The position of the limbs is a matter of individual

"frog" plaster with the hip abducted 90 degrees and laterally rotated 90 degrees, but most, with whom the authors concur, have rejected it on the grounds that it may endanger the blood supply to the femoral head, with consequent risk of Perthes-like changes, and prefer a position of moderate abduction and medial rotation (Batchelor 1951). The plaster is most easily applied if a special box support is made (Fig. 367).

The duration of immobilisation in plaster also depends upon the preference of the individual surgeon. Many would agree that if excessive ante-version has been found—as is usually the case—rotation osteotomy of the upper end of the femur (p. 279) should be undertaken four weeks or so after the open reduction, as recommended by Somerville (1953) and by Somerville and Scott (1957). Thereafter a plaster need be retained only until the osteotomy is united—usually a matter of about six weeks.

Comment

Although the anterior approach described here is usually adequate, nevertheless in cases of special difficulty—for instance, when there have been previous unsuccessful attempts to replace the femoral head in the acetabulum—the McFarland-Osborne postero-lateral exposure (p. 33) offers material advantages, for it enables the hip to be approached both from in front and from behind.

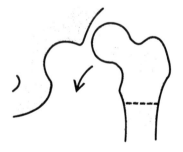 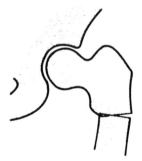

FIGS 368–369. In older children the femoral head may have to be turned down by adduction osteotomy just below the greater trochanter to enable the head to enter the true acetabulum. Alternatively the femur may be shortened at the upper end of the shaft.

preference, for the hip is usually stable both in the laterally rotated (frog) position and in the medially rotated position. Some surgeons still use the

The main essential in the operation is to persist until a clear view of the true acetabulum is gained. Until the position of the acetabulum has been established with certainty it is impossible to identify the nature of any structure that is preventing full reduction. The view of the acetabulum is often impeded by the femoral head itself, but by manoeuvring it into flexion or applying traction and rotation it is possible to get the head out of the way. As noted above, it is sometimes easier in the first instance to locate the true socket by feel rather than by inspection, or by following the ligamentum teres to its origin within the socket. When the socket has been found, the next essential is not to rest until the femoral head is seen to be stable within it.

In older children, 5 or 6 years of age, reduction may be prevented simply by the impossibility of bringing the head low enough to enter the true acetabulum even after division of the psoas tendon. A useful plan then is to divide the femur just below the greater trochanter and to turn the head downwards into varus (Figs 368 and 369). This will usually allow it to enter the acetabulum. Thereafter the osteotomy is fixed with a miniature nail-plate. Alternatively, the femur may be shortened by removal of a section of bone in the subtrochanteric region.

In the after-treatment, the problem of the

"frog" position versus the medially rotated position is still raised and each has its protagonists. Observations suggest, however, that the "frog" position is followed by avascular changes in the femoral head epiphysis much more often than is immobilisation in medial rotation. This is one important reason for preferring the position of medial rotation. Probably the important point is that the extreme limit of either position should be avoided, for extreme rotation either laterally or medially can be shown to constrict the capsular blood vessels.

If anteversion is found to be excessive, it is worth considering whether rotation osteotomy should be carried out at the same time as open reduction. The authors consider, however, that the combined operation is rather too big an undertaking in a small child: they prefer after reduction to immobilise the hip in moderate medial rotation and to undertake rotation osteotomy at a separate operation about four weeks later. In an older child, if varus osteotomy has been necessary in order to bring the femoral head down into the acetabulum the opportunity may be taken to correct anteversion at the same time.

ROTATION OSTEOTOMY OF UPPER END OF FEMUR

The description that follows relates to the operation as carried out in children, usually about 2 years old and usually suffering from excessive anteversion of the femoral neck in association with congenital dislocation of the hip. Similar principles apply to the operation in older children and in adults. The operation to be described is that of lateral rotation of the distal fragment relative to the proximal fragment. Only rarely is rotation in the opposite direction required.

PRELIMINARY STUDIES

It is important to decide before the operation what degree of rotational correction is required. If there has been a previous operation for open reduction of a congenitally dislocated hip the degree of ante-

version will have been noted by direct inspection at the time. If not, reliance must be placed upon estimates based on radiological studies. Radiological methods of determining the angle of anteversion have been described by Dunn (1952) and by Harris (1965). These methods may be a useful guide, but it is difficult to ensure reliable results. As an alternative, antero-posterior radiographs may be taken with the limb rotated medially through 45 degrees and through 60 degrees as well as is the neutral position. If there is marked anteversion, the contour of the upper end of the femur in a film taken with the limb in neutral rotation will suggest a valgus inclination of the femoral neck: in other words the neck-shaft angle appears excessive. This appearance is due to foreshortening of the anteverted femoral neck. In contrast, a film taken with the limb rotated medially will show the neck-shaft angle closer to the normal (Figs 370 and 371). Comparison of the radiographs taken with the limb in, say, 45 degrees of medial rotation and 60 degrees of

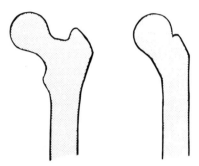

FIGS 370–371. Effect of anteversion on radiographic outline of femoral neck, as seen in antero-posterior projections. Figure 370—Normal profile with limb in neutral anatomical position. Figure 371—Fore-shortening of neck due to anteversion, giving an appearance of valgus inclination. In such a case the outline can be restored to that of Figure 370 by rotating the limb medially.

medial rotation with true antero-posterior radiographs of a normal child of the same age will indicate which rotational position of the upper end of the femur brings the neck-shaft angle most nearly to the normal. This may then be taken as the approximate degree of excessive anteversion, and the rotational correction should be planned accordingly.

TECHNIQUE

The plan is to divide the femur 2 to 3 centimetres below the lesser trochanter, and after the appropriate rotational adjustment has been made to fix the fragments with a four-hole plate.

Position of patient. The child lies supine with a small sandbag under the buttock of the affected side to roll the body slightly towards the opposite side. This brings the greater trochanter of the affected limb into prominence. It is not practicable to use a tourniquet.

Incision. The incision is a vertical one in the mid-lateral plane. It extends distally from the lateral prominence of the greater trochanter for about 8 centimetres.

Exposure of femur. The incision is deepened through the fat to reveal the fascia lata in the distal half of the wound and, continuous with it more

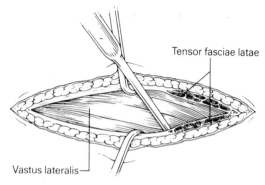

FIG. 372. Seeking the posterior edge of the vastus lateralis after incision of the fascia lata and tensor fasciae latae muscle.

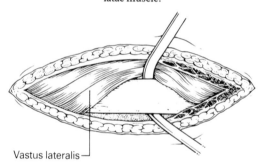

FIG. 373. The vastus lateralis muscle has been levered forwards to expose the femur.

proximally, the tensor fasciae latae muscle. The muscle and fascia are incised vertically in the line of the skin incision and the fibres are separated to expose the vastus lateralis muscle. Rather than divide this, it is better to seek its posterior margin with a curved bone lever and to lift the muscle forwards (Fig. 372). The bone lever is then manoeuvred over the front of the femoral shaft in order to hold the muscle well forward out of the way (Fig. 373). Any remaining muscle fibres overlying the lateral aspect of the femur are now divided by a vertical cut down to the bone. The incision divides also the periosteum, which should be stripped sufficiently from the femur to allow curved bone levers to be inserted round the bone anteriorly and posteriorly. In this way an appropriate length of the upper part of the femoral shaft is presented for the osteotomy and for the subsequent plating procedure. The upper limit of the cleared area of bone should be at about the point where the greater trochanter begins to flare outwards from the shaft.

Selection of site for osteotomy, and insertion of indicator wires. The first step is to mark lightly on the surface of the femur the level selected for the osteotomy. This should be about in the middle of the exposed length of bone, or 3 to 4 centimetres distal to the outward flare of the greater trochanter.

Next, two guide wires are inserted into the shaft of the femur at right angles to it, one wire being proximal to the proposed line of osteotomy and the other distal to it. The proximal guide wire is directed horizontally—that is, in the coronal plane. The distal wire is entered more anteriorly and is directed postero-medially, in such a way that the angle subtended by the two wires is equal to the proposed angle of rotational correction (Fig. 374). The vertical distance between the guide wires where they enter the bone must be equal to the distance between the two inner holes of the four-hole plate that will be used for internal fixation: this is important because the guide wire holes will be used later for two of the screws that will hold the plate (Figs 375 and 376). Each guide wire must be driven just through, but not beyond, the far cortex of the femur (Fig. 374).

The purpose of the two guide wires is to control the proximal and distal fragments of the femur after it has been divided, and to indicate the angle of rotational correction. Since the wires have been inserted in such a way that the angle between them equals the proposed angle of correction, it follows that if after division of the bone the distal fragment is rotated laterally until the wires are parallel, then the degree of correction will automatically be correct.

Division of femoral shaft. The femur is now divided transversely at the site already marked. In

a young child the bone is relatively soft and it may easily be divided either with a thin sharp osteotome or by a combination of fine-pointed bone-cutting forceps and an osteotome. It is important

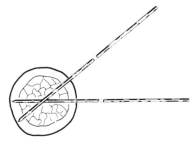

FIG. 374. Rotation osteotomy. Guide wires, one above and one below the site of osteotomy, subtend the required angle of rotation.

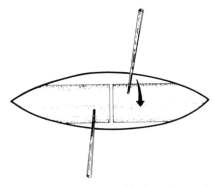

FIG. 375. After division of the bone the distal fragment is rotated laterally to bring the wires parallel.

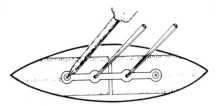

FIG. 376. The plate is slipped over the guide wires, the tracks of which serve for the inner two screws.

to divide the bone cleanly without leaving any projecting spurs.

When the osteotomy is complete the distal fragment of the femur—in other words the lower limb as a whole—is rotated laterally in relation to the proximal fragment, which may be counter-rotated medially. Each fragment is well controlled by handling the protruding guide wire. When rotation has been sufficient to bring the wires parallel it remains only to fix the position with a plate and screws.

Application of plate. The selected four-hole plate is slid down over the protruding guide wires, each of which should engage one of the inner two holes of the plate (Fig. 376). The plate may then be clamped in position upon the bone with a sequestrum forceps or fine bone-holding forceps. Since the inner two holes of the plate are occupied by the guide wires the end holes are used for the first two screws. Through these holes the bone is drilled, and self-tapping screws of appropriate length are driven home. Each guide wire is then removed in turn and replaced by a screw.

Closure. The vastus lateralis muscle is allowed to fall back into position and the fascia lata and tensor fasciae latae muscle are repaired with interrupted sutures. The skin is closed without drainage.

POST-OPERATIVE MANAGEMENT

A plaster-of-Paris hip spica enclosing the affected limb down to and including the foot is retained until the osteotomy is united—usually a matter of four to eight weeks, depending upon the age of the child. In small children walking may be deferred until the plaster is removed. In older children walking with crutches may be encouraged earlier.

Comment

The use of guide wires to indicate the desired angle of correction in the manner described is strongly recommended. It ensures that the surgeon has full control of the fragments at all times. When the fragments are rotated to bring the wires parallel the surgeon knows that the desired angle of correction has been achieved. Care is needed to space the wires correctly at the time of their insertion. It adds to the convenience and neatness of the operation if the distance in level between the

two wires is equal to the distance between the two inner holes of the selected bone plate, for the guide wire holes may then be used for the inner two screws.

Some surgeons prefer to apply the plate on the anterior aspect of the femur rather than on the lateral aspect, on the grounds that the uppermost screw then traverses robust anterior and posterior cortices instead of engaging the medial cortex at the base of the femoral neck, where the bone is apt to be so soft that the screw may pull out.

It sometimes happens that when the fragments are rotated accurate apposition between them is lost: one fragment rotates away from the other and there may be almost total loss of end-to-end contact. This difficulty is especially liable to occur if the osteotomy is not made cleanly right through the bone, so that a spur of cortex remains and acts as a fulcrum. Another cause is inadequate stripping of periosteum on the deep aspect of the femur, so that there is a medial pivot of soft tissue. These defects are easily remedied and the two fragments can then be levered back into full end-to-end apposition.

ALTERNATIVE TECHNIQUES

In adults there are advantages in using a nail-plate rather than a simple four-hole plate: a nail-plate allows better fixation of the upper fragment and it may permit plaster-of-Paris splintage to be dispensed with. Some surgeons use a miniature nail-plate even in small children.

In adults the osteotomy site is best perforated and thus weakened with multiple drill holes before the final division is effected with an osteotome (see p. 52). Alternatively, a reciprocating power-driven saw may be used.

VARUS OSTEOTOMY

If varus angulation is to be combined with rotation, as is sometimes desired in cases of congenital dislocation of the hip, this is easily achieved by appropriately bending the plate before it is applied.

ANGULATION OSTEOTOMY OF ILIAC BONE

(SALTER'S INNOMINATE OSTEOTOMY)

The principle of the angulation osteotomy described by Salter (1961, 1969) is that the lower half of the pelvic bone, bearing the acetabulum, is tilted downwards and forwards. In consequence the roof of the acetabulum covers the femoral head rather more fully than it did before the operation (Fig. 377). The osteotomy is carried out a short

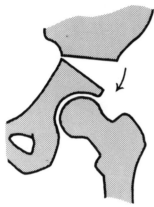

FIG. 377. Salter's innominate osteotomy. The acetabulum-bearing part of the innominate bone is inclined downwards and forwards after osteotomy at the level of the greater sciatic notch.

distance above the acetabulum, and the rotation of the lower half of the innominate bone takes place about the symphysis pubis, which in children is still mobile and acts as a hinge. The operation was devised originally for certain cases of congenital dislocation of the hip, but it has been used by its originator also for the treatment of selected patients with Perthes' disease.

TECHNIQUE

The technique to be described, applicable to a child, is basically that of Salter, with minor differences.

Position of patient. The patient lies supine. The affected side of the pelvis is thrust forward by placing a firm flat sand-bag beneath the buttock.

Incision. The incision begins just lateral to the middle of the crest of the ilium and follows the line of the crest as far forwards as the anterior superior spine. Thence it extends downwards and medially over the lateral half of the inguinal ligament (Fig. 378).

Exposure of iliac bone. The dissection begins in the proximal half of the wound, where the skin edges are reflected to reveal the apophysis of the iliac bone. The crest, comprising the apophysis and the epiphysial plate, is separated from the main part of the ilium by a thin osteotome driven from front to back. By means of slender bone levers, the crest is then displaced inwards on a hinge of periosteum, and the periosteum is stripped from the inner surface of the wing of the ilium (Fig. 380). The periosteum on the outer

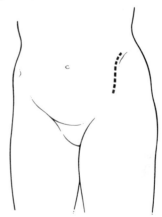

FIG. 378. Salter's pelvic osteotomy. The skin incision.

aspect of the ilium is likewise separated. Packs are inserted on each side of the ilium to hold the periosteum and overlying muscles away from the bone.

Attention is next directed to the lower half of the wound, where the sartorius muscle medially is separated from the tensor fasciae latae muscle laterally. Clearance of the fatty tissue thus exposed reveals the rectus femoris muscle arising by its direct head from the anterior inferior spine of the ilium and by its reflected head from the iliac bone immediately above the acetabulum. The muscle is detached at its origin and reflected distally.

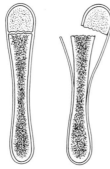

FIGS 379–380. Innominate osteotomy. The iliac apophysis is separated by an osteotome and displaced medially on a hinge of periosteum. The periosteum on the outer side of the ilium is likewise stripped away from the bone.

The stripping of the periosteum from the outer and inner aspects of the wing of the ilium may then be extended downwards and forwards as far as the anterior inferior spine.

Locating the greater sciatic notch. To complete the exposure it now remains only to locate the greater sciatic notch both from the outer and from the inner side. This is done by carefully stripping the periosteum from the bone well back towards the buttock, it being remembered that the greater sciatic notch lies directly posterior to the anterior superior spine of the ilium. Dissection must be strictly between periosteum and bone rather than outside the periosteum. In the final stages the periosteal stripping should be done with a well curved blunt-pointed bone lever. As this is gradually worked backwards from the direction of the anterior superior spine of the ilium the point will be felt to enter the greater sciatic notch.

When the notch has been thus located from the outer side a second curved bone lever is made to enter the notch in like manner from the inner side of the iliac bone. The tips of the bone levers thus meet within the notch (Fig. 381). Provided the levers have been kept strictly in the subperiosteal plane their points are superficial to the sciatic nerve and they protect the nerve from injury during division of the bone.

Division of bone. The osteotomy is conveniently effected by slender osteotomes. The line of division should extend from the anterior inferior spine of the ilium to the greater sciatic notch, already located by bone levers. It is easiest to divide the bone partly from the outer side of the ilium and partly from the inner side (Fig. 381). As the cut nears the greater sciatic notch the bone becomes thicker and harder. At this point great care must be taken to direct the osteotome strictly towards the bone levers in the sciatic notch, which serve to

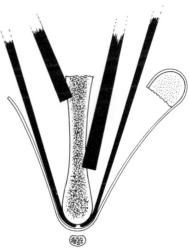

FIG. 381. The points of curved levers meet deep to the bone in the greater sciatic notch, protecting the sciatic nerve. Osteotomes are shown dividing the bone from either side.

protect the sciatic nerve. To facilitate the final stages of the section the osteotomy site may be sprung open with a distractor. Newman's spinous process distractor is ideal for this purpose.

Tilting the distal fragment. The aim should be to tilt the distal fragment outwards and forwards upon the axis formed by the symphysis pubis. This may be done by grasping the lower fragment with a towel clip close to the anterior inferior iliac spine and applying a distracting force to open up the anterior part of the osteotomy site. The posterior (deep) part of the cut bony surfaces should remain in contact. Thus the opening at the site of osteotomy is wedge-shaped. Once the correct direction of tilt of the distal fragment (outwards and forwards) has been established the gap between the bone fragments may be held open by a distractor (Fig. 377).

Propping open the osteotomy gap with bone graft. It is a simple matter to shape a block of bone to fit the anterior part of the opened-up osteotomy site in order to keep it propped open. In young children—say under 3 years of age—the authors prefer to use heterogenous bone (for instance beef bone). For older children a graft obtained from the crest of the patient's own ilium is appropriate. The bed for the graft near the front of the wedge-shaped gap between the bone fragments should be

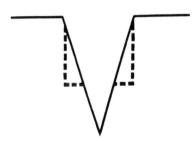

FIG. 382. Conversion of the wedge-shaped gap into a rectangular recess allows a more stable fit of the bone graft.

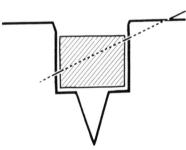

FIG. 383. The block of bone inserted to prop open the gap, and held in position by transfixion with a Kirschner wire.

shaped to take a rectangular graft rather than a wedge-shaped graft (Fig. 382), because a rectangular graft is intrinsically more stable. The dimensions of the bed are measured accurately so that the graft may be shaped precisely to the correct size. The graft is then inserted into the prepared space, being orientated in the way best calculated to resist compression (Fig. 383).

Fixation of graft by Kirschner wire. It is convenient to transfix the graft together with the bone on either side of the osteotomy with a Kirschner wire in order to hold the graft in position. The wire is driven in from above, where it enters the proximal bone fragment close to the anterior inferior spine and is directed distally across the osteotomy gap, through the contained graft, to enter the distal fragment. The wire is cut off and its proximal end is hooked over and made to lie just deep to the skin surface to facilitate its retrieval after the osteotomy has united.

Elongation of psoas tendon. Salter recommended that innominate osteotomy should be supplemented by elongation of the psoas tendon. This may be located through the distal half of the wound as it crosses deep to the inguinal ligament towards its insertion into the lesser trochanter of the femur.

Closure. When the bone levers have been removed the periosteum and muscles on each side of the iliac bone are allowed to fall back into place. Care is taken to ensure that the detached iliac crest is restored to its natural position, where it is held by absorbable sutures through the periosteum. The skin is closed with interrupted sutures, without drainage.

POST-OPERATIVE MANAGEMENT

Gauze dressings are held in place by a crepe bandage firmly applied in spica fashion. Over this is applied a plaster-of-Paris hip spica extended well up on the trunk and including the whole limb on the affected side down to the metatarsal heads. The limb should be in a position of slight flexion and slight abduction. The plaster is retained for five to seven weeks, depending upon the age of the patient. The Kirschner wire transfixing the graft and the adjacent bone should be removed when the plaster is discarded.

Comment

The operation is straightforward and does not present difficulty provided each step is carried out in a deliberate manner. Sometimes it has been commented that the greater sciatic notch is difficult to locate. This is not so if it be remembered that the notch lies directly posterior to the anterior superior spine of the ilium. Thus with the patient supine the bone lever seeking the notch should be insinuated vertically downwards towards the table in a line extending from the anterior superior spine. When the curved point of the bone lever enters the notch the movement is imparted to the hand holding the lever and is unmistakable.

The need to protect the sciatic nerve from injury is obvious and should not require further emphasis. Many surgeons avoid the use of osteotomes, preferring to pass a Gigli saw through the greater sciatic notch and to divide the bone from behind forwards; but the authors have found this method less satisfactory than the method described.

Salter stressed the need to tilt the distal fragment outwards and forwards by pulling upon it with a towel clip rather than by simply opening out the osteotomy site with a distractor. Nevertheless a distractor can be used effectively to open the gap or to hold it open once the correct direction of angulation has been established.

The use of heterogenous bone (usually commercially prepared non-antigenic sterilised beef bone) to prop open the gap between the fragments is not universally approved, but the authors have not seen trouble from its use in this particular situation. In children under 3 years old it is not always easy to obtain a stout enough graft from the ilium, and the use of heterogenous bone obviates the need to disfigure the pelvic contour by taking an autogenous graft. In older children, however, autogenous bone is to be preferred.

Impaction of the graft in the osteotomy gap is made easier if the triangular shape of the space for the graft is converted to a rectangle by trimming the cut edges of the bone fragments as shown in Figure 382. A compression force does not tend to squeeze out a rectangular graft as it does a wedge-shaped graft.

Skewering of the graft together with the host bone to hold the graft in place calls for careful directing of the Kirschner wire, which ideally should traverse the bone in the cancellous layer between the two cortices.

PERICAPSULAR OSTEOTOMY OF ILIAC BONE

(PEMBERTON'S ILIAC OSTEOTOMY)

The "pericapsular" osteotomy of the ilium described by Pemberton (1965, 1974) differs in principle from Salter's iliac osteotomy (p. 283) in that the pelvic ring is not disrupted: instead the osteotomy emerges at the triradiate cartilage of the acetabulum, thus permitting the upper segment or roof of the acetabulum to be deflected downwards about the flexible "hinge" formed by the triradiate cartilage (Fig. 384). Since this hinge is close to the articular segment that is to be turned down, deflection can be through a greater angle than in the case of the Salter osteotomy, in which the fulcrum is at the symphysis pubis and the lever arm consequently much longer. Since adequate deflection of the acetabular roof in Pemberton's osteotomy is dependent upon flexibility of the triradiate cartilage, the operation is not applicable to children over about 6 to 8 years of age, when the cartilage loses its flexibility. In practice the operation is usually done in children aged about 3 or 4 years.

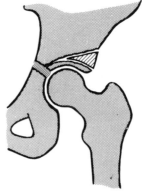

FIG. 384. Principle of Pemberton's pelvic osteotomy. Note that the osteotomy terminates at the triradiate cartilage.

Downward deflection of the acetabular roof inevitably reduces the capacity of the socket, but in the type of case for which this osteotomy is appropriate—that in which the acetabular roof is steeply sloping and is not for the most part in contact with the fully reduced femoral head—this must be regarded as an advantage.

PREREQUISITES

It is important that the femoral head be fully reduced before the osteotomy is undertaken. If necessary the tendon of the ilio-psoas muscle may be divided in order to facilitate the centring of the head in the acetabulum.

TECHNIQUE

The main difference in technique from that of Salter's iliac osteotomy is that the division of bone is at a slightly lower level, only a few millimetres above the site of attachment of the capsule of the hip joint to the ilium. Moreover the osteotomy is curved, following the contour of the acetabulum, a little above it; and instead of emerging at the greater sciatic notch, as in the Salter operation, it arches backwards to meet the triradiate cartilage, which marks the junction of ilium, pubis and ischium.

Exposure. The position of the patient, the exposure, and the clearance of the iliac bone on both its outer and its inner aspects so that well-curved bone levers may be inserted into the greater sciatic notch from without and within in order to hold the soft tissues retracted, are the same as described for Salter's iliac osteotomy (p. 283).

Arthrotomy and inspection of joint. The joint capsule is opened transversely parallel to its attachment to the rim of the acetabulum, to permit inspection of the joint. In this way any obstruction to full concentric reduction of the femoral head may be revealed and corrected.

Osteotomy. The osteotomy is carried out with curved narrow osteotomes, partly from the outer side of the iliac bone and partly from the inner side. The outer table is divided first. The osteotomy begins anteriorly, immediately above the anterior inferior spine of the ilium, and follows the curve of the attachment of the capsule to the iliac bone, about 6 millimetres above it. Care should be taken to ensure that the osteotome does not emerge at the greater sciatic notch. Instead it should be directed to reach the ilio-ischial limb of the triradiate cartilage at a point halfway between the anterior margin of the sciatic notch and the centre of the posterior rim of the acetabulum.

When the outer table of the iliac bone has been divided thus far back, the inner table is likewise divided by a corresponding cut, the deeper part of which cannot be made entirely under direct vision. Orientation is, however, greatly facilitated by reference to a dried skeleton of the pelvis, preferably from a child.

Finally, a somewhat broader osteotome is driven in, midway between the outer and inner tables, to divide the intervening cancellous bone. When this has been done, it will be apparent that the segment of bone below the osteotomy (which includes the roof of the acetabulum) has become loose anteriorly, so that it may easily be deflected by leverage outwards and forwards with the osteotome, thus creating a wedge-shaped gap, open anteriorly, at the site of osteotomy. It is convenient to hold open the gap by a laminectomy spreader while preparations are made to prop the gap open by a block of bone.

Insertion of bone graft. The anterior part of the wedge-shaped gap is made rectangular in the manner described for the Salter operation (Figs 382 and 383), so that a bone graft, usually to be obtained from the crest of the ilium just behind and including its anterior spine, may be jammed securely in the gap without fear of dislodgement. If the bone prop does not seem entirely stable, it may be transfixed together with the adjacent part of the ilium by a short length of Kirschner wire (Fig. 383).

Closure. The incision in the capsule is closed with absorbable sutures. The iliac apophysis is reconstituted and the muscle and superficial layers are closed over it as described in the previous section.

POST-OPERATIVE MANAGEMENT

This is the same as for Salter's innominate osteotomy.

Comment

The performance of the osteotomy is rather more difficult in this operation than in the Salter procedure. This is because the extremity of the cut in the bone cannot be made under direct vision. It is important that suitably curved osteotomes be used, so that they may follow the curve of the acetabulum to enter the triradiate cartilage. It is recommended that at this stage reference be made to a dried skeleton of the pelvis, which makes the understanding and execution of the operation far simpler than could the most detailed description.

ACETABULAR ROOF ADVANCEMENT BY ILIO-PLASTY FOR DYSPLASIA OF ACETABULUM

(WAINWRIGHT SHELF OPERATION)

In this operation a sheet of the outer table of the ilium is turned down to form a bony cover for the previously unsupported upper part of the femoral head and overlying capsule. The essence of the operation is the use of a large flap of iliac bone in order to cover completely the unsupported part of the capsule.

TECHNIQUE

The technique is that of Wainwright (1976).

Position of patient. The patient lies supine but is rolled slightly towards the opposite side by means of a rather flat sand-bag placed beneath the buttock of the affected side. The affected lower limb is draped separately so that it can be moved or manoeuvred easily during the operation.

Incision. The approach is anterior (see p. 26). The skin incision begins just in front of the highest point of the crest of the ilium and follows the lateral margin of the crest as far as the anterior superior spine. Thence it is extended vertically down the upper part of the thigh for approximately 8 centimetres in an adult or correspondingly less in a child.

Exposure of ilium and capsule of hip joint. The key part of the exposure is the stripping back of the tensor fasciae latae muscle and part of the gluteus medius muscle from the outer table of the ilium. The separation is begun anteriorly where the deep fascia (iliac aponeurosis) is first separated from the lateral margin of the crest of the ilium by sharp dissection. The deep fascia is further divided in the upper thigh in the line of the skin incision. Muscle fibres of the tensor fasciae latae are thus exposed at the front of the wing of the ilium, and with a periosteal elevator the muscle is levered backwards together with the periosteum so that the raw bone of the wing of the ilium is exposed. This reflection of muscle is continued as far posteriorly as the incision allows.

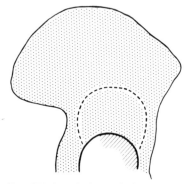

FIG. 385. Acetabular roof advancement. Interrupted line defines the flap of outer table of ilium to be turned down.

By following the rawed ilium distally, the surgeon will immediately encounter the prominence formed by the femoral head with its overlying capsule. In the conditions for which this operation is usually done, the prominence formed by the femoral head is much more marked than it is in the normal hip, because the acetabulum is shallow

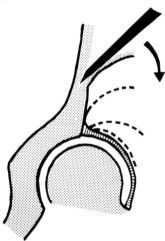

FIG. 386. Successive stages in the downward deflection of the iliac flap. The flexible bone flap is gently coaxed down by leverage with a chisel driven between the outer and inner tables of the ilium, until finally it rests upon the outer surface of the joint capsule.

and the head is often subluxated. Indeed, the prominence formed by the femoral head is often easily palpable through the skin and superficial

confirmed by directing an assistant to rotate the limb, when movement will be detected through the exposed capsule.

It is important that before the definitive part of the operation—that is, the turning down of a sheet of iliac bone—is begun the whole area of the outer table of the ilium be completely cleared right down to the attachment of the capsule of the hip to the upper rim of the acetabulum; and likewise the anterior and superior aspects of the capsule must be thoroughly cleared and cleaned. In many cases the capsule is much thickened, and in such a case it is recommended that the surface layers be thinned away to reduce the thickness by perhaps half—though preferably without making an opening into the hip joint.

Outlining and turning down the iliac flap. The flap of bone that is to be turned down is outlined by light cuts with an osteotome. It is shaped like a horseshoe, with its base corresponding to the anterior and superior attachments of the capsule to the rim of the acetabulum. The curve of the horseshoe sweeps upwards close to the anterior superior spine of the ilium and thence upwards and backwards where in an adult the highest point of the flap extends 5 or 6 centimetres proximal to

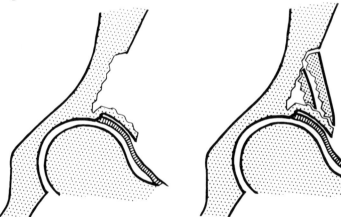

FIGS 387–388. Figure 387—Deflection of the iliac flap completed. An intact hinge of tissue is preserved at the base. The flap is moulded to the contour of the capsule with contained femoral head. Figure 388—The deflected flap of bone retained in position by blocks of bone impacted into the wedge-shaped gap.

tissues before the operation is begun. Thus there should seldom be any difficulty in locating the femoral head, and its identity can be positively

the acetabular margin. Thence the outline of the flap curves backwards and downwards to meet the posterior end of the base of the flap at the postero-superior margin of the acetabulum (Fig. 385).

Next comes the most important and the most difficult part of the operation—namely to turn down the flap of bone until it lies upon the capsule covering the femoral head, conforming faithfully to the domed shape of the prominent head. The bone is levered down little by little by means of an osteotome driven in between the two tables of the ilium, the aim being to split the bone about midway between the outer and the inner table (Fig. 386). In moulding the flap it is a mistake to try to lever it down too quickly. Success comes more easily if the flap is coaxed down little by little, steady leverage being applied through the osteotome each time it is driven on another half centimetre or so.

As the flap is progressively raised and turned down it remains attached eventually only by a bridge of capsule and periosteum at its base, close to the margin of the acetabulum (Fig. 387). It is important to try to preserve this hinge intact, both to safeguard some supply of blood to the flap and also to maintain the flap's stability. Peripheral parts of the flap are moulded to the contour of the capsule covering the femoral head, and it is often an advantage to perforate the bony flap at two or three points to enable its edge to be sutured to the outer surface of the capsule.

Buttressing the flap. When the flap of iliac bone has thus been turned down and moulded to the uncovered part of the femoral head, it is necessary to buttress it in position by means of slivers or chunks of cancellous iliac bone impacted into the space between the down-turned flap and its former bed (Fig. 388). Sufficient bone for this purpose may usually be obtained from the crest of the ilium or from the region of the posterior superior iliac spine.

Closure. It is important to suture the tensor fasciae latae muscle snugly back into position because in this way the loose cancellous grafts are held in place. The superficial layers are repaired with absorbable sutures and the skin edges are closed after the insertion of an appropriate tube for suction drainage.

POST-OPERATIVE MANAGEMENT

Although the originator recommended weight traction on the limb for the first two weeks, the authors prefer to apply a plaster-of-Paris hip spica with the affected hip abducted 20 degrees and with the opposite limb included down to the lower part of the thigh. After two weeks the plaster spica is renewed and at the same time the sutures are removed. The plaster is retained for a total of six weeks, during which the patient may be able to get around to some extent with axillary crutches. When the plaster is removed, mobilising exercises are carried out in recumbency for a further two weeks before walking is resumed, initially with elbow crutches or in the pool, and later with full weight bearing.

Comment

It is remarkable to what extent the newly extended roof of the acetabulum hypertrophies in the succeeding months or years after operation. Presumably this hypertrophy is a response to function— that is, to the transmission of weight-bearing stresses through the transposed bone.

The Wainwright operation is undertaken in the same kind of case as the Chiari pelvic osteotomy (see below)—namely for the shallow dysplastic acetabulum with the femoral head tending to ride outwards and upwards—and to some extent the two operations are in competition. An important advantage of this operation is that it is non-destructive. It is less prone to complications than is the Chiari operation, and it does not prejudice the performance of other operations about the hip later if necessary.

SUPRA-ACETABULAR DISPLACEMENT OSTEOTOMY OF ILIUM

(CHIARI'S OSTEOTOMY)

This operation was described by Chiari of Vienna in 1955. It aims to provide extracapsular bone cover for the femoral head by displacing the lower half of the innominate bone (together with the acetabulum) medially in relation to the upper half

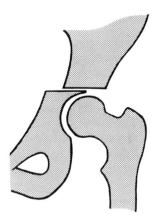

FIG. 389. Diagram showing the principle of the Chiari pelvic osteotomy. The lower part of the ilium is displaced medially, so that the cut surface of the upper part of the bone forms an extension to the roof of the acetabulum.

(Fig. 389). The line of division of the bone is immediately above the attachment of the capsule of the hip joint to the ilium. The operation has been used mainly for acetabular dysplasia with or without subluxation of the hip.

TECHNIQUE

Position of patient. The patient is placed on the orthopaedic table in the neutral anatomical position and the feet are bandaged to the footplates of the table. Provision is made for radiographic monitoring in the antero-posterior plane only, either by films or by the image intensifier.

Incision. The anterior (Smith-Petersen) incision (p. 26) is appropriate in that it permits easy access to both the inner and the outer aspect of the

wing of the ilium. The incision lies over the anterior half of the crest of the ilium, curving downwards from the anterior superior spine for 10 centimetres in a line which, if prolonged downwards, would cross the lateral femoral condyle.

Exposure of iliac bone. After separation of the abdominal muscles from the crest of the ilium by dissection very close to the bone, and detachment of the sartorius from the anterior superior iliac spine, the tensor fasciae latae muscle is stripped from the outer face of the ilium and the iliacus from the inner face. The interval between the tensor fasciae latae and the rectus femoris is then developed and the direct head of rectus is separated from the anterior inferior spine and reflected distally.

With a sharply curved blunt dissector or bone spike the greater sciatic notch is identified and entered from the outer side of the ilium. A similar instrument is made to enter the notch from the inner side of the ilium, so that the two instruments meet each other in the notch and thus protect the sciatic nerve (see p. 284).

The supero-lateral aspect of the hip is now fully exposed and preparation can be made for the osteotomy.

The osteotomy. First the reflected head of rectus femoris is identified and divided close to its attachment to the ilium above the superior rim of the acetabulum, where it is often partly blended with the capsule of the hip joint. The linear junction between the reflected head of the rectus and the capsule is the correct starting point for the osteotomy. A narrow thin osteotome is driven in here in a medial direction with a 10 degrees upward slant, and its position is checked radiographically. From this point the line of the osteotomy curves backwards, following the line of attachment of the capsule to the ilium (Fig. 390), finally to enter the greater sciatic notch. Division of the bone is accomplished most easily by a series of narrow osteotomes.

When the bone cut has been completed right

back to the greater sciatic notch, loosening between the upper and lower halves of the pelvis becomes apparent. At this stage medial displacement of the lower fragment (bearing the acetabulum) is effected by abducting the limb 30 or 40

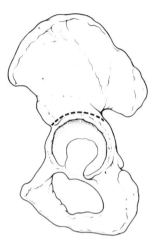

FIG. 390. Chiari osteotomy. The site of the osteotomy in relation to the acetabulum is shown.

degrees and pushing upon the femoral head in a medial direction: a curved lever between the fragments may also be a help. Displacement should be equal to half the thickness of the bone at the site of osteotomy—or about 1.5 to 1.75 centimetres in an adult. The displacement can be observed by direct vision, but a check radiograph should also be obtained.

The bones are usually stable in the displaced position. If there is doubt about this, however, the fragments may be transfixed by a screw driven obliquely from the proximal fragment into the distal—with care to ensure that it does not enter the hip joint.

Closure. The wound is closed in layers with suction drainage.

POST-OPERATIVE MANAGEMENT

At the conclusion of the operation a plaster hip spica is applied. This should include the whole of the limb on the side of the operation and the opposite limb down to the lower thigh. The plaster is retained for three weeks. Thereafter hip and knee movements through a restricted range are practised and walking with elbow crutches is begun.

Comment

The main essential is to ensure that the osteotomy is done at the correct level—that is, immediately above the attachment of the capsule to the ilium. To find the correct site for the osteotomy does not usually present difficulty: nevertheless it is a wise precaution to view the site of proposed osteotomy radiographically after the first osteotome has been driven in. It is also important to slant the line of the osteotomy 10 degrees upwards: this ensures that the outer lip of the bone, after displacement, comes well down over the head of the femur. Furthermore, the line of osteotomy should be curved as viewed from the outer aspect of the ilium; this curve helps to match the contour of the acetabulum, and it also helps to prevent backward displacement of the distal fragment. Finally, one should make sure that the displacement is not excessive. Displacement beyond 50 per cent of the bone thickness has no advantage and may prejudice union.

It should be noted that it was not the intention of the originator that the displaced shelf of bone should bear hard down upon the femoral head. In the post-operative radiographs there is a distinct gap between the overhanging bone and the femoral head. Part of this space is occupied by the capsule, but part fills with fibrous tissue, so that eventually a firm natural extension of the acetabulum is provided.

For comment on the Chiari operation as it compares with the Wainwright shelf operation, the reader is referred to page 290.

SCHANTZ-TYPE ABDUCTION OSTEOTOMY OF FEMUR

Essentially the Schantz osteotomy is an abduction osteotomy of the femur at a site that is not determined by any femoral landmark but by the ischial tuberosity. Since the operation is usually carried out for long-standing congenital dislocation of the hip with a false joint high on the wing of the ilium, the site of the osteotomy is in the femoral shaft well below the trochanters (Fig. 391).

The principle of the operation is that the upper part of the femur should be allowed to lie fully adducted against the sloping side wall of the pelvis, and the angle of osteotomy should be such that with the upper end thus fully adducted the distal part of the femur is directed vertically downwards. Adduction beyond the neutral position is thereafter impossible and a Trendelenburg dip on walking is eliminated.

PRELIMINARY STUDIES

Before the operation it is necessary to establish accurately the range of adduction of the affected hip. This may be determined clinically with a goniometer or protractor, or radiographically. The abduction angulation to be gained at the site of osteotomy should be equal to the fullest range of adduction, so that when the limb is in the weight-bearing position the upper fragment of the femur will be close to the side wall of the pelvis (Fig. 391).

TECHNIQUE

Position of patient. It is most convenient to place the patient upon an orthopaedic table with the feet strapped to the foot-pieces. Provision should be made for antero-posterior radiography, but lateral radiographs are not required. It is not practicable to use a tourniquet.

Exposure. A vertical lateral incision about 10 centimetres long extends downwards from the prominence of the greater trochanter: its centre should be at the level of the ischial tuberosity, which is the level at which the osteotomy is made.

The fascia lata is split in the direction of its

fibres, the posterior margin of the vastus lateralis is sought with a curved bone lever, and the muscle is lifted forwards upon the lever, which is hooked over the front of the femoral shaft, as in the normal lateral exposure of the upper part of the femur (p. 37). Remaining muscle fibres are stripped from the lateral aspect of the femur and the periosteum is incised. The bone is fully displayed throughout the length of the incision by bone levers at each corner of the wound.

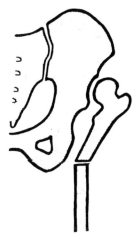

FIG. 391. Schantz osteotomy for old unreduced congenital dislocation of hip. The bone is divided opposite the ischial tuberosity and angled to bring the proximal fragment into full adduction when the limb is in line with the trunk. The bone fragments are fixed by an angled plate held by screws.

Radiographic confirmation of level. It is well to check that the correct site has been chosen for the osteotomy by placing a marker upon the bone (a small drill driven through at the site provisionally selected for osteotomy is appropriate) and then taking an antero-posterior radiograph. From this the correct site for the osteotomy—which should be level with the ischial tuberosity—is easily established.

Division of bone. Before the bone is divided two guide wires should be driven into the femur, each at right angles to the lateral cortex, one about 3 centimetres above the site of osteotomy and the other a similar distance below the site of osteotomy. The guide wires should be parallel to one another (Fig. 392). Their purpose is to serve as markers to indicate the degree of abduction produced at the site of osteotomy (Fig. 393). They also serve to ensure that rotational deformity is not inadvertently created.

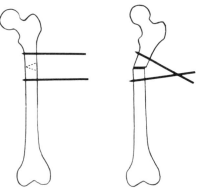

FIGS 392–393. Use of guide wires to control the angulation at site of osteotomy. Figure 392—Parallel wires inserted above and below proposed site of osteotomy. Figure 393—Angle subtended by wires indicates degree of angulation after osteotomy.

The femur may be divided by making multiple drill holes and completing the section with an osteotome, or by a power-operated reciprocating saw. It is best to cut out a wedge of bone with its base laterally, the angle of the wedge being equal to the calculated angle of abduction that is required (that is, equal to the pre-operative range of adduction).

Abduction of lower fragment. When the femur has been divided it is a simple matter to swing the lower section of the limb outwards on the hinged leg-piece of the orthopaedic table. During this manoeuvre care should be taken to ensure that the femoral fragments remain in contact and do not become displaced or over-ride one another. If necessary the fragments may be well controlled with heavy bone-holding forceps.

Internal fixation. When the correct position of abduction has been gained as indicated by the marker guide wires, which should now subtend the calculated angle of abduction required, the position is stabilised by a stout four-hole plate. Usually it is most convenient to bend a plate to the required angle before the operation, but if this has not been done a straight plate may be angled by suitable plate benders. Each half of the plate is held to the femoral shaft with a clamp while drill holes are prepared and screws inserted.

Closure. The vastus lateralis is anchored posteriorly by one or two absorbable sutures. The split edges of the fascia lata are re-united and the skin is closed without drainage.

POST-OPERATIVE MANAGEMENT

If a sufficiently stout plate has been used the patient may lie free in bed without external splintage. Hip and knee flexion exercises are begun within a few days of the operation, and walking with crutches (not weight bearing) may be encouraged as soon as the wound is healed. Partial weight bearing may be resumed after six weeks, but the resumption of full weight bearing must await union of the osteotomy. If the plate used for fixation is slender or if the patient is of heavy build it is advisable to use external support in the form of a plaster spica for the first six weeks.

Comment

The critical part of the Schantz operation is to make sure that the abduction angulation is of the correct degree. It is essential to establish this angle before the operation by measuring the range of adduction at the hip, for once the bone has been divided it is difficult to calculate how much abduction is required. It is also important to choose the site for the osteotomy correctly. It must be exactly level with the tuberosity of the ischium.

DISPLACEMENT OSTEOTOMY OF UPPER END OF FEMUR

(McMurray Osteotomy)

In the operation as originally described by McMurray (1935) the femur was divided just below the greater trochanter and the lower fragment—that is, the shaft of the femur—was forced markedly inwards; the position was held by immobilisation of the limb in a plaster spica with slight abduction. In the modern operation, used mainly for early or moderate osteoarthritis of the hip, medial displacement of the shaft fragment is usually restricted to not more than a quarter of the diameter of the bone, and the bone fragments are held rigidly by a suitable fixation device—usually a nail-plate, spline or compression plate. In the method to be described fixation is achieved by a Jewett nail-plate.

TECHNIQUE

Positioning the patient. The patient is placed upon the orthopaedic table with the pelvis resting on the saddle and the feet strapped to the footpieces of the table. Setting up is similar to that for fixation of a fracture of the neck of the femur (see p. 261). The sound hip should be abducted about 40 degrees to allow the positioning of a mobile x-ray unit for lateral radiography. Anteroposterior radiography is provided for by a second unit centred vertically over the femoral shaft immediately distal to the greater trochanter. Alternatively, an image intensifier may be used.

Incision. A vertical lateral incision is made from the greater trochanter downwards, as in the operation of applying a nail-plate for trochanteric fracture (p. 266). When the fascia lata, and more proximally the tensor fasciae latae muscle, have been divided in the line of their fibres the posterior border of the vastus lateralis is sought (Fig. 394). The muscle is lifted forwards by a bone lever which is hooked over the front of the femur and used to retract the vastus lateralis anteriorly (Fig. 395). The femur is thus exposed in its upper part: it should be further cleared by incising the periosteum vertically onto the bone and reflecting the periosteal sleeve anteriorly and posteriorly with bone levers.

Confirmation of level for osteotomy. The aim should be to divide the femur below the greater trochanter but immediately proximal to the lesser trochanter (Fig. 397). The correct level may be marked upon the pre-operative radiograph, and it

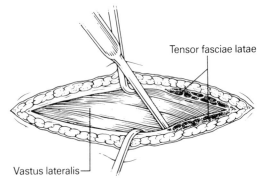

Fig. 394. Seeking the posterior edge of the vastus lateralis after incision of the fascia lata and tensor fasciae latae muscle.

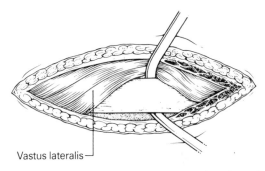

Fig. 395. The vastus lateralis muscle has been levered forwards to expose the femur.

is usually a simple matter to define the lateral starting point of the osteotomy upon the surface of the exposed femur: usually it is just distal to the point where the femoral shaft begins to flare out to form the greater trochanter. When the level has been selected it is a wise precaution to confirm that it is correct by taking an antero-posterior radiograph after a drill or guide wire has been driven across the bone at the level of the proposed osteotomy. If this marker drill is shown to be a little too high or too low a suitable adjustment is easily made when the bone comes to be divided.

Insertion of guide wire in neck of femur. In order to direct the nail-plate correctly into the neck of the femur a guide wire is first inserted and its

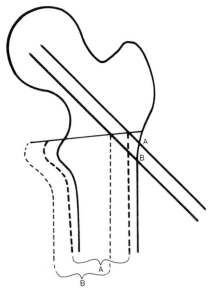

FIG. 396. The lower the guide wire is entered, the greater the displacement entailed by fixation with a nail-plate. Thus position A gives slight displacement, whereas position B gives wider displacement. The thickness of the nail-plate itself must be allowed for.

position is checked by antero-posterior and lateral radiographs. The technique of inserting the guide wire is the same as described for nailing of a femoral neck fracture (p. 261) or of a trochanteric fracture (p. 266). The entrance point for the guide wire is critical, because it governs the degree of medial displacement of the shaft fragment: thus if the nail-plate were to enter the proximal fragment well above the level of osteotomy no medial displacement of the shaft would be possible; on the other hand, if the guide wire were so placed that the nail would enter the cut surface of the proximal fragment displacement could easily be excessive. The authors prefer to enter the guide wire immediately distal to the proposed site of osteotomy (Fig. 396). The displacement achieved will then automatically be approximately equal to the thickness of the Jewett nail-plate (Fig. 397). If a little more displacement is required the guide wire

may be entered a few millimetres more distally. These points will be made clear by reference to the diagrams.

Selection of nail-plate. A Jewett type nail-plate is now selected. It must be of the correct angle and of appropriate length. The angle is determined by direct measurement upon the radiograph with a protractor. If the particular features of the case demand that there be some abduction or adduction as well as displacement of the distal fragment appropriate allowance is made for this when the nail-plate is chosen. The length of the nail is determined by measuring the part of the guide wire still protruding and calculating from this the length of wire within the bone. Appropriate adjustment is made if the radiograph shows that the guide wire is over- penetrated or under-penetrated: ideally the point of the nail after insertion should lie about 1.5 or 2 centimetres short of the articular surface of the femoral head.

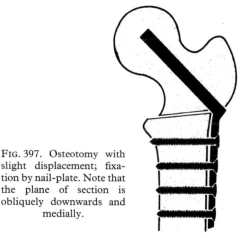

FIG. 397. Osteotomy with slight displacement; fixation by nail-plate. Note that the plane of section is obliquely downwards and medially.

Partial insertion of nail. It is convenient at this stage to drive the nail-plate part-way into the proximal fragment of the femur, though it cannot be driven home fully until the bone has been divided. In driving the nail over the guide wire the surgeon must be sure that the plate section of the device is exactly parallel to the long axis of the femur. Unless the bone is very soft, it is usually wise to make a triangular starting slot for the three fins of the nail by means of a slender osteotome or chisel, or of a specially designed three-flanged starter chisel.

Division of femur. When the nail-plate has been driven in approximately half way—or at least far enough to have obtained a good grip in the proximal fragment—the femoral osteotomy should be carried out at the level already determined. Of the several methods of dividing the bone that are available—Gigli saw, multiple drilling with completion of the division by osteotomes, or reciprocating saw—the authors prefer the last named; but if a suitable power-operated saw is not available the technique of making multiple drill holes and joining them by osteotomy cuts works well. The main point is that the bone should be divided cleanly without any splintering, and with particular care to avoid leaving a medial spur of cortex which may prevent ready displacement of the shaft fragment.

To ensure a clean division it is important that the cortical surface of the femur at the site of osteotomy should be exposed throughout its full circumference by stripping and retracting the periosteal sleeve with bone levers. The plane of the osteotomy should be almost transverse, but with a slight distal inclination from lateral to medial (Fig. 397): this helps to ensure tight coaptation of the fragments when the shaft fragment is pushed medially.

Fixation of fragments with appropriate displacement. At this stage the nail-plate should be driven in to its fullest extent. The distal fragment of the femur is then drawn up against the medial aspect of the plate by a Lowman's clamp. Provided the nail-plate has been placed accurately at the correct level, there will now be slight but appropriate medial displacement of the shaft fragment relative to the proximal fragment of the femur. Before screws are finally inserted to secure the plate to the femoral shaft it is wise to ensure that there is no gap between the fragments. If necessary, it is a simple matter to insert a screw partly into the anterior cortex of the shaft and by hammering upon a punch placed below the screw to impact the shaft into the proximal fragment (Fig. 398): the screw is then removed.

In fixing the plate to the femoral shaft with screws the surgeon should be sure to choose the length of the screws carefully. If self-tapping cobalt-chrome screws are to be used it is wise to select screws that are slightly longer than the diameter of the bone as measured by the depth gauge, so that the fluted self-tapping point of each

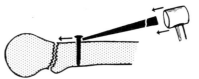

FIG. 398. Method of impacting the fragments by hammer blows upon a screw driven temporarily into the shaft fragment.

screw will lie beyond the bone in the soft tissues (Fig. 399): otherwise bone tends gradually to grow into the flutes, with consequent difficulty in turning the screws if their removal should be required later. An alternative is to use stainless steel screws or to tap the threads first and to use plain-threaded rather than self-tapping screws.

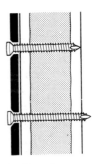

FIG. 399. If self-tapping screws are used they should be slightly longer than the diameter of the bone so that the tapping flutes project beyond the cortex. This prevents the screws from becoming locked by growth of bone into the flutes.

Before closure of the wound it is important to check the position of the nail-plate and of the bone fragments by antero-posterior and lateral radiographs.

Closure. The vastus lateralis falls back into position: its posterior edge may be lightly tacked with two or three absorbable sutures. The fascia lata is repaired with interrupted sutures and the skin with everting mattress sutures. Drainage of the wound is not usually required.

ALTERNATIVE TECHNIQUE OF FIXATION

Medial displacement osteotomy may also be stabilised by the use of a Muller-type nail-plate (Fig. 400). This has a channel section which is driven across the upper end of the femoral shaft, joined in one piece to a plate which is screwed to the femur. The degree of medial displacement of the femoral shaft is dictated by the offset of the nail-plate. A special starter gouge is used to prepare the path for insertion of the nail section. With this gouge in place, the femur is divided 1 centimetre distal to the gouge and parallel to it.

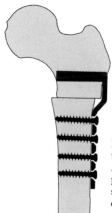

FIG. 400. Fixation of subtrochanteric osteotomy by Muller-type nail-plate. The plate is so shaped that only slight medial displacement of the shaft fragment is permitted.

The gouge is then removed and the nail-plate is fully inserted. This automatically displaces the distal femoral shaft medially. A compression device is inserted in the distal hole of the plate and screwed to the femur. This facilitates compression of the fragments together at the osteotomy site before the plate is screwed to the femur.

POST-OPERATIVE MANAGEMENT

Two or three wide crepe bandages are applied spica fashion over copious gauze dressings. For the first few days the patient lies free in bed and is encouraged to begin active knee and hip flexion exercises under the supervision of a physiotherapist. Walking is usually resumed about a week after the operation, crutches being used at first, with avoidance of weight bearing on the affected limb. Provided good fixation has been secured by the nail-plate, partial weight bearing may usually be begun three to four weeks after operation. Thereafter, progressively more weight may be taken on the limb but the patient must continue to use crutches or elbow crutches until union of the osteotomy is sound, as confirmed radiographically.

Comment

This operation was employed extensively in the two decades that followed the Second World War. Because of the development and widespread adoption of total replacement arthroplasty in the treatment of osteoarthritis of the hip it is now undertaken rather infrequently; but it still has a place. Moreover, it is emphasised by surgeons who recommend the operation that the degree of displacement of the shaft fragment should be small: wide displacement, such as was formerly advocated, may make total replacement arthroplasty—if it should eventually be required—unduly difficult.

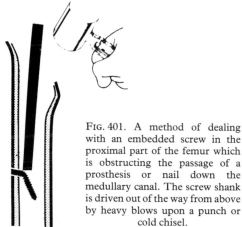

FIG. 401. A method of dealing with an embedded screw in the proximal part of the femur which is obstructing the passage of a prosthesis or nail down the medullary canal. The screw shank is driven out of the way from above by heavy blows upon a punch or cold chisel.

For the same reason, as already noted, the surgeon should avoid using self-tapping screws in such a way that they may become locked in the bone. If the self-tapping points of cobalt-chrome screws remain in the femoral cortex the growth of bone into the flutes may prevent the screws from being turned if their removal is desired later. The head of the screw is often then inadvertently twisted off, the main part of the screw remaining within the bone. If a femoral prosthesis is then to be inserted the most practical method of clearing the broken screw out of the way is usually to strike it from above with a punch or cold chisel driven down the medullary canal after the femoral head and neck have been removed (Fig. 401).

Many surgeons prefer to use a one-piece nail-plate rather than a spline or compression device, because the degree of displacement of the femoral shaft fragment is well controlled and easily varied according to requirements by adjusting the level at which the nail is entered. Moreover a nail-plate gives rigid fixation which permits relatively early weight bearing, and yet there is no bulky mass of metal to cause local discomfort in the trochanteric region when the patient lies upon the affected side. The incidence of delayed union and of non-union with this method is probably no greater than it is after alternative methods of fixation, provided always that the bone is divided in a plane that slopes slightly distally from the lateral to the medial side, as described.

TOTAL REPLACEMENT ARTHROPLASTY OF HIP

This operation was pioneered by McKee of Norwich (McKee 1951, McKee and Watson-Farrar 1966) and by Charnley (1961) after abortive attempts many years earlier (Wiles 1958) had failed largely because suitable inert metals were not then available. The operation entails replacement of the femoral head by a metal prosthesis and lining the suitably enlarged acetabulum with a socket prosthesis of high density polyethylene. The operation has been modified in many ways and a great variety of different prostheses is available. Most of the standard ones give results that are comparable with one another, and the choice is largely a matter of individual preference. So also is strongly advocated by Charnley (1970), as unnecessary in that adequate exposure can easily be gained without it.

PRELIMINARY STUDIES

Careful clinical and radiographic studies are required before operation to determine whether or not the case is a straightforward one or whether any special difficulties are to be expected. For instance, if the patient has previously undergone displacement osteotomy of the upper end of the femur there may be difficulty in directing the stem of the prosthesis down the femoral shaft,

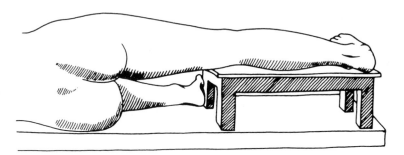

FIG. 402. Total replacement arthroplasty. Position of patient. The easily made platform allows the affected limb to lie in the neutral position and it facilitates exposure of the hip by the postero-lateral route.

the surgical approach. The authors prefer the postero-lateral approach to the antero-lateral approach because access to the medullary canal of the femur is very much easier. On the other hand they regard detachment of the greater trochanter, especially if displacement has been other than slight. Moreover, if the osteotomy was fixed by a nail-plate or spline, much time may have to be spent in removing this before the operation proper can begin. Self-tapping cobalt-chrome screws tend to become locked in the bone, and it is common for the head to twist off rather than for the screw to turn (see p. 60). In consequence the channel for the stem of the prosthesis in the medullary canal may be obstructed.

TECHNIQUE

The method to be described here relates to the insertion of a McKee type femoral prosthesis with plastic socket through the postero-lateral approach. The technique is applicable also to the Stanmore prosthesis and to many other similar prostheses.

Position of patient. The patient lies in the true lateral position with the affected hip uppermost. Preferably, the affected limb should rest from the knee downwards on a platform that rests upon the operation table (Fig. 402). This platform is about 20 centimetres high and serves to keep the limb horizontal. The body must be prevented from

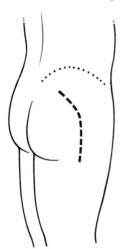

FIG. 403. Postero-lateral exposure of hip. The skin incision.

rolling forwards or backwards by suitable supports clamped to the table. If the other hip is normal, stability on the table can be enhanced by flexing the unaffected hip and knee to a right angle and strapping the limb to the table in this position (Fig. 402).

Exposure. The exposure is that described by Austin Moore (p. 34). The incision begins a little in front of the posterior superior spine of the ilium

and runs from there to the top of the greater trochanter and thence for 10 centimetres vertically downwards over the femur (Fig. 403). The approach entails splitting the gluteus maximus and the gluteal aponeurosis and upper part of the

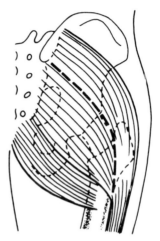

FIG. 404. The gluteus maximus is split in the direction of its fibres. The dotted outline shows the underlying bony landmarks.

fascia lata (Fig. 404). The edges are spread apart and held by a self-retaining retractor. Next, fatty tissue is removed posterior to the greater trochanter to reveal the short transverse rotator muscles of the hip, namely from above downwards the piriformis, the obturator internus and gemelli, and the quadratus femoris (Fig. 405). Crossing the three last mentioned muscles further back is the sciatic nerve; this need not be disturbed. The obturator internus and gemelli muscles, and if necessary the piriformis, are severed close to their attachment to the greater trochanter after the insertion of holding sutures which are then used to turn the muscles backwards over the sciatic nerve, which is thus protected (Fig. 406).

The leg being now medially rotated by an assistant to bring the trochanter forwards, the hip is entered from behind by incising the capsule close to the greater trochanter. The posterior capsule is best removed at this stage. The femoral head and the margin of the acetabulum are thus readily identified, especially if the assistant rocks the hip a few degrees in rotation. Blunt curved bone levers are passed round the femoral neck, one above it and the other below. The back of the femoral neck is then scraped clear of capsule and synovial membrane so that its junction with the greater trochanter is clearly displayed.

the femoral neck. But if the hip will not dislocate easily it is wrong to apply great force in an attempt to dislocate it, because the shaft of the femur may easily be fractured. It is better, and perfectly simple, to divide the femoral neck near its middle with an osteotome or a reciprocating saw, and then to remove the femoral head with a corkscrew

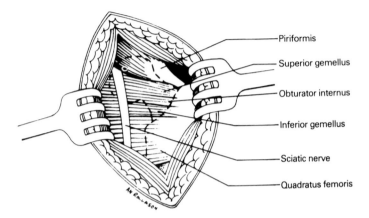

FIG. 405. The short transverse lateral rotator muscles deep to the gluteus maximus. Note that the sciatic nerve lies upon the superficial aspect of the obturator internus, gemelli and quadratus femoris, but deep to the piriformis.

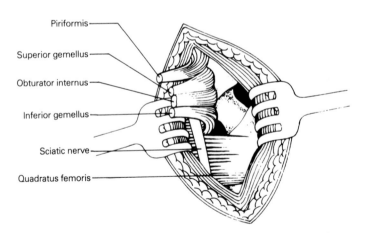

FIG. 406. The piriformis, obturator internus and gemelli have been divided close to the greater trochanter. They are reflected backwards on stay sutures (not shown), thus protecting the sciatic nerve. (In most cases sufficient access can be gained without reflecting the piriformis.)

Dislocation of hip. It may be possible at this stage to dislocate the hip by rotating the limb medially, or by lifting the head out of the socket by means of stout bone-holding forceps gripping

and bone levers. Once the head has been removed there is then no difficulty in rotating the femur 90 degrees medially, so that with the knee flexed to a right angle the tibia is vertical.

Preparation of femur to receive prosthesis. First the femoral neck must be cut at its base at an angle that will match the flange of the prosthesis. To determine the correct line of section a test prosthesis is laid on the surface of the femur, parallel to the position that it will occupy after insertion. The correct line of section of the femoral neck is then marked on the surface. In cutting the femoral neck the surgeon must make allowance for the need for the prosthesis to be anteverted 20 degrees. This means that with the femur rotated 90 degrees medially so that the flexed tibia is vertical, the cut surface must face backwards and slightly downwards.

When the neck has been cut off in the correct plane, either by osteotomes or by a power-driven reciprocating saw, the next step is to prepare a suitable track in the upper part of the femoral

such as a blunt bone lever is thrust by hand through the soft cancellous bone. With this instrument the surgeon can feel that he is within the medullary canal of the femur and has not inadvertently thrust the instrument through the cortex.

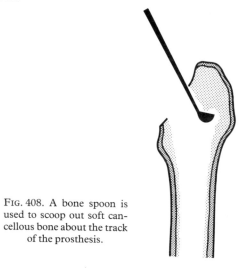

FIG. 408. A bone spoon is used to scoop out soft cancellous bone about the track of the prosthesis.

This preliminary exploration is followed by thorough reaming out with a rough rasp or broach (Fig. 407), of which many varieties are available for this purpose. In using the broach it is important that it be operated in the correct axis, allowing for 20 degrees of anteversion of the prosthesis. The broach is operated partly by hand and partly by tapping with a mallet. The track is thus enlarged until the stem of a trial prosthesis can be thrust down to its full extent.

When the main track for the prosthesis has been prepared, it is wise to scoop out cancellous bone with a bone spoon (Fig. 408) so that the bed for the cement will be largely of firm cortical bone. It is important that the prosthesis be inserted well up under the greater trochanter, and bone should be scooped out from there to allow for this. The prosthesis can then be fitted in a somewhat valgus position rather than in the less stable varus position that is often seen (Figs 412 and 413).

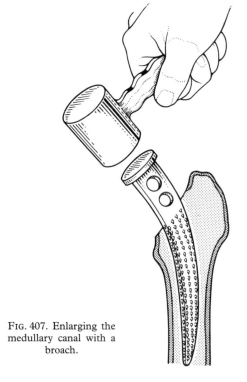

FIG. 407. Enlarging the medullary canal with a broach.

shaft to receive the stem of the prosthesis. It is often convenient to start this track with a chisel, creating a slot in the cut surface of the femur that will mark the correct axis for the prosthesis. Through this slot a slightly curved instrument

Preparing the acetabulum to receive the prosthetic socket. The limb is now laid flat on the platform and rotated in such a way as to give the best possible exposure of the acetabulum. This is facilitated by retracting the femur out of the way by means of a strong bone hook inserted into the medullary cavity. It is usually possible to secure a direct end-on view of the acetabulum, so that working upon it with gouge or reamer presents no difficulty.

First the margins of the acetabulum should be cleaned by pushing the soft tissues away with a periosteal elevator superiorly, posteriorly and anteriorly. The soft tissues may conveniently be held

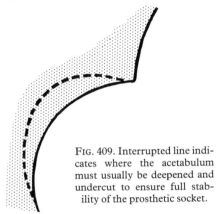

FIG. 409. Interrupted line indicates where the acetabulum must usually be deepened and undercut to ensure full stability of the prosthetic socket.

out of the way by three or four awls or Steinmann pins driven into the bone in an arc about 2 centimetres from the periphery of the socket. A lever retractor of the Hohmann type may also be placed round the anterior margin of the acetabulum—between it and the upper end of the femur—to hold the femur forwards out of the way. An end-on view of the whole acetabulum is thus obtained.

Work now starts on the inside of the acetabulum. First the cavity is cleared of synovial membrane and remnants of the ligament of the femoral head (ligamentum teres). Osteophytes are removed from the periphery. It will nearly always be found that the acetabulum requires deepening considerably, especially in the superior quadrant, to give a rather more horizontal roof which will fully support the artificial socket (Fig. 409). It is usually best to begin the deepening by hand, using a curved gouge of Capener or Müller pattern; but if a powered reamer of suitable cutting capacity is available its use may save time.

When the socket has been sufficiently deepened a trial fit with the selected prosthesis should show that the cup sinks almost completely under the

roof of the acetabulum. At this stage it will be clear which size of cup is required. Only in large individuals is anything other than the smallest cup needed. The final stage in the preparation of the acetabulum is to make three or four drill holes, each about 6 millimetres in diameter, at various points in the superior and medial aspects. These are required to key in the cement and thus to guard against loosening.

Embedding the artificial socket with acrylic cement. When all is ready and the selected high density polyethylene socket is to hand the cement is mixed. When it has reached the required consistency (just firm enough not to adhere to the dry glove) it is placed by hand in the acetabulum and pressed in with two or three sharp thrusting movements of the fingers, to force the cement into the drill holes and crevices. The prosthetic socket is then pushed into the cement with steady pressure.

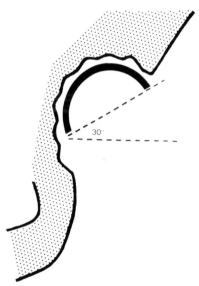

FIG. 410. Diagrammatic coronal section showing orientation of the socket: the plane of its mouth is at an angle of 30 degrees to the horizontal plane.

Orientation of prosthetic socket. It is important at this stage to ensure that the socket is inserted with the correct orientation. The outlet or axis of the socket should face mainly downwards, but with a 30 degrees abduction tilt and 20 degrees forward tilt (Figs 410 and 411). Special directors are available to set this orientation automatically, but with experience it is almost as simple to set the prosthesis by eye. Once the socket has been embedded in the cement in the correct position it must be

enough elasticity of the muscles to allow the artificial femoral head to be distracted 2 or 3 millimetres from the socket when a strong distal pull is applied to the limb. If the head comes away more

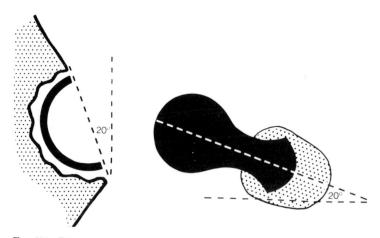

FIG. 411. Diagrammatic horizontal section. The socket should be turned forwards (anteverted) 15 or 20 degrees. The diagram also shows the correct orientation of the femoral prosthesis: it should be anteverted 20 degrees.

held perfectly still until the cement hardens. While the cement is still soft any excess that has extruded round the margins may be cut away with a knife or elevator.

Making a trial fit with the definitive femoral prosthesis. Before the femoral prosthesis is cemented in, it is essential to make a trial fit in order that the right length of prosthesis may be selected. At the same time the surgeon may decide, after testing the tension, whether the prosthesis must be driven fully home or whether it must be left standing a little proud of the cut surface of the femoral neck to give greater length.

The trial is made first with the prosthesis that seems most likely to be of the correct length. More often than not this is the long-necked prosthesis. The trial is made by tapping the prosthesis into place and then reducing the artificial head into the socket, a manoeuvre that is easily accomplished by flexing the hip and rotating it slightly laterally while the head is guided into place by finger pressure. The limb is then straightened, and longitudinal traction is applied to test the tension of the soft tissues. Ideally there should be just

than this the assembly is too loose. If the head cannot be pulled at all from the surface of the socket the assembly is too tight. Appropriate adjustments are made either by selecting a different neck length or by varying the depth to which the stem of the prosthesis is thrust into the femur.

During the trial fitting of the femoral head prosthesis it is also important to move the joint in flexion, extension, abduction, adduction and rotation in order to make sure that the head moves concentrically in the socket throughout the range, and that there is no impingement of any part of the femoral neck or trochanter against any part of the pelvis with consequent tendency for the femoral head to be levered out of the socket. Sometimes such impingement does occur, especially when a short-necked prosthesis is used: excessively large osteophytes round the lower half of the acetabulum are often responsible. Impingement may be prevented by cutting away the offending bone until a free range of concentric movement of the head in the socket is assured.

It is also important to be sure that the length of the leg is normal. Anatomically, the tip of the greater trochanter is at the level of the centre point of the femoral head. Failure to ensure that this is the case at the conclusion of the operation may lead to lengthening or to shortening of the limb, either of which is distressing to the patient and often a cause of complaint.

When attention has been directed to all these points the next step is to cement the definitive prosthesis into the femur.

Embedding the femoral prosthesis in the femur with acrylic cement. While the cement is being mixed a fine polythene catheter (size 8) is passed into the medullary canal of the femur to act as an air vent when the cement is thrust down the canal. At the same time blood and debris are removed from the canal with a sucker.

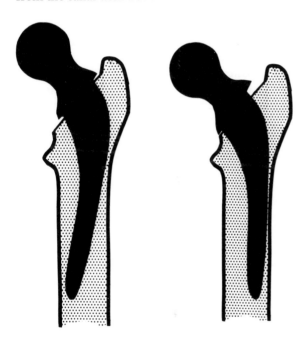

FIGS 412–413. Figure 412—The femoral prosthesis correctly inserted. Note that it has been entered high up on the cut surface of the femur close under the greater trochanter, and that it is inclined in a valgus position, with the tip of the stem abutting against the medial cortex of the femur. Figure 413—Prosthesis inserted incorrectly. It enters too low on the cut surface of the femur and is inclined in a varus position.

Cement of the correct consistency (just stiff enough not to adhere to the glove) is thrust down the medullary canal, preferably by means of a cement gun, which ensures that cement fills the

whole of the recipient cavity. (A double quantity of cement is recommended when the cement gun is used.) If a cement gun is not available the cement must be inserted by a finger or thumb. When sufficient has been inserted the catheter is quickly withdrawn; the prosthesis is then immediately pushed into the cement and driven down to the predetermined level with hammer and punch. Special care should be taken at this stage to ensure that the femoral head is inserted with a valgus rather than a varus inclination (Figs 412 and 413), and that it is anteverted sufficiently—namely through 20 degrees. When the cement has hardened the femoral head is reduced into the socket.

Reconstruction of soft tissues. No attempt is made to suture the short lateral rotator muscles back to their original position. It is better to bring them obliquely upwards and to attach them under the edge of the gluteus medius muscle. In this way they help to obliterate the "dead space" around the neck of the femoral prosthesis. On the other hand, reconstruction of the gluteal aponeurosis is very important. For this, strong interrupted sutures of absorbable material or wire are used. For the skin flaps, deep tension sutures are used together with continuous sutures for the skin edges. The authors' practice is to close the wound without drainage, but many surgeons prefer to use suction drainage for one or two days.

POST-OPERATIVE MANAGEMENT

At the conclusion of the operation a wedge-shaped pillow is placed between the patient's legs and attached by loosely closed Velcro straps to restrain the legs. The pillow is kept in place for two to four days while the patient is at rest in bed. It prevents excessive flexion or adduction at the hip during the early post-operative period: either of these movements may lead to dislocation of the hip. An alternative method of preventing dislocation is by means of a removable knee splint of plaster or plastic, fitted at the conclusion of the operation. By restricting knee flexion the splint also restricts hip flexion. Some patients find this less irksome than an abduction pillow.

Standing and walking (without any restraining harness) are begun on the day after operation, with the aid of elbow crutches. Hip and knee flexion exercises are encouraged under supervision, and the patient may sit out of bed for most of the day. It is important, however, that attempts to squat on a low lavatory seat or on a low chair be avoided because of the excessive hip flexion that these postures demand, with risk of dislocation.

Comment

Four essential rules about total replacement arthroplasty of the hip concern 1) orientation, 2) tension, 3) freedom of movement without impingement, and 4) length of the limb. Emphasis has already been laid on these points.

Orientation of both components of the prosthesis in slight anteversion is particularly important in the case of the McKee assembly here described. Without it, the femoral neck impinges against the rim of the socket during flexion of the hip. This greatly limits the range of flexion and also entails a risk of loosening of the prosthesis from repeated impingement. Beginners sometimes have difficulty in judging anteversion at operation. But this is quite simple if the femoral neck is orientated in relation to the knee flexed to a right angle. The line of the tibia then indicates the true antero-posterior plane. If the femoral neck is at right angles to this it is directed truly medially, and is neither anteverted nor retroverted. When the neck is anteverted it is inclined a little in a direction away from the foot. Similarly there should be no difficulty in orientating the artificial socket. First let the opening in the socket face directly downwards (distally). From this position abduct it 30 degrees, and then in a separate manoeuvre turn it forwards 20 degrees. This gives the correct orientation.

The need to position the femoral head prosthesis in a valgus rather than a varus inclination has also been emphasised (Figs 412 and 413). To ensure a good valgus position it is best to extend the recipient slot for the femoral prosthesis well up into the greater trochanter, so that the prosthesis can be entered high.

The technique for testing for correct tension has already been described. It is important that tension should be right: if the assembly is too tight recovery of a good range of movement may be slow; whereas if it is too loose there is an increased risk of dislocation.

The third rule is that the hip must move freely without mechanical obstruction and impingement, which may tend to lever the femoral head out of the socket. It is most important to examine the movements of the hip during the trial fitting and to make sure that osteophytes are not in contact with the femoral neck in any position of the joint.

To ensure correct length of the limb it is necessary so to fit the prosthesis that the tip of the greater trochanter is level with the central point of the original acetabulum, which usually corresponds to the centre of movement of the prosthetic femoral head.

Dislocation of an artificial hip does not occur if the operation is carried out as described. The risk of the patient's dislocating it by flexing the hip acutely in the stage of recovery from the anaesthetic is prevented by the temporary use of a wedge-shaped pillow strapped between the patient's legs, or by fitting a knee splint which automatically restricts hip flexion, as described. In the early post-operative period there is a definite risk of dislocation if the rules of rehabilitation are ignored. The patient must not be allowed to sit in a chair or on a lavatory seat that is too low. Either of these postures over-flexes the hip, with consequent risk of the femoral head's being levered out of the acetabular socket. In getting out of bed, the patient should be careful to ensure that the legs are kept together, so that the affected leg is not left stranded and forced into medial rotation.

ALTERNATIVE TECHNIQUES

It is not the intention here to give details of the many techniques of total replacement arthroplasty that have been developed by workers in this field. In fact, any of the many prostheses available can be inserted perfectly well by any of the techniques that have been described, and probably the master of one technique can gain results equal to those of the master of any other technique. Those who wish to follow in detail the method of McKee

(1970), who used an antero-lateral approach, or of Charnley (1961, 1970), who described a lateral approach with removal and reattachment of the greater trochanter, or the method of Müller (1970), who used an antero-lateral approach,

should consult the original papers. In recent years much attention has been directed to the development of non-cemented prostheses. Some authorities now commend the use of prostheses coated with hydroxy-apatite.

EXCISION ARTHROPLASTY OF HIP

(Girdlestone Pseudarthrosis)

Excision of the head and neck of the femur was originally used by Girdlestone (1945) as a means of promoting healing in cases of septic arthritis of the hip: excision of the femoral head and neck allowed free drainage and gradual obliteration of the cavity by granulation from its depths. Later the operation was used in non-infective cases as a primary treatment for osteoarthritis of the hip, especially by the Oxford school (Taylor 1950).

Since the advent of total replacement arthroplasty the Girdlestone excision has been used mainly as a salvage procedure, particularly when total replacement arthroplasty has failed irretrievably on account of infection or for other reasons.

Essentially the operation entails excision of the head and neck of the femur, excision of the superior lip of the acetabulum, and interposition of soft tissue (usually gluteus medius muscle) between the raw bones.

TECHNIQUE

Position of patient. The patient lies in the lateral position with the affected hip uppermost. It is convenient to have the limb resting upon a platform (Fig. 402), as described in the section on total replacement arthroplasty (p. 299).

Exposure. A postero-lateral incision such as Gibson's modification of Kocher's incision (p. 30) is appropriate. It begins 5 centimetres below and in front of the posterior superior spine of the ilium and slopes across the buttock to the front of the greater trochanter, where it is angled to proceed vertically down the lateral aspect of the thigh for about 10 centimetres. Splitting of the gluteal aponeurosis and fascia lata below, and of

the gluteus maximus proximally, exposes the lateral surface of the greater trochanter and above it the gluteus medius muscle. The hip joint, or what remains of it, is exposed by detachment of the gluteus medius and the short lateral rotator muscles from the trochanter.

Determining the nature of the pathology. Since excision arthroplasty is nowadays seldom employed as a primary procedure, the hip is likely to be already extensively disorganised either in consequence of infection—often a complication of replacement arthroplasty—or from other causes such as extensive erosion following loosening of a cemented hip prosthesis or extensive destruction of the joint by a gunshot wound.

The first stage of the operation is therefore exploratory, to enable the surgeon to ascertain the true extent of the pathology and to plan the operation accordingly. Thus if in a case of replacement arthroplasty the femoral prosthesis and surrounding cement are found to be loose in the medullary canal it is necessary not only to remove the prosthesis but also, if there is any sign of infection, to get away every fragment of cement. Likewise any excavation of the side wall of the pelvis must be thoroughly cleaned out, and if there are profuse cheesy granulations of the type that form not uncommonly when a cemented prosthesis has worked loose, it is important that all the unhealthy tissue be cleared away.

Removal of prosthesis. A femoral prosthesis, whether or not it has been cemented in, may usually be loosened by a sharp tap with hammer and punch to drive the prosthesis in a proximal direction. Sometimes there may be difficulty in freeing the prosthesis, particularly if it is of the Austin Moore type, which may become anchored by the growth of bone through the openings in the stem. In such a case it may be necessary to insinuate a thin osteotome within the upper part of the medullary canal to divide the bar of bone.

Removal of cement from femoral medullary canal. Removal of all the cement may present formidable difficulty; yet in cases of infection it is vital that

it be loose, on account of a mass of cement that may have penetrated through a hole in the floor of the acetabulum. A sharp tap with hammer and punch often dislodges it, but it may be necessary to break up the cement with a chisel and remove it piecemeal.

Excision of head and neck of femur. If the femoral head and neck have not already been removed as part of a previous operation such as total replace-

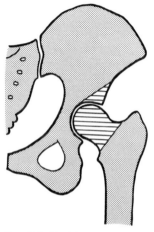

FIG. 414. Excision arthroplasty of hip. Diagram shows the amount of bone to be removed.

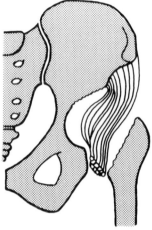

FIG. 415. The operation completed by interposition of muscle between the raw bone surfaces.

the clearance be complete. It is best achieved by cutting a narrow gutter—perhaps 5 or 6 millimetres wide—from the lateral cortex of the femur over the whole length that is occupied by cement. Through this gutter the cement may be broken up with a chisel and removed. Fragments that are still too large to be extracted through the gutter may be pushed upwards with a bone lever and extracted at the upper end of the bone. If pus has been present in the medullary canal the cavity is cleaned out as thoroughly as possible by suction and sponging. Whenever possible a flap of muscle (for instance a strip of vastus lateralis) should be sutured into the cavity to obliterate the dead space.

Removal of acetabular prosthesis. An acetabular prosthesis may be difficult to remove even though

ment arthroplasty, they should now be excised. In the unlikely event that the parts are still articulated the hip should first be dislocated either by lateral or by medial rotation. The line of bone section should run obliquely downwards and medially from the greater trochanter towards the lesser trochanter (Fig. 414). The femoral neck is thus removed right at its base. The bone should be cut cleanly to leave a smooth surface without any spurs.

Resection of upper lip of acetabulum. With a broad chisel driven into the wing of the ilium 2 or 3 centimetres above the acetabulum and driven downwards and medially to emerge at the acetabular floor the upper rim of the acetabulum is excised to leave a smooth sloping surface (Fig. 414).

Postero-lateral transfer of psoas tendon. To help to reduce the lateral rotation deformity that is often a sequel to the operation the psoas tendon is detached from its insertion at the lesser trochanter of the femur and re-routed round the front of the femoral shaft to be sutured to the soft tissues at the postero-lateral aspect of the femur. The tendon should be so sited that it is best able to act as a medial rotator of the thigh in contradistinction to its normal action as a lateral rotator.

Interposition of soft-tissue curtain. The gap between the upper end of the femur and the sloping side wall of the pelvis should be cushioned with a good wad of soft tissue sewn between the bones. In most cases a satisfactory soft-tissue curtain is provided by the gluteus medius muscle (Fig. 415). While the limb is drawn distally by an assistant and the trochanter is pulled laterally to open up the space between the bones, the gluteus medius is drawn down deep to the upper end of the femur and is anchored with absorbable sutures to the soft tissues in the region of the lesser trochanter in such a way that it forms a thick membrane between the femur and the pelvis.

Closure. The fascia lata, the gluteal aponeurosis and the gluteus maximus are repaired with absorbable sutures. The wound is closed with deep tension sutures and interrupted skin sutures. In most cases it is advisable to leave a polythene tube deep to the muscle layer for suction drainage.

POST-OPERATIVE MANAGEMENT

The wound is supported firmly with gauze dressings and crepe bandages applied spica fashion. For the first three or four weeks after operation the limb is supported in a Thomas's splint (or suitable modification thereof) with sustained weight traction of 8 to 10 pounds (3.5 to 4.5 kilograms). Usually it is most convenient to apply traction through a Steinmann pin inserted through the tibia behind its tubercle (see p. 62). The pin may be used to control lateral rotation by attaching a separate cord to the lateral end of the pin and suspending a weight of 0.5 to 1 kilogram (1 to 2 pounds) over a pulley in such a way that a medial rotation force is exerted. Splintage should be so arranged that the knee and the hip rest in 20 degrees of flexion. Each day, however, the patient should lie flat, with the knee and hip fully extended, for at least an hour: this helps to prevent flexion contracture. In this initial stage of post-operative management exercises for the quadriceps and gluteal muscles are encouraged, together with exercises for the foot and ankle.

After three or four weeks, depending upon progress, traction is discontinued and the splint removed. The patient may then lie free in bed and practise hip and knee exercises for one to two weeks before beginning walking—at first with axillary crutches with minimal weight bearing, but two weeks later with elbow crutches and gradually increasing weight bearing. Eventually the patient may progress to using only one stick, held in the hand opposite to the hip that is affected.

Comment

There are a number of technical points in this operation which make the difference between success and disappointment. There is no universal agreement as to the incision of choice: many surgeons prefer an anterior incision. The authors prefer the postero-lateral approach because of the excellent access that it affords and because the sciatic nerve may be identified and protected from harm.

An indifferent result may be due to failure to divide the bones cleanly, to leave smooth sloping surfaces. If a considerable stump of the femoral neck is left, and particularly if the upper rim of the acetabulum is not trimmed away, the bones may impinge and cause discomfort on walking. For similar reasons it is important to interpose a curtain of soft tissue between the trimmed bone ends. If muscle is used it is eventually transformed into fibrous tissue, and in consequence of the extensive scar tissue that forms about the joint a surprising degree of stability is finally achieved.

A troublesome defect of the Girdlestone pseudarthrosis has been the marked tendency for the limb to assume a position of lateral rotation. Transfer of the psoas tendon in order to counteract this tendency is well worth while, although it does not solve the problem completely.

In many centres weight bearing is delayed for up to two months or more, and thereafter a weight-relieving caliper is prescribed for up to six months or even longer. Function seems to be restored just as well, however, if the patient resumes walking as early as four or five weeks after the operation, without the use of a caliper. Even at best, rehabilitation tends to be slow and the fullest recovery of function cannot be expected before six to nine months have elapsed from the time of operation. Most patients need to use a stick (carried in the hand opposite to the side affected) indefinitely.

INTRA-ARTICULAR ARTHRODESIS OF HIP

Intra-articular arthrodesis of the hip entails, firstly, dislocation of the joint to allow access for the removal of diseased articular cartilage; secondly, fixation of the joint in the correct position by a transfixion nail; and thirdly, reinforcement by a cancellous bone graft.

POSITION FOR ARTHRODESIS

The best position for arthrodesis of the hip is with 15 to 20 degrees of flexion, no abduction or adduction, and no rotation.

TECHNIQUE

Position of patient. In the first part of the operation the patient should lie supine, with the entire limb draped to allow free manoeuvring by the assistants. For the second part of the operation, namely the insertion of the transfixion nail across the joint, the patient should be on the orthopaedic table with the limbs strapped to the foot-pieces. It is thus desirable to have a table that allows easy conversion from a flat-topped operation table to an orthopaedic table with adjustable leg pieces.

Exposure. The anterior (Smith-Petersen) approach is recommended. The steps in this were described on page 26. These steps are followed to the point of dislocating the hip by flexion and lateral rotation.

Excision of articular cartilage. Articular cartilage is removed from the whole surface of the femoral head by a chisel, down to raw bone. Hard subchondral bone should then be broken up superficially by multiple small chisel cuts into the surface, in order to promote vascularisation across the joint. If preferred, this denudation of the femoral head may be carried out with a powered oscillating saw or with a coarse burr. The articular surface of the acetabulum is likewise cleared and rawed with suitable gouges or burrs. This completes the first stage of the operation, and the femoral head is now reduced into the socket ready for the second stage, namely transfixion of the hip with a three-flanged nail.

Insertion of nail across the joint. For this second stage of the operation the patient must be positioned on the orthopaedic table with the feet strapped to the foot-plates. The position of the affected hip must be carefully adjusted to the optimal position—that is, with 15 to 20 degrees of flexion but no abduction or adduction and no rotation. It is very important to ensure that this optimal position is achieved: any deviation from it may mar the result.

A separate vertical incision is made over the lateral aspect of the upper end of the femur as for Smith-Petersen nailing (p. 261). The principles of inserting the three-flanged nail are the same as those for the insertion of a nail for fracture of the neck of the femur, except that the nail is directed more steeply upwards and that it penetrates across the hip joint into the iliac bone (Fig. 416). Introduction of the preliminary guide wire is easier than in nailing for fractured neck of femur because the femoral neck and head are exposed to view. It should therefore be possible to direct the guide wire correctly without the aid of radiographs. Nevertheless facilities for radiography should be available in case they are required.

The steps in the insertion of the nail are as follows. First the correct starting point is marked on the lateral aspect of the femur 2 or 3 centimetres below the flare of the greater trochanter, and a drill hole is made through the cortex to permit easy insertion of the guide wire.

Secondly, the guide wire is driven in by hand in a direction that will cause it to emerge from the inner aspect of the ilium through the thick bar of bone that forms the brim of the true pelvis. This implies a rather steeper inclination than is usual in nailing the femoral neck. If part of the iliacus

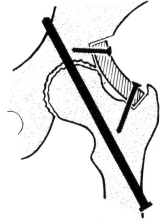

FIG. 416. Intra-articular arthrodesis of hip with ilio-femoral graft.

muscle is stripped from the inner wall of the ilium the point of emergence of the guide wire may be seen, or the tip of the wire may be felt by a freshly gloved finger inserted along the inner wall of the iliac bone from just behind the anterior superior spine.

Thirdly, when the guide wire has been satisfactorily placed, the correct length of nail that will allow it just to emerge through the inner wall of the iliac bone is calculated: this may be as much as 15 centimetres. A triangular starting hole for the nail is prepared in the outer cortex of the femur, and when it has once more been checked that the hip is in the optimal position the nail is driven in across the hip until its point is seen to emerge inside the pelvis.

Application of onlay bone graft. A raw bed is prepared for the reception of a bone graft designed to bridge the greater trochanter to the lateral aspect of the iliac bone just above the hip joint. For this purpose part of the greater trochanter may be cut away, or a slot may be cut into it from above (Fig. 416). Proximally, a bed is prepared in the wing of the ilium by breaching the cortex with a chisel and shaping a flat facet in the plane of the proposed graft. A graft of cancellous bone, with one cortical surface left intact, is taken from a conveniently accessible part of the wing of the ilium and shaped to fit the prepared bed. The graft is secured in place by two screws, one in the ilium and one in the femur (Fig. 416). Further slivers of cancellous bone are placed about the graft and particularly on its deep aspect, between it and the rawed hip joint.

Closure. The wound is closed in layers. Suction drainage is usually to be advised.

POST-OPERATIVE MANAGEMENT
Protection of the hip in a plaster-of-Paris spica is required, usually for twelve weeks. If rigid immobilisation of the hip joint has been secured with a well placed three-flanged nail, it may be permissible to use a single half-length spica—that is, one that encloses the affected side to a point just above the knee and extends well up on the trunk but which leaves the opposite limb free. If there is any doubt about the fixation afforded by the nail, however, a full-length spica is to be preferred. The patient should rest in bed for the first six weeks. Thereafter he should begin to walk with axillary crutches, without putting weight on the affected limb. The correct time at which it is safe to discard the plaster spica depends upon the clinical and radiographic state of the hip when it is examined three months after the operation. Protection in plaster should usually be continued until clinical tests show total immobility of the joint and radiographs show evidence of bony fusion.

Comment

Although this operation does not present particular difficulty many points of detail are of prime importance. Of these the most vital is to ensure that the hip is placed in the optimal position before the transfixion nail is driven in. Securing this position demands careful adjustment of the limbs when the patient is placed on the orthopaedic table. Any imperfection of the position will prejudice the patient's comfort thereafter. Thus, whereas 15 or 20 degrees of flexion are desirable, excessive flexion causes the patient to stand with marked lordosis, and backache is a likely sequel. Likewise, any adduction or abduction throws the spine out of alignment and may lead to persistent discomfort. Moreover, abduction jeopardises the opposite hip and throws abnormal stresses upon the knee of the affected side.

Another detail in which skill and judgement are required is in the correct placing of the transfixion nail to ensure that it grips good solid bone both in the femoral neck and in the pelvis. A nail that lies too horizontally is liable to engage only thin bone in the pelvic wall and may quickly work loose. An arthrodesis nail has to be placed much more vertically than a nail used for fractured neck of femur. It must also be inclined about 15 degrees forwards from the coronal plane. However, the fact that the bony structures are exposed to view makes correct placing of the guide wire and of the nail relatively easy.

It is usually helpful to expose the inner aspect of the iliac bone by stripping muscles down to the brim of the pelvis, as described, so that the point of penetration of the guide wire and nail can be observed or felt. This helps to ensure accurate placement of the nail, and allows the correct length to be determined precisely.

It should be appreciated that it is not always easy to get the hip to fuse. Failure may often be due to inadequate rawing and fitting of the surfaces, or to incomplete immobilisation. In this respect much depends on proper placement of the nail so that it secures a firm grip in solid bone.

EXTRA-ARTICULAR (ISCHIO-FEMORAL) ARTHRODESIS OF HIP

In this method of arthrodesis a tibial graft is inserted through drill holes to bridge the space between the ischium and the upper end of the femur. The hip is held immobile by a screw and a nail while the graft becomes incorporated (Fig. 417). The operation should be undertaken only by experienced hip surgeons who have had tuition in the technique or who have practised it in the cadaver. Consequently a summary rather than a detailed description is appropriate to this book. For a full account of the operation the reader is referred to the senior author's monograph, *Ischio-femoral Arthrodesis* (Adams 1966).

PRELIMINARY STUDIES

It is important to be sure before the operation is undertaken that the hip can be placed in the optimal position for arthrodesis (see previous section). If adduction or abduction deformity is present this may usually be corrected by the use of the Roger Anderson well-leg traction apparatus (Fig. 418) for a week or so before operation. If there is severe flexion or rotation deformity the case may be unsuitable for ischio-femoral arthrodesis and the intra-articular technique may have to be preferred.

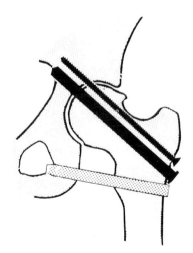

FIG. 417. Ischio-femoral arthrodesis. Diagram showing position of screw, nail and graft.

TECHNIQUES

The operation may be carried out by the so-called closed or blind technique, or by the open method.

CLOSED TECHNIQUE

The "closed" operation is done through a short lateral incision and neither the hip nor the ischium is exposed.

TECHNIQUE

Position of patient. The patient is placed supine upon the orthopaedic table with the feet strapped to the leg-pieces. Provision must be made for antero- posterior radiography: lateral films are not

Placement of guide wire. The first step is to transfix the hip with a screw and a nail. To ensure correct placement of the nail a guide wire is introduced in such a way that it traverses the middle of the femoral neck and head and crosses the hip joint to engage the thick bar of bone that forms the brim of the true pelvis (see section on intra-articular arthrodesis of hip, p. 310). If necessary, part of the iliacus muscle may be stripped from the ilium through a small separate incision made over the iliac crest immediately behind the anterior super-

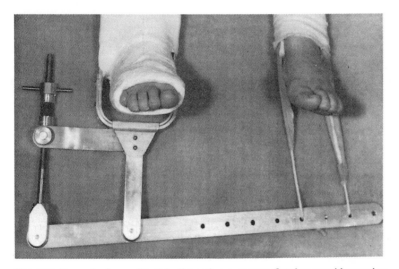
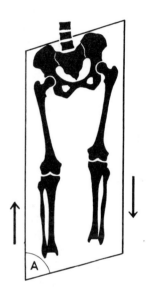
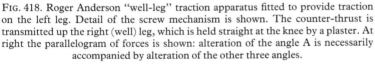

FIG. 418. Roger Anderson "well-leg" traction apparatus fitted to provide traction on the left leg. Detail of the screw mechanism is shown. The counter-thrust is transmitted up the right (well) leg, which is held straight at the knee by a plaster. At right the parallelogram of forces is shown: alteration of the angle A is necessarily accompanied by alteration of the other three angles.

required. The position of the hip is adjusted, the correct position being: flexion 15 to 20 degrees, abduction/adduction nil, rotation nil. A preliminary radiograph is taken after skin markers have been applied, to facilitate placement of the guide wire to be used for directing the nail (see page 262).

Exposure. The incision runs vertically downwards from the greater trochanter for 10 to 15 centimetres according to the size of the patient. The lateral aspect of the upper end of the femur is exposed by splitting the fascia lata and levering the vastus lateralis forwards as described on page 37.

ior spine, to allow the tip of the emerging guide wire to be seen or felt. Its position and length may thus be checked. The position of the wire should also be shown by a radiograph.

Driving of screw across joint. When the guide wire has been correctly placed the next step is to drive a Venable hip screw across the joint in a direction parallel with that of the guide wire. A hole 4 millimetres in diameter is first drilled with a long drill in the proposed direction of the screw. The proximal three-quarters of this hole should be drilled out to the overall diameter of the screw, to allow a sliding fit. A screw of appropriate length, as determined from the penetration of the guide wire, is then driven firmly home. It is important that the screw be inserted before the nail, because one of the main purposes of the screw is to prevent "rebound" of the femoral head from the acetabulum when the nail is hammered in.

Insertion of nail. A three-flanged nail of appropriate length, as determined from the penetration of the guide wire, is driven in over the guide wire with the normal precautions appropriate to this manoeuvre (see p. 310).

Preparation of track for graft. The track for the bone graft is prepared by drilling through the femur from the outer side and penetrating the ischium in the same axis. The initial pilot hole is made with a 9.5 millimetre drill. The starting point for the drill is determined from the radiograph. It is usually about 1 or 2 centimetres below the head of the three-flanged nail. Since the drill is to be directed about 15 degrees backwards as well as medially the starting point is a little in front of the mid-lateral line of the femoral shaft (Fig. 419).

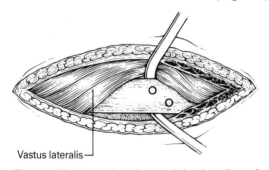

Vastus lateralis

FIG. 419. The vastus lateralis muscle has been levered forwards to expose the (left) femur. The sites chosen for insertion of the nail (posterior and proximal) and of the graft are indicated.

Initially the drill traverses only the femur. It is then removed to allow probing of the ischium, so that the surgeon may be sure that it is in the direct line of the drill. If probing shows that this is not so, the direction of the pilot hole is changed accordingly. When the drill is correctly directed towards the ischium it is driven forwards to penetrate right through the bone. The initial hole is then enlarged to the definitive size—usually 12.5 millimetres in diameter. The drill is left in position and a check radiograph is taken.

Preparation of graft. To form a peg 12.5 millimetres in diameter (equal to the drill hole in the femur) two strips of medial cortex of tibia are taken and wired together cortex to cortex (Fig. 420). Each strip is thus 12.5 millimetres wide and of a length commensurate with the depth

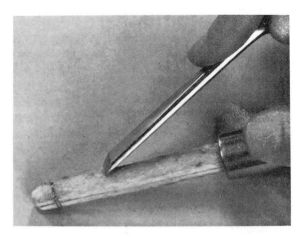

FIG. 420. Preparation of tibial graft, made up from two pieces of bone wired cortex to cortex.

from the lateral cortex of the femur to the deep cortex of the ischium: the length is determined by measuring the depth at which ischium is probed, and adding 2.5 centimetres for the thickness of the ischium. The leading end of the peg thus prepared should be slightly tapered to facilitate its entry into the drill hole. (For the technique of taking a tibial graft see p. 72).

Driving of graft. The 12.5 millimetre drill having been removed from the femur, the graft is inserted through the hole in the same direction and driven in with light hammer blows on a broad punch. The graft can usually be felt to enter the ischium, which offers slightly increased resistance. It is driven on until the outer end is flush with the lateral cortex of the femur. A final check radiograph is taken to ensure that the graft has been correctly placed (Fig. 417).

POST-OPERATIVE MANAGEMENT

The hip is protected by a single plaster spica extended well up on the trunk but including only the thigh of the affected leg, the knee being left free. The patient remains in bed for three weeks, during which knee exercises are practised. Walking is then begun with axillary crutches, at first with limited weight bearing. Six weeks after operation the plaster is removed. By this time the patient is usually able to take full weight on the limb and he may progress to elbow crutches. These should be continued until four months from operation because the graft is fragile during the critical phase of revascularisation, which is active between the sixth and sixteenth weeks.

Comment

Points noted in the commentary upon intra-articular arthrodesis of the hip apply equally to this operation. In particular, it is fundamental to ensure that the hip is fixed in the optimal position.

With this closed or "blind" method of ischio-femoral fusion there is a potential hazard to the sciatic nerve, but this does not become an actual hazard provided due precautions are observed (Adams 1964). A cardinal rule, however, is that the closed technique must not be used when the anatomy of the pelvis and femur is grossly distorted or when the bones are hypoplastic (as in certain cases of poliomyelitis or tuberculosis with onset in early childhood). Nor should the closed technique be used in children under sixteen. In such cases the posterior open method of ischio-femoral grafting (see below) should be preferred, as it should always be by the inexperienced operator.

In slender women or in patients whose bones have become porotic it is advisable to use a nail and plate (for instance, the MacLaughlin two-piece nail-plate) instead of a simple nail, as a precaution against fracture through the drill hole for the graft.

OPEN TECHNIQUE

In the open technique the hip is first transfixed by a screw and a nail with the patient supine upon the orthopaedic table. The patient is then turned to the prone position to allow exposure of the gluteal area from behind and insertion of a bone graft under direct vision.

TECHNIQUE
The steps of the operation are precisely the same as for the closed technique as far as the insertion of the screw and three-flanged nail. When these have been inserted and the hip thus rendered immobile in the correct position, the patient is turned to the prone position upon an ordinary operation table to allow exposure of the ischium and of the sciatic nerve from the back.

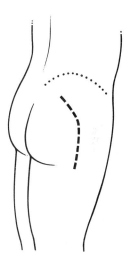

FIG. 421. Ischio-femoral arthrodesis. Incision for open technique.

Exposure. The existing vertical incision is prolonged upwards, curving posteriorly towards a point 2.5 centimetres in front of the posterior superior spine of the ilium (Fig. 421). The large gluteal flap may then be retracted posteriorly to expose the short transverse lateral rotator muscles of the hip. The obturator internus and gemelli above and the quadratus femoris below should be identified and separated while the sciatic nerve, which lies superficial to these muscles, is retracted gently out of harm's way (Fig. 422). Through this gap between the muscles the body of the ischium may be palpated and exposed to view.

Preparation of track for graft and insertion of graft. The subsequent stages of the operation are the same as described in the previous section, except that the penetration of the drill between the femur and the ischium, and its entrance into the

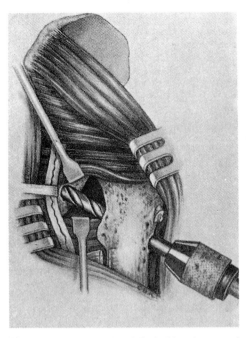

FIG. 422. The tuberosity of the ischium is exposed by separation of the inferior gemellus and the quadratus femoris. A drill hole is made through the femur and on into the ischium under direct vision.

ischium, are observed under direct vision. Thus it is possible to ensure that the sciatic nerve is unharmed.

POST-OPERATIVE MANAGEMENT

This is the same as described for the closed technique.

Comment

It may be thought inconvenient to have to change the patient from the supine to the prone position between the two stages of the operation. Nevertheless the authors believe that this is the price that has to be paid for accuracy, because it is not practicable to adjust the hip to the correct position for arthrodesis with the patient prone. Once the hip has been nailed in the correct position with the patient supine, he may then be turned over without fear of mal-position.

Some surgeons prefer to undertake ischiofemoral arthrodesis routinely by the open method, and this is certainly recommended for the relatively inexperienced operator. But those with experience of the closed technique find that it is simpler and quicker; and if patients are properly selected and due precautions are observed, the sciatic nerve is not endangered.

For additional comments the reader is referred to the section on closed ischio-femoral arthrodesis (p. 312).

PIN FIXATION FOR SLIPPED UPPER FEMORAL EPIPHYSIS

In this operation two, or usually three, pins are driven across the epiphysial cartilage plate into the femoral head to prevent progressive slipping. The pins are slender (usually 2 millimetres in diameter) and pointed at the tip: the base is threaded to grip the bone and thus to prevent the pin from sliding out* (Fig. 423). In most cases the epiphysis is pinned in the existing position of minor slip. If the epiphysis is mobile, preliminary reduction may be attempted either by sustained traction and medial rotation, or by gentle manipulation. Although two pins are probably adequate, most surgeons aim to insert three for extra security.

* The pins designed and used by the authors are manufactured by Messrs Howmedica Ltd of London, England.

TECHNIQUE

The basic technique is the same as that for nailing a fracture of the neck of the femur (p. 260), the description of which should be read in conjunction with this section.

Setting up. The patient is placed on the orthopaedic table in the way described for nailing a femoral neck fracture. Skin clips are applied as markers (Fig. 350) and radiographic units are positioned for antero-posterior and lateral radiography.

Reduction. As implied above, reduction is usually either not required or, in the case of a mobile epiphysis, it has been achieved by gentle manipulation before operation. In the occasional case in which reduction is attempted at the time of

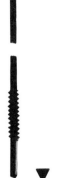

FIG. 423. Crawford Adams's pin for the stabilisation of slipping femoral epiphysis. The threads prevent extrusion of the pin. The base is of triangular section, to allow it to be gripped in the chuck of a drill.

operation it is done by very gently rotating the limb medially, while steady traction is maintained. Great force should never be used for fear of further damaging the blood supply of the capital epiphysis, which is already endangered.

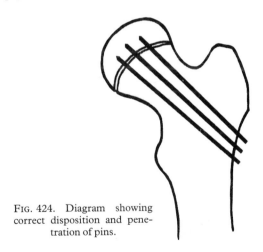

FIG. 424. Diagram showing correct disposition and penetration of pins.

The operation. This proceeds in the way described for nailing a fractured femoral neck, to the point of exposure of the lateral aspect of the femur just below the greater trochanter. The insertion of guide wires follows a similar method. If three guide wires are to be used the entrance holes are grouped in a triangle so that they are spaced about a centimetre apart. The exact disposition of the three wires is not important so long as each tra-

verses the femoral neck and crosses the epiphysial plate (Fig. 424). The wires should be parallel or nearly so, but not so close together as to be almost contiguous. Their position is checked by radiographs.

When the guide wires have been placed satisfactorily each is removed in turn and replaced in the same track by a slipped epiphysis pin, the correct length of which has been calculated from the control radiographs. The threads at the bases of the pins stand proud; so the pins must be twisted in once the threads engage in the bone. This is easily done by a hand drill, the chuck of which grips the triangular base of the pin: an extension tube or box spanner may be used if the chuck tends to foul a pin already inserted.

After the pins have been driven in, check radiographs are taken and any necessary adjustments to the depth of penetration are made. The wound is closed in layers without drainage.

POST-OPERATIVE MANAGEMENT

Splintage is not required: the patient lies free in bed and is encouraged to move the hip and knee. Walking with the partial support of crutches is begun within three or four days, and full weight bearing may be permitted as soon as the wound is healed.

Comment

The main difficulties of this operation are to get the multiple pins satisfactorily directed into the displaced femoral epiphysis, and to ensure correct penetration of the pins. The margin for error in judging correct length and penetration of the pins is small: each pin must cross the epiphysial cartilage and yet it must stop short of the articular surface. Radiographic determination of a pin's penetration is apt to be fallacious even with films in two planes at right angles to each other (Pollen 1965): the point of a pin may in fact have penetrated the articular surface when no such penetration is shown in the radiographs. A margin of safety must therefore be allowed: it should be a rule that the points of the pins should not penetrate closer than 5 millimetres from the articular surface as shown in the radiographs.

PROPHYLACTIC PINNING OF EPIPHYSIS

In certain circumstances pinning of an unslipped epiphysis is advised when the epiphysis on the other side has suffered a severe slip. The technique is the same as that just described. The operation is somewhat easier because, since there is no slip, the full width of the femoral neck is available for the pins and there is consequently some latitude, whereas in the case of a slipped epiphysis great accuracy is required in directing the guide wires.

SUBTROCHANTERIC CORRECTIVE OSTEOTOMY FOR SLIPPED UPPER FEMORAL EPIPHYSIS

This osteotomy, carried out just below the greater trochanter, is designed to compensate for the angulation of the upper femoral epiphysis and thus to restore the epiphysis—that is, the articular component of the upper end of the femur—to a proper relationship with the acetabulum. It is undertaken only when the degree of slip is such that pinning *in situ* is inappropriate and when manipulative reduction is not feasible: this usually means in practice a slip that exceeds 35 or 40 degrees (see below for method of measurement).

PRELIMINARY STUDIES

To give a good and lasting result this operation must be performed with precision. It is necessary first to determine the angle through which the epiphysis has slipped and the direction of the slip. This information is determined from true antero-posterior and lateral radiographs of the neck of the femur.

Care must be taken in obtaining these radiographs, because in a case of severe slip the affected limb may lie in lateral rotation and it may not be possible to rotate it inwards as far as the neutral position, let alone to the position of 15 or 20 degrees of medial rotation that is required to bring the femoral neck into the coronal plane. Thus the standard projections will not provide either a true antero-posterior or a true lateral image. It may therefore be necessary to direct the x-ray beam obliquely, to ensure that for the antero-posterior radiograph it passes at right angles to the plane of the femoral neck and for the lateral radiograph precisely in the plane of the femoral neck.

In nearly every case the direction of slip is strictly posterior—that is, the capital epiphysis slides down the back of the femoral neck in an arc whose axis is horizontal and in the coronal plane (Griffith 1973). Seeming medial displacement, as observed in antero-posterior radiographs that are taken with the limb laterally rotated, is in most cases an illusion.

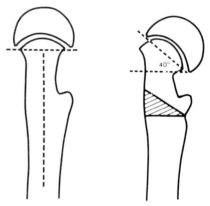

FIGS 425–426. Measurement of angle of posterior slip of epiphysis on true lateral radiograph. Figure 425—Normal position. Figure 426—Posterior slip measures 40 degrees. Shaded area below shows site of compensatory osteotomy.

The extent of the posterior slip may be determined from measurements upon a true lateral radiograph. A line is drawn at right angles to the long axis of the femur, and a second line joins the two "horns" of the capital epiphysis. The angle subtended by these two lines is the angle of slip (Figs 425 and 426). In theory this is the angle of correction required at the site of osteotomy, but in practice if the deformity is severe it is permissible, and compatible with a good result, to under-correct it by up to 20 degrees.

If there is marked lateral rotation deformity—such that correction to the neutral position is not possible—it is advisable to combine an element of medial rotation of the shaft of the femur with the anterior wedge osteotomy that is required to compensate for the backward tilting of the epiphysis. Such rotational correction should be limited to the number of degrees by which lateral rotation is a fixed rotation beyond the neutral position. Thus, for example, if there is fixed lateral rotation of 20 degrees, a rotational correction of 20 degrees is required. It should be remembered that there is a tendency for lateral rotation deformity to be corrected spontaneously in the months or years after operation as remodelling occurs.

Before the surgeon sets out upon the operation, therefore, he should have determined the size of the anterior wedge that is to be removed and also the degree of rotational correction, if any, that is to be made.

TECHNIQUE

The plan is first to correct any excess rotational deformity by dividing the femur transversely just below the greater trochanter and rotating the distal fragment medially; and then to remove a wedge of bone, of predetermined size, from the front of the femur.

Setting up. The patient is placed on the orthopaedic table in the manner described for nailing of a fracture of the neck of the femur, the description of which should be read in conjunction with this section (p. 260). The feet are secured to the footplates and the position of the affected limb is adjusted so that the patella is directed 15 or 20 degrees medially—or, if there is fixed deformity, as near to this position as possible. Radiographic units are brought into position for anteroposterior and lateral radiography. The image intensifier may be used if preferred.

Exposure. The antero-lateral exposure (p. 28) is appropriate. The lower half of the incision extends vertically downwards from the prominence of the greater trochanter for 10 or 12 centimetres according to the size of the patient (Fig. 427). Proximally the incision curves forwards to allow dissection between the anterior

margin of the gluteus medius and the posterior margin of the tensor fasciae latae muscle. Retraction of the muscles with bone levers allows a full exposure of the front of the femoral neck and of the upper end of the femoral shaft.

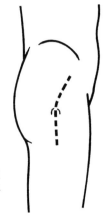

FIG. 427. Antero-lateral exposure of hip. The skin incision.

Rotation osteotomy. If there is excessive rotational deformity the first step in the correction is to divide the femur and to rotate the lower fragment medially upon the upper fragment. The osteotomy should be immediately below the greater trochanter and it should be strictly transverse—that is, at right angles to the long axis of the femoral shaft. Before the bone is divided two guide wires should be driven into the femur to project out at right angles to it, one above and one below the proposed line of osteotomy: their points should just engage the far cortex but need not penetrate it (Fig. 428). These guide wires serve as indicators to show how much the femoral fragments are rotated relative to each other (Fig. 429). It is best to insert the wires in such a way that they diverge from one another through an angle that is equal to the proposed angle of correction. Then, when rotation has been effected through the required angle the wires will be parallel.

When the wires have been placed in position the bone is divided cleanly either by a power-operated reciprocating saw or by making multiple drill holes and completing the section with a thin osteotome. The cuff of periosteum adjacent to the osteotomy must be freed all round the bone, lest it hinder the rotation. When the bone has been divided completely and the periosteum separated, the bone fragments are gripped with bone-holding forceps and, after the foot-plate attachment of the orthopaedic table has been loosened so that it is free to rotate, the distal fragment and with it the whole leg is rotated medially through the predetermined angle. The foot-plate attachment is then locked again to steady the position of the limb.

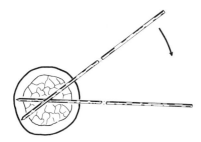

FIG. 428. Guide wires inserted above and below the site of osteotomy subtend the required angle of rotation. When the full amount of rotational correction has been achieved the wires will be parallel.

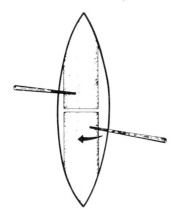

FIG. 429. After division of the bone the distal fragment is rotated medially to bring the wires parallel.

Resection of anterior wedge and correction of angular deformity. It is now a simple matter to excise a wedge of bone of predetermined dimensions from the front of the femur at the level where (if rotation has been deemed necessary) the bone has already been divided (Fig. 426). It is usually best to take the wedge mainly at the expense of the proximal fragment.

When the wedge of bone has been removed the gap is closed by flexion of the distal fragment upon the proximal end of the femur. The manoeuvre is

best accomplished by releasing the clamp on the telescopic leg-piece of the orthopaedic table so that it can be pushed in and thus shortened. This allows the knee to be flexed: at the same time the femur comes up into flexion, closing the osteotomy gap (Fig. 430). The leg is held in this position by an assistant while the bone fragments are secured by internal fixation.

Internal fixation. The application of a suitable fixation device tends to be awkward because of the sharp angulation of the femur resulting from excision of the anterior wedge. Usually the most convenient device is a four-hole plate bent to fit

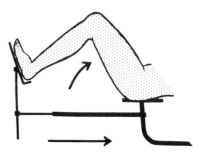

FIG. 430. The leg-piece of the orthopaedic table has been shortened to flex the hip and knee, thus closing the wedge-shaped osteotomy gap.

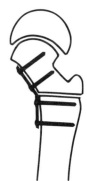

FIG. 431. By compensatory osteotomy the epiphysis is restored to normal relationship with the acetabulum.

the angled anterior cortex of the femur, bridging the site of osteotomy (Fig. 431). The plate may have to be bent as much as 45 degrees or more, depending upon the angle of correction that has been required. The plate is fixed in position with screws. Fixation may be supplemented by two or three wide staples.

Pinning of epiphysis. If the epiphysial plate is still open further slipping of the epiphysis is theoretically possible; so it is wise to prevent this by inserting two or three threaded pins across the epiphysial cartilage. This is done in the manner described on page 316. If the slip is of long duration, however, and the epiphysial plate closed or almost closed, this last step in the operation may be omitted.

Closure. The wound is closed in layers. Suction drainage for twenty-four hours is recommended.

POST-OPERATIVE MANAGEMENT

With the patient still in position on the orthopaedic table and with the affected hip and knee still flexed, a plaster-of-Paris hip spica is applied to include the whole of the affected limb and the sound limb down to the knee. After three weeks the plaster is changed: the new plaster spica immobilises the affected limb with the hip and knee in only slight flexion and with slight abduction, the sound limb being left free. The plaster is discarded when the osteotomy is shown to be well on the way to union—usually about six to eight weeks after the operation. Thereafter the patient begins walking with elbow crutches, and intensive hip and knee exercises are practised under the supervision of a physiotherapist.

Correction of leg length discrepancy. If a large anterior wedge has had to be removed in order to bring the femoral capital epiphysis into the acetabulum, the upper end of the femur is so crooked that substantial shortening—in the order of 3 or 4 centimetres—may be produced. Such shortening may justify epiphysiodesis at the lower end of the femur on the sound side at the appropriate age (see p. 108). Timing of the epiphysiodesis must be accurate, so that correct adjustment is achieved by the time growth is complete.

Comment

This anterior wedge osteotomy, combined if necessary with medial rotation osteotomy, achieves the object of bringing the femoral epiphysis back into its proper relationship with the acetabulum without jeopardising the blood supply of the epiphysis. It is an operation that must be done with great precision after careful study of the pre-operative radiographs to determine the angle of correction that is required. It can be a difficult operation that should not be attempted by the occasional operator in this field.

Not the least of the difficulties that may be encountered is to secure adequate fixation of the fragments after rotational and angular correction has been gained. The authors prefer to rely largely upon a plaster-of-Paris spica to maintain the position of the fragments once they have been held reasonably securely by a plate with screws, aided usually by two or three staples. In these young patients union at the site of osteotomy advances rapidly, and it is safe after three weeks or so to bring the limb down close to the neutral position.

A disadvantage of this compensatory osteotomy is that it may lead to some shortening of the limb, sometimes necessitating subsequent leg equalisation; but this is a price that is justifiably paid for virtual immunity of the femoral epiphysis from risk of avascular necrosis, a complication that is a serious hazard of the alternative operation of intracapsular cervical osteotomy (see below).

INTRACAPSULAR CERVICAL OSTEOTOMY FOR SLIPPED UPPER FEMORAL EPIPHYSIS

In this operation, which in many cases is a possible alternative to the operation described in the previous section, the deformity of the upper end of the femur is corrected by osteotomy through the femoral neck close to the epiphysial plate. The authors prefer no longer to practise this operation, because even in the best hands there is a significant risk of damaging the blood supply to the epiphysis in such a way that avascular necrosis and eventual collapse of the femoral head occur. Those who wish to study this operation further should consult the paper by Dunn and Angel published in 1978.

RELEASE OF GLUTEAL APONEUROSIS FOR SNAPPING HIP

Snapping hip is caused by a vertically disposed thickened band of the gluteal aponeurosis in the outer wall of the trochanteric bursa snapping over the lateral prominence of the greater trochanter when the aponeurosis is under tension (as when

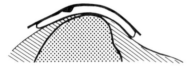

Fig. 432. Transverse section through outer part of greater trochanter and overlying tissues, showing prominent aponeurotic band in outer wall of trochanteric bursa. (Patient in lateral position with affected side uppermost.)

standing on the limb) and the hip is moved into extension or flexion (Fig. 432). The snap cannot be reproduced with the patient relaxed in recumbency, nor on the operation table. Cure of this sometimes disturbing mechanical derangement is best brought about by division of the offending band of tissue from within the trochanteric bursa.

TECHNIQUE

Position of patient. The patient lies in the lateral position with the affected hip uppermost.

Incision. The incision is a vertical one 10 centimetres long, centred over the lateral prominence of the greater trochanter (Fig. 433). It is deepened through the subcutaneous fatty tissue to display the outer glistening surface of the immensely strong gluteal aponeurosis.

Splitting of aponeurosis and location of abnormal band. Over the centre of the greater trochanter the gluteal aponeurosis is first incised vertically with a knife, opening the trochanteric bursa. With strong

scissors the vertically disposed fibres of the aponeurosis are split proximally and distally through the length of the skin incision. At this stage it is possible to locate the abnormally thickened band of aponeurosis by palpation of its under surface

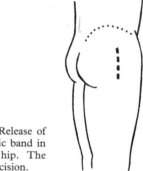

Fig. 433. Release of aponeurotic band in snapping hip. The skin incision.

with a finger introduced into the trochanteric bursa through the split in the aponeurosis (Fig. 434). The band usually lies in the anterior half of the aponeurosis, where it will be felt on the deep surface as a very tight ridge. Indeed, it may be necessary to abduct the hip before the pal-

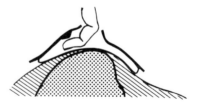

Fig. 434. The tight band palpated by a finger in the trochanteric bursa.

pating finger can be introduced beneath the band. The posterior half of the aponeurosis should also be palpated, but it is usually found to be smooth.

Division of abnormal band. The abnormal band is best divided by a knife with number 10 blade inserted alongside the palpating finger and so directed that the band can be divided transversely

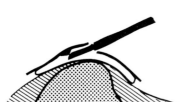

FIG. 435. The abnormal band is severed from within the bursa by a knife directed outwards. The knife is best guided by a finger alongside the blade.

from its deep surface (Fig. 435). Once the band has been severed the tight vertical ridge initially palpated will no longer be felt. In dividing the band it is not necessary to cut through the whole thickness of the aponeurosis: the superficial fibres may be left intact.

Closure. The vertical splitting incision in the gluteal aponeurosis is repaired with strong interrupted absorbable sutures. The skin is closed without drainage.

POST-OPERATIVE MANAGEMENT

Prolonged recumbency is not required, and the patient may be allowed up and about to a limited extent from the beginning. Only a brief stay in hospital is required and the patient should be encouraged to resume a normal life within two to four weeks of the operation.

Comment

The operation described is simple but nevertheless fully effective, and it is well worth while in those few patients in whom the repeated snapping is a source of annoyance or anxiety.

DISARTICULATION OF HIP

Strictly, the term disarticulation implies removal of the entire femur including the femoral head. In practice, however, the term is sometimes used to include a through-thigh amputation so high that the small remnant of femur is functionless and limb fitting is comparable to that after true disarticulation. Any femoral stump that is less than 5 centimetres long from the level of the lesser trochanter may be regarded as functionless and the amputation akin to disarticulation.

TECHNIQUE

Position of patient. The patient lies supine.

Marking out the line of incision. It is well to draw the line of the proposed incision upon the skin with ink, with care to ensure that adequate skin is left intact. The incision will be racquet-shaped, with the handle of the racquet anteriorly (Fig. 436). The outline should be commenced at the anterior superior spine of the ilium. Descend-

ing vertically for a few centimetres, it curves medially to follow the line of the inguinal ligament to the medial side of the thigh, which should be crossed about 5 centimetres distal to the origin of the adductor muscles. The line of incision then sweeps across the back of the thigh 5 to 7 centimetres distal to the tuberosity of the ischium to reach the lateral aspect of the thigh 8 to 10 centimetres distal to the base of the greater trochanter. From this point the incision curves proximally and anteriorly to join the commencement of the incision at the anterior superior iliac spine. When the outline has thus been drawn upon the skin surface a careful estimate is made as to whether sufficient skin has been left to close the stump without tension, due regard being paid to the build of the patient and the bulk of the thigh.

Incision. When the surgeon is satisfied that the outlines have been correctly drawn upon the skin surface he incises the skin and subcutaneous tissue throughout the length of the racquet incision.

Ligation of femoral vessels. Through the proximal part of the incision the femoral artery and vein are identified, doubly ligated with transfixion ligatures, and divided just below the inguinal ligament. At the same time the adjacent femoral nerve is pulled distally, cut cleanly and allowed to retract.

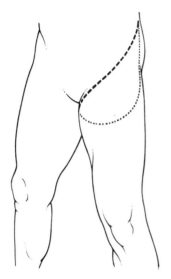

FIG. 436. Disarticulation of hip. Outlines for the skin incision.

Division of anterior muscles. First the sartorius muscle is detached from the anterior superior spine of the ilium and the rectus femoris from the anterior inferior spine, and both muscles are reflected distally. Next the pectineus muscle is detached close to its point of origin from the pubis and turned distally.

Separation of medial muscles. The thigh is flexed and rotated laterally to bring the lesser trochanter into view: the ilio-psoas tendon is detached from it and reflected proximally. Further medially, the adductor muscles and the gracilis are separated from their origin from the ischio-pubic ramus. Next it is necessary to identify the obturator externus muscle, and between this and the short lateral rotator muscles of the hip to isolate and ligate the main branches of the obturator artery. The obturator externus muscle is not divided at this stage.

Separation of lateral and posterior muscles. The limb being now rotated strongly medially, the gluteus medius and the gluteus minimus muscles are severed from their attachment to the greater trochanter and reflected proximally. At the lateral side of the thigh, below the greater trochanter, the fascia lata is divided obliquely in the line of the skin incision and the tendinous insertion of the gluteus maximus is detached from the back of the femur. The whole mass of the gluteus maximus is then reflected proximally. The sciatic nerve is thus brought into view and is ligated and divided cleanly. It now remains only to divide the lateral rotator muscles of the hip (piriformis, obturator internus and gemelli, obturator externus and quadratus femoris) and to separate the hamstring muscles from the ischial tuberosity.

Separation of femur. In a true disarticulation the capsule of the hip joint is now incised circumferentially and the femoral head is prised out of the socket, the ligament of the femoral head [ligamentum teres] being severed. If a short length of femur is to be retained the bone is sawn through at the appropriate point after reflection of a sleeve of periosteum.

Closure. It is important to spend time on securing full haemostasis before the wound is closed. In the closure it is the aim to bring the mass of the gluteal muscles forward beneath the hip joint and to suture its distal margin to the remains of the medial and anterior muscles. Two polythene tubes for suction drainage are inserted deep to the muscle mass. The skin edges are brought together and any obvious excess of skin is trimmed away to allow accurate suture of the edges without undue laxity but without tension, care being taken to avoid wrinkles and "dog ears".

POST-OPERATIVE MANAGEMENT

Soft gauze dressings are held in place by three or four wide crepe bandages applied in spica fashion over the stump and round the waist above the iliac crest. The drainage tubes should be removed after forty-eight hours, when the dressing may be reinforced with further crepe bandages. After two weeks, when the sutures are removed, plaster-of-Paris may be moulded to the stump and round the pelvis: it is held in position by careful shaping above the iliac crest, aided by shoulder straps.

The plaster should also be moulded closely below the ischial tuberosity to help to shape the stump for definitive limb fitting, which may be commenced about six weeks after operation.

HIND-QUARTER AMPUTATION

Hind-quarter amputation (hemipelvectomy or trans-pelvic amputation) entails removal of the lower limb together with the iliac bone on the affected side. It is a formidable operation, calling for intensive supportive measures to combat loss of blood and surgical shock. It is not an operation that the junior surgeon is called upon to undertake, and consequently a full description of the technique is not within the scope of this book.

TECHNIQUE

The operation as described by Gordon-Taylor and Monro (1952) is carried out in two stages, the first with the patient supine and the second with the patient in the lateral position. In the first stage the incision, beginning at the pubic tubercle, extends proximally above the inguinal ligament and the crest of the ilium. Distally, it extends backwards in the crease between thigh and perineum. Abdominal muscles are separated from the iliac crest, and the peritoneum is pushed medially from the iliac fossa. The rectus abdominis muscle is divided distally to expose the symphysis pubis, which is divided after the bladder has been freed and displaced backwards and towards the opposite side. The common iliac artery and vein are exposed, ligated and divided.

In the second part of the operation the patient is placed in the lateral position and the incision is continued distally from the back of the iliac crest to the region of the greater trochanter. Thence it curves round the back of the thigh to meet the medial thigh incision near the tuberosity of the ischium. The iliac bone is divided from the posterior part of the crest to the greater sciatic notch. This allows the pelvis to be opened out. The pelvic viscera are displaced medially and the muscles are separated from the inner wall of the pelvis. The remaining posterior muscles and the sciatic nerve are divided and the limb with the major part of the innominate bone is discarded. The gluteus maximus is brought forward as a flap and sutured to the abdominal muscles. The skin edges are closed with appropriate drainage.

CHAPTER NINE

Thigh and Knee

The thigh and knee are intimately linked: knee function is heavily dependent upon an intact and powerful quadriceps muscle and upon normal alignment of the femur.

The knee area may be regarded as a microcosm of orthopaedic surgical practice, for most disorders and most types of operation are represented—injury, deformity, arthritis, osteochondritis dissecans, loose body formation, cysts and ganglia. In recent years the range of operations has been expanded to include total replacement arthroplasty. This is still in a stage of development, but results are now being obtained that begin to approach the high success rate of arthroplasty of the hip.

Technical refinements in endoscopy have led to the universal acceptance of arthroscopy of the knee as an irreplaceable technique in diagnosis; and there is an increasing body of surgeons who see arthroscopic surgery as the method of choice for many, if not most, of the routine operations upon the knee.

CONTENTS OF CHAPTER

THE PRINCIPLES OF ARTHROSCOPY AND ARTHROSCOPIC SURGERY OF THE KNEE

Arthroscopy has been practised for many years by pioneers in the field, notably in Japan (Takagi 1933). The great upsurge in the use of the technique that occurred in the 1970s was due largely to technological advances, particularly in the field of fibre optics. The perfection if fibre optic illumination revolutionised endoscopy in general, and with it arthroscopy. (For most practical purposes this means arthroscopy of the knee: the technique has been used in other joints, but the advantages are less evident and the incentives correspondingly slender.)

Arthroscopy is now well established as a valuable aid to the diagnosis of knee complaints—indeed it has become virtually indispensable. And arthroscopic surgery has achieved such impressive success in reducing discomfort and accelerating recovery and rehabilitation, that the time cannot be distant when virtually all routine operations upon the knee such as meniscectomy, removal of loose bodies, trimming of osteophytes, etc., will be carried out arthroscopically. Indeed the discerning patient may come to demand this less harassing method.

The credit for advancing the art of endoscopic knee surgery cannot easily be accorded to any one person, for there have been many pioneers. But recognition must be given to two exponents of the technique who have done much to disseminate knowledge on the subject and to instruct others in the art—namely R. W. Jackson of Toronto and D. J. Dandy in Britain (Jackson and Dandy 1976, Dandy 1981).

Arthroscopy and arthroscopic surgery cannot be learnt from books: proficiency can be acquired only by apprenticeship and long practice, which in the early stages may well be upon models of the knee rather than upon patients. Consequently no attempt will be made in this book to cover the details of technique: only general principles will be expounded. The important rule is that the surgeon who sets out to master the techniques—as every orthopaedic surgeon will be required to do in the future—must become skilled in diagnostic arthroscopy before he attempts to undertake arthroscopic surgery.

The arthroscope. The modern arthroscope is made with a wide angle of vision (usually 70 degrees in saline) to facilitate inspection of the joint tissues within the very restricted space available. It also has a 30 degrees fore-oblique telescope, which means that one is not seeing straight ahead but at an angle of 30 degrees. This enables a wider area to be surveyed by rotating the instrument. Chemical sterilisation is normally used, but some arthroscopes can be autoclaved.

Anaesthesia. General anaesthesia is advised. If local anaesthesia is used there may be severe discomfort from the tourniquet.

Tourniquet. A tourniquet is applied on the upper part of the thigh. Full exsanguination by an Esmarch bandage is best avoided because the tissues may appear excessively blanched: structures such as synovial membrane are more easily recognised when they retain reasonable vascularity.

Aseptic precautions. The limb is prepared and draped in the same way as for an open operation.

The use of an arthroscope with a telescope breaks one of the rules of sterility. The telescope becomes unsterile through contact with the eye and yet it is within the sterile field. It must be remembered that the eyepiece must not be touched with the gloved hand that will then be in contact with parts of the telescope or with instruments that will be used within the knee. This is a special problem if the eyepiece becomes misted by condensation. An assistant must be called upon to clean the eyepiece. The problem of an unsterile eyepiece in the operative field is avoided if a miniature television camera is fitted to the telescope.

Irrigation. The synovial cavity is distended by injection of saline through a needle inserted into the suprapatellar pouch. A constant-flow system is set up, fluid entering through the channel in the arthroscope and escaping through the injection needle left in position in the suprapatellar pouch. This enables debris to be washed out. It is easier and less likely to cause damage to the articular surfaces if the arthroscope and instruments are inserted with the knee distended with saline.

Arthroscopic approaches. Correct siting of the arthroscope is essential for success. The approach most commonly used is the antero-lateral approach, which permits visualisation not only of the medial compartment but also of the lateral meniscus. The mid-line approach is also often used. Other approaches—for instance postero-medial—may be required in special circumstances. The information gained through any approach may be enhanced if the part under inspection is moved by a needle or hook introduced at another point, so that the two instruments converge at an angle.

The joint is surveyed in a systematic manner, and the examination should include the suprapatellar pouch, the deep surface of the patella, the medial meniscus and medial femoral condyle, the lateral meniscus and lateral femoral condyle, the intercondylar notch with the anterior cruciate ligament, and if possible the posterior recesses.

Arthroscopic surgery. When the pathological anatomy has been revealed fully by diagnostic arthroscopy the operation must be carefully planned. The commonest arthroscopic operation by far is partial meniscectomy.

Most arthroscopic surgery is carried out by the double puncture technique. In this method the diagnostic arthroscope, usually inserted antero-laterally, is used to monitor the various instruments that may be used, which are inserted through a separate opening to converge upon the arthroscope at an angle. Siting of the entrance point for the cutting and grasping instruments is critical, for clearly it must be so disposed that the point of the instrument can be brought to bear on the lesion, while at the same time this is kept under direct vision through the arthroscope.

There is often difficulty in aligning an operative instrument inserted through a separate incision with the view through the telescope. It may also be difficult to know exactly how much of the telescope is in the joint. If the length of the telescope is measured before insertion and a sterile rule is available to measure the length of the telescope outside the knee, it is easy to calculate the length that is within the knee.

Because an instrument used for an operative procedure inside the knee is usually shorter than the telescope, orientation is helped if the instrument is touched onto the shaft of the telescope near the surface and then run gently deeper along the telescope until it comes into view.

Many different operative instruments are available for use with the arthroscope. Small rongeurs are most commonly used. Small meniscal tags and frayed pieces of articular cartilage from the edge of defects can be freed from their attachments and then washed out of the knee. By the use of arthroscopic scissors a meniscal "bucket-handle" can be cut free at each end and grasping forceps used to withdraw the remnant from the knee through the incision where the grasping forceps enter.

Large irregular areas can be smoothed by using powered shavers. These instruments must be very carefully controlled and kept under close observation so that the cutting end does not stray onto intact articular cartilage.

Special instrument sets are available to allow separated segments of meniscus to be sutured back into place. This is a difficult technique that demands long practice and is not suitable for the inexperienced operator. Moreover it is practicable only under the enlarged vision which the television arthroscope provides.

INTRAMEDULLARY NAILING FOR FEMORAL SHAFT FRACTURES

This section should be read in conjunction with the general description of intramedullary nailing in Chapter 2 (p. 84). A proportion of fractured femora can be nailed by the closed technique—that is, without exposure of the fracture itself. In a far greater proportion closed nailing is impossible because adequate reduction cannot be obtained without exposure of the fracture. In these cases open nailing is employed.

CLOSED NAILING

TECHNIQUE

Position of patient. The patient lies in the lateral position with the affected limb uppermost. The authors prefer to have the limb resting upon a platform which forms a bridge over the sound limb (Fig. 437).

reduction the position is checked with the image intensifier.

If attempts at closed reduction fail to secure an acceptable position of the fragments, closed nailing should be abandoned and the surgeon should proceed to open nailing. If on the other hand the reduction is shown to be adequate, closed nailing proceeds in the following stages.

Incision. For closed nailing only a short incision over the top of the greater trochanter is required.

Exposure of greater trochanter. The skin edges being retracted, the fascia and muscles are incised

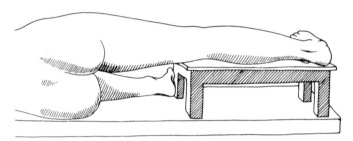

FIG. 437. Position of patient for intramedullary nailing of femur. The platform holds the limb horizontal.

Provision must be made for sustained traction on the limb if this is required to aid reduction. Traction is applied through a Steinmann pin transfixing the upper tibia, by weights suspended either over the end of the operation table or over a pulley attached to the wall. Counter-traction must be provided in the groin. Some operation tables provide for this, but in the absence of such equipment a mechanism for providing counter-traction may be improvised: a well padded transverse bar may be clamped to the table in the appropriate position or a padded sling passed under the groin may be fastened near the head of the table.

Reduction of fracture. Depending upon the shape and position of the fracture surfaces as seen radiographically, reduction may be attempted by manipulation (for instance, for a displaced transverse fracture), by heavy traction alone (as in the case of a spiral fracture without loss of contact between the fragments), or by a combination of manipulation and traction. After attempted

straight down to the lateral aspect and top of the trochanter. With blunt-pointed scissors the muscles are stripped from the apex of the trochanter so that raw bone is exposed. The muscles are held aside with a self-retaining retractor.

Preparation of initial track for guide wire. It is wise to prepare an entrance track for the guide wire so that it will more easily find its way down the centre of the medullary canal. The initial track is best prepared with a rigid instrument such as a Steinmann pin on a holder or, perhaps better, a screwdriver. This is thrust centrally down the medullary canal after being inserted through a hole broached in the cortex of the trochanter with a small gouge.

This starting hole should be made towards the medial side of the trochanter rather than at its tip, for this is where the line of the medullary canal, projected upwards, would emerge (Fig. 438). The advantage of using a rigid instrument such as a screwdriver for starting the track is that the way down the medullary canal can be easily felt, whereas a flexible guide wire, inserted *ab initio*, is much less easily controlled and may deviate from the central axis of the bone.

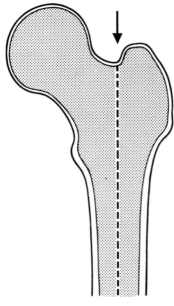

FIG. 438. A line projecting the medullary canal proximally emerges towards the medial face of the greater trochanter rather than at its tip. This is the correct entrance point for guide wire and nail.

Reaming the medullary canal. The medullary canal is widened by the use of flexible reamers driven by a slow-speed motor. The initial reamer should be 9 or 10 millimetres in diameter, and progressively larger sizes should be substituted

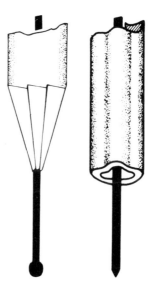

FIG. 439. The olive-tipped guide wire (*left*) is used to guide the reamers. It should be changed for a plain wire (*right*) before the nail is inserted. For explanation see text.

Insertion of guide wire. A long guide wire with a bulbous or olive-shaped tip (to facilitate retrieval of a reamer head should it break off) (Fig. 439) is passed into the track and driven down the medullary canal by twisting with a hand chuck. If it makes easy progress it may be assumed that the wire is taking the correct course down the centre of the medullary canal. The length of the wire being known, and the amount protruding from the trochanter being measured from time to time, the position of the tip of the wire can be calculated. Usually it should be driven on until the tip is within 5 centimetres or so of the femoral condyles. Its position is then checked with the image intensifier. Should the wire seem to get held up at any point immediate checking with the intensifier is required because the wire may be taking a false course.

until the canal will take a large nail: in a man of strong build the aim should be to use a nail 15 or 16 millimetres in diameter. Each reamer is passed over the guide wire in turn and should be pressed on steadily, without haste: the reamer should be allowed to cut its own way down the canal with only moderate pressure from above. If the reamer is not making steady progress it should be withdrawn and the cutting flutes cleared with a sharp hook. If they are left blocked the reamer will heat up and the bone fragments will become burned into the cutting flutes. The reamer may then become stuck in the medullary cavity. Excessive force may cause splitting of bone fragments or even breakage of the reamer. As each reamer is removed care must be taken to ensure that the guide wire remains in position: often it tends to come out with the reamer.

Selection and insertion of nail. The thickness of the nail should usually correspond with the diameter of the final reamer (see p. 86). Its length should be determined from the known length of the guide wire within the bone, and as a double

canal with light hammer blows, its position being checked with the image intensifier at intervals, especially as it nears full penetration. If the length of the nail has been calculated correctly, the upper end of the nail should be flush with the top of the

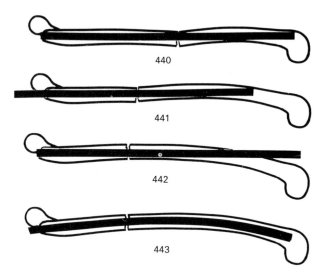

440

441

442

443

FIGS 440–443. The insertion of a straight nail into the curved medullary canal of the femur may present difficulties. If the fracture is near the middle of the shaft, slight angulation at the fracture may allow a full-length nail to be accommodated (Fig. 440). But if the distal, curved fragment is long, a full-length nail often cannot be accommodated and it may become jammed against the anterior cortex (Fig. 441) or penetrate the cortex (Fig. 442). The use of a curved nail (or of a three-quarters length straight nail) obviates this difficulty (Fig. 443).

check by measurement of the thigh from the tip of the greater trochanter to the upper pole of the patella. Usually, the aim should be to allow the nail to penetrate to within 2 or 3 centimetres of the lower articular surface of the femur, but for fractures above the mid-point of the femoral shaft a shorter nail is to be preferred (see p. 87).

Before the selected nail is introduced into the medullary canal it is important that the initial guide wire be removed and replaced by a plain wire—that is, without the olive-shaped bulbous tip, which might hinder removal of the wire after the nail has been hammered in (Fig. 439).

The selected nail is then introduced, preferably with the slot for removal of the nail directed laterally. It is hammered down the medullary

greater trochanter when the point has penetrated to the optimal level. It is a mistake to leave the nail protruding prominently above the trochanter.

POST-OPERATIVE MANAGEMENT

Upon completion of wound closure the Steinmann pin that may have been used for traction is removed from the tibia. Provided the case has been properly selected for nail fixation, and provided a nail of adequate size has been driven in over a sufficient length, external support by plaster or splint should not be required. The patient may lie free in bed and should begin exercises for the gluteal and thigh muscles and knee flexion exercises within a day or two of the operation.

Walking with crutches may be begun within the first week, though it is possibly wise to prohibit weight bearing until the soft tissues have healed. Thereafter progressively increasing weight may be taken upon the limb and the axillary crutches may be discarded in favour of elbow crutches.

Comment

This is not a procedure that should be undertaken by the occasional operator. Whereas it can be a simple and straightforward operation, there are a number of difficulties and hazards that can turn it into a formidable undertaking.

The first difficulty to be overcome is that of obtaining adequate reduction of the fracture, and of maintaining the reduction while the nail is introduced. In only a relatively small proportion of cases is satisfactory reduction achieved by closed methods. In the remainder the surgeon has to be prepared to proceed to open nailing, which is always a major undertaking.

The following are some of the complications that may present difficulty.

1) *Deviation of the guide wire* from the medullary canal. Sometimes the guide wire has strayed from the bone altogether and been driven into the soft tissues at the site of fracture.

2) *Breakage of a reamer* within the bone. Only if an olive-tipped guide wire has been used can a broken reamer head be withdrawn with the guide wire, and even then considerable difficulty may be presented. In the last resort it may be necessary to cut away part of the cortex of the femur overlying the reamer head in order to extract it.

3) *Impaction of nail.* In most cases there is no risk of serious impaction of the nail provided its diameter matches that of the largest reamer used. There are circumstances, however, in which impaction can occur even though reaming has been to adequate width, particularly if an attempt is made to drive a straight nail into a long curved track. In fractures near the mid-shaft of the femur, with fragments of about equal length, neither fragment is long enough to make the normal slight curvature of the femur significant: the nail can follow a virtually straight path through it because slight angulation can occur at

the site of fracture to compensate for the curvature (Fig. 440). If the fragments are of unequal length, however, and especially if there is a long distal fragment, the natural curvature of the bone may cause a straight nail to become jammed (Fig. 441). The surgeon should guard against this either by using an appropriately curved nail or, if only a straight nail is available, by selecting a relatively short nail (see p. 87). If a nail does become seriously impacted its extraction may prove extremely difficult: in the worst cases the nail may refuse to move either in or out. The surgeon must then decide between sawing the nail off and leaving the impacted nail in position, or splitting one cortex longitudinally to allow it to spring open sufficiently to release the nail. If this has to be done the split usually heals without complications, but the patient's recovery is seriously delayed.

4) *Deviation of nail from medullary canal.* Since the femur is bowed slightly forwards, there is clearly a tendency for a straight nail to strike the anterior cortex of the lower part of the femur, and sometimes the cortex is penetrated (Fig. 442). Doubtless this would happen regularly if one were to nail an intact femur. But the presence of a fracture allows the distal fragment to become re-aligned on the axis of the nail so that actual penetration of the anterior cortex seldom occurs. It is more likely to happen in the case of a high fracture than in that of a low fracture, because in a high fracture the long curve of the distal fragment is not able to accommodate a straight nail. In a high fracture, therefore, it is best—if a straight nail is used—to be content with a nail that penetrates down only to within 10 centimetres or so of the femoral condyles. Even such a relatively short nail will give good rigidity if the fracture site is proximal to the mid-point of the femur, provided of course that a stout nail has been used and that its diameter matches that of the track reamed for it. The best safeguard against straying of the nail from the desired axis is to view the progress of the nail repeatedly with the image intensifier while it is being driven in.

Clearly, it is desirable that in the future only nails that conform to the normal slight curvature of the femur should be used (Fig. 443).

ALTERNATIVE TECHNIQUE

The Swiss school of surgeons responsible for the A.O.* technique recommend a special pattern of curved nail that matches the natural curve of the femoral shaft. A curved nail clearly offers advantages over a straight nail. For further details of the A.O. technique the reader is referred to the account published by Müller *et al.* (1991).

OPEN NAILING

If it is not possible to gain adequate reduction by closed methods the fracture site must be exposed to allow reduction to be carried out under direct vision. Thereafter nailing may be carried out in the same way as described for the closed technique, but often it is easier to take advantage of the exposure of the fracture and to introduce the nail into the proximal fragment from the fracture site—the so-called retrograde method.

TECHNIQUE

Position of patient. The patient lies in the lateral position as described for closed nailing. Facilities for mechanical traction should be available, though often it will not be required (see previous section). Facilities for radiography, preferably by the image intensifier, must be available.

Incision. Two incisions are required. That for exposure of the fracture follows the posterior border of the fascia lata, as described on page 35. The incision for exposure of the greater trochanter is the same as that used in closed nailing.

Exposure of bone and reduction of fracture. The route to the bone is as described on page 35. It lies immediately behind the vastus lateralis, which is lifted forwards and stripped from the femur together with the periosteum. As in the exposure of a fracture at any site, it is best to expose normal bone above and below the fracture and then to follow each fragment towards the fracture site.

* See page 66.

When the skin and muscles have been retracted with suitable bone levers the fracture surfaces are cleared of blood clot and the bone ends are freed from adherent soft tissue in the vicinity of the fracture. Thus cleared, the fracture surfaces may be brought into correct apposition, if necessary with the aid of mechanical traction to restore normal length. Care must be taken to fit the surfaces together exactly, and in particular any rotational deformity must be avoided. In a fresh fracture the correct rotational position is ensured automatically when the matching spikes and crevices on the opposed fracture surfaces can be fitted together accurately. In an old fracture, in which accurate interlocking of the fragments is no longer possible, reliance may have to be placed on matching the surface contours of the two fragments.

When reduction has been gained a decision must be made whether to use the direct method of nailing (that is, by introduction of the guide wire and of the nail at the top of the greater trochanter) or whether to employ the retrograde technique. If the direct method of nailing is to be employed the reduction must be held securely by a suitable bone-holding forceps or by a bone clamp, supplemented if necessary by mechanical traction. The special A.O. repositioning slat may be used for this purpose. If retrograde nailing is to be employed the fragments are taken apart again at this stage for introduction of the guide wire and nail into the proximal fragment from the fracture site.

Reaming of medullary canal and introduction of nail. If direct nailing is to be employed the technique is exactly the same as that described in the previous section on closed nailing.

If retrograde nailing is to be used the procedure is as follows. First the fracture surface of the proximal fragment is delivered into the wound, the fragment being held by strong bone-holding forceps. A guide wire is passed into the medullary canal from the fracture surface and driven in a proximal direction so that the guide wire finds its way through the greater trochanter to emerge through a separate incision above the trochanter. In this instance a plain guide wire may be used instead of the normal olive-tipped wire because the bone is open at both ends: the olive-tipped wire would not serve any useful purpose in the event of breakage of the flexible reamer because the reamer head could be retrieved by driving it back with a punch inserted from the proximal end.

With the guide wire in position powered reamers of graduated size, progressing from about from the fracture surface up the proximal fragment to emerge at the greater trochanter (Fig. 444). It is driven out backwards through the proximal incision so that the point of the nail becomes almost flush with the fracture surface: it may be left protruding a few millimetres so as more easily to engage the medullary canal of the distal fragment (Fig. 445). Each fragment is now

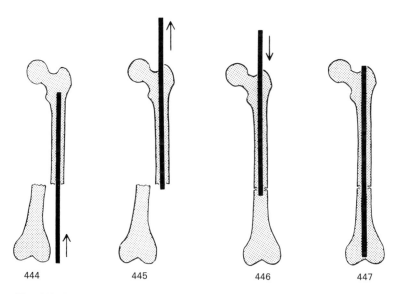

444   445   446   447

FIGS 444–447. In retrograde nailing the nail is first driven into the proximal fragment from the fracture site (Fig. 444) and out through the greater trochanter (Fig. 445). After reduction of the fracture the nail is then engaged in the distal fragment (Fig. 446) and driven home (Fig. 447).

9 millimetres to a final size of 14 to 16 millimetres, are passed through the bone from the fracture surface to emerge at the greater trochanter. The guide wire is then removed from the proximal fragment and attention is directed to the distal fragment. This in turn is delivered into the wound and an olive-tipped guide wire is introduced from the fracture surface and passed distally down the medullary canal almost to the femoral condyles. Powered reamers are driven in over the wire in the same way as for the proximal fragment. When the medullary canal has been reamed to the required diameter the guide wire is removed from the lower fragment.

The proximal fragment is now again delivered into the wound and a nail of the appropriate length and diameter (see p. 86) is passed backwards

gripped with bone-holding forceps and the fracture is reduced, with care once again to secure accurate coaptation of the two cortices: at the same time the tip of the nail is made to enter the reamed medullary canal of the distal fragment (Fig. 446). It remains then to drive the nail from above, down into the distal fragment (Fig. 447). The remaining stages of the operation are the same as for closed nailing.

POST-OPERATIVE MANAGEMENT

This is the same as for closed nailing.

Comment

In so far as the surgeon can reduce the fracture under direct vision, open medullary nailing of the femur is often easier than closed nailing. The operation is, however, more formidable for the patient. There is often considerable loss of blood, necessitating replacement, and the risk of infection is greater than with closed nailing. Every effort must be made to prevent infection by gentle handling of the tissues, by the use of the non-touch technique, and by prevention of haematoma.

Regarding difficulties and complications, many of the comments made on closed nailing of the femur (p. 332) apply equally to open nailing.

It is established that intramedullary nailing gives much more rigid fixation than plating (Laurence *et al.* 1969), and it is widely agreed that nailing has almost supplanted plating so far as fractures of the mid-shaft of the femur are concerned.

THE HUCKSTEP PERFORATED NAIL

The Huckstep nail (Huckstep 1972) was devised in order to gain enhanced fixation in certain difficult cases in which fixation by a plain nail tends to be inadequate—for instance, when one of the fragments is too short to grip the nail securely, or when a nail that was initially secure has worked loose and caused enlargement of the medullary canal in cases of non-union. Although designed initially for femoral fractures the nail also has a place in certain fractures of the tibia or humerus.

The nail, made from titanium alloy, is of square section and is supplied in only two sizes.* The larger size has a diagonal measurement of 12.5 millimetres and the smaller one 10.5 millimetres. The nail is perforated transversely throughout its length at intervals of 15 millimetres. The perforations, not threaded, are designed to accept screws of 4.5 millimetres diameter. These cross-screws, of which any number may be used up to the number of perforations available, traverse both cortices of the bone (Figs 448 and 449) and thus, with the nail, give impressive rigidity even though the nail itself may be no more than a loose fit in the medullary canal; and rotation is entirely prevented.

Nails for fixation of femoral fractures have holes directed obliquely at the upper end, to allow long screws to be driven up the femoral neck. These are additional to the transverse screw holes.

Special but simple equipment is required for the application of this technique. This includes a jig for correct location of the screws: this fits on to

the top of the nail. Also required are screw-cutting taps to match the 4.5 millimetre screws, and a hexagonal screwdriver to fit the screws. The description that follows refers to the use of the nail for a femoral shaft fracture.

TECHNIQUE

Position of patient. The patient lies in the lateral position with the affected thigh uppermost. It is convenient to have the limb resting upon a special platform as shown in Figure 437, but this is not essential.

Exposure of fracture and insertion of nail. The technique of insertion of the nail is the same as that for plain intramedullary nailing by the open technique (p. 333). The perforations of the nail should be so orientated that they allow the insertion of screws from lateral to medial—in other words, they lie in the coronal plane. It is essential that the nail be correctly orientated: otherwise screws through the proximal oblique holes to enter the femoral neck may emerge at the front or back of the neck.

The length of nail required should be calculated before the operation, and the most suitable nail from the 34, 37, 40 and 43 centimetre standard lengths is chosen. (A 60 centimetre nail, designed for arthrodesis of the knee, is also available and may be cut down to an alternative length with a freshly-bladed hack-saw if necessary.)

In reaming the channel for the nail the surgeon must remember that a straight nail is to be driven into a curved femur. If a flexible reamer is used,

*Supplied by Downs Surgical Ltd (division of Aesculap), London, England.

the channel will therefore have to be bored slightly larger than the nail size of 12.5 millimetres, even allowing for some accommodation by angulation of the bone fragments at the fracture site. Alternatively, a very long solid drill 12.5 millimetres in diameter may be used.

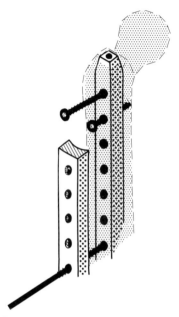

FIG. 448. The Huckstep perforated intramedullary nail shown lying within the ghosted femoral shaft. Note the perforations, with one screw fully inserted and a second screw driven in part way. Lower down, the jig is shown in position: a hole is being threaded in the femoral cortices with a tap.

The nail should be inserted so that its proximal end is recessed slightly below the tip of the greater trochanter. When compression is applied the proximal end of the nail will be extruded a little from the trochanter; so unless it is recessed before compression it may become proud of the trochanter and may cause discomfort.

Fitting of the long jig. When the nail has been inserted the jig is fitted to facilitate insertion of the screws. The jig swivels on an alignment rod which is fixed to the nail by an attachment which is screwed into the threaded upper end of the nail (Fig. 450). Thus mounted, the jig can be folded

over into contact with the bone or, when necessary, swivelled away from it (Fig. 448).

Before using the long jig, it is well to have made a preliminary trial assembly with the nail, in order to be sure that the two line up accurately together and that a drill inserted through a hole in the jig passes smoothly through the nail.

Using the jig to locate the screws. To bring the jig into use it is necessary first to find a hole in the nail that is visible at the site of fracture. To locate such a hole the nail may be hammered a short distance up or down the medullary canal until one of the holes comes into view. When this initial hole has been located it is exposed to full view by nibbling away a small piece of the overlying bone cortex. The jig is now fixed in position by inserting a screw tap (4.5 millimetres diameter) through an appropriate hole of the jig and through the revealed hole in the nail into the far cortex of the femur (Figs 448 and 450). To secure the jig more firmly the femur is drilled through a second, more distal hole in the jig and a further screw tap or screw is inserted.

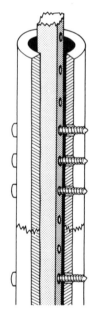

FIG. 449. Cut-away diagram showing the perforated nail within the medullary canal and transfixing screws above and below the fracture.

Insertion of screws in distal fragment. The jig being thus held in position, holes for as many screws as are required are drilled through both cortices of the distal fragment of the femur. Each hole is then tapped with the screw tap, and after the jig has been swung away from the bone screws of appropriate length are driven home. The nail is thus secured rigidly to the lower fragment.

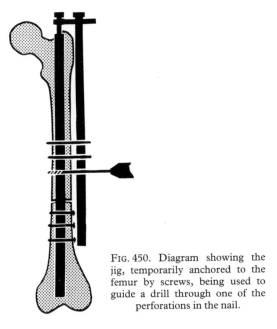

FIG. 450. Diagram showing the jig, temporarily anchored to the femur by screws, being used to guide a drill through one of the perforations in the nail.

Compression of fragments together. If desired, the two fragments may now be compressed together at the fracture site by attaching a special compression device to the upper end of the nail. By a screw action the compressor pulls the nail, and thus the distal fragment, proximally against counterthrust upon the trochanter.

Fixation of nail to proximal fragment. With the jig restored to position and again held by two jig screws (screw taps) in the manner already described, holes for as many screws as are required in the proximal fragment are drilled through the appropriate guide holes in the jig and through both cortices of the femur. The jig ensures that the drills pass through the holes in the nail. Each hole is then threaded by the screw tap, and after removal of the jig, screws of the appropriate length are inserted.

As a general rule, it is recommended that four screws be inserted in each fragment. These provide rigid fixation without undue weakening of the bone cortices.

Closure. The wound is closed with or without suction drainage as desired.

USE OF THE DEVICE FOR SUBTROCHANTERIC FRACTURES

For adequate fixation of subtrochanteric fractures, use of the long oblique screws is obligatory. They are inserted with the aid of the special oblique-holed jig. If it is necessary to use the transverse holes just below the oblique holes, these screws may be inserted before the oblique-holed jig is applied. Alternatively they may be inserted at the end of the operation by re-applying the long jig, which is provided only with transverse holes.

POST-OPERATIVE MANAGEMENT

This is the same as after plain intramedullary nailing (p. 331). Fixation is usually so secure that early weight-bearing with the partial support of elbow crutches may be safely encouraged within two or three weeks of the operation, and often earlier.

Comment

The insertion of this special nail does not present any major difficulties provided the jigs and related equipment are available. The important points to be recapitulated are as follows: 1) The nail is to be inserted with the holes in the coronal plane, to allow insertion of the screws from lateral to medial. 2) The nail must be sawn to the correct length, preferably before it is sterilised. 3) Use of the jig is mandatory in order to direct the screws through the holes in the nail. 4) The first hole for fixation of the jig to the femur must be found at the site of fracture, if necessary by nibbling away a small area of bone. This allows preliminary fixation of the jig to the bone by a tap or screw. 5) A second jig-holding screw or tap is essential to ensure that the jig is correctly aligned on the nail. 6) Holes for screws to hold the lower fragment are drilled and tapped through the jig, but the jig must be swung out of the way before the screws are inserted. If the fragments are to be compressed together it is important that the lower fragment be fixed first. 7) When the lower fragment has been screwed to the nail compression may be applied at the fracture site by means of the special compression screw. 8) The jig is then fixed back in position to guide the drill in the preparation of screw holes in the proximal fragment. 9) When the jig has been finally removed the holes used to fix it to the lower fragment should be filled with screws.

If the jig is fixed carelessly or hurriedly in position, or if only one screw or tap is used to fix it, it may be badly out of line with the nail and in consequence screws passed through the jig may strike the body of the nail instead of passing through the perforations. If this happens it is essential that the jig be reapplied and fixed accurately to the nail.

The number of screws required in each fragment depends upon the nature of each particular fracture. If each fragment is composed of good strong bone not more than four screws in each should be required. On the other hand, if the bone is markedly porotic, with very thin cortex, as many as six or eight screws may be thought desirable.

It should be noted that this technique of nailing may easily be combined with bone grafting, either by sliver grafts or by onlay cortical grafts. If sliver grafts are to be used they are placed about the site of fracture as in the Phemister technique (p. 81). If onlay cortical grafts are to be applied the jig may be used to guide a series of holes through the graft, which is then applied to the lateral surface of the bone and held tightly up to it by the same screws that are used to secure the nail.

REMOVAL OF HUCKSTEP NAIL

As a general rule it is expected that the nail will remain in position permanently. Nevertheless a special nail extractor is supplied with the Huckstep set.

If removal is required for any reason, it should be remembered that bone may have grown into some of the perforations in the nail. The procedure therefore is first to remove all the transfixion screws. If then the nail still appears to be firmly held within the femoral shaft it may be surmised that bone has grown into some of the holes. In order to clear these out by drilling, it is useful to insert drills or screw taps into some of the holes vacated by removing the screws and to apply the floating jig. This permits any or all of the remaining holes in the nail to be drilled out. Those holes that are near the area of the fracture are those most likely to be blocked by new bone, and they should be drilled out first. Of course, only the lateral cortex needs to be drilled to allow the hole in the nail to be cleared: it is a mistake to penetrate the far cortex because this may weaken the femur.

SIGNAL ARM NAILING

(FEMORAL Y-NAILING)

Signal arm nailing or Y-nailing, introduced by Küntscher during the Second World War (Böhler 1948), is an extension of the principle of intramedullary nailing of the femoral shaft for fractures so high that the proximal fragment would not be adequately controlled by a simple intramedullary nail. The nail is therefore interlocked with an extension piece or "signal arm" which grips the femoral neck (Fig. 451). The technique is somewhat demanding, because the extension piece or signal arm must be so placed in the femoral neck that the oblique slot at its base comes into correct register with the canal reamed for the intramedullary nail, so that the nail can be driven through the slot. The stages in the operation are, first, to reduce the fracture if it is displaced; secondly, to prepare a track for the main intramedullary nail in the upper three-quarters of the femoral shaft; thirdly, to prepare a track in the femoral neck to receive the extension piece or signal arm, which is now inserted; and finally to drive the intramedullary nail from the top of the greater trochanter down through the slot in the extension piece into the distal fragment of the femur.

The description that follows should be read in conjunction with the general account of intramedullary nailing in Chapter 2 (p. 84).

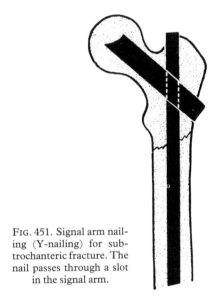

FIG. 451. Signal arm nailing (Y-nailing) for subtrochanteric fracture. The nail passes through a slot in the signal arm.

TECHNIQUE

Position of patient. Although it is possible to carry out this operation with the patient set up on the orthopaedic table as for nailing of a fracture of the femoral neck, the authors have found it easier to have the patient in the lateral position with the affected limb resting upon a platform, as described for intramedullary nailing of the femur (Fig. 437). This arrangement has the disadvantage that lateral radiography of the femoral neck is not practicable. On the other hand the position of the signal arm in the femoral neck is not critical, and it is quite feasible by a combination of antero-posterior radiography and a sense of "feel" imparted by a probing guide wire within the femoral neck to place the signal arm in an acceptable position without lateral radiography.

Incision. The incision is a vertical one at the lateral aspect of the thigh. It extends distally from a point 2.5 centimetres proximal to the greater

trochanter for about 10 or 12 centimetres. If open reduction of the fracture is required the incision may be extended distally as far as is necessary.

Exposure of greater trochanter. Through the upper part of the wound the tip of the greater trochanter is exposed by cutting directly down upon it and clearing a space between the attached muscle fibres for the introduction of the intramedullary nail. Usually, the correct site for the insertion of the nail is towards the medial aspect of the greater trochanter where it begins to slope down towards the femoral neck (Fig. 438).

Exposure of upper end of femoral shaft for introduction of signal arm. The lateral aspect of the femur is exposed just below the greater trochanter by first dividing the fascia lata and, more proximally, the tensor fasciae latae muscle vertically and then lifting the vastus lateralis muscle forwards and retaining it in this position by a bone lever hooked over the front of the femoral shaft (see p. 37).

Exposure of fracture. If the fracture site is to be exposed for the purpose of reduction, or in the case of a pathological fracture for taking a specimen for histological examination, the exposure of the femoral shaft is simply prolonged distally by further splitting of the fascia lata and forward retraction of the vastus lateralis (see p. 37).

Reduction of fracture. If the fragments are not in acceptable apposition and alignment reduction is carried out after full exposure of the fracture surfaces as described on page 333.

Reaming of medullary canal. The technique of introducing a guide wire and of reaming the medullary canal to the required diameter by flexible power-driven reamers is the same as that described on page 333. Signal arm devices are supplied in a range of sizes to accept intramedullary nails up to 16 millimetres in diameter*.

Preparation of channel in femoral neck for signal arm. When the track for the main intramedullary

*Supplied by Messrs Howmedica Ltd, London, England.

nail has been prepared in the femoral shaft a suitable track must be made in the femoral neck for the signal arm attachment. The track must intersect that made for the intramedullary nail at an angle of 135 degrees, which is the fixed angle between nail and extension piece when assembled. A jig to aid the correct placing of the signal arm in the femoral neck has not yet been perfected, and it is best at present to make the track more or less free-hand. Nevertheless it is useful to place a preliminary guide wire along the femoral neck and to check its position by an antero-posterior radiograph. With care, the way along the inside of the neck can be felt reasonably accurately with the guide wire; so lateral radiographs—technically difficult to obtain with the patient in the lateral position—may be dispensed with.

When the preliminary guide wire, inclined at 45 degrees to the line of the femoral shaft, has indicated the general direction in which the signal arm is to be placed, an oval window is cut in the lateral cortex of the upper part of the femoral shaft just below the greater trochanter to receive the base of the signal arm. This window is deepened into a slot, with care to ensure that the track lies at the correct angle of 135 degrees with the line of the femoral shaft. As the slot is deepened the vertical track that has been reamed for the main intramedullary nail will be entered with the gouge. To aid the identification of the track it is useful to leave a guide wire in position in the medullary canal. It is essential that the two tracks—that for the signal arm and that for the intramedullary nail—intersect in the same plane. Inspection of the signal arm will indicate how deeply the oval slot for the base of the appliance must be cut. The point of the signal arm, unlike the base, is of open-U section and it can usually be driven into the soft bone of the femoral neck without preliminary gouging of a track for its whole length.

The correct length of signal arm required may be calculated from the antero-posterior radiograph with the guide wire in position, by determining the length of guide wire within the bone and estimating how much further or how much less far the signal arm should penetrate. As a rule it is well that the point of the signal arm should not penetrate nearer than 3 centimetres or so from the articular surface of the femoral head. Even when this wide margin is allowed, the device gains a good grip on the femoral neck. Three lengths of signal arm are available, namely 8 centimetres, 9 centimetres and 10 centimetres, and the most appropriate one of these three must be selected.

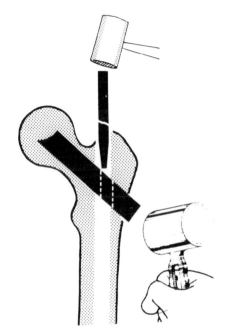

FIG. 452. Signal arm nailing. Getting the signal arm into correct register with the reamed medullary canal by means of a tapered punch.

Insertion of signal arm. When a signal arm of appropriate length has been selected it is inserted into the elliptical slot that has been prepared for it, with care to ensure that it is correctly orientated to bring the slot in its base into line with the vertical axis of the femur. It may be helpful to place a tapered punch in the upper part of the medullary canal of the femur and to drive it down just far enough to strike the upper surface of the signal arm. The signal arm is then driven in slowly, a few millimetres at a time, until light taps upon the tapered punch eventually cause its point to engage in the slot in the signal arm (Fig. 452). In this way the slot in the signal arm is brought into correct register with the track that has been reamed for the intramedullary nail.

Insertion of intramedullary nail through signal arm. The final stage is to drive the definitive intramedullary nail from above so that it passes through the slot in the signal arm to enter the distal part of the medullary canal after traversing the fracture site. Progress of the nail is checked at intervals by the image intensifier. Since signal arm nailing is done only for high fractures of the femoral shaft the distal fragment of the femur is always long, and it is not essential for the medullary nail to penetrate as far as the femoral condyles (see p. 331). It is sufficient to drive the nail to a point 8 or 10 centimetres proximal to the condyles, where the narrow part of the medullary canal ends and the canal begins to widen out.

POST-OPERATIVE MANAGEMENT

In most cases post-operative care is the same as that for intramedullary nailing of femoral shaft fractures without the signal arm attachment (p. 331).

Comment

The technique of signal arm nailing is difficult and the operation should not be attempted by the inexperienced surgeon. Preparation of the track in the femoral shaft for the main intramedullary nail is straightforward: it is in no way different from the technique as described in the section on intra-

medullary nailing for fracture of the shaft of the femur (p. 333).

The main difficulty of the operation is to pass the signal arm accurately along the femoral neck so that its track intersects that of the main intramedullary nail and allows the track for the nail to fall into exact register with the slot in the signal arm through which the nail must pass. Since the opening that must be made in the femur to receive the base of the signal arm is fairly large, the track can be excavated to some extent under direct vision, and it is possible in this way to ensure that the track for the signal arm correctly intersects that for the nail. Nor is it difficult to ensure that the nail is driven in at the critical angle of 135 degrees to the line of the femoral shaft. It is rather more difficult to ensure that the signal arm is driven on exactly to that point at which the slot through its base coincides with the track reamed for the main intramedullary nail, so that the nail will in fact pass through the signal arm. To get the two appliances to interlock it is best to tap the signal arm in a few millimetres at a time, and after each few blows with the hammer to drive a tapered punch down the medullary canal from the greater trochanter to test whether it enters the slot in the signal arm (Fig. 452). Eventually the point will be reached at which the nail enters and passes through the signal arm. It should be noted that the open side or groove of the clover-leaf-section intramedullary nail must be directed laterally, because this is the only position in which the nail will pass through the slot in the signal arm.

FIXATION OF SUBTROCHANTERIC FRACTURE BY ZICKEL NAIL

For patients with a subtrochanteric fracture of the femur a satisfactory method of fixation is by use of the Zickel nail* (Zickel and Mouradian 1976) (Fig. 453). Many subtrochanteric fractures occur in patients who have metastatic tumour deposits. The quality of the bone is poor, and fixation by nail-plate or screw-plate often fails because the screws holding the plate to the femur cut out of the soft bone.

Unlike the signal arm or Y-nail, which is combined with a standard intramedullary nail of clover-leaf section, the Zickel nail is purpose-made in its entirety. The main intramedullary component, a rod of square section, is expanded at the upper end and perforated obliquely by a tunnel that accepts a three-flanged nail or extension arm (Fig. 453). There are three thicknesses of intramedullary rod (11, 13 and 15 millimetres in

*Supplied by Howmedica Ltd, London, England.

cross section) for left and right femora, and four lengths of three-flanged extension nail. Introduction of the three-flanged nail is facilitated by a jig.

TECHNIQUE

Position of patient. Access to the upper end of the femur is most easily gained with the patient in the lateral position. Admittedly, this has the disadvantage that lateral radiography of the femoral neck is not practicable. But provided the trifin nail is inserted only part of the way into the femoral neck, its positioning is not critical; so in fact lateral radiography is not required.

Incision. The incision starts 5 centimetres proximal to the tip of the greater trochanter, and curves posteriorly and distally until it can be continued downwards over the lateral aspect of the femur for 10 to 15 centimetres.

Exposure of greater trochanter. Through the upper part of the wound the tip of the greater trochanter is exposed by cutting directly down upon it and clearing a space between the attached muscle fibres for the introduction of the intramedullary nail.

Exposure of upper end of femoral shaft. If the fracture is displaced, the upper end of the femoral shaft is freed from enclosing muscle by dividing the fascia lata posteriorly and reflecting it forwards. The upper end of the vastus lateralis is also freed from the femoral shaft and reflected forwards. The proximal end of the femoral shaft can then be held in strong bone forceps and presented for testing with the Zickel nails.

Insertion of Zickel nail. A nail of the correct side (left or right) and of the largest diameter that will easily fit into the femoral medullary canal is test fitted into the femur by way of the fracture site. When the appropriate nail has been chosen it is withdrawn to allow the greater trochanter to be reamed proximally with the special reamer included in the instrument set. The fracture is then reduced and the nail inserted at the proximal end of the greater trochanter. It is driven distally across the fracture site.

Insertion of trifin nail. A guide wire is passed along the anterior surface of the femoral neck to aid correct rotational alignment of the nail. With the femoral nail inserted so that its tip is flush with the upper surface of the greater trochanter, the special jig for directing the guide wire for the trifin nail is screwed temporarily to the top of the vertical nail. A guide wire is passed through the hole in the jig. This wire passes through the hole in the nail and up the femoral neck. Its position is checked radiographically to see that it is not above or below the femoral neck. If its position is not satisfactory the femoral nail is inserted further or retracted accordingly. By ensuring that the guide wire is parallel with the wire that has been inserted along the anterior surface of the femoral neck, correct rotation of the nail is achieved.

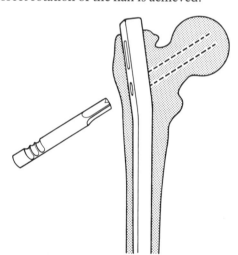

FIG. 453. The Zickel nail. Introduction of the three-flanged nail through the hole in the vertical nail is facilitated by a jig that is screwed temporarily to the top of the vertical nail.

By measurement of the length of guide wire outside the femur, the overall length of the wire being known, a trifin nail of the appropriate length can be chosen.

Both guide wires are now removed. The trifin nail is mounted on the special introducer. It is noted that there are three hollows on one side of the barrel of the trifin nail (Fig. 453). These are to receive the locking screw. The trifin nail is inserted with the barrel hollows facing towards the tip of the greater trochanter. When it has been fully inserted the locking screw is driven home into one of the hollows to prevent the trifin nail from backing out.

Closure. The wound is closed in layers, with suction drainage.

POST-OPERATIVE MANAGEMENT

In most cases post-operative care is the same as that for intramedullary nailing of a femoral shaft fracture (p. 333).

Comment

The main difficulty with this operation is to keep the trifin nail central within the femoral neck. The shorter the trifin nail that is chosen, the easier this is. Any attempt to drive the trifin nail right into the femoral head greatly increases the risk of its coming out of the neck either in front or behind. The method is therefore not suitable for the fixation of combined femoral neck and subtrochanteric fractures.

BONE GRAFTING FOR DELAYED UNION OR NON-UNION OF FRACTURE OF FEMORAL SHAFT

The techniques of bone grafting were described in Chapter 2 (p. 78). This section is therefore confined to comments on the application of grafting techniques to femoral shaft fractures.

Although onlay cortical bone grafting has been used for old ununited fractures of the femur and is still so used occasionally, it has been largely superseded by the technique of cancellous sliver grafting (Phemister 1947), and in most such cases grafting is combined with rigid fixation by a stout intramedullary nail. This combination has much to commend it, and it is regarded by the authors as the method of choice especially for fractures near the middle of the femoral shaft. In some cases the Huckstep perforated nail (see p. 335) may be used in preference to a plain intramedullary nail.

The recommended approach for the application of cancellous sliver grafts to the femoral shaft is through the postero-lateral incision, described on page 35. The route is between the vastus lateralis and the lateral intermuscular septum, behind which lies the biceps femoris. The vastus lateralis and the vastus intermedius are stripped from the femur to expose the site of fracture. The position of the fragments is adjusted if necessary, and fixation is achieved by the insertion of a medullary nail in the manner described on page 333. Finally, thin slivers of cancellous bone are laid around part of the circumference of the femur at the site of fracture, and the muscles are closed over them.

When imperfect union of a fracture of the femoral shaft has been treated by the use of some form of intramedullary nail, the operative procedure involves reaming. If the bone is healthy the reamings can be collected from the flutes of the cutting head and saved for insertion at the fracture site. This may obviate the need to obtain bone grafts from a distant site.

POST-OPERATIVE MANAGEMENT

The programme of management after operation depends upon the rigidity of the fixation afforded by the intramedullary nail. If the fracture is near the middle of the femoral shaft, and if a sufficiently stout nail has been used, it is safe and indeed desirable to encourage weight-bearing with the partial support of elbow crutches as soon as the soft tissues have healed. If internal fixation is not sufficiently firm to permit early weight-bearing, axillary crutches may have to be used until union of the fracture is well advanced.

FIXATION BY NAIL-PLATE FOR SUPRACONDYLAR FRACTURE OF THE FEMUR

The device to be described* is that of Austin Brown (Brown and D'Arcy 1971). It consists of a plate section 12.5 centimetres long, curved to accommodate the lateral condyle of the femur and drilled for five screws. This is in one piece with the nail section, which is either 5 or 6.5 centimetres long, and with a threaded cannulation. When the main part of the device has been applied from the lateral side of the femur, a small rectangular plate fitted over the medial condyle is com-

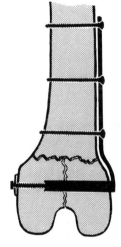

FIG. 454. Austin Brown nail-plate for fixation of supracondylar fracture of femur. The three-flanged nail and the main plate are in one piece. The small medial plate is drawn against the medial condyle by the bolt, which engages a threaded tunnel in the nail.

pressed against the bone by a bolt which engages the internal threads of the nail section (Fig. 454). In the case of a T-shaped fracture, the two condyles can thus be compressed together to restore the normal shape of the lower end of the femur.

TECHNIQUE

Position of patient. The patient lies supine, with the knee slightly flexed over a bulky sand-bag. A tourniquet may be applied on the upper thigh.

The lateral incision. The main incision is a vertical one, a little behind the mid-lateral axis of the lower third of the thigh. It lies over the lateral intermuscular septum, which separates the biceps muscle and tendon behind from the vastus lateralis muscle in front (see p. 35). The fascia lata is

*Supplied by Howmedica Ltd, London, England.

divided immediately in front of the intermuscular septum to expose the vastus lateralis, which is displaced forwards by bone levers hooked over the front of the femur. The lowest quarter of the femur, including the supracondylar region, is thus exposed and the fracture is brought into view.

Correction of displacement. The fragments are cleared in the usual way to allow full reduction of displacement under direct vision, the fragments being held by suitable bone-holding forceps.

Insertion of guide wire. While an assistant holds the bone fragments reduced, a guide wire is inserted transversely from the lateral aspect of the lateral condyle of the femur to emerge through the medial condyle and through the overlying skin. The guide wire should be 2.5 to 3 centimetres above the lowest part of the articular surface of the femur. The position of the guide wire should be checked by antero-posterior radiography or by viewing with the image intensifier.

Application of nail-plate. To facilitate introduction of the nail into the lateral condyle of the femur, the cortex is drilled by a 6 millimetre cannulated drill applied over the guide wire. The nail-plate is then brought into position by passing the cannulated three-flanged nail section over the guide wire and driving it home into the femoral condyles while the plate section is held parallel with the lateral contour of the femur, it having been previously determined from measurements upon the radiograph whether the 5 or the 6.5 centimetre nail is the more appropriate.

The medial incision. A vertical incision 5 centimetres long and centred over the emerging guide wire is made over the medial femoral condyle. The incision is deepened straight down to the cortex of the medial condyle.

Fitting of medial plate and compression bolt. First, the cortex is drilled by a 6 millimetre cannulated drill operated over the guide wire. This allows easy insertion of the bolt carrying the medial rectangular plate and the locking device. The bolt being cannulated, it is applied over the guide wire and driven laterally to meet the threaded cannulation of the three-flanged nail. Before the bolt is tightened home, the position of the small rectangular plate is adjusted to give the best possible coverage of the medial condyle, being placed with its longer axis vertical, horizontal or oblique as best suits the circumstances. While the bolt is being tightened, counter-thrust is applied over the lateral condyle and the plate. When good compression has been obtained, the special locking device is closed over the hexagonal bolt head. At this point, it is convenient to assess again the state of the fracture and the position of the fixation device by radiography.

Securing the plate section. The medial incision is now closed temporarily with towel clips and the lateral skin edges are retracted to expose the plate, which should lie closely apposed to the lateral surface of the femur. While it is held in this position appropriate drill holes are made and screws inserted (Fig. 454).

Closure. After removal of the tourniquet and sealing of any bleeding vessels, the divided edges of the fascia lata are approximated by absorbable sutures. The two skin incisions are closed in the normal way. Suction drainage from the sub-aponeurotic layer may be used if it seems desirable.

POST-OPERATIVE MANAGEMENT

Copious gauze dressings are held in place by wide (15 centimetre) crepe bandages. The patient lies free in bed with the limb supported upon a soft pillow. Quadriceps exercises are begun immediately, and flexion exercises through a small range may be begun after a few days. If a continuous passive motion (CPM) machine is available it may be used to hasten the restoration of mobility to the knee. The patient sits out of bed after four or five days and may begin walking with the partial support of elbow crutches after three weeks.

Comment

This operation greatly facilitates the management of these often difficult fractures, especially in elderly patients. In the post-operative management it is important to concentrate mainly on restoring good quadriceps power, with full extension of the knee. It is more important to restore powerful extension than to strive for early flexion. Flexion exercises are clearly important, but it is wise to exercise patience in the knowledge than many weeks may elapse before flexion to the right angle is regained. As quadriceps strength returns, leg lifting exercises with the knee held fully extended should be encouraged.

FIXATION OF FEMORAL CONDYLAR FRACTURE BY A.O. DYNAMIC CONDYLAR SCREW

When a fracture of the distal end of the femur extends into the knee joint separation of the femoral condyles complicates treatment. The A.O. dynamic condylar screw (Fig. 455) is a versatile system of fixing these fractures.

TECHNIQUE

Position of patient. The patient lies supine. A tourniquet may be applied on the upper thigh.

The lateral incision. The incision is a vertical one, a little behind the mid-lateral axis of the lower third of the thigh. Proximally it lies over the lateral intermuscular septum, which separates the vastus lateralis in front from the biceps muscle and tendon behind. Extending distally, the incision is brought a little more anteriorly over the upper tibia. The fascia lata is divided immediately in front of the intermuscular septum. The vastus lateralis is displaced forwards by bone levers hooked over the front of the femur. This exposes the lowest quarter of the femur and allows good access to the fracture.

Correction of displacement. Any blood clots preventing reduction of the fragments are removed. The exposure allows full reduction of the fragments. They are held reduced with bone-holding forceps. Two guide wires are then inserted into the lateral aspect of the distal femur, close to the anterior and posterior surfaces of the femur. They are inserted across the intercondylar fracture to maintain reduction. Placed close to the anterior and posterior surfaces of the femur, they do not interfere with later stages of the operation.

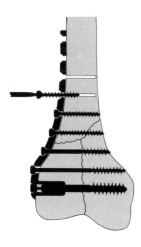

FIG. 455. A.O. dynamic condylar screw used for fixation of complicated supracondylar fracture. The lowest (cancellous) screw draws the separated condyles together.

Insertion of cancellous screws. First the site for insertion of the condylar screw is chosen. This is a point 2 centimetres proximal to the knee joint line and one-third of the way back from the anterior surface of the femur. Next, two cancellous screws are inserted across the intercondylar fracture from the lateral surface of the femur. One is in front of, and the other behind, the site chosen for the condylar screw. The guide wires are then removed and one is re-inserted in the axis of the condylar screw. It is directed parallel to the anterior surface of the femoral condyles and parallel to the distal surface of the femoral condyles. It is pushed in far enough to reach, but not pierce, the medial cortex of the femur. This can be checked radiographically. The direct measuring device is then placed behind the guide wire and the length of pin inserted into the femur read directly.

The dynamic condylar screw reamer is assembled. It is labelled "D C S" to avoid confusion with the reamer for the dynamic hip screw. The reamer is set to 10 millimetres less than the length of the guide wire which has been inserted. The bone is reamed. The bone is then tapped for the special screw threads with the tap centred in a short sleeve. The dynamic screw is assembled by inserting the coupling screw through the hollow guide shaft. The long centering sleeve is slid over the wrench and the assembled condylar screw is slid into the wrench. The condylar screw is then inserted over the guide wire until the 5 millimetre mark reaches the lateral cortex of the femur. The T handle of the wrench must finish in line with the femoral shaft. This aligns the flattened sides of the condylar screw with the flattened inner sides of the dynamic condylar plate. The wrench is removed and the appropriate D C S plate slid onto the screw assembly. The coupling screw is undone and the guide shaft removed. The D C S plate is then gently impacted with the special impactor.

The compressing screw is next inserted to compress the plate onto the D C S screw. Cancellous screws can then be inserted through the two holes in the plate nearest its end barrel to compress further the intercondylar fracture. Compression of the condylar fragments to the shaft of the femur is then done by using the dynamic compression of the oval holes of the plate, or by the separate use of the articulated compression device (p. 71) before placement of cortical screws in the remaining holes of the plate.

Closure. After removal of the tourniquet any identifiable bleeding vessels are sealed. The fascia lata is closed with absorbable sutures. If there is significant oozing from the fracture lines suction drainage is advisable. Superficial and skin closure is done in the normal way.

POST-OPERATIVE MANAGEMENT

The dressings are held in place by crepe bandages. Quadriceps exercises are started immediately. A continuous passive motion machine may be useful in retaining mobility of the knee joint. The fixation is not secure enough to allow even partial weight bearing until at least four weeks after operation.

FIXATION OF SUPRACONDYLAR FRACTURE OF FEMUR BY INTRAMEDULLARY NAIL TRANSFIXING THE KNEE

In severe supracondylar fractures through porotic bone in old persons—especially when there is also severe comminution—there is much to be said for driving a long intramedullary nail throughout the whole length of the femur and across the knee joint into the proximal third of the tibia (Fig. 456). In an old person, in whom prolonged bed rest is clearly undesirable, this may be the only practicable way of supporting the fracture sufficiently to allow immediate or early weight-bearing. Moreover, fixation across the knee joint is not so drastic a measure as it might seem at first, for after union of the fracture the nail may be removed with good prospect of restoring useful mobility and function of the knee.

TECHNIQUE

Basically, the technique resembles that for inserting an intramedullary nail for fracture of the shaft of the femur, except that a much longer nail must be used to allow its penetration across the supracondylar fracture and across the knee joint into the proximal third of the tibia. The section on nailing for fractured femoral shaft (p. 333) should be read in conjunction with the description that follows.

Position of patient. The patient lies in the lateral posture with the affected hip uppermost and the lower part of the limb resting upon a platform (Fig. 437).

Incisions. A vertical lateral incision 5 centimetres long is centred over the tip of the greater trochanter. A second, postero-lateral incision for exposure and reduction of the fracture may be required in the lower part of the thigh (see p. 35).

Reduction of fracture. The fracture may be reduced by closed manipulation or under direct vision through the optional lower incision, as circumstances demand.

Selection and preparation of nail. It is well to determine the optimal length of the nail before the operation, and to procure a suitable nail or to cut

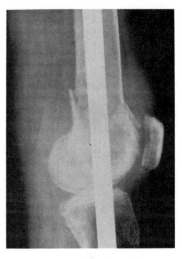

Fig. 456. Immobilisation of a supracondylar fracture of the femur by a long intramedullary nail transfixing the knee.

one down to this chosen length. A nail 14 millimetres in diameter is usually appropriate, but a thicker one may be chosen for a heavy patient, or a thinner one if the patient is slender. It is important that the nail be curved to match the natural curvature of the femur: attempting to drive a straight nail down the intact curved femoral shaft may lead to its becoming impacted. If a suitably curved nail is not available, a straight nail may be shaped in a bending machine or even by holding the ends in suitable iron piping and bending the nail over a rigid fulcrum. It is important, however, that the curve be uniform throughout the length of the nail: otherwise extraction of the nail later may be difficult.

Insertion of nail. The nail is inserted as described in the section on nailing for femoral shaft fracture by the closed technique (p. 329), a long guide wire being inserted first while the knee is held straight at this stage. When the position of the guide wire has been checked radiographically, the knee (and with it the guide wire) is flexed 10 to 15 degrees. The channel for the nail is then reamed to the predetermined diameter (equal to the diameter of the nail) by graduated flexible reamers, and the nail is driven home over the guide wire with radiographic control.

POST-OPERATIVE MANAGEMENT

Provided firm fixation has been secured, early walking may be encouraged, at first with a walking frame. The frame should be discarded in favour of elbow crutches as soon as the patient's physical state permits.

The nail should be removed as soon as radiographs indicate that the fracture is well united.

ALTERNATIVE USE OF LONG HUCKSTEP NAIL

A long Huckstep nail serves well as an alternative to a standard intramedullary nail for trans-articular fixation of difficult supracondylar fractures. Nails 60 centimetres long are available and may be cut down to the appropriate length.

The technique of insertion is broadly the same as that for fixation of a fracture of the femoral shaft (p. 335).

SUPRACONDYLAR OSTEOTOMY OF FEMUR

This osteotomy, which is associated with the name of MacEwen (1878), was formerly demanded frequently for the correction of rachitic deformities. It may be used for the correction of valgus or varus deformity or to correct fixed flexion deformity or extension deformity from whatever cause, when the deformity is in the femur rather than in the tibia. The technique entails removal of a wedge of bone of predetermined size at the appropriate site, and fixation of the fragments usually with staples or with a plate and screws (Figs 457 and 458).

PRELIMINARY STUDIES

Before operation is undertaken the nature and site of the deformity must be analysed, and the angle of correction required, as well as its direction, must be determined from clinical measurements and from measurements upon radiographs. Neglect of this precaution may lead to undercorrection or over-correction of the deformity. In determining the correct dimensions of the wedge it should be remembered that in the normal individual there is valgus at the knee of approximately 7 degrees: this compensates for the lateral cranking of the upper end of the femur. When the opposite knee is normal the angle of valgus should be matched precisely.

TECHNIQUE

The following description applies to the correction of valgus deformity by removal of a wedge of bone with its base directed medially. The correction of other deformities follows the same principles, the only differences being the site of the incision and the position of the base of the wedge.

Position of patient. The patient lies supine. A rolled towel or sand-bag may be placed behind the knee so that it rests in slight flexion. A tourniquet may be used on the upper thigh.

Incision. The incision extends vertically upwards from the medial prominence of the medial femoral condyle over a distance equal to one-fifth or one-quarter of the length of the thigh, depending on the degree of obesity.

Exposure of supracondylar region of femur. The incision is deepened immediately behind the vastus medialis. The femur is exposed first at the lower end of the incision and from this point the bone is traced proximally by blunt dissection. The periosteum is incised vertically in the mid-medial plane and stripped from the anterior and posterior aspects of the femur with a curved elevator. The periosteal flaps are held back by two pairs of bone levers passed between periosteum and bone.

A large part of the circumference of the lower end of the femoral shaft is thus exposed. In children the epiphysial cartilage will be seen as a white line running round the lower end of the femur where the shaft flares out to form the condyles. The epiphysial cartilage should be left undisturbed: the osteotomy is carried out well above this level, just proximal to the point where the parallel sides of the femoral shaft begin to flare out (Fig. 457).

Excision of wedge of bone. From previous measurements upon the radiographs the angle of correction required is already known, as should also be the breadth of the base of the bony wedge that is to be removed. The outlines of the wedge may now be marked upon the femur (Fig. 457), and when this had been done the division of the bone may begin. In a child the femur may be soft enough to be divided easily with sharp osteotomes, or even in part by sharp-pointed bone-cutting forceps. In an adult the wedge should be cut out partly by multiple drill holes, which are then joined by cuts with the osteotome; or alternatively the bone may be cut with a power-driven reciprocating saw.

Both in children and in adults it is important to leave the apex of the wedge—that is, the lateral part of the cortex and the overlying periosteum—intact so that it may form a hinge to stabilise the two fragments when continuity of the bone is broken. If no stable hinge remains it is easy to lose control of the fragments, which may become markedly displaced upon one another.

When the appropriate wedge of bone has been removed the knee is straightened and, one hand being placed over the site of osteotomy to act as a fulcrum, the leg is forced into varus so that the wedge-shaped gap in the lower femur is closed and the cut edges of the medial cortex come into

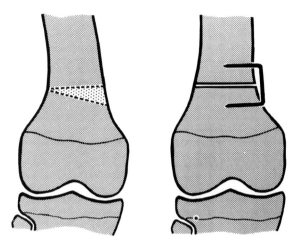

FIGS 457–458. Supracondylar corrective osteotomy of femur. Figure 457—Outline of wedge for correction of valgus deformity. Figure 458—The gap closed after removal of the wedge, and the fragments fixed with a staple.

contact (Fig. 458). At this point the shape of the leg is examined clinically to check that the degree of correction is exactly right. If necessary a radiograph may be taken to confirm this.

Internal fixation. In children fixation by metal staples is usually satisfactory. Two or at the most three staples are required: they are ranged round the antero-medial and postero-medial aspects of the femur. Holes for the legs of the staples are prepared with fine drills in such a way that each staple bridges the osteotomy, with one leg in each fragment. In adults there is a greater tendency for the fragments to become displaced, and better fixation may be achieved by one or two four-hole plates fixed with screws.

Closure. The muscles are allowed to fall back into position, and only a few deep absorbable sutures are required. The skin is closed without drainage.

POST-OPERATIVE MANAGEMENT

A wide crepe bandage is applied snugly over copious gauze dressings, and a plaster-of-Paris knee cylinder extending from the groin to the malleoli is applied with the knee almost but not quite fully extended. The plaster is moulded in such a way as to maintain correction of the valgus deformity: in other words it is moulded to keep the osteotomy gap closed. The plaster is maintained until bony union is well advanced, as shown radiologically. In children this may be a matter of five to six weeks, but in adults correspondingly longer. When bony union has been demonstrated a course of knee mobilising and muscle strengthening exercises is arranged.

Comment

The main essential in this operation is to ensure that exactly the right degree of correction is gained. It is all too easy to under-correct or to over-correct the deformity. Special care must therefore be taken before operation to determine the angle of correction that is required, both from clinical and from radiological measurements. It may even be useful to make a template of the required angle from lead or zinc sheet and to sterilise it for use as a guide during the operation.

Another important point is to ensure that a hinge of intact cortex and periosteum remains at the apex of the wedge. In children the hinge of cortex may bend without complete loss of continuity, but in adults the cortex inevitably breaks when the wedge is finally closed, and stability must depend upon an intact soft tissue hinge.

In children care must be taken not to damage the epiphysial cartilage, lest growth be disturbed.

ALTERNATIVE TECHNIQUE: MOORE'S OSTEOTOMY-OSTEOCLASIS

Moore (1947) described "osteotomy-osteoclasis" in two stages. At the first stage an appropriate wedge of bone was removed, but about a fifth of the circumference of the cortex was left intact at the apex of the wedge, and no attempt was made at this stage to gain correction. The excised wedge of bone was cut up into chips and re-inserted in the wedge-shaped gap. The limb was protected in a plaster splint and at the second stage of the procedure two or three weeks later, when sticky granulations could be expected to have formed about the site of osteotomy, osteoclasis was carried out. By judicious force the remaining cortex at the apex of the wedge was broken or bent to allow closure of the wedge with correction of the deformity. Thereafter a new plaster was worn until union occurred. For further details of this technique the reader is referred to Moore's original paper.

PRIMARY REPAIR OF TORN MEDIAL LIGAMENT OF THE KNEE

Traumatic rupture of the medial ligament of the knee (consisting of tibial collateral and medial capsular components) is commonly associated with rupture of the posterior capsule ("posterior oblique ligament"), the anterior cruciate ligament and the medial meniscus.

Primary repair is to be considered if there is complete rupture with medial rotatory instability, and it should be performed within fourteen days of injury.

The aim is to repair the medial ligament (both components) and the posterior capsule. The joint is inspected to assess damage to the medial meniscus and anterior cruciate ligament, and if the meniscus is torn it should be removed.

TECHNIQUE

Position of patient. The patient lies supine. The hinged lower flap of the operation table is lowered to allow the knee to flex to 30 degrees: or the knee may be supported in the semi-flexed position by a large wedge of plastic foam. A tourniquet may be used on the upper thigh.

Exposure of damaged ligaments. A longitudinal incision is made over the medial aspect of the knee. The superficial layer of the tibial collateral ligament, including its proximal and distal attachments, is exposed. The site of rupture in this layer is usually visible but it may be indicated at first only by a haematoma. Sharp dissection at the site of rupture will reveal the deeper capsular ligament, and by rocking the tibia into valgus a rupture of the medial capsular ligament may be exposed.

Arthrotomy. With the knee now flexed to a right angle, the joint cavity is opened by a longitudinal incision through the capsule at the anterior margin of the tibial collateral ligament. The joint is inspected thoroughly and medial meniscectomy is performed if indicated.

Repair. With the knee restored to a position of 30 degrees of flexion, the tibia is rotated medially.

The medial capsular ligament is repaired first. A rupture through its substance is repaired with interrupted absorbable sutures. If one end has become detached from bone, it should be re-attached by sutures passed through drill holes through the cortex of the bone.

The posterior capsule is repaired and the tibial collateral ligament is re-attached or repaired in a similar fashion to the medial capsular ligament.

Closure. The wound is closed in layers, everting mattress sutures being used for the skin.

POST-OPERATIVE MANAGEMENT

Soft gauze dressings and crepe bandages are applied. An above-knee plaster is applied with the knee in 20 degrees of flexion. This plaster is removed after two weeks and the sutures are removed. A second plaster, applied with the knee again flexed 15 or 20 degrees, but with the foot left free, is worn for a further four weeks, during which walking is encouraged. Thereafter, intensive exercises designed to restore knee movement and to redevelop the quadriceps muscle are practised under the supervision of the physiotherapist.

ANTERIOR TRANSFER OF PES ANSERINUS FOR ROTATORY INSTABILITY OF KNEE

This operation is designed to alter the line of pull of the three muscles, whose insertion into the upper part of the medial aspect of the tibia is termed the pes anserinus from its resemblance in shape to a goose's foot, and thus to prevent forward subluxation of the medial tibial condyle upon the femur in cases of impairment of the anterior cruciate and medial ligaments. The main action of these muscles upon the knee is to flex it. With the knee flexed they act as medial rotators of the tibia upon the femur. When the insertion of the muscles is transferred forwards and proximally their action as medial rotators of the tibia upon the femur is enhanced.

The operation consists essentially in detaching the distal and medial parts of the broad insertion of the conjoined tendons into the tibia and folding it upwards and forwards over the proximal and anterior part of the natural insertion. If necessary the knee may be explored at the same operation for possible internal derangement, and the operation may be combined with the reconstruction of other ligaments about the knee.

TECHNIQUE

Position of patient. The patient lies supine. The hinged lower flap of the operation table is let down to allow the knee to be flexed 90 degrees over the edge of the table, as for meniscectomy. A tourniquet may be used on the upper thigh. The surgeon sits facing the front of the knee with the foot of the affected side resting upon his lap.

Incision. A vertical antero-medial incision is made, extending 10 to 12 centimetres below the upper articular margin of the tibia. If the knee is to be explored at the same operation the incision is made continuous with the antero-medial arthro-tomy incision.

Defining the pes anserinus. It is important to define clearly the margins of the pes anserinus, formed in order from above downwards by the sartorius, the gracilis and the semitendinosus. The lower extremity of the fan-like tendinous insertion of these muscles extends fully 7 or 8 centimetres below the line of the knee joint.

The posterior margin of the muscle group is defined first: the semitendinosus is easily palpated in the lower thigh and the line of its insertion into the tibia is easily defined. The surgeon then works forwards and upwards to clear the fascia from the superficial aspect of the tendinous expansion over the medial aspect of the tibia, as far forwards as the tibial tubercle and patellar tendon, and as far proximally as the point where the tibial condyle begins to flare forwards. Proximally the three tendons are traced to a point level with the supracondylar part of the femur. At the medial side of the knee the medial ligament will be seen lying deep to the anterior edge of the pes anserinus.

Detachment and reversal of lower two-thirds of tendinous attachment. By clean dissection with a knife the lower and posterior two-thirds of the tendinous expansion are severed from the medial aspect of the tibia. The division is made close to the bone. The separated major part of the tendinous expansion is then folded upwards and forwards to cover the remaining undetached part of the membrane. The aim should be to bring the lowermost part of the tendon forwards to lie adjacent to the medial border of the patellar tendon and tibial tubercle, while the posterior margin after being turned up lies horizontally, parallel with the joint line but immediately distal to the part of the tibia that flares forwards and medially

to form the medial condyle (Fig. 459). The membrane is sutured in this new position under moderate tension with the knee flexed 90 degrees and the tibia rotated medially upon the femur. Anteriorly the sutures anchor the membrane to the medial border of the patellar tendon and to the periosteum over the tibial tubercle. Proximally

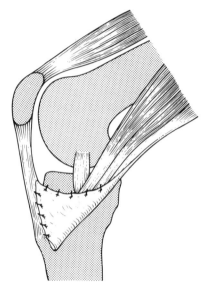

FIG. 459. Pes anserinus transfer. The strong membranous insertion of the conjoined tendons—consisting largely of the semitendinosus tendon—has been folded upwards, to be sutured to the medial edge of the patellar tendon and to the periosteum adjacent to the tibial tubercle. The direction of pull of the conjoined tendons is thus moved proximally, with enhancement of their action as medial rotators of the tibia.

the sutures grip the upper edge of the undisturbed part of the pes anserinus and the adjacent periosteum. At the conclusion of the suture the inverted part of the pes anserinus has the appearance of a tendinous sling wrapped round the upper medial part of the tibia just beneath the flaring condyle.

Closure. Subcutaneous tissue and skin are closed with interrupted sutures.

POST-OPERATIVE MANAGEMENT

Gauze dressings are held in place by a wide crepe bandage over which is applied a full-length lower limb plaster from upper thigh to metatarsal heads, with the knee flexed about 30 degrees and the ankle at a right angle. Leg raising exercises are commenced from the first day.

After two weeks, when the sutures are removed, a new plaster of similar extent is applied. A walking heel is added and the patient resumes full weight bearing under supervision. The plaster is retained for a total of five weeks, after which intensive muscle exercises and knee flexion and extension exercises are instituted.

Comment

Those seeking further details of this operation should consult the original paper of Slocum and Larson (1968). The operation tends now to be much less favoured than it was a decade ago, because in general the results have not matched up to expectations.

FASCIAL STABILISATION FOR ANTERO-LATERAL INSTABILITY OF THE KNEE

(MacIntosh Antero-lateral Stabilisation)

In antero-lateral instability the lateral condyle of the tibia becomes subluxated forwards in relation to the lateral femoral condyle with the knee in slight flexion (lateral pivot shift). As flexion is increased the subluxation is spontaneously reduced, often with a click or jerk. The MacIntosh operation (Galway *et al.* 1972) aims to control this subluxation of the lateral tibial condyle by anchoring a strip of fascia lata, left attached distally to the tibia, to the femur through the medium of the lateral ligament and the tough lateral intermuscular septum.

TECHNIQUE

Position of patient. The patient lies supine with the knee flexed 60 degrees. A tourniquet may be used on the highest part of the thigh.

Incision. The incision begins in the mid-lateral line of the thigh 15 centimetres proximal to the joint line of the knee, and it follows the mid-lateral line to cross over the prominence of the lateral femoral condyle; thereafter it inclines forwards at its lower end to cross the articular margin of the tibia midway between the lateral margin of the patella and the head of the fibula.

The deep dissection: isolating a fascial strip. The posterior skin margin is retracted to allow thorough clearing of the deep fascial layer. A strip of fascia lata not less than 15 millimetres wide and 15 centimetres long is dissected free, being left

attached only at the distal end: this intact base of the flap should lie antero-laterally, over the bony eminence of the tibia known as the lateral tibial tubercle (Fig. 460).

Preparing the track for the new fascial ligament. The small fossa behind the lateral condyle of the femur is cleared to reveal the lateral intermuscular septum, which is easily felt in the semi-flexed knee 2 centimetres in front of the prominent biceps tendon. When this has been cleared of fatty tissue the lateral ligament is also defined where it crosses the joint line from the head of the fibula to the lateral eminence of the lateral condyle of the femur. Before being revealed by sharp dissection this ligament can be palpated more easily than seen.

Routing and anchorage of fascial strip. The next step is to pass the strip of fascia—still attached to the tibia distally—beneath the lateral ligament and to anchor it to the tough tense band that forms the lower attachment of the lateral intermuscular septum to the femur (Fig. 460).

First a tunnel is formed deep to the lateral ligament by a blunt instrument such as an artery forceps. The fascial strip is then drawn up through the tunnel.

The fascia is then brought up towards the insertion of the lateral intermuscular septum and passed deep to it. So that the course of the fascia over the lateral femoral condyle may be straight, a small plaque of bone and periosteum should be turned down on an intact periosteal hinge, and the fascia placed deep to it. The new ligament thus runs in a straight course from its tibial insertion upwards to the femoral attachment of the intermuscular septum (Fig. 460).

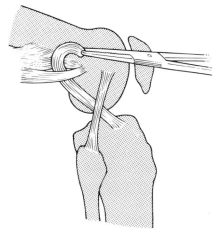

FIG. 460. Antero-lateral stabilisation. The strip of fascia lata, attached distally, is brought up deep to the lateral ligament and anchored to the lowest fibres of the lateral intermuscular septum near the point of their insertion into the femur.

Finally the strip of fascia is pulled taut while the foot and lower leg are rotated laterally by an assistant. This rotation brings the upper and lower attachments of the new ligament closer together and thus ensures maximal tightness. The new fascial ligament is anchored proximally by looping it twice around the taut band of insertion of the intermuscular septum and locking it by strong transfixing sutures. Further sutures are used to unite the fascia to the lateral ligament.

Closure. It should be possible to close the gap in the fascia lata proximally, but in the distal half of the incision the fascial gap must be left open. The superficial layers are closed without drainage.

POST-OPERATIVE MANAGEMENT

It is important that lateral rotation of the foot and leg relative to the thigh be maintained while a plaster-of-Paris splint is applied from the upper thigh to the metatarsal heads with the knee flexed 60 degrees. This flexed position of the knee precludes early weight bearing, but the patient may walk with crutches. The plaster may be changed after two weeks, when the sutures are removed. Plaster splintage should be retained for a total of six weeks. Thereafter mobilising exercises are encouraged and walking is resumed, at first with elbow crutches. The patient should be warned that the newly constructed ligament is unsuitable to withstand severe stress in the early stages, and the resumption of active sporting activities should be delayed for six months.

RECONSTRUCTION OF ANTERIOR CRUCIATE LIGAMENT

In reconstruction of the anterior cruciate ligament it is necessary to introduce new material—tendon, fascia or strands of extrinsic material—accurately in the line of the natural ligament. The technique to be described is based on that of Jones (1963). Essentially, a strip of quadriceps tendon, including a strip of bone from the mid-line of the patella and left attached distally to the tibial tubercle, is re-routed through a deep groove in the intercondylar eminence of the tibia to emerge at the anterior tibial spine, and thence into a drill hole traversing the lateral condyle of the femur, where the free end of the tendon is anchored. A basically similar method of routing other materials through appropriate drill holes may be used as an alternative.

TECHNIQUE

Position of patient. The patient lies supine and the limb is draped in such a way that the knee may rest flexed or extended. A tourniquet may be used on the upper part of the thigh.

Incision. The skin incision is anterior and almost vertical, being arched slightly medially to skirt the medial edge of the patella (Fig. 461). The lower extremity of the incision is at the tibial tubercle.

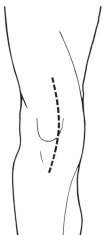

Fig. 461. Reconstruction of anterior cruciate ligament. The skin incision.

Preparation of tendino-osseous strip. After retraction of the skin edges the anterior aspect of the lower part of the quadriceps expansion, of the patella, and of the patellar tendon is exposed and cleared. The joint cavity is opened by a parapatellar incision through capsule and synovial membrane. The joint cavity is inspected, and any ragged remnants of the anterior cruciate ligament are cleared away.

A continuous vertical strip of tissue comprising the central part of the quadriceps expansion, a mid-line piece of the anterior surface of the patella together with overlying aponeurosis, and a central strip of the patellar tendon is now separated by sharp dissection and by powered saw (Fig. 462). The strip of tissue should measure 6 to 10 millimetres in width, according to the build of the patient. It includes the whole thickness of the quadriceps expansion and of the patellar tendon, and about half the thickness of the patella. Distally it is left attached at its normal insertion into the tibial tubercle.

Preparation of channel in tibia. With the knee flexed the front of the upper part of the tibia is exposed by retraction of the patellar tendon laterally and the infrapatellar fat pad upwards. A deep channel is cut in the antero-superior corner of the tibia, emerging on the intercondylar eminence at

the normal point of attachment of the anterior cruciate ligament (Fig. 463). The channel may be cut out with a narrow gouge, or a block of bone may be removed, to be re-attached later with a screw (Lamb 1968).

Drilling the hole in the femoral condyle. In order to anchor the new ligament at the correct point of attachment on the medial aspect of the lateral femoral condyle, it is necessary to drill a hole through the condyle from the outer side. To

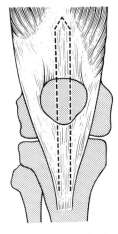

Fig. 462. Reconstruction of anterior cruciate ligament. Outline of strip of tendon and bone used to form the new ligament. The strip of tissue is left attached distally.

ensure that the hole emerges at the correct site it is best to use a special C-shaped guide to direct a preliminary guide wire, though it is possible to insert the guide wire freehand. With the guide wire thus inserted and seen to emerge at the correct point on the medial surface of the lateral femoral condyle, a hole 6 to 10 millimetres in diameter (to match the diameter of the new ligament) is made with a cannulated drill passed over the guide wire. Bone debris from the drilling is carefully removed from the joint.

Insertion of new ligament in prepared track. The tendino-osseous strip, still attached at the tibial tubercle, is smoothed to a uniform diameter and passed beneath the infrapatellar fat pad to lie deeply in the channel that has been gouged out of the tibia. Bone is replaced over it. The proximal part of the strip, including the osseous portion, is then drawn through the drill hole in the lateral femoral condyle by a holding suture of wire or strong silk passed on an eyed probe. The reconstructed ligament is pulled taut with the knee in a position 10 to 15 degrees short of full extension. The part of the tendon that emerges on the outer

sudden stress and that a very easy life should be led. If running and sports are to be resumed, an interval of six months is advisable.

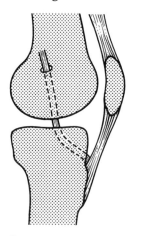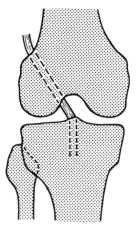

FIG. 463. Showing the direction of the track through the upper end of the tibia and the lateral femoral condyle in which the new ligament will lie.

surface of the femoral condyle is again drawn taut, turned over and fixed to the bone with a staple.

Closure. The linear gaps in the quadriceps expansion and in the patellar tendon are closed with interrupted absorbable sutures. The tourniquet should be removed before closure of the capsule and skin, with or without suction drainage as preferred.

POST-OPERATIVE MANAGEMENT

A plaster-of-Paris splint extending from groin to malleoli is applied over a soft dressing and cellulose padding. The plaster may be changed after two weeks, when the sutures are removed: it is retained for a total of six weeks. Walking on the limb is encouraged after the first few days. Static quadriceps exercises should be arranged under the supervision of a physiotherapist. After removal of the plaster, knee flexion and extension exercises and quadriceps exercises are practised intensively.

The patient should be warned that in the early weeks and months after the operation the reconstructed ligament—and indeed the extensor mechanism of the knee itself—is vulnerable to

ALTERNATIVE TECHNIQUES

Instead of the central strip of quadriceps tendon and patella, the use of a lateral strip comprising joint capsule and patellar tendon—but not part of the patella—may be used for the substitute ligament (Campbell 1939). The method of insertion is basically the same, except that a drill hole rather than a deep channel may be used to convey the material through the tibia to the site of emergence of the ligament on the intercondylar eminence of the tibia.

Artificial ligaments have also been used, but their place has not yet been fully evaluated.

Comment

Reconstruction of the anterior cruciate ligament may be combined if necessary with other stabilising operations on the medial or lateral side of the knee.

The operation should be approached with due circumspection: though worthwhile improvement is to be expected, it is unrealistic to expect restoration to normality in the long term. Improvement rather than cure must be regarded as acceptable.

SYNOVECTOMY OF KNEE

The operation to be described does not set out to be a total synovectomy: some synovial tissue is left posteriorly but the lining membrane is stripped from the inside of the capsule and from the non-articular surfaces of the femur and tibia in the anterior two-thirds of the joint and from the suprapatellar pouch. In other words, as much of the synovial lining as can be reached from the anterior incision is excised.

TECHNIQUE

Position of patient. The patient lies supine with the knee resting upon a rolled towel or sand-bag in slight flexion. A tourniquet may be used on the upper thigh.

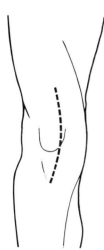

FIG. 464. Medial parapatellar incision for synovectomy of knee.

Incision. The skin incision, almost vertical, is arched slightly medially to skirt the medial edge of the patella (Fig. 464). The upper limit of the incision is about 10 centimetres above the upper margin of the patella and the lower end is level with the tibial tubercle.

Exposure of joint. The skin edges are retracted, and in the upper part of the incision the vastus medialis component of the quadriceps muscle is divided by a cut that skirts the patella about 1.5 centimetres from its medial margin. Deep to this the joint capsule and synovial membrane are incised to open the suprapatellar pouch. The incision through capsule and synovial membrane is extended distally so that the joint is exposed from the upper extremity of the suprapatellar pouch right down to the point where the synovium is attached to the articular margin of the tibia.

With the whole extent of the joint thus opened medial to the patella, it is possible to retract and evert the whole of the lateral flap containing the patella (so that the articular surface of the patella is directed forwards) and thus to gain a clear view of the whole of the interior of the joint. Moreover by flexing the knee fully the intercondylar notch, the menisci and the lateral and medial recesses of the joint cavity may be fully explored.

Excision of synovial membrane. The synovial membrane is now systematically stripped from the inner aspect of the capsule, starting in the suprapatellar pouch. Once the correct plane has been found between synovial membrane and capsule separation of the two layers presents little difficulty: usually it is most easily accomplished with blunt-pointed scissors. The diseased synovial membrane is often boggy and much thickened: in a florid case it may somewhat resemble a placenta.

When the suprapatellar pouch has been cleared attention is directed to the medial and lateral recesses of the joint, where synovial membrane is cut away as far back as can be reached. The membrane is then stripped from the non-articular parts of the femur and tibia and from the intercondylar notch. The patella being fully everted through 180 degrees so that its articular surface is directed forwards, synovial membrane lining the deep surface of the quadriceps tendon is also excised as cleanly as possible.

The medial and lateral menisci are inspected: if they appear soft and ragged they should be excised.

During the operation careful note should be taken of the condition of the articular cartilage of the femur, tibia and patella. If the patello-femoral compartment of the joint is badly damaged by the arthritic process it is permissible to excise the patella at the same operation.

Closure. It is important that the tourniquet be removed and all bleeding points controlled before the wound is closed. The deep suture line unites the cut surfaces of the capsule and quadriceps expansion. The skin is closed with interrupted everting mattress sutures.

POST-OPERATIVE MANAGEMENT

Two crepe bandages 15 centimetres wide are applied snugly over copious gauze dressings so that there is even pressure over the joint. For ten days the knee is immobilised in a plaster splint extending from upper thigh to lower calf. Quadriceps exercises are begun immediately, the patient being taught to practise static contractions within the plaster. When the plaster is removed after ten days, intensive flexion and extension exercises are begun under the supervision of a physiotherapist. The aim should be to gain full extension and to restore flexion approaching the pre-operative range within three weeks of removal of the plaster. If progress is unduly slow, so that only a small range of flexion has been regained four weeks after operation, gentle manipulation under general anaesthetic is recommended. Thereafter exercises should be continued as before.

When it is available, the use of a continuous passive motion machine from an early stage may hasten the restoration of movement.

Comment

Synovectomy of the knee is now recommended less frequently than it was in the past, for it has come to be accepted that the operation does little to retard the progress of rheumatoid arthritis.

Nevertheless it is of definite benefit when a bulky mass of inflamed synovial membrane causes marked discomfort.

In general, it is appropriate to remove as much synovial tissue as can be made accessible through a straightforward parapatellar approach with displacement of the patella. Although the greater part of the membrane is removed, the operation is by no means a total synovectomy.

Post-operative treatment is important. Some surgeons prefer to encourage active joint movements immediately after the operation. Others, with the authors, prefer to immobilise the knee at first to promote healing of the soft tissues and to reduce pain and discomfort. Restoration of movement does not seem to be significantly slower after an initial period of immobilisation than it is with immediate exercises. Whatever technique is used, and whatever the post-operative programme, manipulation under anaesthetic will be required in a proportion of cases in which recovery of knee flexion is slow.

Arthroscopic Synovectomy

Synovectomy of the knee is now often carried out arthroscopically in preference to making a formal incision into the joint. A powered cutter is used. The synovectomy is of necessity only partial, only the exuberant folds of inflamed membrane being removed and not the whole thickness of the tissue.

The great advantage of arthroscopic synovectomy is that recovery from the operation and rehabilitation are much more rapid than after open synovectomy, which usually entails a long programme of after-treatment.

REMOVAL OF MEDIAL MENISCUS

The commonest lesion of the medial meniscus is the bucket-handle tear. This necessitates the removal either of the whole meniscis or (much more often) of the displaced body of the meniscus, depending upon the state of the remaining rim (Fig. 465). Anterior horn tears, posterior horn tears and cysts usually necessitate removal of the whole meniscus.

Excision of Whole Meniscus

Excision of the whole meniscus necessitates a peripheral sharp dissection in the plane between the avascular meniscus and the soft, vascular synovial membrane.

TECHNIQUE

Position of patient. The patient lies supine upon the table, the end flap of which should be dropped to allow both lower legs to hang vertically with the knees flexed 90 degrees. The surgeon sits on a low stool with the foot of the affected limb on his lap. At the outset, precautions should be taken to ensure that there is no pressure contact between the neck of the fibula and the corner of the operation table; otherwise the common peroneal nerve may suffer damage. To this end many surgeons protect the lower part of the hamstring area with a small soft cushion placed between the thigh and the lower end of the table. A tourniquet should always be used on the upper thigh.

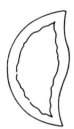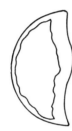

FIG. 465. The common longitudinal ("bucket-handle") split of the medial meniscus. *Left*—Large remaining rim. *Right*—Small remaining rim: almost the whole meniscus displaced.

Incision. A vertical skin incision is made 1.5 centimetres medial to the patella. The incision begins at the level of the junction of the upper and middle thirds of the patella and extends distally to a point one centimetre below the prominent ridge formed by the anterior margin of the upper articular surface of the tibia (Fig. 466). The incision exposes the capsule of the knee joint. Its surface is cleared of overlying areolar tissue over a width of about a centimetre on each side of the incision to facilitate subsequent suture.

Exposure of joint. The capsule is incised in the same line as the skin incision. The underlying synovial membrane is then opened. It is easiest to open it first at the upper end of the incision by grasping the membrane with forceps and pulling it forwards to separate it from the underlying

femoral condyle. Once the initial opening has been made it is easy to extend the synovial incision distally either by knife or with scissors. The opening should be sufficiently long to expose at the

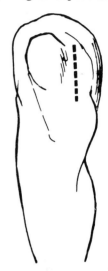

FIG. 466. Incision for medial meniscectomy.

lower end the anterior margin of the tibial articular surface. The cut margins of the synovial membrane are retracted to expose the interior of the joint. Often there is an excess of synovial fluid which at first obscures the view: this should be squeezed out by firm pressure applied behind the knee.

Inspection of joint. Although the joint will almost always have been studied by arthroscopy or arthrography, or both, in order to confirm the clinical diagnosis, it is nevertheless important that upon opening the joint the surgeon carry out a full visual survey of the accessible parts of the joint. If a bucket-handle tear of the meniscus is present the displaced body of the meniscus will be seen lying in the intercondylar space, hugging the lateral margin of the medial femoral condyle: the split between this displaced part and the remaining rim of meniscus will be clearly evident. A pedunculated tag tear of the anterior horn of the meniscus will also be easily identified, but a posterior horn tear cannot always be seen at this stage of the operation.

When the meniscus has been carefully inspected attention should be directed to the medial femoral condyle. This should be inspected and palpated with a blunt instrument for the possible presence of an area of softened articular cartilage which might indicate osteochondritis dissecans. Next the intercondylar space is examined, with particular reference to the integrity or otherwise of the cruciate ligaments. Attention is next directed to the lateral compartment of the joint, part of which can be seen through the intercondylar space. It is possible to see the medial aspect of the lateral femoral condyle, and if there is a displaced bucket-handle tear of the lateral meniscus the displaced body of the meniscus may be seen. Finally, the deep surface of the patella is inspected by first straightening the knee and then lifting the patella forwards with a bone hook. Areas of chondromalacia of the patella may thus be revealed.

If no abnormality is found within the accessible parts of the joint, either in the menisci or elsewhere, meniscectomy may proceed provided the diagnosis of torn meniscus has been established by arthroscopy or arthrography, because a posterior tear may not become evident until the anterior two-thirds of the meniscus have been mobilised.

Excision of meniscus. The first step is to clear the anterior end of the meniscus. This should be displayed first where it lies upon the front of the tibial condyle, by separating synovial tissue from its anterior margin. It is also useful to open up the space between the under surface of the meniscus and the upper surface of the tibia by incising synovial membrane at the lower edge of the meniscus. The meniscus can then be easily pulled forward with a button hook (Fig. 467).

With a knife passed under the anterior end of the meniscus the anterior horn is easily detached. The free anterior part of the meniscus is then grasped firmly in two Kocher's or Martin's forceps; pulling these forwards will display clearly the junction between the peripheral margin of the meniscus and the synovial membrane. The assistant retracts skin and capsule medially while this junction is divided either with a small knife or with scissors. In this way there is no difficulty in extending the separation of meniscus from synovial membrane half way round to the back of the joint.

At this point the separation becomes more difficult. A slightly larger retractor may have to be inserted to display the peripheral margin of the

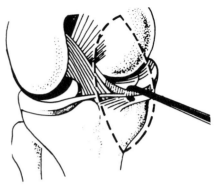

FIG. 467. Total medial meniscectomy. Anterior rim of meniscus defined and secured with button-hook to facilitate division of the anterior horn. The margins of the incision are outlined.

meniscus adequately, and a new grip may have to be obtained on the meniscus by Kocher's or Martin's forceps to enable a firm forward pull to

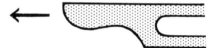

FIG. 468. In separation of the meniscus from the synovial membrane the knife should be pushed forward into the junctional tissue so that the cut is made with its anterior edge.

be sustained. The separation of meniscus from synovial membrane from this point round to the posterior horn should be done with a small

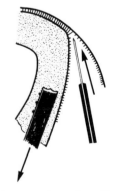

FIG. 469. As the separation proceeds, the meniscus, held firmly in Kocher's forceps, is pulled towards the intercondylar space while the knife divides the junctional tissue under direct vision.

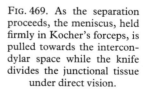

rounded (size 15) knife blade on a long handle. The correct technique is to push the knife forwards into the gap between meniscus and synovial membrane, cutting with the front edge of the knife (Figs 468 and 469). Any twisting of the knife is to be avoided because it will assuredly lead to breakage of the blade. As the division proceeds a firm pull upon the front of the meniscus is maintained to keep it on the stretch (Fig. 469), but with care to avoid excessive force which might easily tear the meniscus across. Each forward thrust of the knife should cause a characteristic tearing sensation as the meniscal fibres give way. When the separation has proceeded to within 2 or 3 centimetres of the posterior horn of the meniscus the remaining peripheral attachment may be torn by pulling the meniscus across laterally towards the centre of the joint.

It remains now to detach the posterior horn of the meniscus. To display this more clearly the retractor is removed from the medial side of the incision and placed in the lateral side. The intercondylar region of the knee is thus displayed, and the posterior horn of the meniscus comes into view far back behind and medial to the anterior cruciate ligament. The correct procedure is to cut the posterior horn through from above downwards with a short sawing action of the knife, the cut being directed downwards and medially, parallel to the fibres of the anterior cruciate ligament. As the knife cuts are made the meniscus is pulled forward firmly with Kocher's or Martin's forceps: the last fibres of attachment may tear and the meniscus is free.

Retrieval of posterior part of meniscus after accidental rupture. If the meniscus is handled injudiciously and is pulled forward too forcibly it may tear in half, so that the posterior part of the meniscus is left partly detached in the back of the joint. It may be impossible to obtain a new grip on the remaining fragment from the anterior incision, and in that event a second incision has to be made to open the posterior compartment of the joint for removal of the broken fragment.

To make this new incision the surgeon abducts the thigh in order to gain access to that part of the joint that lies behind the medial ligament; or alternatively, the flap of the operation table may be raised level and the foot planted upon it with the knee held flexed 90 degrees. In either case the surgeon must face directly the medial aspect of the knee. To locate the correct site for the incision, the depression between the femoral condyle and the tibial condyle is palpated to define the level of the joint. A vertical incision extends 2 centimetres

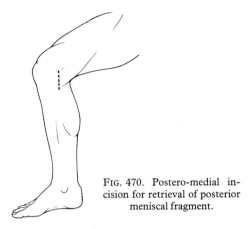

Fig. 470. Postero-medial incision for retrieval of posterior meniscal fragment.

above and 2 centimetres below this point, about 1.5 or 2 centimetres behind the medial ligament (Fig. 470). Capsule is exposed and opened, as is the underlying synovial membrane. It is often helpful to pass a curved blunt bone lever from the

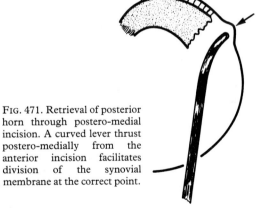

Fig. 471. Retrieval of posterior horn through postero-medial incision. A curved lever thrust postero-medially from the anterior incision facilitates division of the synovial membrane at the correct point.

anterior incision to push the synovial membrane medially from within: this facilitates its identification and division (Fig. 471).

Once the joint has been opened the edges of the synovial membrane are retracted with blunt hooks to expose the posterior rim of the meniscus. Again this may be identified more easily if the stump of the meniscus at the point of rupture can be grasped with an artery forceps and moved to and fro from the anterior incision. Once the fragment of meniscus has been identified there should be no difficulty in grasping it through the posterior incision and separating its posterior edge from the remaining synovial attachment round to the posterior horn. This dissection is best done with blunt-pointed scissors. Finally, the posterior horn is severed under direct vision and the fragment of meniscus is discarded.

Closure. There is no need to suture the synovial membrane as a separate layer. A single line of fine interrupted absorbable sutures including capsule and edge of synovial membrane is to be preferred. Usually not more than five or six sutures are required. The skin is closed with interrupted everting mattress sutures. In contradistinction to most operations carried out under tourniquet, in meniscectomy it is best to defer release of the tourniquet until the wound is closed and the dressings and bandages have been applied. Provided the tissues are cut in the correct plane bleeding is minimal, and ligation or cautery of vessels is not required.

POST-OPERATIVE MANAGEMENT

Copious gauze dressings are used in order to fill the concavities between the various bony landmarks of the knee and thus to make more effective the firm crepe bandages that are next applied. For this purpose bandages 15 centimetres wide are best.

Many rules of post-meniscectomy management have been advocated. The authors' firm conclusion is that the best method is to apply a cylinder of plaster-of-Paris from groin to malleoli over a generous lining of cellulose cotton, with the knee very nearly straight but nevertheless flexed 2 or 3 degrees to prevent the troublesome pain that may accompany immobilisation of the knee in forced extension.

Intensive supervision by a physiotherapist is of great importance in reducing the period of convalescence to the minimum. Exercises should be begun as soon as the patient regains consciousness. Even while he is still drowsy he should be encouraged repeatedly to lift the leg, encased in

the plaster, in order to initiate the return of active quadriceps contractions. The earlier leg lifting is begun, the more easily is the post-operative inhibition of quadriceps contraction overcome.

In the succeeding days static quadriceps exercises are progressively increased and hip and ankle exercises are practised regularly. Walking within the confines of the ward is permitted in the plaster from the day of operation. Indeed this facility is one of the advantages of using plaster immobilisation. The plaster is removed on the tenth day after operation, and thereafter knee flexion exercises as well as continued extension exercises are practised. Final rehabilitation may be carried out in the gymnasium. Prolonged treatment is usually needed to build up the wasted quadriceps muscle to the same bulk as that of the normal limb.

Comment

Meniscectomy can be a difficult operation for those not accustomed to it. The main difficulties for the novice are to find the correct plane of division between peripheral rim of meniscus and synovial membrane, and more particularly to separate and detach the posterior part of the meniscus. These problems become lighter if the best possible view of the relevant part of the joint is obtained. This means skilful retraction by the assistant, who should be given a full view of what he is retracting, and by adjustments of the position of the limb as it rests upon the surgeon's knee: a little more flexion, a little rotation one way or the other, and particularly a little abduction of the tibia upon the femur may help to give a better view.

In detaching meniscus from synovial membrane at the periphery, the surgeon should acquire the knack of pushing forward with the knife blade rather than cutting downwards (Fig. 468). For this purpose a nicely rounded end to the blade is essential: the normal size 15 blade is ideal for the purpose. If the art of using this blade is learnt there is no need to resort to special end-cutting knives, which in any case have certain dangers (Patrick 1962) and which can seldom be kept as sharp as a disposable blade. It is very important that the division between meniscus and synovial membrane should not be made at the expense of synovial membrane. If the knife is allowed to wander too much into the membrane, away from the meniscus, there is a risk of damaging sizeable blood vessels or even the popliteal artery itself. The rule is never to cut where one cannot see what one is cutting. What one is cutting should always be the exact junction between the periphery of the meniscus and the synovial membrane.

The use of a plaster cylinder or splint to support the knee after operation offers the advantages that local discomfort in the knee is reduced, the knee is kept virtually straight, and interference with the dressings is discouraged.

Strenuous rehabilitation after operation is of vital importance in meniscectomy. The patient must be exhorted to practise vigorous muscle exercises every hour of the day and repeatedly to lift the leg with the knee straight. As strength improves weights may be added to the foot to intensify the effort needed to raise the leg. Neglect of proper post-operative management prolongs the period of recovery and may lead to persistent weakness of the knee from inadequate quadriceps action.

EXCISION OF DISPLACED BODY OF MENISCUS ALONE

When in a case of bucket-handle tear the peripheral rim of meniscus appears healthy, and when the displaced "bucket-handle" fragment comprises a large part of the meniscus, removal of the displaced part alone without the peripheral rim is recommended (Fig. 472). The procedure is simpler than that of removing the entire meniscus, and trauma to the joint is much reduced.

Although the open operation is to be described, it must be recognised that in most of these cases the operation is now carried out arthroscopically, without the need for formal opening of the joint (see p. 365).

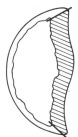

FIG. 472. Excision of displaced meniscal fragment without the peripheral part, which in most cases may safely be left undisturbed. Shaded area shows the extent of the excision.

TECHNIQUE

The meniscus is exposed from the front as already described. Instead of detaching the anterior horn entire, only the bucket-handle fragment of meniscus is grasped in Kocher's or Martin's forceps and its anterior end is cut from the rim of meniscus. The meniscus is now free except for its posterior attachment. With a retractor in the lateral side of the wound the intercondylar area of the joint is exposed and the junction of displaced body of meniscus with the posterior horn is displayed. It remains to sever the meniscus at this point by a small knife blade directed downwards and medially.

POST-OPERATIVE MANAGEMENT

This is the same as for removal of the entire meniscus.

REMOVAL OF LATERAL MENISCUS

The lateral meniscus is excised either because it has been torn or because of cystic degeneration.

LATERAL MENISCECTOMY FOR TEAR OF MENISCUS

This operation is similar to medial meniscectomy as described in the previous section. The preliminaries are precisely the same. The surgeon sits facing the antero-lateral aspect of the affected knee.

Incision. The incision slopes downwards and slightly forwards from a point 2.5 centimetres lateral to the top of the patella, to end just below the prominence of the anterior margin of the superior articular surface of the tibia (Fig. 473). The capsule is cleaned and divided in the line of the skin incision, which is also the direction of the capsular fibres. The synovial membrane is opened to expose the lateral compartment of the knee joint.

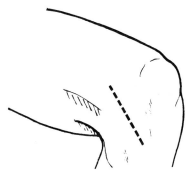

FIG. 473. Incision for lateral meniscectomy.

Inspection of joint. After any excess fluid has been squeezed out by pressure behind the knee the various components exposed to view are inspected to ascertain the nature of the pathology, which will previously have been assessed by arthroscopy, arthrography or both. The lateral meniscus may show a bucket-handle tear or an anterior or posterior horn tear similar to those of the medial meniscus. Occasionally the meniscus appears intact at first glance, for a postero-lateral peripheral tear may not become obvious until the front of the meniscus has been mobilised.

Excision of whole meniscus. Removal of the meniscus follows the same stages as described for removal of the medial meniscus. The anterior horn is easily identified and severed from its attachment. The front of the meniscus is then gripped by Kocher's or Martin's forceps and drawn lightly forwards to display the junction between meniscus and synovial membrane. This junctional tissue is divided around the periphery of the meniscus. Anteriorly scissors may be used but further back the division must be made with a small (size 15) knife blade as described for medial meniscectomy.

Freeing of the posterior rim of the meniscus may present some difficulty, but if a forward pull on the meniscus is maintained the correct plane for incision can be kept in view right round to the posterior horn. Separation of the posterior horn is somewhat easier than in the case of the medial meniscus because it is further forward and more accessible.

Excision of bucket-handle fragment alone. As in the case of the medial meniscus, it may be unnecessary to remove the rim of the meniscus if it is healthy: the displaced bucket-handle fragment only is excised.

Closure. This is the same as for medial meniscectomy.

POST-OPERATIVE MANAGEMENT
This is the same as for medial meniscectomy (p. 362).

Comment
The capsule over the lateral compartment of the knee tends to feel tighter than that over the medial compartment, and this fact sometimes makes separation of a lateral meniscus from its peripheral junction with synovial membrane relatively difficult. On the other hand, freeing of the back of the lateral meniscus and separation of the posterior horn from its attachment are often easier in lateral than in medial meniscectomy. Equal emphasis must be given in both procedures to clear definition of the plane of incision between the periphery of the meniscus and the synovial membrane. It is dangerous to allow the knife or scissors to stray too far into the synovial membrane. It is better if anything to err on the side of cutting too close into the meniscus.

LATERAL MENISCECTOMY FOR CYSTIC DEGENERATION

A cyst of the lateral meniscus usually involves the antero-lateral part: it bulges forwards just below the front of the lateral femoral condyle, stretching the antero-lateral part of the overlying capsule. For this condition removal of the entire meniscus is advised: attempted removal of the cyst alone with preservation of the meniscus is impracticable, except in occasional instances (Flynn 1976).

TECHNIQUE

Incision of the skin and capsule is the same as in lateral meniscectomy for torn meniscus. The next stage is rather different because the synovial mem-

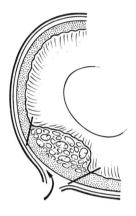

FIG. 474. Diagram shows plane of separation in removal of meniscal cyst. Part of the synovial membrane may have to be sacrificed because the cyst may be blended with it.

brane tends to be involved in the cystic process and part of the membrane overlying the cyst has to be removed with the meniscus. To this end, once the joint has been opened, the peripheral wall of the cyst, blended with synovial membrane, should be separated by dissection with scissors from the inner wall of the capsule (Fig. 474). This dissec-

tion will involve the sacrifice of that area of the synovial membrane that overlies and is blended with the cyst. Once the cyst has been separated from the inner wall of the capsule, subsequent stages in the removal of the meniscus are as described above.

POST-OPERATIVE MANAGEMENT

This is the same as for medial meniscectomy (p. 362).

Comment

Removal of a cystic meniscus can be difficult, especially if the cyst is large. It bulges the antero-lateral capsule very tightly, and it is not always easy to define the plane between the outer wall of the cyst and the inside of the capsule. An area of synovial membrane almost inevitably has to be removed with the cyst, and this leaves a gap in the synovial lining. This is of little significance because the deficiency is soon made good by the formation of a new lining membrane.

ARTHROSCOPIC MENISCECTOMY

Meniscectomy—nearly always partial rather than total—is increasingly being carried out arthroscopically, and the time cannot be far distant when to open the knee for removal of a meniscal fragment will be exceptional rather than commonplace. The overriding benefit of arthroscopic meniscectomy is the greatly increased speed of recovery from the operation and of rehabilitation. Thus it is usually possible for a patient to leave hospital on the day after the operation and to return to work within one or two weeks.

Before arthroscopic meniscectomy is undertaken it is essential that the full extent of the pathological anatomy be established by diagnostic arthroscopy, with the use of a hook or needle inserted through a secondary approach to probe

the lesion as necessary. Only when the detailed anatomical situation has been determined can the steps in the removal of the meniscal fragment or fragments be planned.

The arthroscopic approach is usually anterolateral. The secondary incision for passage of instruments must be sited according to the requirements of each case, as determined from the diagnostic survey.

After the meniscal fragment has been removed, a careful examination of the affected compartment is carried out to make sure that the remaining rim of meniscus is smooth and that there are no residual tags of tissue large enough to cause further trouble.

REMOVAL OF LOOSE BODY FROM KNEE JOINT

Loose bodies, formed most commonly in osteo-chondritis dissecans and in osteoarthritis, may lie 1) in the suprapatellar pouch, 2) in the anterior intercondylar region, or 3) in the posterior compartment. Loose bodies are often removed with the aid of the arthroscope, without formal opening of the joint (p. 368). The description that follows relates to the open operation.

PRELIMINARY STUDIES

Because of the tendency for loose bodies in the knee to move about the joint it is wise to obtain a fresh radiograph immediately before the operation commences. Alternatively, the joint may be viewed with the image intensifier.

Bodies that are entirely free tend to lodge for most of the time in the suprapatellar pouch: when seemingly loose bodies are shown radiographically in other parts of the joint, especially in the posterior compartment, the possibility of their being embedded in synovial membrane and not truly loose must always be borne in mind. Many such bodies do not in fact cause symptoms and do not need to be removed.

REMOVAL OF LOOSE BODY FROM SUPRAPATELLAR POUCH

This is the simplest of all operations for removal of loose bodies.

TECHNIQUE

Position of patient. The patient lies supine with the affected knee slightly flexed over a sand-bag or cushion: the knee is not flexed over the end of the table as it is for meniscectomy. A tourniquet should be used on the upper thigh.

Procedure. The skin incision is vertical: it extends proximally from a point just lateral to the supero-lateral corner of the patella for a distance of 3 centimetres (Fig. 475). The capsule, blended here with the quadriceps aponeurosis, is incised in the line of its fibres and the synovial membrane is opened. The edges of the incision are retracted

and a spotlight is directed into the cavity of the suprapatellar pouch while the patella is lifted forwards with a bone hook. Usually the loose body is immediately evident and can be squeezed out or grasped with forceps. Before the wound is closed

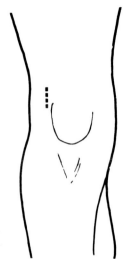

FIG. 475. Incision for removal of loose body from suprapatellar pouch.

the interior of the pouch should be searched for any further loose bodies. The capsule and synovial membrane are sutured as a single layer and the skin is closed with interrupted eversion sutures.

POST-OPERATIVE MANAGEMENT

This simple operation causes very little trauma to the joint and consequently protection in a plaster splint (as used after meniscectomy) is not required. Bulky gauze dressings should be held in place firmly by one or two wide crepe bandages. Exercises, especially for the quadriceps muscle, are encouraged but walking should be restricted to the confines of the ward until the wound is healed.

REMOVAL OF LOOSE BODY FROM INTERCONDYLAR REGION

TECHNIQUE

Position of patient. The patient lies supine with the knee flexed over the end of the table as for meniscectomy (p. 359). A tourniquet should be used on the upper thigh.

Procedure. The incision is either antero-medial or antero-lateral, according to whether the loose body is situated in the medial or the lateral compartment: if it is in the mid-line an antero-medial incision is usually made. The incision is the same as for meniscectomy (Fig. 466). When the joint cavity has been opened the wound edges are retracted. The loose body should be found without difficulty: it is grasped with forceps and removed. Capsule and synovial membrane are sutured as one layer and the skin is closed with interrupted sutures.

POST-OPERATIVE MANAGEMENT

This is the same as for meniscectomy (p. 362).

REMOVAL OF LOOSE BODY FROM POSTERIOR COMPARTMENT

This operation is seldom required because loose bodies that are truly mobile within the joint cavity seldom lodge persistently in the posterior compartment. Mobile bodies move freely about the joint and in serial radiographs they are likely to be shown in different positions at different times. A body that is seen repeatedly in the same position in the posterior compartment is likely to be enclosed in a fold of synovial membrane: it seldom causes symptoms and should not need to be removed.

TECHNIQUE

In the exceptional case in which a truly loose body is lodged posteriorly it should be removed through a postero-medial incision. The exposure is the same as that described for removal of a torn-off posterior horn of the meniscus in medial meniscectomy (p. 361).

REMOVAL OF LOOSE BODIES IN SYNOVIAL CHONDROMATOSIS

Because of the very large number of loose bodies that form in synovial chondromatosis it is not practicable to remove them all through a small incision. It is necessary to open the knee widely in order to make sure that all the loose bodies are removed.

An almost vertical incision, arched slightly medially to cross the medial edge of the patella, is appropriate (Fig. 476). The skin edges are retracted, and the quadriceps expansion and capsule are divided in a curved line that skirts the

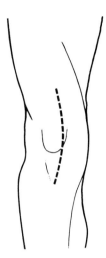

FIG. 476. Arthrotomy for removal of loose bodies in synovial chondromatosis. The skin incision.

patella about a centimetre from its medial margin. The underlying synovial cavity is opened to expose the suprapatellar pouch above and the knee joint proper below.

As the joint cavity is opened a mass of small white glistening faceted bodies extrudes from it. Those that remain and that are immediately accessible are removed. The patella is then lifted forwards with a bone hook and displaced to the lateral side to allow access to the lateral recess of the joint. When all the visible loose bodies have been removed the joint may be irrigated with saline through a bladder syringe.

When the joint cavity has been emptied the surface of the synovial membrane is inspected. Commonly, pedicled cartilaginous bodies that have not yet separated are seen attached to it. Because of the tendency of the synovial membrane to continue to form loose bodies synovectomy may often have to be advised. This may be carried out at the same time that the loose bodies are removed or, preferably, at a subsequent operation dictated by actual recurrence of the synovio-chondromatous proliferation.

REMOVAL OF LOOSE BODY BY ARThROSCOPIC TECHNIQUE

With the technical refinements that have been made in arthroscopic surgery it is nearly always possible to remove a loose body from the knee arthroscopically and thus to avoid opening the joint, with corresponding benefit to the patient in the form of more rapid rehabilitation.

The free mobility of loose bodies in the knee can make arthroscopic removal more difficult than might seem likely. The technique is relatively simple if the loose body is in the suprapatellar pouch, and if it can be retained there by finger pressure applied to the side of the knee. The use of an antero-lateral approach for the arthroscope and a lateral suprapatellar approach for the grasping instrument is then satisfactory. If the loose body is in the intercondylar region or in one of the posterior compartments the approach must be modified accordingly.

When multiple loose bodies are present, as in synovial chondromatosis, open operation is required.

CLEARANCE OF CAVITY IN FEMORAL CONDYLE IN OSTEOCHONDRITIS DISSECANS

Policies in the treatment of osteochondritis dissecans of the knee vary. In the young adolescent an expectant policy is generally adopted. In the older adolescent or young adult the stage may be reached when spontaneous regression of the lesion will not occur. A cavity, almost always in the lateral aspect of the medial femoral condyle, is occupied by a discrete disc-shaped fragment which radiologically appears loose but in reality is anchored for a while longer by a hinge of intact articular cartilage. It is the treatment of this type of lesion that is to be described below. Unless the fragment is exceptionally large the usual treatment is to remove it and to bevel the edge of the cavity but not to attempt to fill it.

In many cases the extent and maturity of the lesion will have been determined before operation by arthroscopy. Clearance of the cavity by arthroscopic control is also often undertaken by those experienced in the technique. The description that follows relates to clearance by open operation.

TECHNIQUE

Position of patient . The patient is positioned as described for medial meniscectomy (p. 359), with a tourniquet on the upper thigh and the knee flexed over the end of the table so that the foot rests upon the knees of the seated surgeon.

Incision. The incision is antero-medial, midway between the medial margin of the patella and the prominence of the medial femoral condyle. It begins opposite the junction of the upper and middle thirds of the patella and extends vertically down to the level of the upper margin of the tibia (Fig. 477). The skin edges are retracted and the

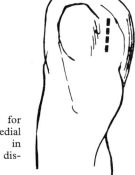

FIG. 477. Incision for exploration of medial femoral condyle in osteochondritis dissecans.

underlying capsule is cleaned and incised in the same line as the skin incision. The underlying synovial membrane is lifted forwards with dissecting forceps and incised so that the cavity of the knee joint is entered. This initial opening is best made in the upper part of the incision and then extended distally as far as the upper margin of the tibia.

Defining the lesion. When suitable retractors have been placed, a thorough inspection of the accessible parts of the joint is made. Particular attention is directed to the postero-lateral aspect of the medial femoral condyle, which is the common site for osteochondritis dissecans (Fig. 478). The lesion may or may not be obvious:

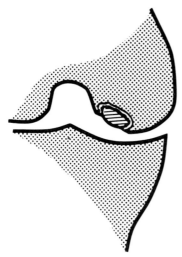

Fig. 478. Osteochondritis dissecans of medial femoral condyle. Diagram shows the common site of the lesion.

if a covering of virtually intact articular cartilage remains over the separating fragment of bone the glistening articular surface may look almost unblemished. Palpation with a blunt dissecting forceps, however, may reveal softening of the cartilage and perhaps a fissure outlining part of the circumference of the lesion. More often, if the correct time for operation has been chosen, the articular cartilage over the separating fragment is defective and the fragment is found unattached round a large part of its circumference, though often a hinge of intact cartilage remains.

The procedure is first to define the limits of the lesion and then to clear out the necrotic fragment and to clean up the edges of the cavity. The limits of the lesion are defined by palpating articular cartilage adjacent to the defective area with a blunt dissecting forceps. A zone of marked softening of the cartilage may denote a secondary lesion adjacent to the main fragment. If the articular cartilage is firm and unyielding the underlying bone may be presumed to be healthy.

Removal of fragment. Attention is now directed to removing the necrotic fragment. Usually it may be easily levered up from its bed by a blunt dissector, and any remaining hinge of articular cartilage is severed with a knife. The bed of the cavity is usually smooth and does not require further attention. The edges however may be ragged, and fringes of the circumferential articular cartilage may have lost their attachment to the underlying bone. With a fine knife these edges should be trimmed and slightly bevelled all round the margin of the lesion, so that the cartilage that remains is healthy, firm and well supported by normal bone. Often the diameter of the cavity that remains is in the region of 1.5 to 2 centimetres.

Closure. The capsule and synovial membrane are closed as a single layer with interrupted absorbable sutures and the skin edges are closed with everting mattress sutures.

POST-OPERATIVE MANAGEMENT

In this operation, as in meniscectomy, it is convenient to apply the dressing and crepe bandage before the tourniquet is removed. A plaster-of-Paris knee cylinder from groin to malleoli is worn over the crepe bandage and protective cotton for ten days, short walks within the ward being permitted. Active knee flexion and extension exercises and quadriceps development exercises are practised vigorously under the supervision of a physiotherapist.

Comment

It may seem unsatisfactory to leave a raw cavity in the femoral condyle, but in practice the results are usually satisfactory, provided that the cavity is not too large and that it does not extend to the part of the condyle that bears weight when the knee is in the straight position. Nearly always, the defect is on the postero-lateral aspect of the condyle rather than on its inferior weight-bearing aspect. Sufficient intact cartilage remains around the lesion to allow smooth action of the knee. To some extent the cavity fills with fibro-cartilaginous tissue, though the contour remains flattened.

RE-ATTACHMENT OF LOOSE FRAGMENT

For an account of the alternative operation of reattaching the loose fragment in its bed with pins the reader is referred to the description by Smillie (1957, 1960, 1980).

EXCISION OF PATELLA

The patella may be excised for fracture or for non-traumatic conditions such as degenerative arthritis. There are slight differences in the technique of excision of the patella in these two categories. Excision for non-traumatic conditions will be described first, and therafter the manner in which the technique should be varied in cases of fracture will be mentioned.

EXCISION OF PATELLA FOR NON-TRAUMATIC LESIONS

TECHNIQUE

Position of patient. The patient lies supine. A high thigh tourniquet is used, but it is recommended that the tourniquet be released before the sutures in the patellar tendon are tied.

Incision. The skin incision is S-shaped (Fig. 479). A transverse cut over the middle of the patella is curved proximally a little beyond the lateral margin of the bone, forming a vertical limb of the incision about 5 or 6 centimetres long. At the medial end of the transverse cut the incision curves distally a centimetre beyond the medial margin of the patella to end just distal to the upper margin of the tibia. The two triangular skin flaps thus outlined are retracted to reveal the anterior surface of the patella, with the adjacent parts of the quadriceps tendon above and the patellar tendon below.

Shelling out the patella. In order to preserve the continuity of the vertical fibres of the quadriceps expansion where it overlies the patella the aponeurosis is incised longitudinally down the midline of the patella, the cut extending a little way into the quadriceps tendon above and into the

patellar tendon below. Medial and lateral flaps of aponeurosis are reflected from the bone by sharp dissection. It is important to keep the knife close to the bone throughout, because the aponeurosis is thin and as much as possible of it must be preserved.

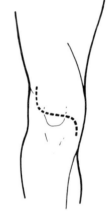

FIG. 479. Excision of patella. The skin incision.

At the sides of the patella the aponeurosis becomes thicker as it blends with the lateral expansions of the quadriceps tendon. Here again the bone must be hugged closely as the knife turns posteriorly over the lateral and the medial edges. Once this stage is reached the synovial lining is opened and the joint is entered. The upper and lower poles of the patella are treated in similar manner, the aponeurosis being peeled back by sharp dissection close to the bone until the joint is entered. The patella is now free and is discarded. Deep to it is a fatty synovial membrane partly occluding the joint proper.

Reconstruction of quadriceps tendon. In non-traumatic lesions of the patella the lateral expansions of the quadriceps tendon remain intact. Even though the patella has been shelled out there is some continuity of the quadriceps mechanism.

Nevertheless it is important to draw together the raw surfaces left by excision of the patella. The flaps of aponeurosis should be bunched together in the position of the knee cap by mattress sutures of strong absorbable material. Before the sutures are tied it is important to release the tourniquet

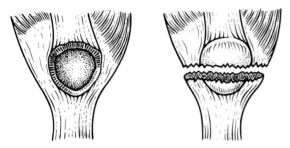

FIGS 480–481. When the patella is excised for a non-traumatic lesion it is simply shelled out from its aponeurotic capsule: the tendinous expansion on either side and the aponeurosis over the front of the bone are intact (Fig. 480). In contrast, in a case of fracture with separation of the fragments, the lateral and medial expansions of the quadriceps tendon are ruptured (Fig. 481); so repair is more difficult.

lest part of the quadriceps muscle be drawn up above it, preventing a tight repair. After these main sutures have been tied further sutures are used to approximate the flaps of quadriceps aponeurosis. The skin wound is then closed without drainage.

POST-OPERATIVE MANAGEMENT

At the conclusion of the operation wide (15 centimetre) crepe bandages are applied firmly over copious gauze dressings. A plaster-of-Paris cylinder from groin to malleoli is applied over cellulose wool with the knee straight.

After excision of the patella active quadriceps contractions are inhibited reflexly, and since excessive muscle action could tear open the suture line it is recommended that instruction in quadriceps contractions be deferred until one week after operation. Static quadriceps exercises are then begun, and continued throughout the second week. In the third week straight leg lifting exercises are practised.

At the conclusion of the third week the plaster is removed and static exercises and straight leg lifting are continued. Provided there is good power of

straight leg lifting at this stage the patient may be allowed to walk with sticks or elbow crutches, taking weight upon the limb. In this fourth week flexion exercises are begun.

One of the problems may be to restore a full range of flexion. It is equally important, however, to ensure that full extension is achieved and that the leg can be lifted straight without any lag (that is, dropping of the lower leg with slight knee flexion when the limb is elevated). Thus whereas flexion exercises must be encouraged, extension exercises with vigorous quadriceps contractions must not be neglected. The use of a continuous passive motion machine may be helpful at this stage. Usually flexion is restored gradually over eight or ten weeks from the time of operation. If at six or eight weeks there is still marked restriction of flexion the formation of flimsy fibrous adhesions within the joint must be suspected. Sometimes it may be appropriate to divide the adhesions arthroscopically. Alternatively, gentle

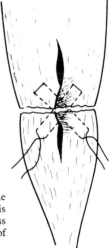

FIG. 482. Suturing the ruptured aponeurosis by diagonal mattress sutures after excision of patella.

manipulation under anaesthesia will often tear the adhesions and lead to dramatic improvement. Needless to say, excessive force should not be used; otherwise the newly joined quadriceps mechanism may be ruptured.

Comment

Although excision of the patella is not a difficult operation unsatisfactory results are often seen.

The most common deficiency is lack of ability to keep the knee fully straight when the leg is lifted from the couch—the so-called extension lag. This may result from inadequate suture of the raw surfaces of tendon, and possibly a contributory factor in this is failure to release the tourniquet before the sutures are tied: part of the quadriceps muscle may be locked above the tourniquet and thus the quadriceps tendon cannot be drawn down fully until the tourniquet is released.

Another reason for failure of adequate redevelopment of quadriceps power may be a lack of proper supervision after operation. The quadriceps muscle wastes very rapidly after knee injuries and operations, and unless vigorous exercises are continued for a long period recovery may be incomplete.

Failure to regain a full range of flexion may be an additional problem, though not a common one: steady increase in the range is nearly always achieved with progressive exercise. Occasionally it is found that the range of movement, having reached a certain stage, remains stationary and is not improving. This may denote the formation of intra-articular adhesions, and the advisability of arthroscopic division of adhesions or of judicious manipulation under anaesthesia may then have to be considered. The best time at which to undertake manipulation, should it become necessary, is probably about two months after the operation.

Excision of Patella for Fracture

Excision of the patella is undertaken commonly for fracture—usually a comminuted fracture with irreparable damage to the articular surface. The technique is essentially the same as that for non-traumatic lesions but there is an important difference: namely that the lateral and medial expansions of the quadriceps tendon, which are not disturbed when the patella is removed for non-traumatic lesions, are ruptured. There is thus total loss of continuity of the quadriceps mechanism (Figs 480 and 481).

Procedure. After the fragments of patella have been removed by sharp dissection close to the bone, in the manner described above, careful reconstruction of the quadriceps tendon and adjacent aponeurosis by strong mattress sutures is required. It may be best to insert the main sutures diagonally in order to bunch up the flaps in the front (Fig. 482), and to reinforce the anterior repair with two or three further mattress sutures in each lateral expansion of the aponeurosis.

POST-OPERATIVE MANAGEMENT

This is the same as after excision of the patella for non-traumatic lesions.

Comment

The comments in the previous section apply equally here.

If a patellar fracture is such that excision is demanded, all the fragments should be removed: there is no place for partial excision. Operations that aim to leave the main fragment and to unite the tendon to it—though seemingly attractive—have nearly always given disappointing results.

REPAIR OF QUADRICEPS TENDON AVULSED FROM PATELLA

The quadriceps tendon is avulsed from the upper pole of the patella only when it is degenerate, and the injury is thus seen almost exclusively in elderly people.

Because the tissues to be repaired are of rather poor quality, it is important that the reconstruction be meticulous and that intimate contact between the tendon and the margin of the patella be assured. The most reliable method is to prepare a series of drill holes through the patella near its margin, and to secure the quadriceps tendon to the bone by strong mattress sutures.

TECHNIQUE

Position of patient. The patient lies supine. If a tourniquet is used it should be applied high on the thigh, and the surgeon should be prepared to release the tourniquet to give full freedom to the quadriceps muscle before the main sutures are tied.

Incision. A transverse incision over the upper margin of the patella is curved proximally at the lateral side to extend 5 centimetres into the thigh, and distally at its medial extremity to run 5 centimetres or so near the medial margin of the patella (Fig. 483). The incision is deepened through the

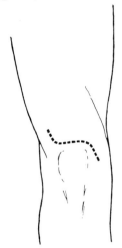

FIG. 483. Repair of quadriceps tendon avulsed from patella. The skin incision.

deep fascia, and the supero-lateral and infero-medial flaps are retracted by stay sutures to expose the site of the injury, which is marked by bruising, oedema and maceration of the tissues and the presence of some clotted blood.

Preparation of margins of rent and drilling of holes in patella. When blood clot has been cleared away the elliptical rent in the quadriceps expansion will be obvious. The avulsed tendon is freshened by excision of shredded tissue to give a clean-cut edge. Likewise, the upper margin of the patella is cleaned up by removal of tags or shreds of tendon, which are cut away close to the bone. A series of holes ranged round the upper crescentic margin of the patella is next prepared (Fig. 484). Usually five or six holes should be drilled. Each hole should be oblique from below upwards and backwards: beginning on the anterior surface of the patella about 8 millimetres below the superior margin, it is so directed as to emerge on the

postero-superior corner of the upper border, just clear of the articular surface (Fig. 485). It is important that the holes be not too close to the

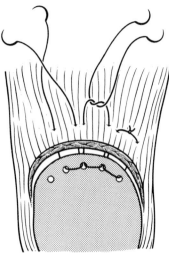

FIG. 484. Diagram showing the method of repair, by mattress sutures passed through holes drilled near the margin of the patella.

margin of the patella lest the sutures cut through the bone—in other words there must be a good solid bridge of bone between the entrance and exit holes of the drill. If five holes are drilled they will be approximately 8 millimetres apart.

At this stage attention should be directed to the medial and lateral slips of the quadriceps expan-

FIG. 485. Each drill hole should emerge from the postero-superior margin of the patella just clear of the articular surface, as shown in this sagittal section.

sion on either side of the patella. These may be found intact, but if they are partly or widely ruptured the edges should be cleaned ready for suture.

Insertion of mattress sutures. The authors use stainless steel wire (gauge 30) for the repair, but sutures of strong catgut or of man-made material may be used if preferred. The sutures are inserted mattress-fashion as shown in Figure 484. In this way, each drill hole in the bone except the end ones transmits two sutures, and firm approximation of the tendon to the bone is assured when the knots are tied. Before the sutures are tied, however, it is important that the tourniquet be released in order to relax the quadriceps muscle: if some of the muscle were to remain bunched-up above the tourniquet there could be difficulty in drawing the tendon down fully into contact with the bone.

When the main sutures have been tied, additional sutures, through soft tissue only, may be inserted to strengthen the medial and lateral expansions of the quadriceps apparatus.

Closure. The skin edges are closed in the usual way without drainage.

POST-OPERATIVE MANAGEMENT

First a dressing of dry gauze and crepe bandage is applied, and over this a plaster-of-Paris case is constructed to extend from the upper thigh to the malleoli, with the knee flexed about 5 degrees. The patient may sit out of bed with the limb supported on a couch or stool, but since these patients are nearly always elderly and perhaps unsteady it is better to defer walking for two or three weeks.

At first the quadriceps muscle is reflexly inhibited and the patient will find it difficult to initiate quadriceps contractions; but after a week or ten days the power to contract the muscle actively should be regained, and by the end of

three weeks it should be possible for the patient to begin lifting the leg from the bed. At that stage walking may be resumed with full weight upon the injured limb, elbow crutches being used to provide stability.

The plaster should be retained for six weeks, after which cautious knee flexion exercises are begun. Even at this stage, however, the emphasis should be on restoring full active extension and good quadriceps power rather than on hurrying to regain flexion.

Comment

Although this is a seemingly straightforward operation, and would indeed be so if the quadriceps were of normal quality, it may nevertheless present difficulties because the avulsed tendon is often thin and a little friable, and moreover the bone of the patella may be rather spongy. In order to get a firm approximation of tendon to bone, it may therefore be necessary to take rather large "bites" of tissue in the sutures in order to avoid cutting through. It is important that the coaptation between tendon and bone be very close: preferably the tendon should be "bunched-up" against the bone edge.

Because of the degenerate nature of the tendon, often associated with some flabbiness of the muscles, rehabilitation under supervision may have to be continued for many months before good function is restored, and it may be wise for the patient to use a walking stick (cane) thereafter for an indefinite period.

QUADRICEPSPLASTY

This operation—not very aptly titled—is designed to release tethering of the quadriceps muscle or knee joint capsule, wheresoever it may have occurred, and thereby to increase the range of knee movement when this has been badly impaired, usually after fracture of the femoral shaft.

TECHNIQUE

Position of patient. The patient lies supine, with a rolled towel or sand-bag behind the knee to give

slight flexion. A tourniquet may be used on the highest part of the thigh.

Exposure. The quadriceps muscle is exposed from the front by a mid-line vertical or serpentine incision extending from the mid-point of the thigh to a point 4 centimetres below the distal pole of the patella (Fig. 486). Skin edges and deep fascia are retracted laterally and medially to expose the main tendon of the quadriceps below, with the bulky vastus lateralis and vastus medialis blending with the tendon in the lower third of the thigh. Above this the rectus femoris is displayed.

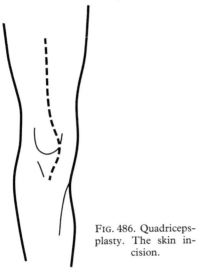

FIG. 486. Quadriceps-plasty. The skin incision.

Investigation of pathology and release of tight structures. The first essential is to find out in which part of the quadriceps mechanism knee movement is being impeded. This may be: 1) the joint itself, which may be partly obliterated by intracapsular adhesions (these may already have been seen through the arthroscope); 2) the vastus intermedius, which may be scarred and adherent both to the underlying femur and to the overlying rectus femoris tendon; 3) the expansion of the vastus medialis or of the vastus lateralis, which may be adherent to the corresponding femoral condyle; or 4) the rectus femoris, which may be scarred and adherent high up in the thigh, with consequent restriction of the normal excursion of the tendon.

To find out which of these pathological features is responsible for the stiffness the joint is first opened by an incision through the lateral quadriceps expansion and capsule just lateral to the patella. With the knee straight, the patella is then lifted forwards with a hook to allow full inspection of the interior of the joint. Any visible fibrous adhesions are excised. The knee is then flexed to its limit, when any tight bands of the quadriceps expansion in the region of the femoral condyles may be noted and divided. For this purpose it may be necessary to open the joint antero-medially as well as antero-laterally.

If the division of tight structures in or about the knee leads to an adequate gain of knee flexion, nothing further is required. If on the other hand the pathology does not seem to be related to the knee joint itself, the exploration must be extended upwards and is next directed to the vastus intermedius. To explore this, the vastus lateralis is detached from the quadriceps tendon along the line where they unite. Through this opening the quadriceps tendon is lifted forwards so that any adherence of its under surface to the vastus intermedius and through that to the femur itself may be revealed. If these structures are found matted together the rectus tendon must be freed from the underlying vastus intermedius by sharp dissection. If the vastus intermedius is extensively scarred it may be advisable to excise it, but care must be taken in doing this not to damage the main tendon of the quadriceps. Again knee flexion should be repeatedly tested during the procedure, so that those parts where the mechanism seems to be tethered may be dealt with in turn.

If no cause for the stiffness is demonstrated in or about the knee, nor between the quadriceps tendon and the femur, it is likely that there is contracture of the rectus femoris muscle high up in the thigh. This will be suggested by extreme tightness of the quadriceps tendon, best demonstrated by placing a freshly gloved finger deep to the tendon as the knee is flexed to its limit. Provided the patient has good vastus muscles, it is then permissible to make shallow releasing incisions into the deep surface of the tight rectus tendon at or above the middle of the thigh, the knife being inserted between the lateral margin of the quadriceps tendon and the vastus lateralis and directed forwards. Each incision will allow a gain of a few degrees of knee flexion. As a rule, no further incision should be made when 30 degrees of added flexion have been gained.

Closure. The vastus lateralis is united to the quadriceps tendon with closely spaced interrupted sutures. All incisions about the knee are closed and the skin is sutured without drainage.

POST-OPERATIVE MANAGEMENT
A combination of rest with intervals of passive

exercises is recommended. At the conclusion of the operation crepe bandages are applied over copious gauze dressings, and the knee is immobilised in a position of 60 degrees of flexion or, if a range as great as 60 degrees has not been achieved, in maximal flexion. The plaster is bivalved by cutting down each side, and the halves are bandaged together. The limb, thus encased, is elevated on pillows or on an appropriate well padded frame.

On the third day the limb is removed from the knee as to improving flexion. Once good extension has been restored, then intensive efforts may be made gradually to increase the range of flexion. Vigorous physiotherapy should be continued for several months to ensure the greatest benefit from the operation.

Comment

Quadricepsplasty should never be undertaken lightly and never before intensive treatment by

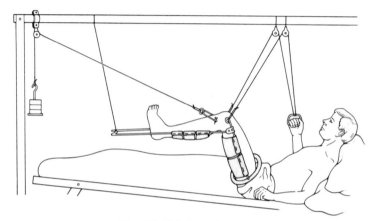

FIG. 487. Fisk dynamic traction.

plaster case and Fisk dynamic splinting is set up (Fisk 1944), with provision for the patient to flex his knee by pulling upon cords attached to the end of the splint and brought over pulleys conveniently placed for the patient's grasp (Fig. 487). Passive exercises are then continued daily under the supervision of a physiotherapist, but for the first ten days the limb should be restored to the bivalved plaster case at night, for greater comfort. At the end of two weeks from operation all splintage may be discarded and the limb allowed to rest free in bed.

Where the necessary apparatus is available, an alternative to the Fisk technique of dynamic splinting is the use of a continuous passive motion (CPM) machine.

In the early days attention should be directed just as much to restoring active extension of the exercises has been tried for many months, and preferably for as long as a year. It is not an operation that can be approached with full confidence, for the results are unpredictable. Moreover it is easy to do more harm than good by injudicious attempts to free the knee. The most important point is that the surgeon should not be over-ambitious. It is best to warn the patient in advance that only a limited improvement can be expected and to be content with a moderate gain in flexion—for instance something in the order of 30 or 40 degrees. If too much is attempted the patient's ability to extend the knee strongly against gravity may be seriously impaired. Contrary to what has been stated (Nicoll 1963) impairment of active extension is a serious handicap: in the authors' opinion any loss of active extension is too high a price to pay for a gain in flexion.

LATERAL RELEASE FOR HABITUAL DISLOCATION OF PATELLA

In habitual dislocation of the patella, as distinct from recurrent dislocation, the patella slips laterally over the femoral condyle every time the knee is flexed. The condition is present from an early age, if not from birth, and the patients are often brought for treatment in early childhood. The underlying cause is often a pathological fibrous or tendinous band anchoring the lateral part of the quadriceps expansion, and through this the lateral border of the patella, to the ilio-tibial tract (Jeffrey 1963). The operation entails division of the band or of any other abnormal tight structure at the lateral side of the joint.

TECHNIQUE

Position of patient. The patient lies supine, with a rolled towel or sand-bag behind the knee to support it in slight flexion. A tourniquet may be used on the upper thigh.

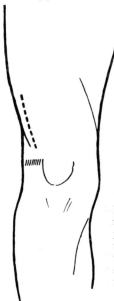

FIG. 488. Lateral release for habitual dislocation of patella. Diagram shows the line of incision through the quadriceps expansion and (shaded) the common site of an abnormal fibrous band.

Incision. The initial exploratory incision extends proximally from a point just lateral to the upper lateral corner of the patella along the lateral margin of the quadriceps tendon (Fig. 488). The incision may be about 10 centimetres long in an adult or proportionately shorter in a child. The incision is deepened through the lateral part of the quadriceps expansion to enter the suprapatellar pouch of the knee. The surgeon must be prepared to extend the incision distally or proximally if the pathological features in a given case demand it.

Locating the pathological band. It is essential to establish the precise cause of the dislocation by palpation of the quadriceps mechanism with a freshly gloved finger during flexion-extension movements of the knee. First the finger is passed distally, deep to the quadriceps expansion at the lateral margin of the patella. The finger is introduced with the knee straight and then an assistant slowly flexes the knee while the tissues are palpated from within. Commonly, as the knee flexes towards the right angle a tight band is felt to compress the finger and at the same time to draw the patella laterally as flexion continues. The band runs almost horizontally towards the ilio-tibial tract at about the level of the middle or upper part of the patella (Fig. 488).

Division of the band. The simplest method of dividing the band is to pass a knife with the palpating finger deep to the lateral part of the quadriceps expansion with the cutting edge directed antero-laterally. The band being then tightened by flexing the knee, it is easily divided from the deep aspect by feel, in the manner of a tenotomy. This method has the disadvantage of dividing the synovial membrane and leaving a raw area within the joint cavity. The alternative method is to extend the skin incision distally so that the band may be divided from without inwards and the synovial membrane left intact.

After division of the band further tests are made by flexing the knee. If the pathological band has been correctly located and released the patella will no longer dislocate even when the knee is fully flexed. If this result is not achieved by the first releasing incision a further search must be made by palpating from within the joint to ascertain where the remaining tight tissues are situated. The release of tight lateral tissues must proceed until the knee can be flexed without dislocation; otherwise the operation is certain to fail.

POST-OPERATIVE MANAGEMENT

A wide crepe bandage is applied snugly over copious gauze dressings and a plaster-of-Paris knee cylinder is applied from groin to malleoli with the knee flexed about 5 degrees. Weight bearing within the confines of the ward may be permitted from the first or second day after operation. After two weeks the plaster is removed and graduated flexion and extension exercises for the knee are practised.

Comment

The success of this operation depends upon finding the causative contracture at the lateral side of the patella. As noted above, the abnormal band is detected most easily by palpation from within the joint, and in the initial stages of the operation it is better to make only a short incision into the suprapatellar pouch, to enable digital palpation to be carried out. If the initial incision extends too far distally the pathological band may be divided with the incision through the aponeurosis, and its true localisation and extent may then be impossible to define. Clearly no procedure must be accepted as adequate that does not allow the knee to be flexed fully without dislocation of the patella.

In the occasional case supplementary operative procedures may be needed to help to provide stability of the patella. Thus if there is severe genu valgum this may be corrected by supracondylar osteotomy of the femur or by upper tibial osteotomy, as appropriate. If the insertion of the patellar tendon into the tibia seems too far lateral, transposition of a block of bone comprising the tibial tubercle and the patellar tendon insertion may be undertaken, as for recurrent dislocation of the patella (see below). This operation must however be confined to adolescents or adults: in children interference with the growth epiphysis may lead to genu recurvatum.

Reefing of the medial part of the quadriceps expansion is sometimes recommended in an attempt to hold the patella in its groove. However, if adequate release is carried out at the lateral side of the joint medial reefing is unnecessary; and conversely, if the lateral band is not adequately divided reefing the medial part of the aponeurosis will not lead to lasting stability of the patella.

TRANSPOSITION OF QUADRICEPS INSERTION FOR RECURRENT DISLOCATION OF PATELLA

Downward and medial transposition of the tibial tubercle together with the insertion of the patellar tendon is the standard operation for recurrent dislocation of the patella after the age at which the upper tibial epiphysis is closed. In this connection the distinction between recurrent dislocation of the patella and habitual dislocation must be emphasised. Recurrent dislocation, in which dislocations occur only sporadically, and usually in adolescents, is characterised by an unusually high and often hypoplastic patella whereas habitual dislocation, which becomes evident at a much earlier age, is characterised by shortening or tethering of the vastus lateralis or of the lateral quadriceps expansion. The treatment required is correspondingly different in the two types of case.

Transposition of the tibial tubercle for recurrent dislocation was described by Hauser (1938) but the operation has been variously modified. The aim is to bring the patella distally so that when the knee is straight its lower pole is about level with the upper articular surface of the tibia. This usually means drawing the insertion down about 1.5 to 2.5 centimetres. At the same time the point of insertion is moved medially in order to redirect the pull of the quadriceps towards the medial side.

TECHNIQUE

Position of patient. The patient lies supine. A tourniquet may be used on the upper thigh.

Incision. The incision is S-shaped. It begins over the tibial tubercle about a centimetre distal to the upper border of the tibia. Extending downwards for 3 centimetres, it then curves medially in an almost horizontal direction before curving downwards again midway between the anterior crest of the tibia and its postero-medial border (Fig. 489). This lower vertical limb of the incision is about 3 centimetres long.

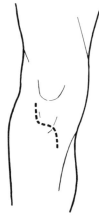

FIG. 489. Transposition of tibial tubercle for recurrent dislocation of patella. The skin incision.

Isolation of bone fragment to be transplanted. When the skin flaps have been turned back the periosteum is incised and reflected to expose raw cortical bone in the vicinity of the tibial tubercle. Fascia is incised at each side of the patellar tendon so that its edges may be clearly defined. Areolar tissue is also cleared deep to the tendon, starting proximally near the upper margin of the tibia and working down to the point where the tendon blends with the tibial tubercle. In this dissection care must be taken not to divide any of the tendon fibres.

With the tibial tubercle and the tendon insertion thus defined, a diamond-shaped block of bone is marked out as an island, usually about 18 millimetres long by 12 millimetres wide (Fig. 490). This island of bone is then cut from the surrounding bone with a high-speed dental burr or with a small circular saw aided by osteotomes. Clean separation of the fragment from the main bone is essential. When the fragment has been thus isolated it is left in its bed for the time being.

Preparation of new bed to receive transplant. The outline of the new bed for the patellar tendon insertion is marked on the antero-medial surface of the tibia after reflection of the periosteum. The bed should be midway between the anterior crest

of the tibia and its postero-medial margin, and it should be so positioned as to bring the transplanted fragment of bone 1.5 to 2.5 centimetres distally according to pre-determined measurements. A diamond-shaped panel is outlined on the bone, of exactly the same dimensions as those of the island of bone to be transplanted (Fig. 490). This diamond-shaped piece of cortical bone is then cut out with a combination of dental burr, osteotome and chisel. The opening should extend right through the cortex, which is relatively thin at this point, into the subcortical spongy bone, and a recess is excavated under the proximal apex of the cortex with a curved dissector, to receive the apex of the fragment of bone now to be transplanted into it.

Transposition and locking of bone island. The separated bone island, comprising tibial tubercle and patellar tendon insertion, is lifted from its bed and held lightly in a towel clip. Care must be taken not to macerate and weaken the tendon. Thus held, the bone fragment is lifted forwards and stretched medially and distally. With scissors any restraining tissue at the lateral and medial margins of the tendon and deep to it is divided as far proximally as the level of the knee joint. The tendon is thus mobilised, and with the aid of downward pressure upon the patella the bone island is easily drawn distally and placed in its new

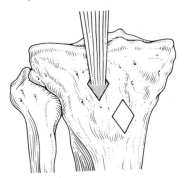

FIG. 490. The diamond-shaped island of bone to be transposed is outlined. The recipient area is also shown.

bed. It is pushed through the recipient diamond-shaped opening into the soft subcortical cancellous bone and then it is pushed upwards deep to the tibial cortex so that it locks under the overhanging edge of the ∧-shaped opening (Figs 491 and 492). As the transplanted bone fragment slides proximally deep to the cortex the tendon slips to the apex of the ∧ and cannot escape.

walking. In the first two weeks walking should be restricted to short journeys within the ward or home, but thereafter, when the wound is healed and a new closely fitting plaster has been applied, unrestricted walking is permitted. During this

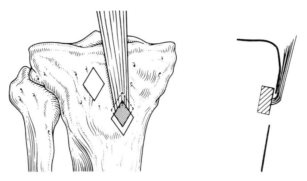

FIGS 491–492. Transposition of quadriceps insertion. Figure 491—The transposed island of bone has been transplanted downwards and medially, and is locked under the ∧-shaped cut edge of the tibial cortex. Figure 492—Detail of technique shown in sagittal section.

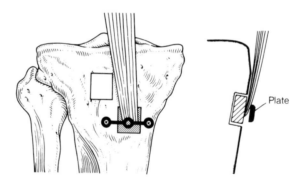

FIGS 493–494. Figure 493—Alternative technique of attaching the transferred island of bone, with the patellar tendon, to its new bed in the tibia. The island of bone is retained in its new bed by a short overlying plate. Figure 494—Method of fixation shown in sagittal section.

Closure. The diamond-shaped cortical fragment from the recipient area is placed in the matching cavity of the donor area. Periosteum is repaired and the skin is closed without drainage.

POST-OPERATIVE MANAGEMENT

Despite satisfactory locking of the transposed fragment of bone, it is advisable to protect the knee in a plaster cylinder from groin to malleoli for six weeks. Splintage in plaster reduces post-operative pain and gives greater confidence for

time intensive static quadriceps exercises and leg lifting exercises must be practised.

After removal of the plaster at the end of six weeks from operation rehabilitation is intensified under the care of a physiotherapist, with special emphasis on quadriceps development and restoration of knee flexion.

Comment

This technique demands delicate precision if a reliable hold on the bone is to be ensured. Pulling away of the transferred tendinous insertion is a complication that must be avoided at all costs, for it necessitates further operation which may be difficult if the tendon has torn away from the bone or if the recipient cortex at the site of the new insertion has given way. Great care must therefore be taken to match the island of bone that is to be transferred accurately to the recipient opening in the tibial cortex, and to ensure that the transferred fragment is pushed deeply enough into the opening to allow it to ride up beneath the cortex (as shown in Figure 492), thus becoming securely locked.

The distance that the transplanted island of bone is to be moved should be determined before the operation from clinical measurements of the position of the patella and from the radiographs.

A much more extensive incision than that described is often advocated, sometimes with release of the lateral part of the quadriceps expansion and reefing of the medial side. In the authors' experi-ence such extensions of the fundamental operation of re-aligning the patellar tendon are usually un-necessary.

ALTERNATIVE TECHNIQUE

If the technique as described above proves diffi-cult and the transposed fragment fails to lock properly in its new bed—usually from imprecise fashioning of the island of bone and of the recipi-ent bed—it is a simple matter to stabilise it by spanning it with an overlying three-hole plate, screwed to the tibia on either side of the re-embedded bone fragment (Figs 493 and 494).

The plate, which may be suitably bent to fit the contour of the tibia, is effective in retaining the fragment rigidly in position, so that early quadri-ceps contractions and leg exercises may safely be encouraged at an early stage.

PROXIMAL TRANSFER OF HAMSTRING TENDONS FOR SPASTIC FLEXION OF KNEE
(EGGERS'S OPERATION)

Transfer of the hamstring tendons from the upper end of the tibia to the lower end of the femur, as described by Eggers (1952), has a double object-ive. Most importantly, the flexing action of the contracted or spastic muscles upon the knee is removed, with the consequence that the flexion deformity is gradually corrected. Secondly, re-attachment of the transferred muscle to the back of the lower femur to some extent reinforces extension power at the hip.

TECHNIQUE

Position of patient. The patient lies prone. A tourniquet may be used on the upper thigh: it should be applied with the patient supine just before he is turned to the prone position.

Incisions. Two incisions are used, one over the lower end of the medial hamstring muscles and the other correspondingly placed over the lateral hamstrings (Fig. 495). The medial incision, 10 centimetres long, follows the medial border of the tendon of the semitendinosus. Three-quarters of the incision are proximal to the line of the knee joint and one quarter is distal. The lateral incision, of similar length, follows the line of the biceps tendon as far as its insertion into the head of the fibula.

If preferred, an S-shaped incision (Fig. 495) may be used.

Exposure of hamstring tendons. The dissection is first carried out on the medial side. Blunt dissec-tion with scissors is used to expose the tendons of gracilis, semitendinosus and semimembranosus close to their insertions into the head of the tibia. Two of the tendons, those of gracilis and semi-membranosus, are detached from their insertions and freed proximally into the lower part of the thigh. Unless the contracture is very tight it is usually wise to leave one of the muscles—preferably the semitendinosus—attached to the tibia so that the power of knee flexion is not too drastically reduced. The tendon may however be lengthened

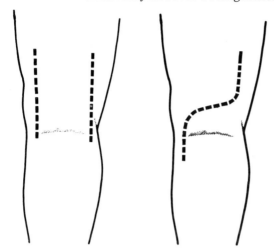

FIG. 495. Proximal transfer of hamstring tendons. Alternative skin incisions.

appropriately by splitting it longitudinally in Z-fashion and suturing the ends side to side after sufficient lengthening has been allowed.

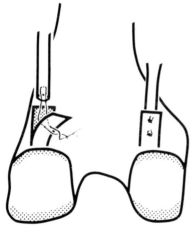

FIG. 496. Technique of securing the tendons beneath flaps of periosteum. On the left the tendon of biceps is shown being sutured deep to a raised flap of periosteum. On the right, reattachment of the tendon of semimembranosus has been completed.

In the lateral incision the first step is to identify the common peroneal nerve where it lies deep to the lower end of the biceps tendon. The nerve is

freed for an appropriate distance in a proximal direction and held out of harm's way while the tendon of the biceps is severed close to its insertion. The tendon is then mobilised proximally into the lower thigh.

Attachment of tendons to back of femur. In the proximal part of the medial wound the postero-medial aspect of the lower part of the femoral shaft is exposed immediately proximal to the medial condyle. A small flap of periosteum is raised with its base distally, and the underlying cortex of the femur is scarified with a small chisel (Fig. 496). The tendons to be transferred are trimmed appropriately and laid upon the rawed surface of the bone. The periosteal flap is folded back to cover the tendons and sutured to them (Fig. 496), with care to ensure that the muscles are drawn reasonably taut. The attachment of the tendons to their new bed may be reinforced by additional sutures through adjacent soft tissues.

In the lateral wound the tendon of the biceps is attached to the postero-lateral aspect of the lower femur in like manner.

Closure. The fascial layers and the skin are closed with interrupted sutures, usually without drainage.

POST-OPERATIVE MANAGEMENT

The limb is encased in a full-length plaster splint in a position about midway between the original angle of fixed flexion and the fully extended position. A useful guide to the best position for splintage is to straighten the knee as far as it will go under moderate pressure and then to relax the posterior tissues by flexing the knee 5 or 10 degrees from this position. When the plaster has set it should be split throughout its full length along each side, the two halves being then held together with soft bandages. The state of the circulation and of nerve function must be watched with the greatest care: any sign of impairment of function, suggesting excessive stretching, necessitates immediate removal of the plaster and renewed splintage in a more flexed position.

After the first week, further plaster splints from

upper thigh to ankle should be applied with the knee in progressively greater extension.

After the first two weeks the patient is encouraged to walk with elbow crutches, taking full weight upon the limb. Plaster splintage may be discarded at the end of four weeks, and thereafter intensive exercises are practised under the supervision of a physiotherapist in order to build up the power of extension of the hip and knee.

Comment

Eggers's operation often gives strikingly good results, especially in patients with spastic paresis. Once the spastic or contracted hamstring muscles are detached from the upper end of the tibia, or elongated, the main deforming force is eliminated and marked improvement in the flexion deformity is immediately apparent.

It is wise to accept moderate correction of the deformity at the time of operation and to gain further correction gradually during the course of the next few weeks. Attempts to gain complete extension at the time of operation entail a serious risk of damage to the main nerve trunks or of impairment of circulation by traction upon the main vessels: thus it is rash to attempt to force the knee straight and to immobilise it in the straight position at the conclusion of the operation. Loss of nerve or vessel function may be immediate, and by the time the surgeon realises what has happened irreparable damage may have occurred. Correction by serial plasters is far safer and the final result is in no way prejudiced.

The contribution that re-implantation of the transferred muscles into the femur makes to the improvement in function is problematical. It seems clear that release of the deforming force upon the knee is the most important feature of the operation and that reinforcement of the power of hip extension is a relatively lightweight bonus.

A long course of physiotherapy is usually advisable after removal of the plaster. Worth-while improvement may continue for as long as a year after the muscle release, but continuing improvement depends upon intensive exercises to redevelop the quadriceps and gluteal muscles.

REPLACEMENT ARTHROPLASTY OF KNEE

Replacement arthroplasty of the knee has not yet become standardised: it is still in a state of development. At present it is unreliable as compared with arthroplasty of the hip, and accordingly it is undertaken only in cases of severe disability, and seldom in the young. Nevertheless improvements in design and in operative technique have led to increasing rates of success, and it is clear that in the future the indications for total knee arthroplasty will be widened.

The earliest methods employed the principle of the hinge, the stems of which were driven into the medullary canal of femur and tibia (Shiers 1954, Walldius 1960). Such devices are still in use (Lettin *et al.* 1978). A different approach was that of MacIntosh (1958, 1967), who replaced one or both of the tibial condyles by blocks of metal (originally of acrylic compound) let into the upper surface of the tibia, and so shaped as to match the normal tibial condyles. The cartilage of the femoral condyles thus articulates directly with the metal insert. The method has the disadvantage that the metal inserts tend to loosen and to become displaced in the course of time.

Recently, the trend has been towards the use of the two-component total condylar prosthesis, in which the convex femoral condyles and the slightly concave tibial condyles are reproduced in metal and in high density polyethylene respectively. The modern prosthesis of this type has virtually no intramedullary stems but is located in position by short lugs that engage with holes prepared in the recipient bone. In most cases fixation is supplemented by acrylic cement; but some prostheses are designed for use without cement, and they may be manufactured with porous coating on the embedded surfaces, into which it is hoped that new bone may penetrate, thus ensuring permanent firm fixation.

With a formidable array of different prostheses now available, and with trends constantly changing, it is clearly impracticable to provide a description pertaining to the fitting of every type of prosthesis. Nevertheless the basic steps in the insertion of representative prostheses of a particular group are very similar in each case, differences being only of detail. With most of the systems that are available today the manufacturers also supply appropriate instruments, including jigs, to facilitate the insertion of their particular prosthesis. It is necessary in this section, therefore, to describe only the basic steps in the fitting of a total knee prosthesis. The description that follows will relate mainly to the total condylar prosthesis—now the type most commonly used. A brief description will also be given of the Charing Cross prosthesis and of the hinged prosthesis.

THE IMPORTANCE OF CORRECT ALIGNMENT

In arthritis of the knee, whether it be rheumatoid or degenerative, the alignment of the tibia relative to the femur is often disturbed. The deformity may be one of varus or of valgus, and an important requirement in any operation for total replacement of the knee is that the alignment of the bones must be restored to normal.

It is important to understand, in this connection, that normal alignment at the knee does not mean that the shaft of the femur and the shaft of the tibia are on the same straight line. There is a natural angle of valgus of the tibia in relation to the femur, because of the fact that the femoral shaft is set outwards at its upper end by the femoral neck. The basic necessity is that the line of weight bearing should pass through the centre of the hip joint, the centre of the knee joint, and the centre of the ankle joint (Fig. 497). This natural angle of valgus at the knee, due to the outward slope of the femoral shaft, is approximately 6 or 7 degrees.

In addition, it should be appreciated that when a person stands, the feet are normally closer together than the hips. In other words the line of weight bearing slopes inwards. The angle that this line makes with the vertical is about 3 degrees; it may be slightly greater in women. Thus the tibia is not quite vertical, and in theory the tibial component of a knee prosthesis should not be set exactly at right angles to the long axis of the bone, but at an angle of 3 degrees to that plane.

The inward slope due to stance should also be taken into account in fitting the femoral component if, as is desired, the line joining the two femoral condyles is to be parallel with the ground.

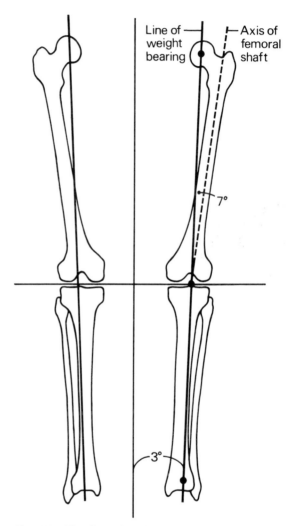

FIG. 497. The line of weight bearing should pass through the centre of the hip joint, the centre of the knee joint, and the centre of the ankle joint. In a standing person this line is not quite vertical, because the ankles are closer together than the hips: the deviation from the vertical is about 3 degrees. The long axis of the femoral shaft forms an angle of about 7 degrees with the line of weight bearing.

In the study of alignment at the knee which should always precede knee arthroplasty there is a need for long radiographic films, to enable the hip and the whole length of the femoral shaft to be included on a single film with the tibial shaft and the ankle. If the radiograph before operation shows that the centre of the hip, knee and ankle are not in a straight line—the true line of weight bearing—it is necessary at operation to ensure, by correctly trimming the bones, that this correct alignment is restored.

TOTAL CONDYLAR REPLACEMENT

The usual prosthesis consists of a femoral condylar component made in metal, and a tibial component of high density polyethylene (Fig. 498). A patellar component may or may not be used.

The femoral component may have twin condyles that match more or less closely the natural condyles; or the condyles may be merged into a single drum-shaped articular surface. The under

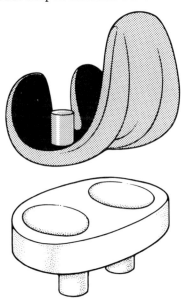

FIG. 498. A typical condylar prosthesis. Lugs to aid positive location of the implant are shown. Acrylic cement is usually used to enhance fixation, but some models are designed for use without cement.

surface of the metal is hollowed out to fit over the re-shaped natural femoral condyles. To aid positive location, they are fitted with short lugs that engage in matching holes drilled in the femur, usually one in each condyle.

The tibial component is usually flat on its under surface, to lie horizontally upon the trimmed upper surface of the tibia. Its upper surface is hollowed out into twin articulating surfaces in which the femoral condyles glide; or in some cases the twin bearing surfaces may be merged into a single concavity.

In the use of some condylar prostheses it is intended that the collateral ligaments and perhaps also the posterior cruciate ligament be preserved; but in other systems the ligaments are discarded.

Jigs provided for a particular prosthesis are designed to ensure that the femur and the tibia are trimmed precisely as required, and that the drill holes to receive the lugs of the prosthetic components are correctly placed. Thus the main areas in which judgement and skill are required are in making sure that alignment is correct, and in adjusting tension to the optimum: the joint must be neither too loose, nor so tight that full extension is prevented.

BASIC TECHNIQUE

Position of patient. The patient lies supine. A tourniquet may be used on the highest part of the thigh.

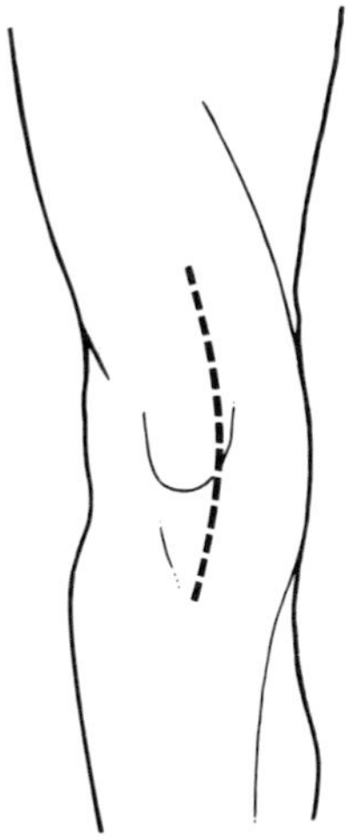

FIG. 499. Total condylar replacement of the knee. The skin incision.

Incision. An almost vertical incision is generally used. It may be curved slightly medially to skirt the medial border of the patella (Fig. 499); but too wide a sweep, creating a flap based laterally, is to be discouraged because the viability of the edge of the flap may be prejudiced.

The deep exposure. The skin edges are retracted to expose the patella, quadriceps expansion, capsule, and patellar tendon down as far as the tibial the patella and quadriceps mechanism displaced across the lateral femoral condyle to lie out of the way at the lateral aspect of the joint.

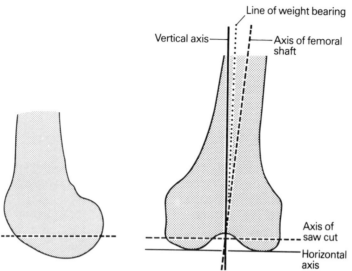

FIGS 500–501. Figure 500—The transverse femoral saw cut, as seen from the side. Figure 501—As seen from the front, the femoral saw-cut is transverse (that is, parallel to the ground) but not at right angles to the femoral shaft, which slopes downwards and inwards at an angle of about 7 degrees to the line of weight bearing, and slightly more than this to the vertical axis. (For explanation see text.)

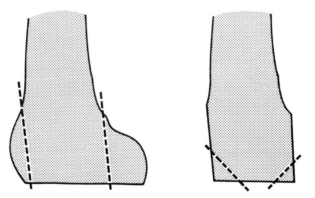

FIGS 502–503. Figure 502—Secondary saw-cuts remove the anterior and posterior protruberances of the lower end of the femur. Figure 503—The prominent anterior and posterior corners are bevelled away at an angle of 45 degrees, to allow the femoral component of the prosthesis to be fitted over the condyles.

tubercle. The joint is opened by a medial parapatellar incision through the quadriceps expansion and joint capsule, and deep to these the synovial membrane. The knee may now be fully flexed and

Clearance of diseased tissue. When arthritic disease has progressed to the point at which arthroplasty is required, the inside of the knee is usually badly disorganised, often with masses of inflamed synovium not only within the joint cavity proper but also in the suprapatellar pouch. All this diseased tissue, together with the menisci and disposable ligaments, is removed to give a clean exposure of the femoral and tibial condyles.

Preparation of femur. The lower end of the femur is next shaped according to the requirements of the particular prosthetic system that is to be fitted. Here the use of the appropriate jigs is helpful, though not mandatory. Usually, five distinct saw-cuts are required in shaping the femoral condyles to receive the prosthesis. 1) The first and most important cut is the transverse distal femur saw-cut—that is, the removal of the inferior weight-bearing convexities of the femoral condyles. This cut must be strictly in the transverse plane—that is, it would be parallel with the ground if the patient were standing (Fig. 500). Because of the natural obliquity of the femoral shaft (see above) this cut should be made not at right angles to the axis of the shaft but at a valgus angle of 9 or 10 degrees from that line as seen from the front (Fig. 501). Special guides are often provided to facilitate making the saw-cut at the correct angle. 2) and 3) The next cuts remove the anterior and posterior protruberances of the lower femur, approximately in line with the anterior and posterior cortices of the femoral shaft (Fig. 502). 4) and 5) Finally the anterior and posterior corners are bevelled away at an angle of 45 degrees by further saw-cuts (Fig. 503).

The femoral condyles, thus prepared, allow a matching fit of the shell-like femoral component of the prosthesis. The only remaining step is to drill holes to receive the lugs provided in most models of prosthesis to locate the prosthesis accurately in position. These drill holes are usually positioned by a jig.

Preparation of tibia. A single saw-cut is usually required to create a flat upper surface to receive the plate-like tibial component of the prosthesis. This saw-cut is usually also in the transverse plane (parallel with the floor if the patient were standing) (Fig. 504). However, because of the slight (3 degrees) inward inclination of the tibia on standing (see above), the cut should not be exactly at right angles to the long axis of the tibia, but deviated 3 degrees from the right angle. A guide may help to ensure that the saw-cut is made in the correct plane.

Finally it is necessary to prepare a hole or holes in the upper surface of the tibia to receive the corresponding locating lug of the tibial component of the prosthesis.

At this stage care should be taken not to place the tibial component too far forward. Within the limits of the design, it should be positioned posteriorly rather than anteriorly, in order to favour the restoration of the fullest range of knee flexion.

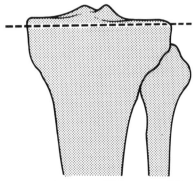

FIG. 504. The upper tibial saw-cut. This is parallel with the ground. It is almost at right angles to the long axis of the tibia but, strictly, allowance should be made for the fact that the tibia is about 3 degrees out of the vertical in normal stance, because the feet are closer together than the hips (see text).

Preparation of patella. If a patellar prosthesis is to be fitted it is necessary only to prepare the appropriate bed on the articular surface with a purpose-made reamer.

Trial fit. In most systems trial femoral and tibial components are provided. The tibial component, and then the femoral component, are placed in position, without cement, and the new articular surfaces are articulated. It is necessary to check that optimal alignment has been secured, that rotational alignment is correct, and that tension in the soft tissues is correct, allowing full extension at the knee. In the light of the trial fit any necessary adjustments are made, either to the prosthesis itself (in many systems graded thickness of tibial component are available) or to the bones, where further trimming may be carried out.

Fitting the definitive prosthesis. The trial components are removed to allow preparation of the raw bone surfaces by clearing away any remaining debris and mopping the surfaces dry. The definitive tibial component is cemented in place first, and then the femoral component. If the patella is to be resurfaced, the patellar prosthesis is cemented into the prepared socket. The components are articulated and the wound is closed.

POST-OPERATIVE MANAGEMENT

Gauze dressings are applied and held in place by one or two broad (15 centimetre) crepe bandages. In the early days after operation activity of the affected limb is confined to static muscle contractions, particularly for the quadriceps muscle and the calf muscles, and to active flexion and extension exercises of the knee through a limited range—a range of 15 or 20 degrees of flexion is a reasonable objective for the first week. (A continuous passive motion (CPM) machine may be used.) Thereafter flexion exercises are progressively increased with the aim of achieving at least 90 degrees of flexion. Meanwhile the power of extension must be restored by intensified quadriceps exercises. Provided the knee is comfortable, walking with full weight on the limb may be begun a day or two after the operation. Rehabilitation under the supervision of a physiotherapist should be continued for many weeks because in the type of case for which this operation is undertaken the muscles are usually markedly wasted in consequence of long-standing disease of the joint, and intensive muscle exercises are well rewarded.

NOTE ON SOFT-TISSUE BALANCING
AND MECHANICAL ALIGNMENT

Some types of total knee prosthesis are designed to ensure re-alignment of the leg with balanced tension in the collateral knee ligaments. The AGC ("anatomically graded components") system is one that uses this principle. A special distractor is inserted between the cut ends of the femur and tibia. The knee is flexed 10 or 20 degrees so that the posterior capsule is relaxed. The distractor is then tensioned equally on each side and to no more than 40 pounds. (A slightly lower setting is to be preferred because over-tensioning has been known to promote delayed rupture of a ligament.) The alignment guide rod is then fitted to the distractor. If it is not accurately centred over the ankle joint the tibia will need to be re-trimmed. At the upper end the guide rod should centre over the femoral head. If it does not, then a further adjustment is necessary to ensure correct alignment.

REPLACEMENT BY THE CHARING
CROSS PROSTHESIS

The Charing Cross prosthesis* (Fig. 505) is suitable for knees in which the medial and lateral ligaments are intact and provide adequate stability. It is also essential that there be adequate bone, particularly at the upper tibial plateau. Any serious deficiency could lead to instability of the tibial component.

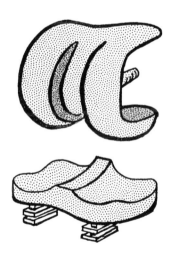

FIG. 505. The Charing Cross knee prosthesis.

Incision. A straight incision on the medial parapatellar line is made.

Procedure. The patella is dislocated laterally with adequate dissection of the lateral tissues to allow this. The intercondylar region is cleared.

*Supplied by Biomet Ltd, Swindon, England.

With a narrow gouge a hole is made as far back as possible on the intercondylar notch of the femur. The cutting template (No. 7311) is then inserted into this hole with the driving rod exactly in line with the femur. This ensures that there is 30 degrees of anteversion of the femoral component. The slots on the surface allow cuts to be made with a mechanical saw to give a proper outline for the shape of the femoral component. When this is removed the femoral template (No. 7310) is inserted into the same hole and its margin used to outline the area of femoral bone which needs to be left in place. The femoral test component can then be applied, and it is important to ensure that sufficient bone has been removed posteriorly for it to seat.

A transverse marking cut is made half way between the upper surface of the tibia and the tibial tubercle and the bone is resected. This should leave adequate space for insertion of the tibial component. With the tibia vertical the tibial template (No. 7309) is put in place with the slotted area on the upper surface of the tibia. It is essential that the vertical rod of this is exactly in a vertical alignment; otherwise the tibial component will be left at an angle. With this tibial template in place small osteotomes are used to excise areas of bone from the upper surface of the tibia to allow insetting of the ribs on the under surface of the tibial component. It is important to see that the tibial component is placed as far backwards as possible, and the raised intercondylar lip should be posterior. With these cuts made it is now possible to articulate the definitive femoral and tibial components and to check that the knee extends fully.

The components are cemented into position. (It may be necessary to mix a double quantity of cement though this is not usually so.) It is essential that all cement be removed from the posterior aspect. With the cement still wet and the components in place the knee is extended and the cement allowed to harden with the knee in this position. This allows final correction of any minor fault in alignment, whether varus or valgus.

Closure. The extensor mechanism is repaired and the subcutaneous tissues and skin are sutured. A suction drain is used.

POST-OPERATIVE MANAGEMENT

The limb is placed on a continuous passive motion machine immediately upon completion of the operation, while the patient is still anaesthetised. The machine is set to flex the knee to 30 degrees, with a cycle rate of once per minute. The flexion is gradually increased, so that 90 degrees is reached by the time the sutures are removed two weeks after the operation. From the third post-operative day the patient is mobilised off the machine, and is encouraged to take full weight on the limb as early as possible.

REPLACEMENT BY HINGED PROSTHESIS

The hinged prosthesis is usually made entirely in metal—commonly a chrome-cobalt alloy. The limbs of the prosthesis are elongated, and so designed that they fit snugly into the medullary canal of the femur and of the tibia, where fixation is usually aided by acrylic cement. The two limbs of the hinge are joined by a metal pivot, fitted after the femoral and tibial components have been separately inserted (Fig. 506).

BASIC TECHNIQUE

Position of patient. The patient lies supine. A tourniquet may be used on the highest part of the thigh.

Exposure of knee. The incision, the deep exposure of the knee, and the clearance of diseased tissue from the interior of the knee, are the same as described in the section on total condylar replacement (p. 385). Division of the anterior cruciate ligament allows the head of the tibia to be drawn forwards away from the femur, so that the whole of its upper surface is exposed.

Trimming of bone ends. The amount of bone to be cut away from the femur and tibia to create the appropriate gap necessary to accommodate the hinge of the prosthesis varies with the particular model that is to be used. The gap should be made mainly at the expense of the femur, and very little at the expense of the tibia. If guides are provided, they should be used to ensure that the saw-cuts are made in the correct plane. As seen from the side, the plane of the saw-cut should be at a right angle to the long axis of the bone. As seen from the front, the plane of the bone section may have to be a few degrees away from a line that is at a right angle to the long axis of the shaft, in order to ensure correct alignment of the tibia relative to the femur (see p. 384). Details vary for the different types of prosthesis.

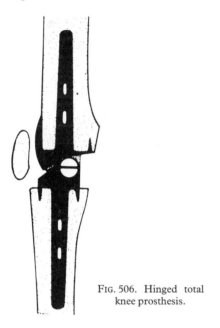

Fig. 506. Hinged total knee prosthesis.

Preparation of femur for reception of prosthesis. The lower end of the femur requires further trimming in order to match the bearing surface of the femoral component of the prosthesis. The surface will at present be too deep antero-posteriorly, and it is necessary to trim off the posterior part of each femoral condyle by a vertical cut at right angles to the sawn surface.

The sawn-off lower surface of the femur is now almost rectangular, and from the centre of the rectangle a vertical hole is prepared along the medullary canal of the femur. The initial track may be made by thrusting a screwdriver or similar semi-blunt instrument proximally through the soft cancellous bone. The hole is then enlarged to a diameter equal to that of the stem of the prosthesis by a suitable hand reamer or by a long narrow osteotome or chisel. The stem of the femoral component of the prosthesis is introduced along the hole into the medullary canal of the femur and tapped in lightly until the bearing surface approximates to the sawn surface of the femur.

Preparation of tibia for reception of prosthesis. The tibia is prepared in like manner by thrusting a semi-blunt instrument such as a screwdriver or hand reamer down the medullary canal from the centre of the sawn surface and then enlarging the hole to the appropriate diameter. The stem of the tibial component of the prosthesis is then thrust down the medullary canal of the tibia to bring the bearing surface of the prosthesis into contact with the sawn surface of the tibia. To seat the prosthesis fully it may be necessary to tap it downwards so that the projecting flanges of the prosthesis are embedded in the cancellous bone.

Trial fit. At this stage, with both components of the prosthesis temporarily in position, the knee is straightened and the components are locked together by the pivot to test their position, particularly with regard to any rotational deformity. If the femur and the tibia are not quite correctly lined up the necessary correction may be made by slightly twisting one or other component of the prosthesis in its bed. The correct rotational position of each component of the prosthesis should now be indicated by making marks upon the cortex of femur and tibia to correspond with fixed points on the prosthesis. The hinge is then dissembled and the two components are removed from their respective channels.

Fixation of components with acrylic cement. Acrylic bone cement is mixed to the appropriate consistency (it is ready for use when it just ceases to adhere to a rubber glove) and is pressed into the medullary canal of the tibia, into which should previously have been placed a size 8 polythene catheter to serve as an outlet for air and blood as the cement is pressed in. When an adequate quantity of cement has been thrust into the medullary canal the polythene catheter is withdrawn. Further cement may be applied to the stem of the tibial component of the prosthesis, which is then thrust down into the cement and tapped in lightly until the bearing surface comes into intimate contact with the sawn surface of the tibial condyles. As the prosthesis is being tapped in care should be taken to ensure that its rotational position is correct, as indicated by the mark previously made upon the tibial cortex. The prosthesis is then held immobile until the cement sets.

When the tibial component of the prosthesis has thus been fixed in position the femoral component is treated in like fashion, care being taken again to ensure that the prosthesis is correctly aligned as regards rotation.

Assembly of component parts of prosthesis. When both components have been satisfactorily placed and fixed in position, the knee is straightened and the two components of the hinge are interlocked. The pivot is inserted and locked in position.

Closure. The patella and the lower part of the quadriceps tendon fall back into place upon the front of the femoral component of the prosthesis. The medial incision in the joint capsule and in the vastus medialis muscle is repaired with absorbable sutures. The skin is closed with interrupted eversion sutures, without drainage.

POST-OPERATIVE MANAGEMENT

This is similar to that described for total condylar replacement (p. 388).

COMPRESSION ARTHRODESIS OF KNEE

Compression arthrodesis of the knee was devised by Key (1932) and refined by Charnley (1948). The principle is to cut away the opposing articular surfaces to expose raw cancellous bone, and to maintain compression contact between the cut surfaces by transfixing each bone end with a Steinmann pin and drawing the protruding ends of the pins together by a screw compression device (Fig. 509).

TECHNIQUE

Position of patient. The patient lies supine. A folded towel or sand-bag may be placed under the knee to maintain slight flexion. A tourniquet may be used on the upper thigh.

Incision. An anterior "lazy S" incision is the most convenient. The central part of the incision lies transversely over the middle of the patella. Laterally the incision curves proximally along the outer border of the quadriceps muscle; medially it curves distally to extend down the antero-medial aspect of the leg to a point level with the tibial tubercle (Fig. 507).

Excision of patella and exposure of joint. When the skin flaps have been reflected the anterior aspect of the extensor mechanism of the knee is

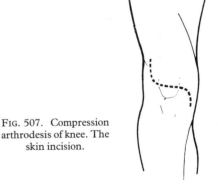

FIG. 507. Compression arthrodesis of knee. The skin incision.

exposed, and the patella is shelled out by dissection close to the bone after a midline incision has been made in the quadriceps aponeurosis. The patellar tendon is detached from its insertion into the tibial tubercle and the entire quadriceps expansion is turned proximally after division of the capsule and synovial membrane longitudinally at each side of the joint. The femoral condyles and the femoro-tibial compartment of the joint are thus fully exposed.

Clearance and resection of articular surfaces. First, as much of the synovial membrane as can conveniently be reached is cleared away, and the medial and lateral menisci are removed. The knee is then flexed fully and the cruciate ligaments are excised by careful dissection in the intercondylar notch of the femur. The collateral ligaments and lateral folds of the capsule are incised horizontally well back behind the axis of movement.

With the knee held fully flexed it is now possible to draw the tibia forwards and thus to dislocate the tibial articular surface more or less completely from its contact with the femur. To hold the tibia forwards a blunt lever may be introduced in the intercondylar notch of the femur and slipped over the posterior margin of the head of the tibia.

The next step is to trim off the articular ends of the tibia and femur with a small tenon saw or hacksaw, or with a powered oscillating saw. The tibial cut should be made first. To do this the knee is flexed to its full extent so that the sole of the foot is planted firmly upon the operation table, with the heel close to the buttock and the shaft of the tibia vertical. A transverse saw cut is made through the entire thickness of the bone just distal to the articular surface of the tibial condyles. The saw cut should be made strictly horizontally—that is, at right angles to the long axis of the tibia in both planes (Fig. 508). The resulting cut surface should be flat and should be composed of cancellous bone without any remnant of articular cartilage or subchondral bone.

The saw cut across the femoral condyles is made in similar manner. The angle of this cut is critical. The plane of the cut should be transverse from side to side (that is, at a right angle to the line of weight bearing though not to the axis of the femoral shaft* (see Fig. 497)), but should slope slightly upwards from before backwards in order

*The line of weight bearing is a straight line that passes through the centre of the hip joint, the centre of the knee joint and the centre of the ankle joint. The axial line of the femoral shaft forms a valgus angle of 7 to 9 degrees with the line of weight bearing.

to give an angle of 15 or 20 degrees of flexion at the knee when the cut surfaces of tibia and femur are brought together (Fig. 508). In order to judge this angle accurately the knee should temporarily be extended from the fully flexed position to the

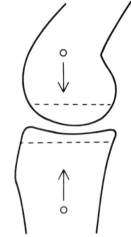

FIG. 508. The cut surfaces outlined. Position of Steinmann pins and direction of compression are shown. Note that the knee is to be fused in slight flexion.

desired final position of 15 or 20 degrees of flexion, so that the line of the saw cut through the femoral condyles may be marked out parallel to the tibial cut. The saw cut should be made with the knee again fully flexed. The level of the section is about 1 to 1.5 centimetres proximal to the lowest point of the femoral condyles.

Coaptation of cut surfaces and insertion of Steinmann pins. If the articular ends of the tibia and femur have been sawn correctly, when the cut surfaces are brought into apposition the knee should be in 15 to 20 degrees of flexion and there should be about 7 to 9 degrees of valgus between the axis of the femoral shaft and that of the tibia— the normal valgus angle* (see Fig. 497). If necessary, one or both of the cut surfaces may be adjusted by further trimming with the saw to ensure that the optimal position for fusion is attained.

The cut surfaces now being held in apposition, a rolled towel is placed behind the knee to maintain the chosen angle of flexion while Steinmann pins are inserted and the Charnley compression device is applied. First the skin incision is temporarily closed by towel clips. Then, with the limb steadied by an assistant, the lower end of the femur and the upper end of the tibia are each transfixed horizontally by a Steinmann pin 20 centimetres long. Each pin should be driven from the lateral side to emerge at the medial side. The two pins are horizontal and strictly parallel to one another. To aid their penetration of the skin without carrying epidermal cells on their points, tiny stab incisions may be made with a fine blade at the point of insertion.

The femoral pin should traverse the condylar part of the femur about 4 centimetres proximal to the sawn surface. The tibial pin should traverse the upper end of the tibia about 4 centimetres distal to the sawn surface. The two pins are thus about 8 centimetres apart.

Closure and application of compression device. When the tourniquet has been removed and all bleeding points controlled the quadriceps expansion is secured back in position with light absorbable sutures and the wound is closed with interrupted eversion sutures. The blocks of the Charnley compression device are now fitted over the protruding ends of the Steinmann pins on each side and are drawn together by tightening the

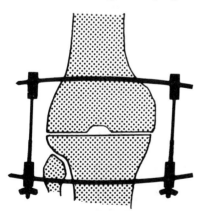

FIG. 509. The compression clamp is tightened sufficiently to cause bowing of the Steinmann pins. (The bowing shown here is somewhat exaggerated.)

wing nuts. Tension should be such that the pins, which have some degree of springiness, are slightly bowed (Fig. 509). With this degree of compression the sawn surfaces of femur and tibia are held immobile in intimate contact.

Alternative use of external fixator. Although the compression device recommended by Charnley serves its purpose well, there are many surgeons now who would prefer to use one of the many types of external fixator that have come onto the market since the operation was first described. The use and fitting of such appliances was described on page 93.

POST-OPERATIVE MANAGEMENT

Despite the rigid fixation provided by the clamped Steinmann pins it is recommended that additional external support from a plaster-of-Paris splint be provided. The plaster should extend from the upper thigh to the malleoli. Foot and toe exercises and leg lifting are encouraged.

The pins are left in position for six weeks; they are then removed and a further full-length plaster cylinder from groin to malleoli is applied. The patient is encouraged to walk in this plaster, which is retained for a further four to six weeks according to progress of the fusion as observed radiologically.

Comment

The first requirement is to gain a complete exposure of the condyles of the femur and tibia. It is important to detach and turn up the quadriceps expansion and it is convenient to remove the patella before this is done, as described. It is important also to divide the collateral ligaments and adjacent parts of the capsule by transverse cuts to allow the tibia to be drawn forwards upon the femur, and to excise the cruciate ligaments by sharp dissection in the intercondylar notch of the femur. Only in this way can the upper end of the tibia and lower end of the femur be delivered in turn into the wound to allow a clean saw cut through the whole thickness of each bone from before backwards.

The next essential is to make sure that the plane of each saw cut is correctly orientated. There is no particular difficulty with the tibial saw cut because this is made strictly at right angles to the long axis of the bone. The saw cut is horizontal. Finding the correct plane in which to saw the femur is a little more difficult, but the line can be judged fairly accurately if the knee is first placed in the desired degree of flexion and the line of the saw cut is then marked out parallel with the cut surface of the tibia. With the line thus marked, the knee is again flexed fully to deliver the femoral condyles from the wound to allow a clean cut to be made with the saw.

The only remaining problem is to place the Steinmann pins to the best advantage. If the bone ends are very soft—as is often the case in long-standing rheumatoid arthritis—it may be wise to place the pins somewhat further apart than usual if in that way they can be made to engage more substantial bone. The pins must not be further apart than 10 centimetres, however, because that is the greatest separation of the blocks of the Charnley compression device. If necessary, the compression clamps may be tightened every few days by adjusting the wing nuts.

One hazard of compression arthrodesis by the method described is the risk of pin track infection, which in rare cases has led to osteomyelitis and failure of fusion. Every care must be taken to ensure sterility by meticulous cleansing of the skin at the points of insertion of the Steinmann pins and by the maintenance of occlusive dressings throughout the period of pin fixation.

NAIL AND GRAFT ARTHRODESIS OF KNEE

Whereas compression arthrodesis of the knee is satisfactory in the great majority of cases there are occasions when the bone is so soft that the trans-fixation pins tend to pull through it, with con-sequent loosening. In these circumstances an alternative method is to immobilise the slightly flexed knee by a stout intramedullary nail intro-duced through the anterior cortex of the femur about 10 centimetres above the condyles and driven downwards into the tibia, and to supple-ment this fixation with medial and lateral bone grafts bridging the joint.

TECHNIQUE

Position of patient. The patient lies supine. A rolled towel or sand-bag is placed behind the knee to flex it 15 or 20 degrees. A tourniquet may be used very high on the thigh.

Incision. The skin incision is S-shaped. The central horizontal part crosses the joint at the lower pole of the patella. A lateral vertical limb of the incision passes upwards over the antero-lateral aspect of the thigh. The medial vertical limb passes downwards over the medial border of the tibia (Fig. 510). Skin flaps are turned back and held with towel clips.

Preparation of opposing bone surfaces. The joint cavity is cleared of all diseased synovial membrane and fibrous tissue. If necessary the patella is removed. The opposing surfaces of femur and tibia are trimmed down to raw vascular bone with chisels and gouges, in such a way that they fit

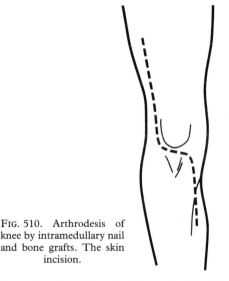

FIG. 510. Arthrodesis of knee by intramedullary nail and bone grafts. The skin incision.

together closely with the knee in the desired degree of flexion (usually 15 or 20 degrees).

Insertion of intramedullary nail. The anterior cortex of the femoral shaft 10 centimetres or so above the condyles is cleared with a periosteal elevator. The exact level of the opening to be made in the cortex depends upon the degree of knee flexion required. It should be so placed that a nail entering at the opening in the cortex will pass vertically downwards across the middle of the joint into the centre of the medullary canal of the tibia (Fig. 511). The initial, pilot opening is made

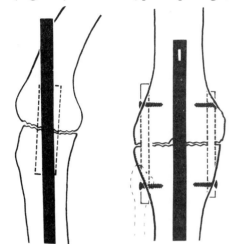

FIGS 511–512. Nail and graft arthrodesis of the knee. Figure 511—Diagram shows position of nail, and of the bed for a bone graft. Figure 512—Showing position of the medial and lateral bone grafts.

with a drill about 6 millimetres in diameter, and the drill is driven down in the intended direction of the nail. Its position is checked with the image intensifier or by radiographs. When the pilot drill has been placed satisfactorily the channel is enlarged to take a nail of appropriate diameter— usually 10 to 14 millimetres. The nail is driven at least 15 centimetres down the tibia. Its position is checked with the image intensifier.

Alternative use of Huckstep nail. A good case may be made for the use of a Huckstep nail in preference to a standard intramedullary nail in this situation. Since the nail thickness is only 12.5 millimetres the hole required in the front of the femoral shaft is comparatively small, and the risk of fracture of the femoral shaft is correspondingly reduced. The added fixation provided by multiple screws also makes for great rigidity.

Preparation and fitting of bone grafts. The joint line is exposed first at the medial side. With a chisel, osteophytes and other irregularities are removed to form a flat bed for the graft about 6 or 8 centimetres long and 2 centimetres wide. The bed may take the form of a slot, cut to a depth of 5 or 6 millimetres at the centre but shallower proximally and distally where the femoral and tibial condyles shelve away (Fig. 512).

In the lower part of the medial limb of the incision the subcutaneous surface of the tibia is exposed and cleared over a length of 6 or 8 centimetres. Periosteum is incised and stripped. With a motor-driven saw a graft of appropriate dimensions is cut (see p. 72). Before it is removed from its bed four holes large enough to provide a sliding fit for screws are drilled. The graft is then transferred to the prepared bed, bridging the medial side of the knee joint. Holes are drilled in the host bone, and the graft is secured with screws, which are driven home firmly but with care not to strip the thread in the soft bone. A similar procedure is next carried out at the lateral side of the joint (Fig. 512), the graft being obtained from the lateral cortex of the femoral shaft, well clear of the condyle. The graft is screwed into position and the wound is closed.

POST-OPERATIVE MANAGEMENT

Firm crepe bandages are applied over plentiful gauze dressings. A full-length thigh-to-forefoot plaster is applied over a cellulose lining, with careful moulding round the upper thigh to ensure the best possible protection against movement imparted from without. The plaster is changed as necessary, but should be retained until there is clinical and radiographic evidence of bony fusion. In the latter part of this period walking with crutches may be permitted, but full weight bearing on the affected limb is discouraged until union is secure.

Comment

This is seemingly a rather elaborate method of arthrodesing the knee, but it works well in practice even when the bones are very soft. It is important to site the anterior window in the femoral cortex for introduction of the nail carefully, because this is critical in relation to the chosen angle of knee flexion: the lower the nail is inserted, the greater will be the angle of knee flexion.

UPPER TIBIAL OSTEOTOMY FOR CORRECTION OF ANGULAR DEFORMITY

Upper tibial osteotomy is usually undertaken for correction of genu varum—occasionally for genu valgum—in adults with rheumatoid or degenerative arthritis. The principle is to remove a wedge of bone with its base so placed that when the gap is closed the deformity is fully corrected. Thus for genu varum the base of the wedge is lateral, whereas for genu valgum it is medial. Similar principles apply to the correction of fixed flexion deformity by removal of a wedge of bone based anteriorly. The recommended level of the osteotomy is about 2 centimetres below the articular surface of the upper end of the tibia.

PRELIMINARY STUDIES

Before the operation is undertaken it is important to determine accurately the degree of correction that is required and where the base of the wedge should be located. To calculate the required angle of correction careful measurement is made of the angle of the deformity by means of a long-armed protractor. If desired, the central axis of the limb may be marked upon the skin surface with a felt pen to facilitate measurement of the angle. The angle subtended by the thigh and the shin should likewise be measured on the unaffected side, for in the normal state the lower leg is not always seemingly in line with the thigh: a few degrees of valgus deviation may be present, especially in women. If the normal side can be measured, the angle of deformity at the affected knee can be determined accurately, and the size of the wedge to be removed from the upper tibia must correspond to this angle.

If measurements are made on the radiographs, it should be remembered that the shaft of the femur normally forms a valgus angle of 6 to 7 degrees with the axis of the tibia: this is because the femoral shaft is cranked away from the line of weight bearing at the upper end. The key point to remember is that the line of weight bearing normally passes through the centre of the femoral head, the centre of the knee joint and the centre of the ankle joint (Fig. 497), and the aim should be to restore this state of affairs.

In deciding the location of the base of the wedge it is necessary to observe whether the deformity is a pure medial or lateral deviation or whether there is an added flexion or recurvatum deformity. Thus, for example, if a varus deformity were combined with a flexion deformity the base of the wedge would be directed antero-laterally, whereas in a knee with pure varus deformity the base of the wedge would be strictly lateral.

LATERAL WEDGE OSTEOTOMY FOR GENU VARUM

PRE-OPERATIVE ASSESSMENT

It is necessary to study the limb as a whole both clinically and radiographically to determine the exact angle of deformity and thus the angle through which the tibia must be abducted upon the proximal fragment after the bone has been divided. It is well to aim for full correction, giving a valgus angle of 6 to 7 degrees between the femoral and tibial shafts, as in the normal limb. This should ensure that weight is transmitted correctly through the centre of the hip joint, the centre of the knee and the centre of the ankle.

TECHNIQUE

Position on table. The patient lies supine, but is rolled a little towards the opposite side by means of a large sand-bag placed under the buttock on the affected side. This allows easier access to the lateral and postero-lateral aspects of the knee. A tourniquet may be used high up on the thigh.

Incision. The incision begins at the postero-lateral aspect of the knee over the biceps tendon about 3 centimetres proximal to its insertion into the head of the fibula. From this point it sweeps downwards and forwards in a gentle curve to cross the anterior border of the tibia immediately distal to the tibial tubercle. Thence it curves medially to end over the subcutaneous surface of the tibia about 2 centimetres medial to its anterior border (Fig. 513).

Exposure and protection of common peroneal nerve. The first step in the operation is to expose the common peroneal nerve as it lies just deep to the biceps tendon near its insertion. From this

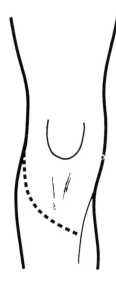

FIG. 513. Upper tibial osteotomy with excision of lateral wedge. The skin incision.

point the nerve is followed and uncovered more distally, where it crosses the neck of the fibula beneath the strong aponeurosis that encloses the proximal fibres of the anterior muscles of the leg. Once it has been exposed the nerve, because it is in full view, can easily be protected from damage during the subsequent stages of the operation.

Shortening of neck of fibula. Unless the wedge to be removed from the tibia is no more than a few degrees it is wise to excise an appropriate length of bone from the neck of the fibula in order to facilitate closure of the gap in the tibia after removal of the laterally based wedge.

The head and neck of the fibula are invested by thick aponeurotic tissue whose fibres run mainly in a vertical direction. To expose the bone these fibres should be separated by an antero-lateral vertical incision, and by knife dissection close to the bone the neck of the fibula is easily cleared in the greater part of its circumference. A section of bone about 1.5 centimetres long is then removed by cutting it across at two levels with an osteotome, gripping the intervening fragment of bone with nibbling forceps, and freeing the remaining deep attachments with a fine knife or scissors. By

thus shelling out the fibular neck from within its aponeurotic "capsule" the integrity of the lateral ligaments of the knee is preserved.

Determining the level for osteotomy. First the surgeon should establish unequivocally the exact position of the upper articular margin of the tibia, so that he knows exactly where the joint lies. This upper articular margin of tibia is not easily palpated with the knee straight, and accordingly the knee should be flexed 90 degrees or more so that the bony ridge formed by the articular margin of the tibia may be felt. It is well to mark the position of the ridge upon the surface with ink before the knee is straightened again. With this landmark identified the level of the osteotomy can now be determined. The upper limit of the insertion of

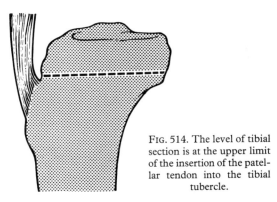

FIG. 514. The level of tibial section is at the upper limit of the insertion of the patellar tendon into the tibial tubercle.

the patellar tendon into the tibial tubercle is a useful guide to the correct level, which is about 2 centimetres below the upper articular surface of the tibia (Fig. 514). If the inexperienced surgeon is still in doubt, it is a reasonable precaution to drive a guide wire transversely across the upper part of the tibia from the medial aspect of the medial tibial condyle at the level of the proposed osteotomy and then to take an antero-posterior radiograph with the wire in position. The radiograph will indicate whether or not the marker wire is at the correct level for the osteotomy: it is a useful safeguard against dividing the bone too close to the articular surface of the tibia.

Clearance of tibia in preparation for osteotomy. The next step is to expose thoroughly the cortex of the upper end of the tibia on its antero-lateral and antero-medial aspects. A zone of tibial cortex is cleared first on the antero-lateral aspect of the bone by incising the uppermost fibres of the tibialis anterior and its overlying aponeurosis transversely, and then peeling periosteum proximally and

flexion deformity is also to be corrected. It is important to be sure that a hinge of intact tibial cortex, with overlying periosteum, is left undamaged at the medial (or postero-medial) aspect of the tibia: it is wrong to complete the osteotomy round the whole circumference of the bone.

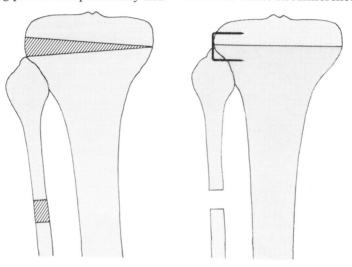

FIGS 515–516. Upper tibial osteotomy for varus deformity. Figure 515— Outline of the wedge of bone to be removed. Figure 516—After closure of the gap the fragments are held closely coapted by staples. Resection of a length of the fibula would usually be at a higher level, through the neck of the bone.

distally with an elevator to expose raw tibial cortex.

The zone of bared cortex is then extended medially round the front of the tibia deep to the patellar tendon. The insertion of the tendon is not disturbed, but immediately proximal to its insertion the tendon is lifted from the bone after division of flimsy intervening attachments. In this way the cortex is cleared deep to the tendon and round to the antero-medial surface of the tibia, where periosteum is incised transversely and reflected proximally and distally.

The osteotomy. The limits of the wedge to be removed—its dimensions should have been worked out beforehand—are now outlined upon the anterior and lateral aspects of the tibia by light taps upon an osteotome. Clearly, the base of the wedge to be removed must be strictly lateral if the deformity is one of pure varus (Fig. 515), but it should be placed antero-laterally if slight fixed

The wedge cut is now begun, preferably with a slender thin osteotome not more than a centimetre wide. It is best to take the wedge in piecemeal fashion, removing first the lateral and antero-lateral cortex to expose the interior of the bone. The cancellous interior is easily cut with a fine chisel on both sides of the wedge, and the soft bone is then scraped out with a small spoon or gouge. It is important to ensure that the sides of the wedge are straight and that they taper accurately to the apex of the wedge, where intact cortex and periosteum must be preserved (Fig. 515).

The most difficult step in the osteotomy is to remove the posterior cortex. If this is to be divided with an osteotome or chisel extreme care is required in order to avoid risk of damaging the popliteal vessels, which lie close behind the bone. Indeed, there is much to be said for removing this part of the cortex with fine bone nibblers or for fragmenting it with a slender punch so that it will buckle when the angular correction is made. It is also important that at this stage the knee be flexed to a right angle so that the vessels are relaxed and fall backwards to some extent.

Correction of deformity and fixation by staples. When the osteotomy has been completed round three-quarters or four-fifths of the circumference of the upper tibia, corrective force is applied to close the wedge-shaped gap. If the wedge has been accurately cut the raw surfaces should come into contact over the whole width of the bone (Fig. 516).

It remains to keep the osteotomy gap closed by the insertion of staples (usually three) into the antero-lateral and lateral aspects of the tibia, bridging the osteotomy site.

Closure. After removal of the tourniquet and control of any bleeding vessels, the skin is closed with interrupted eversion sutures, without drainage.

POST-OPERATIVE MANAGEMENT

Copious gauze dressings are held in place by a crepe bandage applied snugly but not too forcibly. Over this a plaster-of-Paris cylinder from upper thigh to malleoli is applied with the knee almost fully extended. The plaster is well moulded to maintain correction of the deformity.

Walking in the plaster with full weight upon the limb is encouraged within the confines of the ward, the patient using sticks or elbow crutches for support. After two weeks the plaster is bivalved and the anterior half is discarded. The back half is removed two or three times daily for knee flexion and extension exercises but is re-applied for walking and for sleeping. Splintage may usually be discarded finally at the end of six weeks from operation.

Comment

The paramount necessity is to safeguard the common peroneal nerve. The nerve has often been damaged during this operation when the head or neck of the fibula has been divided blindly without exposing the nerve. This is a mistake that should not be made. To expose the nerve and to protect it adds but a few minutes to the duration of the operation, and it should be a routine step whenever the fibular head or neck is to be trimmed.

Apart from this, the main essentials are to ensure that the wedge is of exactly the right dimensions to give full correction of the deformity. The importance of determining before the operation the angle of correction required is obvious. It is equally important to be sure that the angle of the wedge of bone removed corresponds to this angle.

Siting of the osteotomy is important: in general, a high osteotomy is more satisfactory than osteotomy below the tibial tubercle because union is more rapid. Moreover at the higher level the popliteal vessels are in less danger of being accidentally damaged than they are lower down where the anterior tibial artery leaves the main trunk to pass forwards between tibia and fibula. On the other hand the osteotomy must not be so high that the articular surface of the joint is breached, whether by an osteotome or by the leg of a staple.

After this type of osteotomy there is no need for recumbency, nor for prolonged immobilisation. Walking may safely be allowed within a day or two of the operation and knee movements should be commenced after two weeks. Disruption of the osteotomy is almost unknown, and the broad expanse of the cancellous cut surface makes for speedy union. Nevertheless it is a wise precaution to insist on the use of a plaster back splint for walking and sleeping until six weeks or so from the time of operation.

MEDIAL WEDGE OSTEOTOMY
FOR GENU VALGUM

Medial wedge osteotomy is performed less frequently than lateral wedge osteotomy and is less well favoured. So far as technique is concerned, the operation is in many details a mirror image of lateral wedge osteotomy for genu varum, described above, the wedge of bone to be excised being medial instead of lateral. It is somewhat easier to perform than lateral wedge osteotomy because the problem of exposing and safeguarding the common peroneal nerve does not arise.

TECHNIQUE

Position of patient. The patient lies supine. The whole limb must be draped in such a way that the knee may readily be held flexed or extended at different stages of the operation. The drapes should be close-fitting like a stocking, so that the alignment of the limb may be assessed visually. A tourniquet may be used on the upper thigh.

Incision. The incision begins well medial to the inner border of the patella and runs at first vertically downwards. It then curves laterally across the tibial tubercle to end 2 or 3 centimetres lateral to it (Fig. 517).

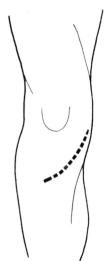

FIG. 517. Upper tibial osteotomy with excision of medial wedge. The skin incision.

Exposure of tibia. The skin edges are reflected and retracted to reveal the subcutaneous aspect of the upper part of the tibia. The periosteum is incised transversely about 2 centimetres below the upper margin of the tibia (this may be more easily palpated if the knee is semi-flexed) and is stripped from the bone a short distance proximally and distally, where necessary by sharp dissection.

Towards the lateral edge of the wound the patellar tendon is encountered. With a fine-bladed knife the tendon is separated from its loose attachments to the tibia immediately proximal to its insertion into the tibial tubercle, so that a transverse tunnel is created deep to the tendon, between it and the bone (Fig. 514). Attention is next directed to the tibia lateral to the patellar tendon, which is cleared and stripped of periosteum over a distance of 3 or 4 centimetres.

On the medial side the dissection should extend round the medial aspect of the medial condyle of the tibia almost onto its posterior surface. The medial edge of the wound is retracted by a curved bone lever passed behind the medial tibial condyle, the point lying between periosteum and bone. The whole of the anterior and medial aspects of the medial tibial condyle and the anterior part of the lateral condyle are thus clearly exposed to view.

Determining the level for osteotomy. As already noted, osteotomy is usually carried out about 2 centimetres below the upper articular surface of the tibia. This level is not always easily determined by palpation alone. A useful guide is the insertion of the patellar tendon. The level of osteotomy should be precisely at the proximal limit of the tendinous insertion (Fig. 514).

Marking the outline for the osteotomy. The desired angle of the osteotomy wedge being known from the pre-operative studies, a pattern of the wedge is cut from paper or sheet lead, the angle being carefully measured with a protractor. This pattern is placed over the tibia with the apex of the wedge over the lateral cortex and its base over the medial cortex. The outline of the wedge to be resected may then be marked upon the cortex of the tibia by scratching the surface with an awl or fine osteotome. The level of the upper margin of the wedge has already been determined (see above). If the deformity is strictly a valgus one, with no flexion or recurvatum element, the base of the wedge must be strictly at the mid-medial axis—that is, at the medial convexity of the medial tibial condyle. The apex of the wedge must be at the cortex of the lateral tibial condyle in the mid-lateral line.

Resection of bone wedge. The wedge is best resected piecemeal by osteotomes and chisels; nibbling forceps may be used for the posterior cortex. It is convenient first to lift off the anterior "roof" of the wedge and then to scoop out the canellous bone. The aim should be to cut the wedge cleanly and accurately, with straight sides that will meet in close apposition when the wedge-shaped gap is closed (Fig. 515). In working deep to the patellar tendon the surgeon should lift the tendon forwards so that the tibial cortex may be cut cleanly beneath it without damaging the tendon.

After patient excavation of the wedge from within the bone in this fashion, the only part that remains to be divided is the peripheral shell of cortex. The lateral cortex should be left intact to serve as a hinge, but the medial cortex and the posterior cortex must be removed to complete the excision of the wedge. At this stage it is important that the knee be flexed beyond a right angle to allow the popliteal vessels to fall backwards. This ensures a margin of safety when the posterior cortex is divided. Even with this precaution, extreme care must be taken in dividing the posterior cortex lest any cutting instrument or a spike of bone be thrust too far posteriorly. Usually it is safest to divide the posterior cortex under direct vision with bone nibblers, and whenever possible the periosteum should be left intact.

Closure of wedge-shaped gap and internal fixation. When the wedge of bone has been removed the remaining proximal and distal surfaces are checked to ensure that they are smooth and flat and that the wedge tapers evenly from base to apex. The knee is then straightened, and by firm pressure in a lateral direction over the tibia near the base of the wedge, with counter-pressure over the lateral malleolus, the wedge-shaped gap is closed so that the cut surfaces come into close apposition. While an assistant holds the gap closed, staples are inserted across the site of osteotomy at the medial and antero-medial aspects.

Usually two or three staples suffice. Because of the outward flare of the tibial condyle at this point it is advisable to use "stepped" or offset staples: these may be improvised by bending the angles of ordinary staples. In driving the staples care should be taken to ensure that the proximal leg of each staple is parallel with the plane of the osteotomy and does not deviate proximally towards the joint surface; otherwise there is a risk that the joint may be penetrated. If desired, check radiographs may be taken at this stage.

Closure. Only the fascia and the skin need to be sutured. Drainage is not required.

POST-OPERATIVE MANAGEMENT

This is the same as for lateral wedge osteotomy as described in the preceding section.

Comment

The comments made in relation to lateral wedge osteotomy are largely relevant to medial wedge osteotomy.

ANTERIOR WEDGE OSTEOTOMY FOR FLEXION DEFORMITY OF KNEE

The same basic technique as described in the previous two sections may be used for correction of a flexion deformity. If the deformity is purely one of flexion the base of the tibial wedge to be excised must be directed strictly anteriorly. If, however, flexion deformity is combined with valgus or varus deformity the base of the wedge must be sited antero-medially or antero-laterally respectively. It should be noted that a marked fixed flexion deformity of the knee may be better corrected by supracondylar osteotomy of the femur than by osteotomy of the upper tibia.

ABOVE-KNEE AMPUTATION OF LEG

Above-knee amputation—usually in the lower half of the thigh—is done less commonly than below-knee amputation but it is next in order of incidence for all major amputations. In a high proportion of cases it is undertaken for ischaemia from arterial disease, and in many of these patients there has been a previous below-knee amputation marred by necrosis of skin.

LEVEL OF AMPUTATION

The thigh stump should be as long as possible, with the proviso that room must be allowed to accommodate the mechanism of the prosthetic knee joint. About 10 centimetres should be allowed for this; so the bone section should generally be made this distance above the level of the knee joint, provided of course that there is sufficient intact skin from which to fashion adequate flaps. A length of at least 5 centimetres of femoral shaft distal to the lesser trochanter is essential if the stump is to have any active function. An amputation giving a stump shorter than this is tantamount to a hip disarticulation.

TECHNIQUE

Position of patient. The patient lies supine. In non-ischaemic cases a tourniquet may be used high up on the thigh, provided that the proposed level of section allows sufficient room. In ischaemic cases a tourniquet should not be used.

Marking out the skin flaps. It is well to mark out the skin flaps with ink before the operation is commenced. If the availability of intact skin permits, a posterior flap slightly longer than the anterior flap, in the ratio of 3 to 2, is recommended; but flaps of equal length may be used if necessary (Fig. 518). The base of each flap should be immediately proximal to the proposed level of bone section. It is well to mark this point upon the skin and to establish this position by measurements from the tip of the greater trochanter as well as from the level of the knee joint. The combined length of the two flaps should be about

25 per cent greater than the diameter of the thigh at the proposed level of bone section: this allows for trimming of excess skin from the flaps during closure of the wound. It is safer to have too much skin than too little.

Beginning in the medial line of the thigh 1.5 centimetres proximal to the planned level of bone section, the outline of the anterior flap sweeps downwards and laterally in a convex curve over the front of the thigh, and then proximally on the

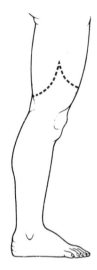

FIG. 518. Above-knee amputation. Outline of anterior and posterior flaps.

outer side to end in the mid-lateral line opposite to the starting point (Fig. 518). The outline of the posterior flap forms a similar convex sweep on the posterior aspect of the thigh.

Reflection of skin flaps. An incision is made in the outline of the anterior flap through skin, fascia and quadriceps muscle. These layers are reflected as a single composite flap. If the amputation is being made through the upper thigh the superficial femoral artery must be identified and ligated at this stage. If the amputation is through the lower thigh and if a tourniquet is being used, ligation of the vessels may be deferred until the limb has been separated.

The hip now being flexed, an incision is made in the outline of the posterior flap and the skin is reflected with the superficial fascia to expose the hamstring and adductor muscles. These muscles, with the deep fascia, are divided 5 centimetres distal to the planned level of bone section. At this stage the profunda femoris artery must be dealt with if a tourniquet is not being used.

Division of femur and separation of leg. The anterior musculo-cutaneous flap being turned well proximally, the planned level of bone section is freshly marked, this time upon the femur, after checking the measurement both from the tip of the greater trochanter and from the level of the knee joint. The periosteum is incised circumferentially and stripped proximally for a centimetre or so. The remaining soft tissues, including nerves and vessels, are now divided; the femur is cut through with a hand saw and the leg is discarded.

Treatment of vessels and nerves. If the major vessels have not already been dealt with—they will have been if a tourniquet is not being used—they are now identified and doubly ligated by transfixion ligatures well proximally. The major nerve trunks and also the cutaneous nerves are individually drawn downwards, cut cleanly across as high as possible, and allowed to retract: before division of the sciatic nerve or of its two main divisions ligation is recommended because the nerve trunks are accompanied by sizeable blood vessels.

Myodesis. To stabilise the stump of the femur in the surrounding cuff of muscles, attachment of the muscles to the end of the bone (myodesis) is recommended. This entails drilling five or six holes at intervals round the circumference of the femoral shaft about 5 millimetres from the cut edge. Mattress sutures of strong catgut are then used to anchor each individual hamstring and adductor muscle to the bone in slight tension, excess muscle being trimmed away as necessary. At this stage the tourniquet (if used) should be removed and all bleeding points should be well controlled.

Myoplasty. The layer of quadriceps muscle contained in the anterior flap is thinned if necessary and slightly tapered to form a muscle flap not more than a centimetre thick to cover the end of the stump. The muscle flap is turned posteriorly and sutured to the deep fascia of the posterior flap.

Closure. The skin flaps are folded into position and any surplus skin is trimmed away to allow a smooth suture line, not too lax but not under tension, and without any "dog ears". Immediately before the skin is sutured a perforated tube for suction drainage is inserted deep to the muscle flap. The skin edges are closed with interrupted eversion sutures.

POST-OPERATIVE MANAGEMENT

Soft gauze dressings are held in place by wide crepe bandages carried well into the groin and round the waist in spica fashion. The bandages may be covered by a thin layer of plaster-of-Paris bandages, the plaster being well moulded over the end of the stump and around its circumference. The drain is removed after thirty-six or forty-eight hours. The initial dressing is removed after two weeks: the skin sutures are then removed and frequent stump bandaging is begun. Supervised exercises especially for the gluteal muscles are practised from an early stage.

AMPUTATION THROUGH KNEE

Amputation through the knee provides a stump that is well suited for end bearing because the skin of the infrapatellar region, accustomed to bearing weight during kneeling, is used to cover the femoral condyles, which are left with the articular cartilage intact.

TECHNIQUE
Position of patient. The patient lies supine. The whole limb is draped in a stockingette tube to facilitate manoeuvring of the knee during the operation. A tourniquet should be used on the upper thigh unless the limb is ischaemic.

Marking out the skin flaps. It is well to outline the skin flaps in ink before the incisions are made. A rather long anterior flap (equal to the diameter of the limb at knee level) and a shorter posterior flap (equal to half the diameter of the limb) are recommended. The outline should be begun just behind the medial ligament, about a centimetre above the joint line. From this point the anterior flap sweeps in a convex curve, crossing the front of the tibia 4 centimetres distal to the tibial tubercle. Thence it curves upwards on the outer side of the limb to end opposite the starting point—that is, a centimetre proximal to the joint in the vertical line of the fibula. The outline of the posterior flap begins at the same point as the anterior flap and sweeps convexly round the back of the knee, extending distally for a maximum of 5 centimetres below the flexor crease of the popliteal fossa.

Incisions. When the flaps have been carefully marked out the anterior and posterior incisions are made. The anterior incision cuts right down to bone, the posterior one to the deep fascia.

The medial dissection. From the medial side of the knee, which at this stage should be held semi-flexed, the edge of the posterior flap is reflected to reveal the medial hamstring tendons. These are divided close to their attachment to the tibial tuberosity. The space thus created allows identification of the popliteal artery, which should be doubly ligated by transfixion ligatures and divided distal to the superior genicular branches. Behind the artery the tibial nerve is identified, drawn distally, ligated and divided cleanly across so that it retracts proximally.

Reflection of anterior flap. Attention is now turned to the anterior flap, which is reflected upwards with the underlying fascia until the patellar tendon is revealed at its insertion into the tibial tubercle. The tendon is severed from its insertion and the whole anterior flap, including the patellar tendon, the deep fascia, and the lower part of the capsule and synovial membrane of the knee, is reflected proximally as far as the joint line. The patella is left undisturbed.

The lateral dissection. The knee being flexed, attention is now directed to the lateral side of the joint. The biceps tendon and the ilio-tibial tract are divided. At this stage the common peroneal nerve is easily identified where it lies deep to the biceps tendon. The nerve is drawn downwards, divided cleanly as high as possible, and allowed to retract proximally.

Separation of leg. The posterior flap is now reflected proximally, and division of the capsule and ligaments of the knee is completed round the whole circumference of the joint. The attachments of the medial and lateral heads of the gastrocnemius muscle are severed close to the femoral condyles and the limb is separated.

Closure. If a tourniquet has been used it is important that it be released at this stage so that full haemostasis may be secured before the wound is closed. When all bleeding has been controlled the patellar tendon is drawn posteriorly into the intercondylar notch of the femur and sutured to the hamstring tendons under tension. The long anterior flap is then folded into position to meet the short posterior flap. The scar should be just behind the weight-bearing surface. If there is an excess of skin and fascia the flap is trimmed appropriately so that it fits snugly without tension but on the other hand without excessive bagginess. A suction drainage tube is inserted deep to the fascia, and the wound is closed by suture of the fascial layer and of the skin.

POST-OPERATIVE MANAGEMENT

Copious gauze dressings are held in place by a smoothly applied crepe bandage. The drainage tube is withdrawn after thirty-six to forty-eight hours. Exercises for the hip are encouraged—particularly gluteal exercises to maintain powerful extension. The stump is re-dressed after two weeks, when the sutures are removed. Thereafter the stump is bandaged frequently with wide crepe bandages applied in oblique turns carried right up to the groin.

Comment

Through-knee amputation provides a sound end-bearing stump with a long lever for muscle control. In these respects it has advantages over the above-knee amputation in non-ischaemic cases. It presents problems to the artificial limb maker, particularly from the cosmetic point of view.

ALTERNATIVE TECHNIQUE

In the technique of Mazet and Hennessy (1966) the femoral condyles are trimmed both at the sides and posteriorly and the patella is removed. The resulting stump is cosmetically more acceptable. The originators designed a new type of prosthesis suitable for this less bulbous stump.

CHAPTER TEN

Leg, Ankle and Foot

Disorders of the lower leg and foot are probably second in frequency only to those of the spine, and they form a considerable proportion of orthopaedic practice. When operation is required in this area it is often on account of injury—particularly for fractures of the tibia or about the ankle. In the foot itself much orthopaedic work is occasioned by deformity—especially of the toes—which though often seemingly trivial to the outside observer may nevertheless be far from trivial to the patient herself, who indeed may become demoralised from unremitting pain on standing and walking.

CONTENTS OF CHAPTER

INTRAMEDULLARY NAILING OF TIBIA

This section should be read in conjunction with the general description of intramedullary nailing in Chapter 2 (p. 84). The following description is not complete in itself but is complementary to the general account of the subject.

CLOSED NAILING

Only a proportion of tibial fractures lend themselves to closed nailing—that is, without exposure of the fracture site to secure reduction. Successful closed nailing presupposes that reduction either is not required or that it can be achieved by closed manipulation.

is intact the advisability of dividing it should be considered. Often an intact fibula makes accurate reduction of a tibial fracture difficult, and the management becomes much easier after division of the fibula.

TECHNIQUE

Position of patient. The patient lies supine. Provision must be made for the knee to be flexed at least 130 degrees to facilitate the introduction of a straight nail. Provision should also be made for mechanical traction to be applied through a Steinmann pin transfixing either the lower end of the tibia or the calcaneus. The authors have found the simple hinged platform illustrated in Figure 519

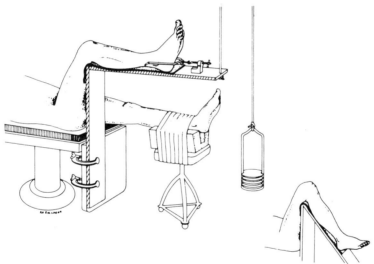

FIG. 519. Hinged platform clamped to flap of operation table for intramedullary nailing of tibia. The platform is counter-balanced by a weight to allow the knee to be flexed acutely (inset) for insertion of the nail. Provision is made for screw traction to facilitate closed nailing.

PRELIMINARY STUDIES

The nature of the fracture should be carefully scrutinised in the radiographs to determine its suitability for nailing. In this respect the degree of comminution is important. In particular, if there is a large "butterfly" fragment nailing may be deemed inappropriate or it may be thought necessary to fix the loose fragment with circumferential wires in conjunction with the nailing: this of course precludes the closed method. If the fibula

satisfactory. Basically the platform consists only of two boards hinged together. The upright board is clamped with G-clamps to the lowered table end, its height depending upon the length of the patient's thigh. The other board, which supports the calf and should be appropriately padded, is suspended at its free end by a cord and balancing weight slung over a pulley. Below the foot is attached a screw traction device to which cords secured to the ends of a Steinmann pin transfixing the tibia or heel may be attached. The hinge and counterbalancing system allow the knee to be held in varying degrees of flexion as required during the various stages of the operation. This arrangement lends itself well to the use of the image intensifier—preferably one with memory-sustained image—which is virtually an essential piece of equipment for this operation. A tourniquet may be used on the upper thigh.

Reduction of tibial fracture. An attempt is made to reduce the fragments by appropriate manipulation, aided if necessary by mechanical traction. Progress of the reduction should be checked by short viewings with the image intensifier. If satisfactory reduction cannot be secured, closed nailing must be abandoned in favour of the open method. It being assumed that reduction has been obtained, the operation proceeds in the following stages.

Preparation of entrance point for nail. A vertical incision 5 centimetres long is made immediately medial to the patellar tendon: its lower end is level with the tibial tubercle. The fascia is incised and the patellar tendon is retracted laterally so that the intercondylar ridge of the upper end of the tibia may be exposed by blunt dissection through the anterior fat pad. The knee joint proper is not

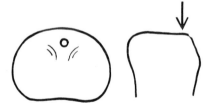

FIG. 520. Upper end of tibia showing site for entry of nail.

entered: the approach lies between the medial and lateral compartments of the joint. The wound edges are held apart with a self-retaining retractor, and the site for entrance of the nail is marked on the anterior end of the intercondylar ridge about 2 centimetres behind the anterior border of the tibia (Fig. 520).

Preparation of pilot track for guide wire. The starting point for the nail track is made with a

small gouge which penetrates the cortex of the intercondylar ridge at the selected site. When the surface has been breached down to cancellous bone a rigid director or rod (a screwdriver serves the purpose well) is thrust down the medullary canal of the tibia, being directed down the central axis of the bone in both the frontal and the lateral planes (Fig. 521). A rigid instrument such as this can force a track in the desired direction, whereas if a flexible guide wire is introduced direct it tends to strike the posterior cortex of the tibia and is likely to come out of the bone at the back, through the fracture site.

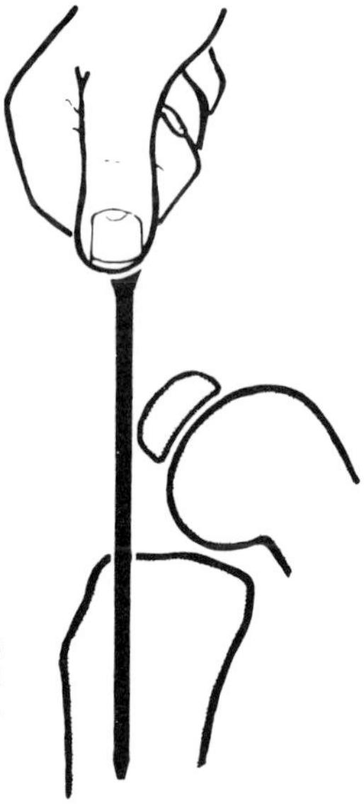

FIG. 521. The starting track for the guide wire is best made with a rigid instrument such as a screwdriver.

Introduction of guide wire. Once the first 15 or 20 centimetres of the track have been prepared by a rigid instrument the guide wire may be introduced on a hand chuck and driven down the medullary canal, across the fracture, to penetrate almost as far as the ankle. Note that the first guide wire should be olive-tipped—that is, with a small rounded knob at the end—in order to facilitate retrieval of a reamer head should it break off during reaming (Fig. 522). The position of the guide wire is checked by the image intensifier, and the length within the bone is calculated by subtracting the amount still protruding from the known total length of the wire.

Reaming of medullary canal. The canal is reamed out by successively larger cutting heads attached to a slow-speed power-operated flexible reamer. Usually it is best to start with a reamer of 8 or 9 millimetres diameter (these may require a thinner guide wire) and to work up to 13 or 14

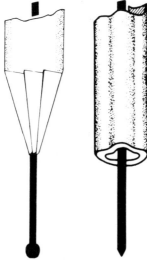

FIGS 522–523. An olive-tipped guide wire is used to guide the reamers (Fig. 522), so that in the event of a reamer's breaking the broken fragment may be retrieved. In contrast, a plain guide wire is used for guiding the nail (Fig. 523), so that there is no obstruction to removal of the wire when the nail has been driven home.

millimetres. Clearly the final size will depend upon the build of the patient, but the object should be to fit a stout nail, provided always that the cortex at the thinnest part of the tibia is not cut away to excessive thinness.

Preparation and driving of nail. Although a straight intramedullary nail can be passed easily with this technique it is an advantage to have the proximal 5 centimetres of nail inclined forwards at an angle of 20 degrees or so to the main axis (Fig. 524). This is simply to make retrieval of the nail easier if it should eventually have to be removed. Nails with the appropriate angulation of the upper end may be prepared before operation, or a nail may be bent at the time of operation by a sterilised bending machine: two lengths of stout steel piping just wide enough to accept the nail may be used if a purpose-built machine is not

available. Some patterns of nail have a gentle curve, convex posteriorly, as a safeguard against the risk of inadvertent penetration of the posterior cortex of the tibia.

The correct length of nail is determined from the length of the guide wire within the bone or by direct measurement of the tibia externally.

Before the nail is introduced it is important to remove the olive-tipped guide wire and to substitute a plain one (Fig. 523). The nail is then introduced into the reamed canal over the guide wire and hammered down by light blows with a mallet. Its progress is checked periodically by viewings

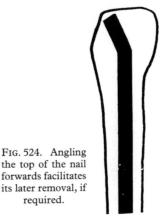

FIG. 524. Angling the top of the nail forwards facilitates its later removal, if required.

on the image intensifier. The penetration of the nail should be such that its tip is within a few millimetres of the ankle: if the length has been calculated correctly the proximal end of the nail should then lie a few millimetres deep to the upper surface of the tibia.

Finally the guide wire is withdrawn and the wound is closed.

POST-OPERATIVE MANAGEMENT

The first prerequisite is to monitor the arterial circulation closely, particularly during the first two days after operation. Because of the potential for swelling within the closed spaces of the lower leg, in consequence both of the fracture itself and of the surgical intervention, there is a risk of the development of compartment syndrome, with possible obstruction of the arterial circulation. If any evidence of arterial deficiency arises the surgeon must therefore be prepared immediately to counter it by opening up the affected closed fascial space by fasciotomy.

If good fixation with a stout nail is achieved—and this presupposes that each fragment has been penetrated over an adequate length—there is no need for external support by a plaster-of-Paris case. Knee and ankle movements may therefore be begun within a day or two of the operation. In the case of a transverse or short oblique fracture weight bearing with the aid of elbow crutches may be resumed as soon as the soft tissues have healed.

If fixation by the nail is not rigid—as may happen if one of the fragments is short—additional support from a plaster-of-Paris case from upper thigh to metatarsal heads should be provided. Again early weight bearing may usually be encouraged.

Comment

Introduction of a nail at the upper surface of the tibia presents little difficulty provided the knee is fully flexed and the tibia drawn well forward. It is important that the starting point for the nail track be made on the central ridge of the upper surface of the tibia midway between the medial and lateral compartments of the knee. This ridge is virtually extra-articular. Difficulty arises only if the knee cannot be flexed as far as 130 degrees: in that event an alternative method of internal fixation may have to be considered (see below).

The question whether an intact fibula should be divided to facilitate closed reduction of the tibia has already been raised. There should be no hesitation in dividing the fibula if it seems to offer some advantage: there is no particular merit in retaining the fibula intact.

A thick strong nail is always to be preferred to a thin nail because of its greater rigidity. Moreover, on account of the greater area of contact with the reamed cortex a thick nail is more effective than a thin one in preventing rotation of the fragments.

OPEN NAILING

If it proves impossible to obtain acceptable reduction by closed manipulation, with or without traction, it is necessary to expose the tibia at the site of fracture and to gain reduction under direct vision. Two incisions are thus required, one to expose the fracture site and the second to expose the upper surface of the tibia for insertion of the nail, as already described in the previous section.

When complete reduction of the fragments has been gained and held by a suitable bone clamp, the subsequent steps in the technique of nailing are precisely the same as those already described in the previous section and in the general section on intramedullary nailing (p. 84).

TIBIAL NAILING BY THE TECHNIQUE OF THE SWISS SCHOOL

The Association for Osteosynthesis (A.O.) in Switzerland has modified the technique of medullary nailing of the tibia. The Swiss surgeons use a specially designed nail which has a slight even curve, concave anteriorly, throughout its length: the proximal end is sharply angled forwards. This nail is introduced by special instruments through the anterior cortex of the tibia just below the upper articular margin. A full description of the technique has been published by Müller, Allgöwer, Schneider and Willenegger (1991).

REMOVAL OF TIBIAL INTRAMEDULLARY NAIL

Removal of a tibial nail should not present difficulty if the nail has been angled forwards at the upper end, which is thus easily accessible through a window cut in the uppermost part of the anterior tibial cortex and in the anterior part of the intercondylar ridge of the upper end of the tibia. Difficulty may arise, however, if a straight nail has been used without any forward inclination of its upper end, and also if flexion of the knee is markedly restricted.

The technique of extraction depends upon the type of nail that has been used and upon the extraction apparatus available. In the case of the commonly used Kuntscher-type nail it is necessary to expose the slot near the upper end of the nail and to insert the hook of a suitable extractor in the slot, preferably from within the channel of the nail.

In the case of a nail of the type used by the Swiss (A.O.) school, a special extractor which screws into the upper end of the nail should be used: slots are provided at the upper end of the nail, but the mechanical efficiency of the hook type of extractor leaves much to be desired, and if the nail is tight extraction of the Swiss nails may be very difficult with the hook device.

When a nail is particularly tight and resistant to extraction, additional measures may have to be used. A method that often works is to expose the tibia at the lower end of the nail and to cut out a window in the cortex to expose the tip of the nail. With an angled punch it may then be possible to drive the nail up from below until a better grip can be obtained at its upper end.

Comment

Extraction of a medullary nail may prove much more difficult than expected. It is a mistake to embark on the operation unless a full range of extraction equipment is at hand. Many of the extraction instruments available on the market are quite inadequate for their purpose. All too often the hook of an extractor bends or breaks off because it is too slender for the job. Instruments for this purpose should be very carefully chosen and duplicates should be available. Removal of a Swiss (A.O.) tibial nail should never be undertaken unless the special extractor, with conical threaded attachment that screws into the top of the nail, is available.

PLATE FIXATION FOR FRACTURE OF SHAFT OF TIBIA

The technique of plating bones for fracture was described in Chapter 2 (p. 82). The application of a plate to the tibia follows the same general lines. It is important that the plate be applied to a submuscular surface of the tibia rather than to the subcutaneous surface, where it may cause discomfort and may prejudice healing of the wound. In general, it is recommended that the lateral submuscular approach be used (p. 40), but if the skin of the leg antero-laterally is in poor condition due to extensive scarring it is better to approach the tibia from behind (p. 41) and to apply the plate to the posterior surface.

POST-OPERATIVE MANAGEMENT

Unless exceptionally rigid plates have been used external support from a plaster-of-Paris splint is recommended until union of the fracture is well advanced.

FIXATION BY TRANSFIXION SCREWS FOR OBLIQUE FRACTURE OF TIBIA

Long oblique or spiral fractures of the tibia (usually with a fibular fracture also), provided there is no comminution, lend themselves to fixation by transfixion screws driven obliquely across the fracture. Such fractures are commonly situated in the lower half of the tibia at about the junction of the middle and lowest thirds.

TECHNIQUE

Position of patient. The patient lies supine. A tourniquet may be used on the upper thigh.

Incision. The incision is mainly a vertical one over the antero-lateral muscles of the lower leg about a centimetre lateral to the anterior crest of the tibia. The line of the incision may sweep medially at the upper end and at the lower end to cross the crest of the tibia, but any sharp angle must be avoided (Fig. 525).

Exposure of fracture and reduction of displacement. The medial edge of the incision is retracted to expose the crest and subcutaneous (anteromedial) surface of the tibia. As is usual if a fracture is to be exposed, the surgeon should display normal bone above and below the fracture and then follow each fragment distally or proximally as the case may be until the fracture site is encountered. In this particular type of fracture this initial step presents little difficulty because the bone is superficial and displacement is seldom severe.

The next step is to clear the fracture surfaces by removal of all blood clot and fibrin in order to allow exact coaptation of the fragments. Obtaining anatomical reduction may present some difficulty, especially if the fracture is several days old,

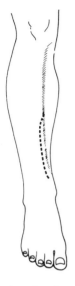

FIG. 525. Fixation of oblique fracture of tibia by transfixion screws. The skin incision.

because the elastic pull of the muscles may have caused shortening of as much as 2 centimetres or more; and the longer the delay the more resistance there is to drawing the bone out to full length. Nevertheless, it is essential that exact anatomical coaptation be secured. This must be achieved by a combination of longitudinal traction and manipulation of the fragments held in bone-holding forceps. In many cases initial sharp angulation of the fracture will permit engagement of matching edges of the cortex, and then the limb may be straightened to secure a true fit of the fracture surfaces. Once this has been achieved the position must be held by gripping the bone across the fracture with a suitable bone-holding forceps or clamp to hold the two fragments together.

Fixation by screws. The drill holes for the screws must be carefully sited so that they traverse sound bone of each fragment. Screws that are placed too close to the broken edge may cut out, with fragmentation of the cortex. Care must therefore be taken to establish the precise outline of each fragment, which may not at first be clear, especially on the deep surface. As a rule, two screws should be inserted, and the drill holes should be located to give these screws the best advantage. In general direction the screws are more or less transverse, but usually with some obliquity in the opposite direction to the obliquity of the fracture (Fig. 526). The exact point at which the drill for each screw should be entered will depend upon the pattern of the fracture: often it can be entered on the subcutaneous (antero-medial) surface near the anterior crest. The holes for the two screws should be more or less parallel. It is important that the hole in the anterior fragment should allow a sliding fit for the screw, whereas the hole in the posterior fragment should be no wider than the core diameter of the screw. It is best therefore to use first a drill corresponding to the core diameter of the screw and then to enlarge the hole in the anterior fragment appropriately. If the screw head will lie subcutaneously it is important that the hole be countersunk to receive the screw head and thus prevent undue prominence.

When the screw holes have been thus correctly drilled, the correct length of screw is determined by measurement with a depth gauge (see p. 55), and screws of corresponding length are driven home firmly but with care not to over-tighten them and strip the thread in the posterior fragment.

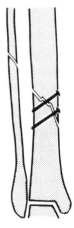

FIG. 526. The fracture reduced and transfixed with two oblique screws.

Closure. If practicable, a few absorbable sutures should be used to approximate the edges of the periosteum or lateral muscles to cover the bone so far as is possible. The skin edges are closed with everting mattress sutures, without drainage.

POST-OPERATIVE MANAGEMENT

The fixation afforded by two screws is somewhat tenuous, partly because of the rather fragile nature of the oblique tongues of bone that are transfixed. Thus the limb must be handled with great caution lest a secondary fracture be produced, with recurrence of displacement; and for the same reason it is essential that the limb be encased in plaster-of-Paris from upper thigh to metatarsal heads with the knee flexed 25 to 30 degrees.

The first plaster should be changed for a closer-fitting plaster when the swelling has subsided after two weeks, and at this time the sutures should be removed. It is wise to caution against full weight-bearing until six weeks have elapsed from the time of operation: in the meantime the patient may usually walk with elbow crutches, putting only a little weight on the injured limb. Plaster immobilisation, or in appropriate circumstances cast bracing, is continued until radiographs show sound union of the fracture.

Comment

Much care is needed to ensure that the fracture is fixed with precise coaptation of the fragments. It is not wise to accept anything short of full anatomical reduction, because if the fragments are ill-fitting the screws necessarily impart far less rigidity and they are liable to break out. It is important in gaining full reduction to avoid unnecessary stripping of periosteum from the bone with consequent impairment of its blood supply.

Fixation by transfixion screws is appropriate only for fractures without comminution. If there is a butterfly fragment—unless it be very small—it is difficult to ensure good stability by transfixion screws and it is better to employ an alternative method of fixation.

BONE GRAFTING FOR DELAYED UNION OR NON-UNION OF FRACTURE OF TIBIA

The techniques of bone grafting were described in Chapter 2 (p. 78), and a further detailed description is not required here.

In cases of delayed union or non-union of a fracture of the tibia the choice has to be made between circumferential sliver grafting (Phemister 1947), onlay cortical bone grafting, and sliding bone grafting. Often, sliver grafting with cancellous bone from the iliac crest is combined with rigid internal fixation of the tibia by an intramedullary nail. This method should usually be preferred to onlay cortical bone grafting, especially when the fracture is in the middle half of the bone or when there has been previous infection. Nevertheless there is still an occasional place for onlay cortical bone grafting or sliding bone grafting, especially for fractures near the upper end of the tibia.

For bone grafting, whether by cancellous slivers or by cortical onlay graft, the tibia should be approached on a submuscular surface rather than on the subcutaneous surface. As a general rule the antero-lateral approach, exposing the lateral submuscular surface of the tibia, is the most convenient route; but if the skin antero-laterally is unhealthy it is better to select the posterior route (p. 41).

POST-OPERATIVE MANAGEMENT

It is usually advisable to provide external support for the limb by a plaster-of-Paris splint until union is well advanced. If rigid internal fixation by a stout intramedullary nail has been secured, however, it may be possible to dispense with external support and to allow unprotected weight bearing as soon as the soft-tissue wound has healed.

SCREW FIXATION OF FRACTURED MEDIAL MALLEOLUS

Open reduction and internal fixation of a separated medial malleolus are often required because a fold of periosteum tends to fall in between the bone fragments, preventing accurate closed reduction (Fig. 527). Even without soft-tissue interposition closed reduction is often imperfect because of the usually smooth fracture surfaces which allow of no interlocking.

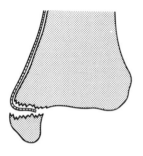

FIG. 527. Infolding of a fringe of periosteum often prevents closed reduction of fractures of the medial malleolus.

TECHNIQUE

Position of patient. The patient lies supine, with the limb rotated laterally so that the foot rests upon its outer border. A tourniquet may be used on the upper thigh.

Incision. The incision is mainly vertical. It lies over the junction of the anterior third and the posterior two-thirds of the medial malleolus, curving slightly backwards in its distal third to

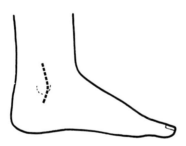

FIG. 528. Internal fixation of fractured medial malleolus. The skin incision.

end just below the tip of the malleolus (Fig. 528). The incision thus lies a little behind the saphenous vein and the accompanying nerve.

Clearance of fracture gap. The oedematous periosteum is incised vertically down to bone. Over the proximal fragment it is stripped from side to side to expose raw cortex. It should not be stripped widely from the distal fragment lest its blood supply be imperilled, but just enough to allow the fracture surface to be seen in its entirety. The fracture being thus exposed, the gap is opened up by light distal distraction of the malleolar fragment with a bone hook. This allows inspection of the fracture surfaces and removal of fibrin, blood clot and interposed periosteum.

Reduction and internal fixation. Under direct vision the fragments are now fitted together, with care to ensure perfect apposition without any shift or rotation. The position is held by an assistant,

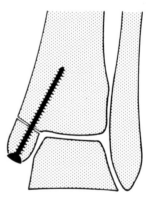

FIG. 529. Position of screw for fixation of fractured medial malleolus.

who pulls proximally upon the malleolar fragment with a sharp bone hook applied near the tip of the bone. While the reduction is thus maintained, a suitable point near the tip of the malleolus is defined for insertion of the screw. At this point a small starting hole is prepared with an awl. A drill, equal in diameter to the core diameter of the screw to be used, is driven proximally and almost vertically—inclining only a little laterally—through the malleolar fragment into the main body of the bone. The drill track in the malleolar fragment is enlarged by a drill equal in diameter to the overall diameter of the screw, to ensure a sliding fit for the screw: the malleolar fragment will thus be drawn tightly up to the main fragment when the screw is driven home (Fig. 529). After insertion of the screw—usually about 5 centimetres long—its position is checked by the image intensifier or by a radiograph before the wound is closed.

Closure. Only the periosteal layer and the skin need to be repaired.

POST-OPERATIVE MANAGEMENT

The authors prefer to protect the ankle and foot in a right-angled below-knee plaster for six or eight weeks. In most cases weight bearing in the plaster may be permitted after removal of the sutures and application of a close-fitting plaster two weeks from the time of operation.

Comment

This operation is usually simple and straight-forward but there are pitfalls to be avoided. Common errors are, first, to fail to maintain full anatomical reduction while the screw is being inserted; and secondly, to fail to locate the screw correctly. Clearly, perfect reduction is essential if the risk of later osteoarthritis is to be eliminated. A sufficiently good view of the malleolus and of its bed on the main fragment must be gained so that the surgeon may be sure that the fracture surfaces are fitting together accurately.

If the malleolar fragment is large it may be worth while to use two drills. The first, a little way from the centre of the malleolar fragment, is left in position to hold the reduction while the second drill is used to make the definitive track for the screw down the middle of the malleolar fragment. If the fragment is small, however, there is not enough room to allow the use of a temporary stabilising drill, and reliance must be placed on coapting the fracture surfaces by proximal traction upon the malleolar fragment with a sharp bone hook, as described.

It is important that the drill hole for the screw be made down the central axis of the malleolar fragment. Particular care must be taken that it does not encroach upon the articular cartilage of the ankle joint. The correct direction for the screw is nearly vertical (Fig. 529), with only a very slight obliquity towards the outer side. All too often one sees screws that have been inserted too obliquely or that lie too close to the ankle mortise.

INTERNAL FIXATION OF FRACTURE OF LOWER END OF FIBULA

Isolated fractures at or just above the lateral malleolus seldom require internal fixation. The operation is usually undertaken for fibular fractures associated with damage to other components of the ankle joint—often a fracture of the medial malleolus with lateral shift of the talus. Fixation of lower fibular fractures is usually effected by a long screw driven in from below or by a suitable plate held by screws.

It should be noted that in a case of combined fractures of the medial malleolus and lateral malleolus, it is appropriate to fix the lateral malleolar fracture first.

TECHNIQUE
Position of patient. The patient lies in the semi-lateral position with the foot resting on its medial border. A tourniquet may be used on the upper thigh.

Exposure. A vertical skin incision follows the posterior margin of the fibula as far as its distal end, where it turns forwards below the tip of the lateral malleolus. The incision is usually 5 to 8 centimetres long according to the site of fracture. The fracture is exposed to view by removal of blood clot and fibrin and by judicious stripping of periosteum immediately adjacent to the fracture. It is important that this clearance of clot and debris be thorough, so that there is no obstacle to perfect coaptation of the fragments.

Reduction and internal fixation. Reduction of the fracture seldom presents difficulty: it is usually effected by direct pressure over the lower fragment with, if necessary, slight adjustment of the position of the foot to centre the talus in the ankle mortise.

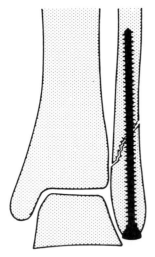

FIG. 530. Use of a long vertical screw for fixation of fracture of lower end of fibula. Fixation of a fractured fibula is seldom undertaken in isolation: it is usually part of a more extensive procedure to stabilise multiple ankle fractures with displacement.

While the reduction is maintained by an assistant, who may press the lower fragment into position with a bone hook, awl or clamp, a small area of bone at the tip of the lateral malleolus is cleared of soft tissue to allow the insertion of a drill. A starting point for the drill should be made with an awl or small gouge. A long drill, equal in diameter to the core diameter of the screw to be used, is driven in to prepare a track for the screw, which should penetrate well proximal to the site of fracture (Fig. 530): a screw 7.5 to 10 centimetres long

is usually required. If a screw of adequate length is not available a threaded slipped epiphysis pin (p. 317) will often serve the purpose well. The screw is driven firmly home, but excessive torque should be avoided lest the soft cancellous bone of the malleolus be entered too deeply by the screw head.

As an alternative to fixation by an internal screw, lateral malleolar fractures may be immobilised by a suitable small plate held by screws. An A.O. plate from the small fragment set, with the small screws designed to match it, is often appropriate. Use of an over-heavy plate, with multiple screws, may hinder union, and is to be deplored.

Closure. Skin sutures only are required.

POST-OPERATIVE MANAGEMENT

After operation the ankle is protected in a below-knee plaster with the foot at 90 degrees. The duration of plaster splintage depends upon other components of the ankle injury. For the fibula alone a period of four to six weeks would be adequate, but associated injuries at the medial or posterior aspect of the joint may demand support for a longer period.

Comment

Since internal fixation of lateral malleolar fractures is usually only part of a wider operation upon the ankle, details of the procedure may have to be modified to meet the problems posed by other components of the injury. For instance, if there is an associated fracture of the posterior articular margin of the tibia (posterior malleolus), the skin incision may be curved further backwards towards the calcaneal tendon so that both fractures may be exposed through the one incision.

INTERNAL FIXATION OF DISPLACED FRACTURE OF POSTERIOR MALLEOLUS

The posterior articular margin of the lower end of the tibia may be displaced slightly upwards in a posterior vertical fracture that enters the joint. The separated fragment of bone—the so-called posterior malleolus—may be displaced upwards through a distance of 1 to 5 millimetres. If the

displaced fragment carries no more than a small part of the articular surface the articulation of the talus with the tibia is not significantly disturbed, and reduction is not required. If the displaced fragment carries a quarter or more of the articular surface, however, accurate replacement of the fragment is necessary; otherwise persistent posterior subluxation of the talus is liable to occur. As pointed out by Perkins (1958), reduction must be perfect: if any step remains the surgeon has failed in his task and the operation might as well not have been attempted (Fig. 533).

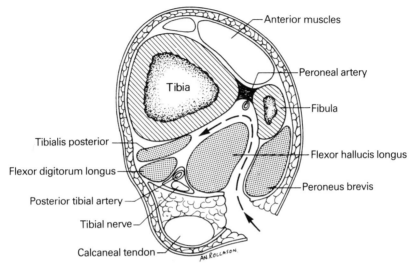

FIG. 531. Exposure of posterior surface of lower tibia. The approach is lateral to the calcaneal tendon, between the flexor hallucis longus and the medial surface of the fibula. Flexor hallucis longus is retracted medially.

TECHNIQUE

Position of patient. The patient lies prone, or in the lateral posture with the affected foot uppermost. A tourniquet may be used on the upper thigh.

Incision. A vertical postero-lateral incision is made between the posterior margin of the fibula and the calcaneal tendon. It may be 6 to 8 centimetres long according to requirements, and its distal limit is about a centimetre above the tip of the lateral malleolus.

Exposure of fracture. In the upper part of the wound the flexor hallucis longus muscle is encountered lying upon the back of the tibia (see p. 42). The muscle is stripped from the bone and displaced medially to reveal the posterior surface of the tibia, which is cleared with an elevator (Fig. 531). The displaced fragment is thus immediately accessible.

Reduction and internal fixation. In most cases there is little comminution and the raw bed where the displaced fragment should lie is easily identified after clearance of blood clot and fibrin. Once any obstructions in the fracture gap have been removed firm downward and forward pressure upon the fragment should restore it to its bed without difficulty.

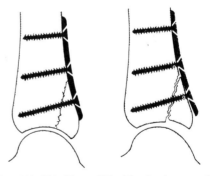

FIGS 532–533. Figure 532—Fixation by curved plate and screws for fracture of posterior articular margin of tibia. Perfect apposition of the fragments is essential. Any residual step in the articular surface (Fig. 533) may lead to persistent subluxation and degenerative arthritis.

Fixation is best effected by a small plate with screws (Miller 1974). The plate should be bent to fit accurately the curved contour of the lower end of the tibia. The plate is held in position while screw holes are drilled and the screws are driven home (Fig. 532). Usually a three-hole plate is appropriate, with two screws proximal to the fracture and one transfixing it. The plate serves to hold the displaced fragment in place rather more effectively than a single screw across the fracture, such as is often used.

The position of the fragments is checked by lateral radiography or by the image intensifier, and if reduction is imperfect the plate must be removed and a fresh start made.

Closure. Usually skin sutures only are required.

POST-OPERATIVE MANAGEMENT

Protection in a below-knee plaster with the ankle held at a right angle is recommended. The plaster should be retained for a total of eight weeks; after the first four weeks weight bearing may be permitted.

Comment

This is a difficult fracture to treat and it is probably the one among all other ankle fractures that is often treated unsuccessfully. The main problem is to gain full anatomical reduction and to hold this while the plate and screws are applied. Miller (1974) described a special clamp designed to press the displaced fragment into position while the plate is secured with screws. Whatever method is used it is vital that the articular surface of the tibia be left smooth: if any step remains, even though it be a small one (Fig. 533), slight persistent subluxation of the ankle is likely to occur and the eventual outcome is osteoarthritis. This is one of the many situations in orthopaedic and fracture surgery in which the perfectionist's approach to the operation is required.

SCREW FIXATION OF LOWER END OF FIBULA TO TIBIA

This operation is undertaken when the inferior tibio-fibular ligament has been ruptured, allowing lateral displacement (diastasis) of the lower end of the fibula and lateral shift of the talus. The principle is to secure the fibula to the tibia by a transverse screw to prevent displacement while the ruptured ligament heals.

TECHNIQUE

Position of patient. The patient lies supine. A large sand-bag is placed under the buttock of the affected side to roll the patient slightly towards the opposite side. A tourniquet may be used on the upper thigh.

Incision. The skin incision, at the lateral side of the ankle, follows a curve convex anteriorly. It begins one centimetre proximal to the tip of the lateral malleolus, arches forwards beyond the anterior border of the fibula, and then curves upwards and backwards to end over the shaft of the fibula 7 or 8 centimetres proximal to the tip of the malleolus (Fig. 534).

Preparation of bones for insertion of screw. The skin flap is retracted posteriorly to reveal the antero-medial border of the fibula and immedi-

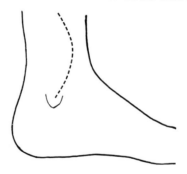

FIG. 534. Screw fixation for diastasis of inferior tibio-fibular joint. The skin incision.

ately medial to this the inferior tibio-fibular joint. In the case of a recent rupture of the interosseous ligament the tissues adjacent to the joint will be found oedematous and thickened, and the lower end of the fibula will be mobile in relation to the tibia. Firm pressure over the lateral malleolus should give full reduction of the tibio-fibular subluxation, and the accuracy of the reduction may be checked by direct inspection.

An assistant maintains the reduction either with a bone hook or with an appropriate clamp while a hole is drilled through the fibula and tibia to receive a screw. The drill track should be almost horizontal and should lie about a centimetre prox-

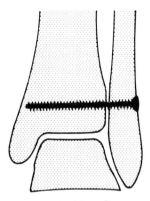

FIG. 535. Position of screw for stabilisation of diastasis of the inferior tibio-fibular joint.

imal to the lower articular surface of the tibia (Fig. 535). Since the tibia lies a little anterior to the fibula the drill should be directed slightly forwards. The drill should just penetrate the medial cortex of the tibia but care must be taken not to drive the drill point on through the skin. The initial drill hole should be equal in diameter to the core diameter of the screw, but the hole in the fibula should then be enlarged sufficiently to allow a sliding fit for the screw, so that the bones will be drawn together as the screw is driven home. Alternatively, a lag screw may be used.

Driving the screw. It is important that a screw of exactly the right length be selected. The depth of the drill track is easily determined with a depth gauge (Fig. 67, p. 55), allowance being made for

slight countersinking of the head of the screw into the lateral cortex of the fibula. The length of the screw should be such that its tip engages the medial cortex of the tibia but does not protrude beneath the skin (Fig. 535). The screw must be driven firmly home while a check is made that the tibio-fibular subluxation is held fully reduced. Excessive force is to be avoided, however, because the outer cortex of the lower fibula at this level is soft and may easily be crushed by the head of the screw.

After the screw has been tightened home its position should be checked with the image intensifier or by radiographs. If the position is found satisfactory the wound is then closed.

POST-OPERATIVE MANAGEMENT

It is recommended that the ankle be protected for about eight weeks in a below-knee plaster holding the foot at a right angle. Weight bearing may usually be permitted after the skin wound has healed, when a new closely fitting walking plaster should be applied.

Comment

The authors believe that the assertion commonly made to the effect that rigid fixation of the inferior tibio-fibular joint by a screw impairs ankle function and that the screw should therefore always be removed is unfounded. The purpose of the screw is to hold the bones together until the interosseous ligament heals. No screw can ever maintain rigidity permanently against a counter-force. The screw will therefore automatically loosen sufficiently to allow what slight tibio-fibular movement is required, and there is no necessity to remove the screw unless it causes local discomfort either on the lateral or on the medial side.

REPAIR OF RUPTURED CALCANEAL TENDON

Although many surgeons now treat ruptures of the calcaneal tendon conservatively (Gillies and Chalmers 1970), there are still those who believe that a rather more certain result is achieved by repairing the tendon, especially in young active individuals.

TECHNIQUE

Position of patient. The patient is usually placed prone, but equally good access is obtained with the patient in the lateral position with the affected limb uppermost. A tourniquet may be used on the upper thigh.

Incision. A vertical incision is placed over the lateral border of the injured tendon. The incision is about 7 to 10 centimetres long, with its lower limit about a centimetre proximal to the insertion of the tendon (Fig. 536).

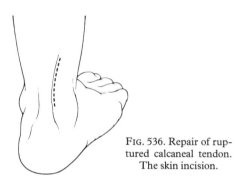

FIG. 536. Repair of ruptured calcaneal tendon. The skin incision.

Defining and repairing the tendon. In ruptures of more than a few hours' duration the paratenon that invests the calcaneal tendon—normally no more than a very flimsy membrane—will be found greatly thickened and oedematous. It must be preserved because it contributes significantly to the healing process. This covering membrane is incised vertically and the edges are separated by holding stitches to reveal the shredded fibres of the calcaneal tendon embedded in blood clot. Blood clot is cleared away and the proximal and distal stumps of the ruptured tendon are defined. Almost invariably the tendon fibres are shredded, so that the repair has been likened to sewing together two horses' tails.

By flexing the knee and plantarflexing the ankle the calf muscles may be relaxed sufficiently to bring the tendon ends easily together without tension. The shredded fibres are "combed out" and laid together end to end: some interdigitation of the ends may be possible in irregular tears but not in incised ones such as those made by broken glass. The tendon ends are repaired by mattress sutures of fine stainless steel wire, the knots being well buried away from the surface. The thickened paratenon is sutured with fine catgut, and after removal of the tourniquet the skin is closed without drainage.

POST-OPERATIVE MANAGEMENT

Wide crepe bandages are applied snugly over copious gauze dressings, with care to fill the hollows behind the malleoli. A light plaster-of-Paris case is then applied from thigh to metatarsal heads with the knee flexed 60 degrees and the ankle plantarflexed 30 degrees. The limb is kept elevated for the first two weeks, though walking with crutches may be allowed immediately for toilet purposes.

After two weeks the initial long plaster is discarded in favour of a below-knee plaster, which again holds the foot plantarflexed 20 or 25 degrees. A high walking heel is added and full weight bearing is encouraged. After a further two weeks a third plaster is applied with the foot held at a right angle.

At the end of six weeks from operation all splintage is discarded and walking in shoes—preferably with a slightly raised heel—is permitted. At this stage gradually increasing exercises are begun, the main object of which is to develop the power of plantarflexion against resistance. These exercises may have to be continued for three or four months if full calf power, permitting the patient to leap off the toes of the affected foot, is to be restored. In the later stages of rehabilitation skipping is perhaps the best exercise. Climbing and descending stairs rather than taking the lift should also be encouraged.

Comment

Complications from repair of a torn calcaneal tendon have been too frequent in the past. Indeed it is largely for this reason that operative repair of the tendon has in many centres been abandoned in favour of conservative management in a walking plaster (Gillies and Chalmers 1970). If due precautions are taken, however, complications should not arise, and suture may still have advantages, especially in young active persons.

The most serious complications have been infection, necrosis of tendon, and sinus formation with discharge of suture material. It should be possible to avoid infection by a delicate technique and by ensuring full haemostasis after the tourniquet has been removed. Furthermore, fancy methods of repair such as intertwining the tendon ends with the plantaris tendon or with a strip of fascia should be avoided: they serve no useful purpose and leave an excessive amount of devitalised tissue in a bed that is poorly vascularised. For this same reason the authors strongly deprecate the use of silk sutures. Often these have led to local necrosis, mild liquefaction and the eventual formation of sinuses through which fragments of silk may be discharged at intervals for months or even years. Sutures of stainless steel wire, or alternatively of absorbable plain catgut, are to be preferred.

Holding the knee flexed in plaster for the first two weeks after operation may be thought an unnecessarily severe precaution, but it effectively relaxes the gastrocnemius muscle and allows the frayed tendon ends to lie in close apposition, eliminating tension on the sutures. Light suture material may thus be used.

Healing of the tendon and of the thickened paratenon may be assumed to be sound enough after six weeks to allow unprotected walking, but resistance exercises should be carefully graduated so that the tendon is spared from the most severe stresses until ten or twelve weeks have elapsed from the time of operation.

Despite an intensive programme of rehabilitation, some wasting of the calf muscles is likely to persist for many months, or even permanently.

TRIMMING OF CALCANEAL TUBEROSITY FOR POST-CALCANEAL BURSA

Permanent relief of post-calcaneal bursa or "winter heel" demands the excision of a substantial piece of bone from the tuberosity of the calcaneus, immediately above the insertion of the calcaneal tendon.

TECHNIQUE

Position of patient. The patient is placed in the lateral position with the affected limb uppermost. The affected foot rests upon its medial border upon a folded towel or sand-bag. A tourniquet may be used on the thickest part of the calf or on the upper thigh.

Incision. A vertical incision about 6 centimetres long is made immediately in front of the lateral margin of the calcaneal tendon. Its upper end is level with the prominence of the lateral malleolus. The lower end is prolonged downwards over the lateral aspect of the calcaneus to a point one or two centimetres distal to the insertion of the calcaneal tendon (Fig. 537).

Exposure of postero-superior corner of calcaneal tuberosity. The skin edges are retracted to allow

dissection deep to the calcaneal tendon just above its insertion. Fat is cut away or reflected until the superior surface of the calcaneal tuberosity is well exposed. It is next necessary to separate the lower part of the calcaneal tendon from the posterior

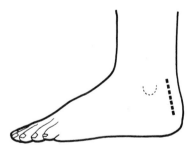

Fig. 537. Trimming of calcaneal tuberosity. The skin incision.

surface of the tuberosity without impairing the continuity of the tendon. This separation is best done by sharp dissection with a fine-bladed knife, the cutting edge being kept always close to the bone. It is well to continue this sharp separation of tendon from bone over about half the area of the tendinous insertion (Fig. 538). This may be done without fear of disrupting the continuity of the tendon fibres, for they are continuous with the aponeurosis that sheaths the back of the calcaneus and is prolonged forwards as the plantar aponeurosis. The aim should be to denude the uppermost 10 to 15 millimetres of the posterior surface of the calcaneal tuberosity.

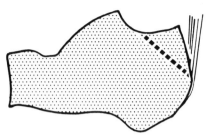

FIG. 538. Trimming of calcaneus for posterior bursitis. Broken line shows amount of bone to be removed. Note that the anterior fibres of the calcaneal tendon have been detached from the bone to allow the line of osteotomy to emerge well down on the back of the calcaneal tuberosity.

Removal of triangular fragment of bone. While the calcaneal tendon is retracted posteriorly the postero-superior corner of the calcaneal tuberosity is separated cleanly with a thin osteotome. The excision should be generous, as shown in Figure 538. When the fragment has been removed the cut surface of the calcaneus is examined to make sure that no projecting spurs of bone remain.

Closure. Provided full haemostasis is secured after the tourniquet has been removed it is sufficient to suture the skin alone, preferably with everting mattress sutures.

POST-OPERATIVE MANAGEMENT

Copious gauze dressings are applied to fill the concavities about the ankle and heel and held in place with a crepe bandage. In the interests of comfort it is advisable to apply a well padded below-knee plaster and to retain this for the first two weeks. The leg should be kept elevated for much of each day, though the patient may be allowed up for toilet purposes. After the plaster and sutures have been removed at the end of the second week, ankle and foot exercises are encouraged to restore full mobility.

Comment

The commonest mistake in the performance of this operation is to remove too little bone. If only a few shavings are taken from the posterior aspect of the calcaneus the operation is likely to be unsuccessful in eliminating the bursitis. The key to success is to strip part of the actual insertion of the calcaneal tendon and then to remove a large triangle of bone, the apex of which extends well down on the tuberosity. This radical excision has no adverse effect and it ensures the full relief of symptoms.

ELONGATION OF CALCANEAL TENDON

The calcaneal tendon may be lengthened by a Z-cut technique, with the longitudinal split of the tendon either in the coronal or in the sagittal plane. Unless it is intended that the line of pull be shifted towards the lateral or the medial side (as for instance in talipes equino-varus: see p. 424) the authors prefer to split the tendon in the coronal plane, and this is the method to be described.

TECHNIQUE

Position of patient. The patient may be placed prone, or in the lateral position with the affected limb uppermost. A thigh tourniquet may be used.

Incision. A vertical incision is made adjacent to the lateral border of the calcaneal tendon. It extends proximally from the level of the insertion of the tendon for a distance equal to about one fifth of the length of the calf (Fig. 539).

Division of tendon. The calcaneal tendon is defined by stripping away paratenon and fatty tissue by blunt dissection. The clearance should

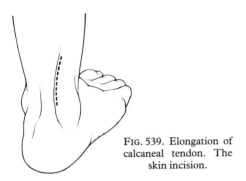

FIG. 539. Elongation of calcaneal tendon. The skin incision.

extend proximally almost to the musculo-tendinous junction, and distally as far as the insertion of the tendon.

While the tendon is steadied by an assistant, the fibres are split midway between the front and back

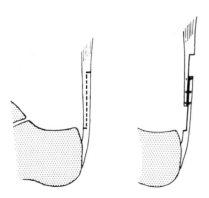

FIG. 540. Technique of lengthening the calcaneal tendon. The tendon is split by a Z-cut in the coronal plane and re-united after appropriate lengthening has been gained by dorsiflexion of the ankle.

by a knife inserted in the coronal plane at the distal end of the tendon and carefully worked proximally as the fibres are split. The length of the longitudinal split will depend upon the size of the

patient, but it should be long enough to allow overlap of the ends by at least 1 centimetre in small children and 3 centimetres in adults, with the ankle in the right-angled position. When the longitudinal split has been completed over a sufficient length the posterior half of the tendon is divided at the proximal end of the split and the anterior half is divided at the distal end of the split, near the insertion of the tendon (Fig. 540).

Repair. With the foot held in the right-angled position the severed proximal and distal ends of the tendon are drawn respecively distally and proximally with mosquito forceps and held in moderate tension while interrupted sutures of fine catgut are inserted at the medial and lateral edges of the tendon. The paratenon is pulled together over the tendon and the skin is closed with interrupted everting mattress sutures.

POST-OPERATIVE MANAGEMENT

A crepe bandage is applied snugly over copious gauze dressings and over this a light plaster-of-Paris case is applied with the ankle at 90 degrees. The initial plaster is changed after one or two weeks according to the age of the patient, and thereafter walking is permitted in the plaster, which should be retained for four weeks in children and seven or eight weeks in adolescents and adults.

Comment

This simple operation demands care especially in two respects. First, it is easy to over-lengthen the tendon, with the consequence that spring-off by calf action is impaired. As a rule the foot should not be dorsiflexed above the right angle during repair of the tendon with moderate tension. Secondly, silk sutures should be avoided in favour of absorbable material. A cellular reaction and persistent discharge from small sinuses are all too frequent after the use of silk sutures in this relatively avascular area.

RELEASE OF TIGHT MEDIAL STRUCTURES FOR CONGENITAL TALIPES EQUINO-VARUS

This operation aims to divide or elongate all those tissues at the back and medial side of the ankle and foot that may be preventing the foot from assuming the plantigrade position. These structures include the calcaneal tendon, the tendons of tibialis posterior, flexor digitorum longus and flexor hallucis longus, and the capsular ligaments of the subtalar, talo-navicular and calcaneo-cuboid joints. The technique to be described is basically that of Clark (1968). Typically the operation is done in infants 2 to 4 months old, and it is to this type of case that the following description relates. Similar principles apply, however, if the operation is undertaken in somewhat older children.

TECHNIQUE

Position of patient. The patient is placed in the lateral semi-prone position with the affected limb next to the table. The unaffected limb is held forwards out of the way so that the affected foot, lying upon its lateral border, is presented medial side upwards. A miniature tourniquet cuff may be applied to the upper thigh but should be inflated only just beyond the arterial pressure.

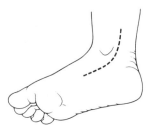

FIG. 541. Medial release for talipes equino-varus. The skin incision.

Incision. A curved medial incision is made with its convexity downwards and backwards. The upper part of the incision is disposed vertically in the lower third of the calf, lying between the medial malleolus and the calcaneal tendon but closer to the tendon. Passing distally below the level of the tip of the medial malleolus, the incision curves forwards on the medial border of the foot to extend half way along its length (Fig. 541).

The deep exposure. The incision is developed first in its upper half—that is, in the lower part of the calf—where the deep fascia is divided to reveal the postero-medial tendons and the neurovascular bundle. Behind the medial malleolus these structures lie in the following order from before backwards: tibialis posterior, flexor digitorum longus, posterior tibial artery with accompanying veins, tibial nerve, flexor hallucis longus. Each structure is defined by cautious dissection, and the neurovascular bundle may be retracted backwards with a loop of tape (Fig. 56, p. 48).

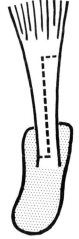

FIG. 542. Z-incision of calcaneal tendon for lengthening. The lateral half remains attached to the calcaneus: the new line of pull thus helps to counteract the inversion deformity.

Attention is next turned to the anterior part of the incision, where the artery and the nerve, which divides here into the medial and lateral plantar nerves, may be identified as they enter the sole of the foot distal to the medial retinaculum. The distal extensions of the three tendons should also be identified. While the vessels and nerves are held out of harm's way the bulk of the tissues of the sole is separated from the osseo-ligamentous framework by sharp dissection, as described below.

Elongation of tendons. The calcaneal tendon is divided in Z-cut fashion. The vertical part of the incision splits the tendinous fibres in the midline. At the lower end of this vertical incision the medial half of the calcaneal tendon is separated from the bone by a horizontal cut. At the upper end of the incision, near the musculo-tendinous junction, the lateral half of the tendon is likewise severed (Fig. 542).

Similar Z-cut divisions are made of the tendons of the tibialis posterior, the flexor digitorum longus and the flexor hallucis longus if they seem tight. The distal ends of these tendons may be temporarily withdrawn into the foot to facilitate the subsequent stages of the operation.

Division of ligaments and joint capsules. Since in talipes equino-varus the navicular bone is subluxated medially upon the head of the talus (this is the most notable feature of the pathological anatomy) it is necessary to divide all the medial and inferior ligaments of the talo-navicular joint in order to allow replacement of the navicular bone in its proper relationship to the head of the talus. Furthermore, it is necessary to divide the medial ligaments of the talo-calcaneal (subtalar) joint in order to allow the heel to be set in normal relationship with the talus. The navicular bone (wholly cartilaginous in small infants) is easily identified by following the tendon of tibialis posterior as far as its insertion into it. After opening the talo-navicular joint the surgeon may then work backwards to identify and open the subtalar joint throughout its length. Attention is next directed towards the more lateral part of the sole of the foot, where the soft tissues and capsule on the lateral side of the neck of the talus are divided and the calcaneo-cuboid joint is opened.

Re-alignment of foot. With the subtalar and midtarsal joints thus freed at the medial and plantar aspects it is now possible to realign the forefoot and heel upon the talus, with full correction of the inversion and equinus deformity. In difficult cases it may be advantageous to fix the bones in the correctly aligned position by transfixing them with a Kirschner wire.

Repair of tendons. The distal ends of the tibialis posterior, flexor digitorum longus and flexor hallucis longus tendons are threaded back through the medial retinaculum and reunited to the proximal stumps with appropriate lengthening, which has been allowed for in the Z-cut divisions of the

tendons. The cut ends of the calcaneal tendon are likewise united with appropriate lengthening to allow the foot to rest in the plantigrade position.

Closure. When full haemostasis has been secured after release of the tourniquet only the skin edges require repair. Interrupted eversion mattress sutures are recommended because there is sometimes a little difficulty in approximating the wound edges.

POST-OPERATIVE MANAGEMENT

It is best not to attempt to hold the foot in the fully corrected position in the immediate post-operative period. Attempts to do so may lead to delayed healing of the skin from tension upon the sutures. After gauze and crepe bandages have been applied, therefore, the foot is supported by a light posterior and plantar plaster splint in the position that it assumes at rest. Two weeks later, or as soon after that as the skin wound is soundly healed, the leg and foot are re-splinted in the fully corrected position. This definitive plaster, renewed as often as is necessary, is retained until three months from the time of operation.

Comment

If complete correction of the inversion deformity is to be gained the essential requirement is that all those structures at the medial side of the foot that help to tether it in the position of deformity must be divided or elongated. It is important to expose thoroughly the ligaments of the subtalar and midtarsal joints. Until these are divided, together with the joint capsules, it is not possible to realign the tarsal bones in their normal relationships. It is particularly important to ensure that the navicular bone is moved forwards from its subluxated position to lie directly in front of the head of the talus.

Elongation of the calcaneal tendon in the manner described, with separation of the medial half of the tendon from the calcaneus, transfers the line of pull to the lateral half of the tendon. Any invertor action of the tendon is thus changed to an evertor action which may help to maintain correction of the heel deformity.

As already noted, skin healing may present a problem because correction of the inversion deformity means that the skin on the medial side of the foot inevitably becomes taut. Skin necrosis is liable to occur if the foot is immobilised after operation in the fully corrected position. If a little inversion is allowed until the skin is well healed, the risk of breakdown of the wound with consequent granulation and rigid scarring is reduced, with a better prospect of a supple foot.

TENDON TRANSFER: TIBIALIS POSTERIOR TO DORSUM OF FOOT

This operation is appropriate both to children and to adults. In children it is usually performed for incompletely corrected talipes equino-varus. The principle is to detach the tendon of the tibialis posterior from its normal insertion, to re-route it between the two bones of the leg and then to reinsert it near the lateral side of the dorsum of the foot.

TECHNIQUE

Position of patient. The patient lies supine. A tourniquet may be used on the upper thigh.

Incisions. Four separate incisions are used—one medial, one posterior and two anterior (Fig. 543). These will be described in the relevant subsections that follow.

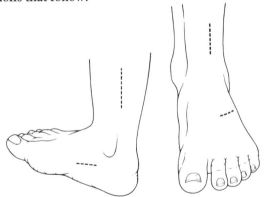

FIG. 543. Tibialis posterior transfer. The skin incisions.

Isolation and detachment of tibialis posterior tendon. The first incision extends backwards from the prominence of the navicular bone for 2 or 3 centimetres, according to the size of the patient (Fig. 543). Through this incision the tibialis posterior tendon is identified as it runs forward from below the medial malleolus to gain insertion into the navicular bone and adjacent tissues. The tendon is cleaned to define its edges and divided close to its insertion. The tendon is then freed proximally as far as the incision allows.

Withdrawal of tendon at calf. The second incision, about 3 to 6 centimetres long according to the size of the patient, is a vertical one in the calf, a centimetre behind the medial border of the tibia (Fig. 543). Its centre is at the junction of the lowest quarter and the proximal three-quarters of the leg. Deep fascia is incised in the line of the incision to open the postero-medial compartment of the leg. The tendon of the tibialis posterior is identified as it lies deep in the compartment, close to the tibia and in front of the flexor digitorum longus. The identity of the tendon is confirmed by pulling upon the divided end of the tendon through the distal incision below the medial malleolus. When its identity has been confirmed the tendon is pulled up through the second incision and delivered from the wound.

Re-routing of tendon. The third incision, of similar length to the second, is a vertical one at the antero-lateral aspect of the lower leg, over the gap between the tibia and the fibula (Fig. 543). Its distal end extends down to about the level where the shaft of the fibula flares out to form the lateral malleolus. The deep fascia is opened. A long artery forceps is now thrust from the second incision behind the tibia, through the interosseous membrane, to emerge from the third incision lateral to the tibialis anterior tendon. The track thus formed in the interosseous space is enlarged by repeatedly opening the artery forceps within it, so that finally the forceps slides freely between the two incisions. The free end of the tibialis posterior tendon is then passed through the interosseous track to emerge through the third incision.

Re-insertion of tendon. The fourth and final incision is made transversely across the antero-lateral aspect of the dorsum of the foot at the level of the base of the fifth metatarsal. It is long enough to extend approximately from the third metatarsal to the fifth metatarsal (Fig. 543). The incision is deepened to expose the lateral tendon of extensor digitorum longus and that of peroneus tertius. The peroneus tertius tendon is cleaned so that its edges are clearly defined. From the third incision—that over the antero-lateral aspect of the lower leg—a long artery forceps is thrust subcutaneously to emerge from the fourth incision. The track is widened by opening the forceps within it, and the free end of the tibialis posterior tendon is passed down through the track and brought out through the fourth incision.

It remains now to suture the free end of the tibialis posterior tendon to the tendon of peroneus tertius. The junction should be made with the ankle dorsiflexed a little above the right angle and with the tibialis posterior tendon drawn down fairly taut. The junction is made by the interlacing technique (see p. 98), the interlaced tendons being sewn through with fine stainless steel wire.

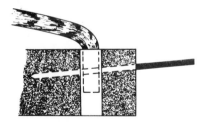

FIG. 544. A technique of attaching the transferred tibialis posterior tendon to the cuboid bone. The tendon is drawn into a drill hole and transfixed within the bone by a fine Kirschner wire.

If the peroneus tertius tendon is considered unsuitable as an anchorage for the tibialis posterior, the transferred tendon may be attached as an alternative to the cuboid bone. First a drill hole 4 millimetres in diameter is made in the dorsum of the cuboid to receive the tendon. The hole should be at right angles to the surface, and should penetrate right through the bone to the plantar surface. A loop of strong nylon or thread is then passed through the transferred tendon close to the cut

end, and by means of a straight needle at each end the thread is passed through the drill hole and out through the soft tissues to emerge through the skin of the sole. Tension upon the thread draws the tendon into the drill hole. When the tension has been correctly adjusted, the tendon where it lies in the drill hole in the cuboid bone is transfixed from the side by a fine Kirschner wire, which is then cut off to leave about 5 millimetres projecting from the bone to facilitate its subsequent removal (Fig. 544). The tendon is further anchored by sutures of fine stainless steel wire through periosteum and adjacent soft tissues at the point where the tendon enters the bone. The holding stitch in the sole is then removed.

Closure. The various wounds are closed without drainage.

POST-OPERATIVE MANAGEMENT

A below-knee plaster is applied. After two weeks the plaster is changed for a below-knee walking plaster and at the same time the sutures are removed. The second plaster is retained until the end of the fourth week from operation. If a Kirschner wire has been used to anchor the tendon it may then be removed. Thereafter active mobilising exercises are practised.

Comment

It is not always easy to obtain sufficient length of the tibialis posterior tendon to allow easy suture at the new point of insertion. In the first stage of the operation the tendon must therefore be severed as far distally as possible. It is wise even to take a small strip of periosteum continuous with the tendon where it joins the tuberosity of the navicular bone.

The second important point is that the tendon should be re-routed in as straight a line as possible from the postero-medial compartment of the leg through the interosseous membrane to the antero-lateral aspect of the dorsum of the foot: any sharp angulation should be avoided. It is necessary also to ensure that the tendon glides freely through the interosseous tunnel created for it; in other words, to ensure that the tunnel is wide enough.

The final point is that the tendon must be anchored firmly at its new insertion, under moderate tension. Considerable care is required to ensure a firm junction, whether this be with the peroneus tertius tendon or with the cuboid bone.

TENDON TRANSFER: TIBIALIS ANTERIOR TO OUTER SIDE OF FOOT

This operation, carried out usually for mobile inversion deformity, is appropriate both to children and to adults. It is wise not to transfer the tendon too far laterally, because it is possible in this way to cause over-correction of the deformity. Usually it is appropriate to implant the transferred tendon into the cuboid bone just proximal to the fourth tarso- metatarsal joint.

TECHNIQUE

Position of patient. The patient lies supine. A tourniquet may be used on the upper thigh.

Incisions. Three incisions are required (Fig. 545). The first incision follows the line of the tibialis anterior from the level of the ankle joint to the medial aspect of the base of the first metatarsal. The second incision, in the lowest third of the leg, follows the lateral margin of the anterior crest of the tibia, extending distally as far as the supra-malleolar level. The third incision extends proximally from the proximal part of the shaft of the fourth metatarsal nearly to the ankle level.

Mobilisation of tibialis anterior tendon. Through the first incision the tendon of the tibialis anterior is defined and separated from its insertion at the base of the first metatarsal. Subsidiary attachments to adjacent tissues are severed and the tendon is mobilised proximally as far as the anterior retinaculum of the ankle.

Through the second incision in the lower part of the leg the tendon of the tibialis anterior is identified where it lies close to the lateral border of the tibia. It is freed distally as far down as the retinaculum, and the distal end of the tendon is then pulled up through the retinaculum and delivered out of the upper wound.

Re-routing and re-insertion of tendon. With blunt dissecting scissors a subcutaneous tunnel is made from the upper wound to emerge in the third incision over the outer side of the dorsum of the foot. The tunnel passes superficially to the extensor retinaculum. A long haemostat is then passed proximally along the tunnel from the distal wound to emerge in the leg wound: with this the end of the mobilised tendon is drawn through the tunnel and brought out through the lateral foot incision.

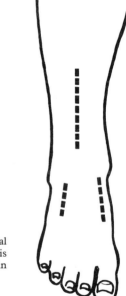

FIG. 545. Lateral transfer of tibialis anterior. The skin incisions.

The part of the cuboid bone that is adjacent to the base of the fourth metatarsal is exposed by sharp dissection and a small area of bone where the tendon is to be re-implanted is bared. A vertical tunnel is then drilled through the bone, and the tendon is drawn into the hole by a stitch passed through the sole, and anchored in the manner described in the previous section (p. 427). Tension is correct when with the ankle and foot dorsiflexed the implanted tendon shows no slack: it is a mistake to draw it excessively taut.

Closure. Each wound is closed with interrupted skin sutures.

POST-OPERATIVE MANAGEMENT

A well padded below-knee plaster is applied with the foot in moderate dorsiflexion and eversion. After two weeks in an adult, or earlier in a child, the sutures are removed and a new below-knee walking plaster is applied. The plaster is discarded four weeks from the time of operation. At that time, if a Kirschner wire has been used to transfix the tendon in its tunnel it is removed under local anaesthesia. Thereafter a course of mobilising and muscle-strengthening exercises is arranged.

Comment

As with other tendon transfers, an important key to success lies in handling the tendon gently and mobilising it cleanly without traumatising the surface. In re-routing the tendon to its new insertion the surgeon must ensure that it runs in a straight line through the new subcutaneous tunnel. Difficulty is sometimes experienced in judging the correct tension under which to suture the tendon at its new insertion. Provided the foot and ankle are fully dorsiflexed there is no need to draw the tendon as taut as possible. It may be anchored with just sufficient tension to ensure that all slack is taken up.

WEDGE OSTEOTOMY OF CALCANEUS FOR INVERTED HEEL

This operation, described by Dwyer in 1963, aims to correct inversion of the heel, such as may be found in relapsed club foot, by dividing the calcaneus obliquely from above downwards and forwards, angling the bone to bring the tip of the heel into the line of weight bearing, and inserting a wedge-shaped bone graft in the medial gap thus opened up. The patient is usually a child under 10.

TECHNIQUE

Position of patient. The patient lies prone with the affected foot resting upon a firm sand-bag. A tourniquet may be used on the upper thigh.

Incision. The incision extends vertically downwards parallel with the medial margin of the calcaneal tendon, as far as its insertion. It then curves forwards to cross the inner side of the heel obliquely, to end at the medial border of the foot just behind the mid-tarsal joint (Fig. 546).

Z-cut division of calcaneal tendon. The calcaneal tendon is cleared down to its insertion and is split vertically into two equal halves in the sagittal plane (Fig. 547). The medial half of the tendon is detached from its insertion into the calcaneus and turned upwards. The lateral half is divided higher up, close to the musculo-tendinous junction, and turned distally.

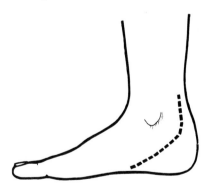

Fig. 546. Wedge osteotomy of calcaneus.
The skin incision.

Exposure of calcaneus. With the calcaneal tendon thus reflected out of the way the superior surface of the tuberosity of the calcaneus is easily exposed by removal of fatty tissue. At this stage the tendons, vessels and nerve lying behind the medial malleolus are identified and protected. The distal half of the incision is then opened up, with care to reflect the deeper tissues with the skin rather than turning aside flaps of skin alone. In

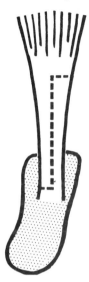

FIG. 547. Z-cut division of tendon allows elongation during repair.

exposing the medial surface of the calcaneus the surgeon may follow the line of the flexor hallucis longus tendon, with care to preserve the neurovascular bundle. Fascia is cleared from the medial aspect of the bone and from the plantar surface.

The osteotomy. The calcaneus is divided with an osteotome just below the line of the flexor hallucis

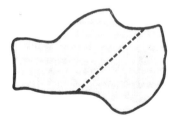

FIG. 548. Diagram showing the line of osteotomy of the calcaneus.

longus tendon and parallel with it (Fig. 548). The bone is divided right through, but the lateral periosteum is left intact to serve as a hinge.

Correcting the varus deformity. An awl or guide wire is thrust into the lower (posterior) fragment of the calcaneus from below and is used to lever

the bone laterally so that a wedge-shaped gap is opened up at the site of osteotomy, with the base medially. Correction should be sufficient to bring the under-surface of the heel directly into the line of weight bearing.

Insertion of bone wedge. Through a separate incision over the upper end of the tibia a wedge-shaped piece of bone of appropriate dimensions is removed. The graft is carefully tailored to fit snugly into the wedge-shaped gap in the calcaneus (Fig. 549). After insertion it is driven home with a punch.

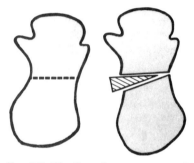

FIG. 549. The line of osteotomy seen in the axial plane, and (*right*) insertion of wedge-shaped bone graft to maintain the lateral tilt of the heel.

Repair of calcaneal tendon with elongation. The flaps of calcaneal tendon are approximated and the two halves are sutured with sufficient elongation of the tendon to allow the foot to be dorsiflexed a little beyond the right angle.

Closure. It is important to suture the skin carefully because the opening up of the calcaneus and the consequent lengthening of the inner side of the heel make closure difficult. Suture under some tension is often unavoidable.

POST-OPERATIVE MANAGEMENT

A below-knee plaster is applied over copious dressings with the ankle at 90 degrees. After two weeks the sutures are removed and a new, closer-fitting plaster is applied. Delay in wound healing, which is not uncommon if the wound has been sutured under tension, may necessitate further changes of plaster, with wound dressing as required. The plaster must usually be retained for about eight to ten weeks, depending upon the age of the child. After the first four weeks walking in the plaster may be permitted.

Comment

In this operation calcaneal osteotomy to correct excessive varus of the heel is combined with any necessary lengthening of the calcaneal tendon to allow good dorsiflexion of the foot. In addition, splitting of the calcaneal tendon with detachment of the medial half from its insertion into the calcaneus causes the line of pull of the calf muscles to

be transferred towards the lateral side of the heel, for calf action is now transmitted only through the intact lateral half of the tendon (Fig. 547).

Opening of the medial side of the calcaneal osteotomy increases the height of the heel as well as bringing the under surface of the calcaneus directly under the line of weight bearing. There is the penalty, however, that skin is relatively short at the medial side of the heel, with the consequence that wound closure may be difficult, and primary healing is not always obtained. Special care is therefore required in the handling of the skin flaps and in suturing the edges.

CALCANEO-CUBOID ARTHRODESIS FOR PERSISTENT EQUINO-VARUS DEFORMITY

This operation was described by Dillwyn Evans in 1961 for the correction of residual varus and inversion deformity of the foot in children of about 4 to 8 years of age. The operation is designed to shorten the lateral pillar of the foot and thus to allow the navicular bone to assume a more normal relationship with the head of the

side to roll the patient slightly towards the opposite side. A tourniquet may be used on the upper thigh.

The medial incision. The medial incision extends proximally in the line of the tibialis posterior tendon from a point just in front of the tuberosity

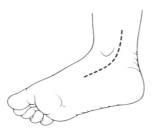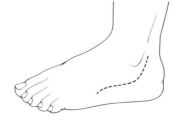

FIG. 550. The medial and lateral incisions for Dillwyn Evans's operation.

talus, so that the first metatarsal is brought into line with the long axis of the talus. The operation on the bones is combined with release of tight soft tissues at the medial border of the foot and behind the ankle. Before it is undertaken, as much correction of the deformity as is possible should have been obtained by serial plasters, each applied in such a way as to maintain the fullest possible correction of the deformity.

TECHNIQUE

Position of patient. The patient lies supine with a firm sand-bag under the buttock of the affected

of the navicular bone to sweep upwards beneath and behind the medial malleolus, thence following the antero-medial margin of the calcaneal tendon for 5 to 8 centimetres (Fig. 550).

The lateral incision. The lateral incision, slightly serpentine, begins on the lateral border of the foot at about the level of the base of the fifth metatarsal and extends proximally in the line of the peroneus brevis tendon to end a little below and behind the tip of the lateral malleolus (Fig. 550).

The medial dissection. Through the medial incision tight ligamentous structures that are tethering the foot in the deformed position are divided or excised, tight tendons are lengthened and the capsule of the talo-navicular joint is opened widely. This dissection is similar to that described on page 424 for much younger children.

Attention is first directed to the tibialis posterior tendon, which should be defined and freed as far forwards as its insertion into the navicular bone. The tendon is then divided by a long Z-cut to allow later suture with lengthening. For the moment the divided ends of the tendon are reflected to allow free access to the talo-navicular joint. Excess fibrous tissue is cut away and the joint is opened freely on the superior, medial and inferior aspects by division of the capsule. This will allow the navicular bone to slide forwards and laterally upon the head of the talus into a more normal relationship.

Attention is next directed to the proximal part of the incision, where the calcaneal tendon is exposed and divided by a long Z-cut to allow subsequent suture with lengthening (see p. 424). This should allow some improvement in the equinus deformity, but if it is still impossible to bring the foot up to the right angle it is necessary to divide the posterior part of the capsule of the ankle joint to enable this to be done. Repair of the divided tendons with elongation should be deferred until the operation on the lateral side of the foot has been completed.

Excision of calcaneo-cuboid joint. Through the lateral incision the calcaneo-cuboid joint is exposed and the capsule is cut away. The objective now is to excise the joint by a wedge-shaped cut with removal of just sufficient bone to allow the deformity to be fully corrected and the foot placed in the neutral position, the forefoot hingeing upon the hind foot at the talo-navicular joint (Fig. 551).

Much care is required to excise a wedge of bone, including the joint, of exactly the right dimensions. The base of the wedge is predominantly lateral, but it should be placed towards the dorsal aspect if there is an element of cavus deformity or towards the plantar aspect if the sole is convex (rocker-bottom foot). When the appropriate wedge has been excised and the raw surfaces of the calcaneus and cuboid have been brought together

the position is fixed by two staples bridging the site of osteotomy.

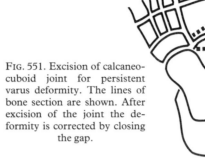

Fig. 551. Excision of calcaneo-cuboid joint for persistent varus deformity. The lines of bone section are shown. After excision of the joint the deformity is corrected by closing the gap.

Closure. When the deformity has been thus corrected and the position stabilised by internal fixation with staples, attention may be turned again to the medial incision, where the amount of lengthening that is required in the tendon of tibialis posterior and in the calcaneal tendon can now be ascertained. The tendons are repaired by side-to-side suture with the appropriate amount of lengthening. Both incisions are then closed by interrupted sutures without drainage.

POST-OPERATIVE MANAGEMENT

A crepe bandage is applied with moderate tension over copious gauze dressings. Plaster splintage is required, but because of the risk of swelling in the first few days a complete encircling plaster is not recommended. Instead, a plaster back splint only may be applied, or an encircling plaster may be put on and immediately divided through its length on its medial and lateral aspects.

After two weeks the skin sutures are removed and a closely fitting below-knee plaster is applied. Provided full healing of the skin has been secured a walking heel may be added and weight-bearing in the plaster encouraged. Immobilisation in plaster should be continued for two to three months according to the age of the patient.

Comment

There are three essentials for success from this operation. First, it is important that the medial border of the foot be thoroughly mobilised by excision of the scarred ligamentous tissues, by elongation of tight tendons, and by thorough opening up of the talo-navicular joint. Only if this is done is it possible for the navicular bone to glide forwards and laterally upon the head of the talus, and this is an essential prerequisite for full correction of the deformity.

Secondly, it is essential that equinus deformity be sufficiently corrected to allow the ankle to be placed at least at a right angle, and preferably in a little dorsiflexion beyond this. Division of the calcaneal tendon may not give sufficient release, and it may be necessary to divide the posterior part of the capsule of the ankle joint freely.

Thirdly, the size of the wedge of bone that is to be removed at the lateral side of the foot, and which must include the calcaneo-cuboid joint, is critical. Removal of too large a wedge can result in over-correction of the deformity, whereas removal of insufficient bone gives incomplete correction. It is important also to correct excessive concavity or convexity of the sole by appropriate positioning of the base of the wedge, and to overcome any rotational deformity so that the foot is plantigrade. Determination of the exact amount of bone to be removed is a matter of precise judgement. If there is doubt it is best to err on the side of removing too little bone, and then to see how the foot lies when the raw surfaces are brought together. If correction is incomplete further bone may have to be removed. Fixation by staples ensures accurate apposition and thus obviates the need for a close-fitting plaster in the early days after operation.

TRIPLE ARTHRODESIS OF TARSAL JOINTS

(COMBINED SUBTALAR AND MID-TARSAL ARTHRODESIS)

This operation aims to fuse the subtalar joint, the calcaneo-cuboid joint and the talo-navicular joint: hence the term triple fusion.

TECHNIQUE

Position of patient. The patient lies supine, slightly rolled towards the opposite side by a large sand-bag under the buttock of the affected side. A tourniquet may be used on the thickest part of the calf or on the upper thigh.

Incision. The incision extends obliquely forwards and medially across the dorsum of the foot from a point 3 to 4 centimetres distal to the tip of the lateral malleolus, ending about a centimetre proximal to the base of the first metatarsal (Fig. 552). Skin-thickness flaps are not reflected: instead the cut is made straight through the deep tissues, which are dissected from the bones and reflected with the skin. This is important because skin-thickness flaps in this area are liable to slough at the edges. At the dorsum of the foot care must be taken to preserve the extensor tendons of the toes, which cross the line of incision near its

anterior end. The tendons should be mobilised and retracted medially.

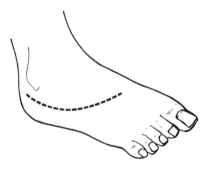

FIG. 552. Skin incision for triple tarsal arthrodesis.

Exposure of joints. By dissection of the deep tissues from the bones on either side of the incision the outer sides of the calcaneus and talus, with the subtalar joint between them, are exposed in the posterior half of the incision. More anteriorly the dissection reveals the lateral end of the sinus tarsi, the contiguous superior surfaces of the front of the calcaneus and of the cuboid bone, and further medially the talo-navicular joint.

The field is thus clear for the essential part of the operation—namely the clearance of all articular cartilage from the subtalar, calcaneo-cuboid and talo-navicular joints (Fig. 553). This is best done with thin chisels and osteotomes. Cartilage and subchondral bone should be sliced off thinly, parallel to the joint surface, to expose the underlying cancellous bone. This decortication should extend right through to the medial side of the foot so that a slice of even thickness is removed from the whole area of the three joints concerned.

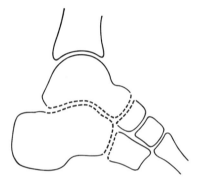

FIG. 553. Triple arthrodesis. The extent of the denudation of the joints is shown by the interrupted lines.

Coaptation and internal fixation. The raw cancellous surfaces are now pressed together: if they do not fit well, further slices of bone may have to be removed selectively to enable them to do so; and to ensure more intimate bone-to-bone contact the raw surfaces may be roughened by multiple small cuts with the osteotome.

Contact between the raw surfaces is maintained by inserting staples across the joints, usually one each for the talo-navicular, calcaneo-cuboid and subtalar joints. (For technique of stapling, see p. 64.)

Closure. Deep interrupted skin sutures are usually all that are required. Drainage of the wound is not recommended.

POST-OPERATIVE MANAGEMENT

A crepe bandage is applied over copious gauze dressings with only light tension. Over this it is wise to wrap a thick layer of surgical cotton (cotton wool) as a lining for a below-knee plaster. To forestall any constriction from swelling within the plaster it is wise to split the plaster right through longitudinally immediately after its application: close protection by a plaster is not essential at this stage if adequate fixation by staples has been secured.

The plaster is changed at two weeks, when a close-fitting below-knee plaster is applied. Thereafter the patient walks with crutches, avoiding weight bearing until the end of the fifth week, when a walking heel is added. Protection by plaster-of-Paris is usually continued for eight to ten weeks, depending upon the radiological progress towards union.

TRIPLE FUSION WITH ANTERO-LATERAL WEDGE TARSECTOMY

This operation is used for the correction of fixed varus deformity of the foot, usually a consequence of talipes equino-varus that has been incompletely corrected. The operation differs from that just described only in that an appropriate wedge of bone is removed in order to bring the foot into a plantigrade position. The wedge to be removed is based antero-laterally. The wedge includes the articular cartilage of the related joints. When a wedge of appropriate size has been excised the gap is closed, thus correcting the deformity. At this stage a careful clinical check is made of the appearance of the foot to ensure that a good plantigrade position has been gained. If this is confirmed staples are inserted as already described.

TRIPLE FUSION WITH ANTERIOR WEDGE TARSECTOMY (LAMBRINUDI'S OPERATION)

The operation to be described is based on that reported by Lambrinudi (1927, 1933) for paralysis of the extensor (dorsiflexor) muscles of the foot and consequent drop-foot. Essentially it is a triple arthrodesis (see p. 433) combined with excision of a wedge of bone, with its base directed anteriorly, from the talo-calcaneal complex (Fig. 554). The wedge is taken largely at the expense of the talus but partly also of the calcaneus, and it includes the subtalar joint.

PRELIMINARY STUDIES

It is important to determine accurately the size of the wedge that is to be removed from the tarsus. First it is necessary to obtain a true lateral radiograph of the ankle and foot with the foot in full equinus. Upon the radiograph lines are drawn to indicate the size of wedge that must be removed in order to bring the foot up to an acceptable position

aspect of the talus and on the superior aspect of the calcaneus. The apex of the bone wedge is at the back of the subtalar joint. Anteriorly the wedge emerges into the midtarsal joint, the cartilaginous surfaces of which are excised (Fig. 554).

When the wedge-shaped gap is closed by forcing the foot up into dorsiflexion the navicular bone rides up over the pointed remains of the head of the talus. To facilitate this the midtarsal joint must be thoroughly mobilised and a notch may also have to be cut in the lower half of the navicular bone to allow it to fit over the tapered head of

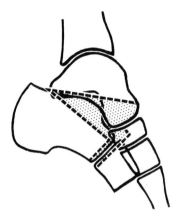 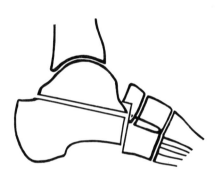

FIGS 554–555. Lambrinudi's tarsal arthrodesis. Figure 554—Broken line shows the anteriorly-based wedge of bone to be excised. When the gap is closed the notch in the navicular bone hooks over the remaining anterior beak of the talus. Figure 555—The wedge-shaped gap has been closed, correcting the equinus deformity. Note how the notch in the navicular bone accommodates the anterior beak of the talus.

of equinus. This will vary between men and women. In men, residual equinus of about 10 degrees is usually acceptable; in women rather more, depending upon the height of heel to which the patient is accustomed.

TECHNIQUE

The exposure is the same as that for triple fusion as described on page 433, the description of which should be read in conjunction with this section. The operation differs only in so far as a wedge of predetermined size is removed from the talocalcaneal complex. The wedge of bone should be cut cleanly with a chisel, the aim being to fashion a flat surface of cancellous bone on the inferior

the talus (Fig. 555). Care must be taken to fit the trimmed surfaces of talus and calcaneus accurately together, with the foot neither inverted nor everted. The position is best held with two or three staples as described for triple arthrodesis.

POST-OPERATIVE MANAGEMENT

The foot is immobilised in a well padded belowknee plaster which is moulded with the foot dorsiflexed. The initial plaster is split immediately after its application to allow for post-operative swelling. After two weeks a new and more closely fitting plaster is applied and two weeks later still a walking heel is added. Support in plaster is usually continued for a total of eight to ten weeks from the time of operation.

Comment

It should be appreciated that although this operation can be done in the presence of a stiff ankle it was used originally for mobile equinus deformity, the ankle joint being healthy and the calf muscles active, but the dorsiflexors paralysed. In such circumstances the effect of the operation is to ensure that the foot drops only to an acceptable degree of equinus when the talus is fully plantarflexed in the ankle mortise. From this position the foot may be dorsiflexed passively. The preservation of passive dorsiflexion allows an almost natural gait.

It will be clear that the critical part of the operation is to excise a wedge of the correct dimensions, just enough to allow an acceptable degree of equinus with the foot at rest—that is, with the talus fully plantarflexed.

Lambrinudi relied upon plaster for fixation of the bone fragments. The use of staples gives rather more precision to the procedure: if they are placed carefully they ensure close contact between the cut surfaces of the bones and thus help to promote rapid bone fusion.

ARTHRODESIS OF ANKLE

In the method to be described the ankle is approached both from the lateral and from the medial side. The contiguous surfaces of tibia and talus are denuded of cartilage, and bone grafts are applied across the joint on both sides.

PRELIMINARY STUDIES

Before the operation the most useful position for the fused joint in the particular patient concerned should be determined. The optimal angle depends mainly upon the type of shoe that the patient intends to wear, and particularly upon the height of the heel. In men the correct angle is about 5 to 8 degrees below the right angle. In women rather more plantarflexion is usually desirable. The point should be discussed with the patient so that her wishes concerning height of heel may be known.

TECHNIQUE

Position of patient. The patient lies supine. A tourniquet may be used on the upper thigh.

Incisions. The lateral incision, about 10 or 12 centimetres long, is made first. It lies over the lowest quarter of the fibula, extending distally about 2 centimetres below the tip of the lateral malleolus. The medial incision matches the lateral one in length and direction, lying over the lowest

quarter of the tibia. Each incision is deepened to the underlying bone.

Exposure of joint and removal of articular cartilage. The first step is to expose the ankle joint from the lateral side. This entails removal of the lowest quarter of the fibula, which will subsequently be used as an onlay graft. Care must be taken not to fragment the fibula during its removal. First the outer aspect of the bone is displayed by peeling back the periosteum with an elevator. When this has been done the surgeon should continue the stripping of soft tissue from the bone round the anterior border and on the medial surface. For stripping the medial surface a well curved elevator should be used, and it should be kept always close to the bone.

When the lower part of the fibula has been thus isolated from the investing soft tissues the bone is divided about 10 centimetres proximal to the tip of the lateral malleolus. It may be divided with a flexible wire saw (Gigli saw), but usually it is just as quick and rather simpler to use nibbling forceps. Bone-cutting forceps should not be used because they tend to crush and split the brittle bone. When the fibular shaft has been divided the upper end of the lower fragment is pulled laterally, and with a knife directed close to the inner surface of the bone the remaining attachments, which include the interosseous ligament and the capsule and lateral ligaments of the ankle, are severed. The lower part of the fibula is lifted from the wound and placed on one side for use as a bone graft.

In the bed of the fibula the ankle joint is now clearly exposed, and it is a simple matter to lever the talus slightly away from the tibia and to cut away the diseased articular cartilage from the upper surface of the talus and from the concave lower articular surface of the tibia. At the same time the hard subchondral bone should be broken up superficially to help to promote vascularisation across the joint.

and removed. Access is thus gained to the medial side of the ankle joint, from which any remaining remnants of articular cartilage should be removed. At the same time the medial articular surface of the talus is denuded of cartilage and shaved away down to raw bone. With a chisel the medial cortex of the lower 5 centimetres of the tibia is smoothed off to form a flat surface in the same plane as the rawed medial surface of the talus (Fig. 556). This flat bed, like that already prepared on the lateral aspect of the joint, is designed to receive an onlay bone graft.

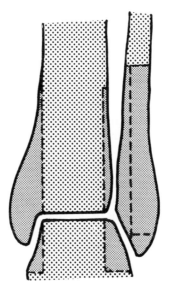 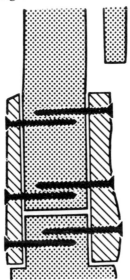

FIGS 556–557. Arthrodesis of ankle. Figure 556—Closely stippled area outlines the bone to be removed. The part of the fibula demarcated by the broken line is preserved for use as an onlay graft. Figure 557—The operation completed. The lower part of the tibia and the talus are sandwiched between the two bone grafts.

Preparation of bed for lateral graft. Attention is now directed to the lateral aspect of the tibia and of the talus. Articular cartilage is chiselled away from the lateral articular surface of the talus to expose subchondral bone. The lateral surface of the tibia is likewise pared down with a chisel so that the surface is in one plane with the lateral surface of the talus (Fig. 556).

Preparation of medial side of joint. Through the medial incision the lowest quarter of the tibia is exposed and the periosteum is stripped from its medial aspect. The medial malleolus is next divided obliquely at its base with an osteotome

Preparation of bone grafts. On the lateral side of the joint the graft is fashioned from the excised piece of fibula. This is prepared by carefully removing the deep cortex and smoothing the underlying cancellous bone into a flat surface to match the bed that has been prepared for it. Great care is required to avoid fragmenting the rather fragile graft.

On the medial side of the joint the graft is obtained from the medial cortex of the tibia immediately proximal to the area that has been prepared as a bed for the graft. The graft is cut in the manner described on page 72. It need not be more than about 6 to 8 centimetres long. The cancellous surface of the graft is smoothed off with a chisel to match the flat bed on which it will lie.

Application and fixation of grafts. The lateral (fibular) graft is placed in position so that it bridges the tibio-talar joint (Fig. 557). Care must be taken to ensure that there is as much contact with the lateral surface of the talus as is possible. The medial (tibial) graft is applied to the medial surface of the lower tibia and talus. At this stage care is taken to ensure that talus and tibia are in intimate contact and that the ankle is in the required angle of plantarflexion: any lateral or medial tilt of the talus must be avoided. The two grafts are then compressed against their beds by gripping them in a wide bone-holding forceps. In this way the lower tibia and the body of the talus are sandwiched between the two grafts.

It remains to fix the grafts firmly in position. To do this the surgeon may drill right through the bones from the lateral graft to the medial and fix the parts with appropriate bolts and nuts (usually two transfixing the tibia and one the talus); or alternatively each graft may be secured to the underlying bone with three screws, two in the tibia and one in the talus (Fig. 557). If this method is used, the drill holes in the grafts should allow a sliding fit for the screws whereas the holes drilled in the tibia and talus should be equal to the core diameter of the screws: when the screws are driven home the grafts are thus tightened up against the recipient bone. In the insertion of the screws care should be taken to ensure that the screw heads are not left prominent: they should be recessed into the grafts by countersinking.

Closure. Only the skin requires suturing. Interrupted eversion mattress sutures are recommended. Drainage of the wound is not required.

POST-OPERATIVE MANAGEMENT

In the immediate post-operative period the calf and foot are supported in a strong plaster-of-Paris backslab, well moulded over copious dressings held by a crepe bandage: a full encircling plaster is not recommended at this stage because of the liability to swelling. If necessary the bandage and dressings should be split anteriorly during the danger period, which is usually within the first forty-eight hours after operation.

After two weeks the sutures are removed and a close-fitting encircling plaster from upper calf to metatarsal heads is applied. Walking is then encouraged, but the patient should use crutches and not take weight on the affected limb.

At the end of the sixth week from operation a further close-fitting plaster may be applied and fitted with a walking heel, and thereafter increasing weight bearing with elbow crutches should be encouraged. The plaster must be retained until bony fusion is demonstrated radiologically, usually twelve to fourteen weeks after operation.

Comment

As with all arthrodeses the first essential is to ensure that the joint is fixed in the correct position. It is important to choose the right amount of equinus for each individual patient. It is also important to ensure that there is no inversion or eversion of the talus. Neglect of these requirements may prejudice the patient's comfort for the rest of his or her life.

The next essential is to make sure that the rawed joint surfaces fit together in intimate contact and that the beds for the grafts are so shaped that the grafts will sandwich the tibia and talus with equal pressure. In preparing the grafts the surgeon must use extra care with the fibula, which is soft and easily fragmented. He must remove the medial cortex cautiously, taking the minimum of surface bone. Likewise the fibula must be drilled very cautiously: otherwise it may easily be fractured.

ALTERNATIVE TECHNIQUE

For a description of the compression technique used by Charnley (1951), which is based on the principle propounded by Key (1932) for arthrodesis of the knee, the reader is referred to Charnley's original paper.

FOREFOOT ARTHROPLASTY

(Excision Arthroplasty of Metatarso-phalangeal Joints)

The operation to be described follows with minor modifications that reported by Fowler (1959). The operation aims to correct fixed clawing and dorsal subluxation or dislocation of the metatarso-phalangeal joints with prominence of the metatarsal heads in the sole and underlying callosites. The operation consists in excision of the bases of the

pair of lesser toes and a separate incision is used for the big toe; so there is a total of three dorsal incisions (Fig. 558).

The plantar incision outlines an ellipse of skin beneath the necks and distal parts of the shafts of the metatarsals (Fig. 559). At its widest point the ellipse of skin outlined by the incision measures

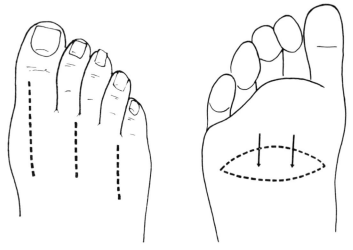

FIGS 558–559. Forefoot arthroplasty. Figure 558—The dorsal incisions. Figure 559—The elliptical plantar incision. The ellipse of skin is excised and the gap closed to draw the anteriorly displaced fibro-fatty pad of weight-bearing tissue back beneath the metatarsal heads. (After Fowler 1959.)

proximal phalanges and trimming and re-shaping of the metatarsal heads. At the same time the anteriorly displaced plantar pad of weight-bearing fibro-fatty tissue—a characteristic feature of these cases—is drawn back to its normal position beneath the metatarsal heads by excision of an ellipse of skin from the sole beneath the metatarsal necks and closure of the gap.

TECHNIQUE

Position of patient. The patient lies supine. A tourniquet may be used on the thickest part of the calf or on the upper thigh.

Incisions. On the dorsum of the foot longitudinal inter-metatarsal incisions are used for each

about 2 to 2.5 centimetres, depending upon the severity of the deformity and the amount of forward displacement of the fibro-fatty weight-bearing pad.

Excision of bases of proximal phalanges. The dorsal incisions are deepened anteriorly to expose the proximal half of each proximal phalanx, including that of the hallux. Often the metatarso-phalangeal joint will be found dislocated, so that the base of the phalanx lies dorsal to the head of the metatarsal. Each phalanx is divided with bone-cutting forceps at the junction of the proximal third with the distal two-thirds: more bone may be removed if necessary. The base of each proximal phalanx is then dissected free and discarded.

Trimming and re-shaping of metatarsal heads. The heads of the metatarsals are now delivered from the wound in turn. Trimming—that is, shortening—of the metatarsals should be carried out in such a way that the trimmed ends of all five metatarsals are lined up in a smooth curve that

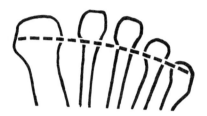

FIG. 560. Diagram to show the clean curve formed by the trimmed metatarsal heads. (After Fowler, 1959.)

extends laterally and slightly proximally from the head of the first metatarsal (Fig. 560). This means that the longer metatarsals, often the second and third, must be trimmed more than those whose heads are relatively recessed. This smooth sweep of the fronts of the metatarsal heads is designed to allow even pressure upon the metatarsals in weight-bearing.

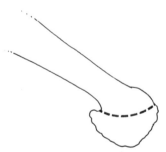

FIG. 561. Diagram to show how the metatarsals are trimmed to provide a smooth convex weight-bearing surface. (After Fowler, 1959.)

Re-shaping of the metatarsal heads is done mainly on the inferior surface. The aim is to remove all irregularities and to provide a smoothly curved surface that will sustain even pressure when in the weight-bearing position (Fig. 561). The trimming is best done with sharp-pointed bone-cutting forceps. Each dorsal incision is then closed by interrupted sutures.

Excision of ellipse of skin from sole and repositioning of weight-bearing fibro-fatty pad. In consequence of the clawing and dorsal subluxation of the toes, the weight-bearing skin that should lie beneath the metatarsal heads is displaced forwards, with the result that weight is borne upon unspecialised skin. The weight-bearing pad is relatively mobile, and it is easily drawn proximally again by excision of the plantar ellipse of skin already outlined, and closure of the resulting gap. The skin is excised through the subcutaneous plane. The elliptical gap is then closed by interrupted eversion mattress sutures uniting the skin edges.

POST-OPERATIVE MANAGEMENT

At the conclusion of the operation the shape of the foot should already be dramatically improved: the metatarsal heads are no longer prominent in the sole and the toes are lined up in normal relationship to the rest of the foot.

It is recommended that the toes be held in the correct position by a well padded plaster-of-Paris boot, which should be moulded to form an arch under the metatarsal heads and projected anteriorly above and below the toes to splint them in the straight position. The plaster should enclose the toes as a group and not individually: this entails less risk of constriction and consequent embarrassment of the circulation. Even so, the circulation in the toes must be carefully watched, especially in the first three days, and the plaster may be split or adjusted as required.

The initial plaster remains in place for two weeks, after which the sutures are removed and a new closer-fitting below-knee plaster, extending well forward above and below the toes, is applied. To this is added a walking heel, and thereafter the patient is encouraged to get about with sticks.

It is usually sufficient to retain the plaster for a total of four weeks from the time of operation. Upon its removal a course of ankle and foot exercises is arranged under the supervision of a physiotherapist. Improvement is likely to continue for several months and the patient should be advised accordingly. For a while there may be some persistent swelling of the toes but this tends gradually to subside.

Comment

This operation is a descendant of that originally described by Hoffmann (1912), which consisted in removal of the metatarsal heads without trimming of the phalanges. Hoffmann's operation has been variously modified by other surgeons, as exemplified by the later reports of Kates *et al.* (1967) and of Barton (1973). In the authors' experience Fowler's modification has given gratifying results. The authors believe, however, that Fowler's long transverse dorsal incision, which inevitably interferes with lymphatic drainage, should be replaced by multiple longitudinal incisions as described here.

Excision of the ellipse of skin from the sole and closure of the gap has the double advantage of bringing specialised weight-bearing skin beneath the metatarsal heads and at the same time of correcting the dorsal displacement of the proximal phalanges. All the elements of the original deformity are thus eliminated and the foot is restored to a shape that approximates to the normal.

DORSAL DISPLACEMENT OSTEOTOMY OF METATARSAL SHAFT

Prominence of one or more of the three central metatarsal heads in the sole, with painful underlying callosities and clawing of the corresponding toes but without dislocation of the metatarsophalangeal joints, may be corrected by the oblique dorsal displacement osteotomy described by Helal (1975). It is suitable for the patient with deformity that is not severe enough to justify the more radical operation of forefoot arthroplasty described in the previous section.

TECHNIQUE

Position of patient. The patient lies supine. A tourniquet may be used on the thickest part of the calf or on the upper thigh.

Incision. If only one metatarsal is to be divided the incision is made longitudinally over the dorsum of the distal half of the metatarsal. If two or three metatarsals are to be divided individual incisions may be used for each, or an incision over the intermetatarsal space may be used for exposure of a pair of adjacent metatarsals.

Procedure. Overlying soft tissues are cleared from the distal half of each affected metatarsal. The periosteum is incised longitudinally and stripped from the bone up to the neck of the metatarsal. The osteotomy should be sited at the junction of the proximal two-thirds with the distal

third of the metatarsal. The bone may be divided with a reciprocating saw or with a rapidly revolving dental burr. The line of osteotomy should be inclined at 45 degrees to the long axis of the bone, sloping from the dorsal surface plantarwards and

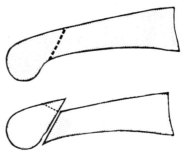

FIGS 562–563. Anterior oblique metatarsal osteotomy for protruberant metatarsal head. Figure 562—The line of the osteotomy. Figure 563—After the bone has been divided the distal fragment is allowed to ride upwards and proximally. The dorsal spike formed by the distal fragment may be trimmed away as indicated by the dotted line.

distally (Fig. 562). The bone fragments are separated and freed so that the distal fragment rides up proximally and dorsally on the proximal fragment (Fig. 563). If the proximal sharp end of the distal fragment forms a marked dorsal prominence it may be trimmed away.

Closure. The skin alone is sutured.

POST-OPERATIVE MANAGEMENT

Splintage is not required if the operation is confined to one or more of the central three metatarsals: the bone fragments are supported sufficiently by the adjacent metatarsals. Gauze dressings with a firmly applied crepe bandage are therefore adequate. Walking in a suitable slipper or sandal may be resumed within a few days of the operation.

Comment

This operation has the merits of simplicity and speedy convalescence. Dorsal displacement of the head fragment reduces its prominence in the sole, and the slight shortening of the metatarsal relaxes the taut tendons, with some relief of the claw deformity.

The originator has used a similar procedure for plantar prominence of the first and fifth metatarsals with underlying callosities.

RE-DOMING AND BONE GRAFTING OF METATARSAL HEAD FOR FREIBERG'S OSTEOCHONDRITIS

The operation to be described is based on that of Smillie (1960), the originator of active surgical intervention for Freiberg's disease of a metatarsal head in its very early stage with the aim of restoring the joint to normal. Unless it is carried out soon after the initial radiographic change is evident the likelihood of success is small. The object of the operation is to scoop out what is presumed to be avascular bone from the distal convexity of the metatarsal head through a dorsal window cut in the neck of the metatarsal, and to push the depressed segment of articular cartilage out to its normal domed shape by pressure with a blunt instrument from within. Normal doming of the cartilage is then maintained by a rigid strut in the form of a small cortical bone graft driven along the neck of the metatarsal into the head and maintained in position by a cross pin transfixing the neck of the metatarsal. Nearly always the second or the third metatarsal is the one affected.

TECHNIQUE

Position of patient. The patient lies supine. A tourniquet may be used on the thickest part of the calf or on the upper thigh.

Incision. A longitudinal dorsal incision is made over the distal third of the affected metatarsal and over the proximal third of the corresponding toe (Fig. 564). In the proximal part of the incision the

wound is deepened directly onto the dorsal surface of the metatarsal, the long extensor tendon being retracted laterally.

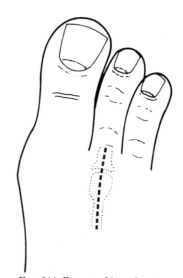

FIG. 564. Bone grafting of metatarsal head in Freiberg's disease. The skin incision.

Exposure of joint for examination of articular cartilage. In the distal part of the incision the wound is deepened to expose the dorsal part of the capsule of the metatarso-phalangeal joint, and the capsule and synovial membrane are incised to allow inspection of the interior of the joint. Particular attention is directed to the articular surface of the head of the metatarsal, where characteristically a fairly large segment of the articular cartilage—usually towards the dorsal part of the surface—is found to lack deep support. It tends to be flattened rather than conforming to the normal convexity of the remainder of the articular surface, and when pressed with a probe it feels soft and may be indented. This segment of cartilage is often almost loose, being held only by a remaining hinge of intact cartilage (Fig. 565).

Fenestration of metatarsal neck and clearance of sub-articular bone from metatarsal head. Attention is next directed to the distal part of the shaft of the metatarsal where it tapers into the neck. The bone is exposed and periosteum is stripped on each side to allow suitable curved dissectors to be passed round the metatarsal neck medially and laterally to hold the soft tissues away. With a slender very sharp osteotome a dorsal window is cut in the cortex of the metatarsal (Fig. 565). The window should be about 15 millimetres long and 3 or 4 millimetres wide. The distal end of the window

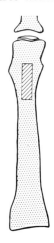

FIG. 565. The dorsal window cut through the cortex of the metatarsal neck. Note flattening of contour of metatarsal head.

should be about 12 or 13 millimetres from the convexity of the articular surface of the metatarsal. It is important to cut out the cortical fragment cleanly without breaking it, because it will be used subsequently as a graft to hold the softened articular cartilage out to its normal domed contour.

When the cortical lid of the window has been removed and set safely aside, the cancellous bone of the neck and head of the metatarsal is scooped out from within, either by a very narrow chisel or by means of a miniature curette. Bone should be

scooped so thoroughly that in the area of the articular defect only a thin layer of subchondral bone remains: in effect the articular surface is reduced to a shell.

Re-doming of articular surface and packing with cortical and cancellous bone. With a Watson-Cheyne dissector inserted through the window in the dorsal aspect of the metatarsal, the shell of articular cartilage is pushed forwards from within

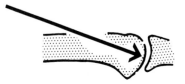

FIG. 566. Pushing the flattened articular cartilage out from within the metatarsal head, to restore the normal dome.

(Fig. 566) while the effect is observed through the distal part of the incision that has opened the joint. With care it is possible to push the shell of cartilage forwards to form, with the remaining intact cartilage, a smooth convex articular surface closely approximating to the normal.

It remains now to hold this position by inserting the bone graft cut from the dorsal cortex of the metatarsal and pushing it forwards as a strut so

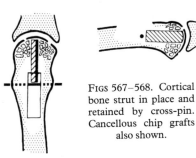

FIGS 567–568. Cortical bone strut in place and retained by cross-pin. Cancellous chip grafts also shown.

that its anterior extremity maintains the normal convexity of the articular surface as did the Watson-Cheyne dissector. While the bone graft is thus pushed forwards with a fine punch the distal part of the neck of the metatarsal is transfixed with a fine Kirschner wire immediately proximal to the graft to prevent it from sliding back (Figs 567 and 568). The wire is inserted from the lateral side sufficiently far to pass through the medial cortex of the metatarsal, and it is then cut off at a point that will allow it to be easily located for removal at a later date. Finally, the remaining cavity in the metatarsal head is packed with cancellous bone removed from the head and from the adjacent part of the shaft of the metatarsal.

Closure. After removal of the tourniquet it is usually sufficient to close the skin alone, preferably with everting mattress sutures.

POST-OPERATIVE MANAGEMENT

For the first ten days after operation the forefoot is kept dressed with dry gauze and a crepe bandage. Walking on the heel within the confines of the

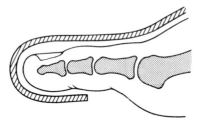

FIG. 569. Splint formed from a strip of plaster-of-Paris, used to protect the toe after re-doming of the metatarsal head.

ward may be permitted. Ten to fourteen days after the operation the sutures are removed and a dorsal plaster splint, hooked anteriorly over the tip of the toe and held in place by ribbon gauze (Fig. 569) is applied. Thereafter, walking in strong-soled sandals is encouraged for a further four weeks. All splintage is then discarded and arrangements are made to remove the Kirschner wire through a small stab incision. If desired, this may be done under local rather than general anaesthesia. Finally, intensive toe exercises must be practised to restore flexion and extension movement.

Comment

The main essential is that the excavated shell of articular cartilage should be held out to its normal convexity, and this is the main function of the small cortical graft. The transfixing cross-pin is a great advantage in preventing this graft from sliding back into the shaft of the metatarsal.

The rationale of this operation is to some extent conjectural: it is supposed that the damaged articular cartilage, nourished largely by synovial fluid, can survive long enough to allow revascularisation of the subjacent bone, and that this revascularisation is hastened by re-packing the partly avascular head with cortical and cancellous grafts. The operation by no means always succeeds, but in the event of failure little or nothing is lost because the natural course of Freiberg's disease is towards osteoarthritis, which often becomes disabling in early adult life and may necessitate excision of the metatarsal head. If this can be avoided, even in a proportion of cases, the operation is well worth while.

EXCISION OF PLANTAR DIGITAL NEUROMA FOR MORTON'S METATARSALGIA

The operation entails exposure of the affected common plantar digital nerve just proximal to its division into proper digital nerves, and excision of the affected part of the nerve.

TECHNIQUE

Position of patient. The patient lies supine. The surgeon should be seated at the end of the table, facing the sole of the foot. The table may be tilted slightly into the head-down, leg-raised position to make the sole more accessible. The foot may be held dorsiflexed by an assistant or by a bandage looped round the sole at the mid-foot level and held taut by a weight suspended over the head end of the table. A tourniquet may be used on the thickest part of the calf or, if preferred, on the upper thigh.

Incision. The incision is made vertically in the sole opposite the base of the affected interdigital cleft. This is usually the cleft between the third and fourth toes but may occasionally be that between the second and third toes. The incision begins a centimetre behind the web and extends proximally for 3 or 4 centimetres (Fig. 570).

Exposure of common plantar digital nerve. As the skin is incised fibro-fatty tissue, characteristic of the subcutaneous layer of the sole, pouts out rather profusely and little can be seen until the edges of this tissue have been cut back. The edges

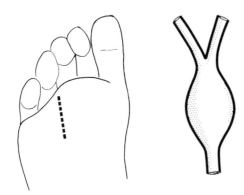

FIGS 570–571. Excision of plantar digital neuroma. Figure 570—The skin incision. Figure 571—A typical plantar digital neuroma after excision.

of the skin and subcutaneous tissue are retracted with a self- retaining retractor. Blunt dissection with scissors then proceeds until the thin basal layer of fascia is encountered. This is incised vertically in the line of the skin incision to reveal immediately deep to it the common plantar digital nerve, which is disposed longitudinally and directed towards the base of the interdigital cleft.

The trunk of the nerve should be cleared of adherent areolar tissue by blunt dissection with scissors, and working forwards the surgeon will see that the nerve divides about 1.5 centimetres behind the web into the proper digital nerves for the adjacent sides of the toes concerned. These nerves are followed forwards for half a centimetre or more towards the toes.

By this time the lesion of the nerve will have become apparent. It is seen as a fusiform swelling of the trunk of the nerve, just proximal to its division into two proper digital nerves (Fig. 571).

This ovoid thickening presents a glistening surface.

Excision of affected part of nerve. The nerve trunk is gripped immediately proximal to the neuroma and divided. Traction upon the distal stump of the nerve brings the proper digital divisions into better view, and each nerve is divided just distal to the point of division of the main trunk (Fig. 571).

Excision of associated ganglia. As well as the nerve trunk swelling there may also be ganglion swellings arising from the metatarso-phalangeal joints. If such a ganglion is tense it may be contributing to the patient's discomfort and should also be excised.

Closure. After release of the tourniquet any bleeding points are secured and the fibro-fatty subcutaneous tissue is sutured with two or three light absorbable sutures. The skin is closed with everting mattress sutures.

POST-OPERATIVE MANAGEMENT

A crepe bandage is applied snugly over a thick pad of gauze in order to give good support under the front of the sole. The patient may be allowed to walk within the confines of the ward, putting weight mainly upon the heel. Excessive dependence of the foot should be avoided, and long periods of elevation should be enjoined during the first two weeks. At this time the sutures are removed and thereafter progressively more walking may be permitted.

Comment

The pain from even a small neuroma can be very disabling and the relief after its removal is dramatic. The operation is straightforward but care must be taken to gain a clear view of the affected nerve, which tends to be obscured by the abundant overlying fibro-fatty tissue. It is well to clear some of this away before the thin basal layer of fascia is incised. The nerves are superficial in the sole. Care must be taken not to damage the blood vessels that lie on a slightly deeper plane.

TENDON TRANSFER: EXTENSOR HALLUCIS LONGUS TO NECK OF FIRST METATARSAL

This operation, described by Robert Jones in 1916, is used mainly for dorsiflexion deformity of the big toe from over-action of the extensor hallucis longus in the absence of an active tibialis anterior muscle, the usual predisposing cause being poliomyelitis. The aim of the transfer is to use the extensor hallucis longus to dorsiflex the foot directly, instead of through the big toe. Since the interphalangeal joint of the big toe is thus deprived of the power of active extension it is usual to arthrodese the joint at the same operation.

TECHNIQUE

Position of patient. The patient lies supine. A tourniquet may be used on the upper thigh.

Incision. The skin incision begins transversely over the dorsum of the big toe just distal to the interphalangeal joint. From the lateral extremity

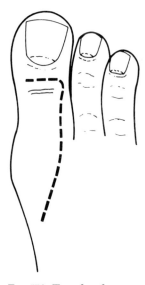

FIG. 572. Transfer of extensor hallucis longus to neck of first metatarsal. The skin incision.

of this cut the line of incision turns proximally to follow the lateral side of the extensor hallucis longus tendon as far as the metatarso-phalangeal

joint. It then curves medially towards the inner border of the foot, ending about 4 centimetres proximal to the metatarso-phalangeal joint (Fig. 572).

Mobilisation of tendon. Through the distal part of the incision the insertion of the extensor hallucis longus tendon is cleared and the tendon is divided close to its point of attachment to the base of the distal phalanx. The tendon is then dissected free in a proximal direction as far as the middle of the first metatarsal and brought out through the proximal part of the wound.

Preparation of metatarsal neck. The neck of the first metatarsal is cleared and the periosteum is stripped to expose the medial and lateral sides. With an awl, a starting notch is made in the bone at the medial side, and a hole is drilled transversely across the neck of the metatarsal with a 4-millimetre drill.

Re-attachment of tendon. An eyed probe bearing a silk thread is passed through the drill hole from

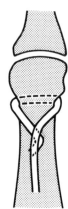

FIG. 573. Method of attaching the tendon to the metatarsal by passing it through a drill hole in the neck.

the medial to the lateral side. The thread is drawn out through the wound and attached securely to the end of the divided extensor hallucis tendon. The thread and with it the tendon are then pulled back through the drill hole to emerge at the medial side. The end of the tendon is looped up proximally to meet the body of the tendon over the dorsum of the metatarsal (Fig. 573). At this point a slit is made in the trunk of the tendon and the cut end of the tendon is drawn through the slit. If there is sufficient length the tendon end may be passed through a second slit at right angles to the first. Sutures of stainless steel wire are inserted through the interlaced tendon, securing the loop. The suture is made with the foot dorsiflexed just beyond the right angle and the tendon drawn moderately taut.

Arthrodesis of interphalangeal joint. The interphalangeal joint is fused in the manner described on page 457.

Closure. Only the skin edges need be sutured.

POST-OPERATIVE MANAGEMENT

A light plaster-of-Paris splint is applied below the knee to hold the ankle at a right angle and the toe straight. After two weeks the sutures are removed and a walking plaster is applied. This is worn for a further four weeks. Thereafter a course of mobilising exercises for the ankle, foot and toes is arranged.

Comment

The main point of difficulty is to judge the correct tension under which the tendon should be sutured. A useful guide is to pull the tendon to the mid-position between the extremes of its excursion, and to make the tendon suture with this amount of tension while the foot is dorsiflexed about 10 degrees above the right angle.

DISPLACEMENT OSTEOTOMY OF NECK OF FIRST METATARSAL FOR HALLUX VALGUS

The operation to be described is based on that of Mygind (1952, 1953) which in turn was essentially that of Thomasen (unpublished). In principle the operation consists simply in dividing the neck of the first metatarsal and then shifting the metatarsal head laterally through at least two-thirds of the diameter of the bone. Lateral displacement of the head eliminates the medial "exostosis" and relaxes the deforming forces that acted upon the hallux, so that the subluxation of the metatarsophalangeal joint that is the essence of the deformity is spontaneously corrected. The joint itself is left undisturbed: there is no need to trim the bony prominence or "exostosis", or to shorten or reef the capsule at the medial side of the joint.

PRELIMINARY STUDIES

Before this operation is undertaken careful examination is required in order to make sure that the conditions are suitable. In particular, it should be remembered that the operation is not appropriate when valgus deformity of the toe is extreme

(40 degrees of valgus is regarded as the outside limit), when the patient is over 65, when degenerative arthritic changes are already present in the metatarso-phalangeal joint as shown radiographically, or when the subluxation of the joint is not correctable passively. This last point can easily be determined by gripping the forefoot in one hand so that the first metatarsal is approximated towards the second, and moving the big toe towards the varus position with the finger and thumb of the other hand. In cases likely to respond to displacement osteotomy the toe can be brought into line with the first metatarsal without force when this test is applied.

As these criteria suggest, the operation is applicable mainly to the adolescent and to adults under about 60 years of age.

TECHNIQUE

Position of patient. The patient lies supine. A tourniquet may be used on the thickest part of the calf or on the upper thigh.

Incision. The incision lies over the dorso-medial aspect of the distal half of the first metatarsal. It is made slightly convex dorsally, where it comes close to the medial margin of the extensor hallucis longus tendon (Fig. 574).

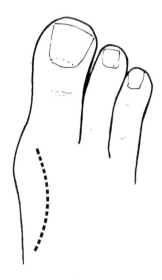

FIG. 574. Displacement osteotomy for hallux valgus. The skin incision.

Exposure of metatarsal neck. The skin flap is reflected medially and a vertical knife cut is made directly onto the dorsum of the metatarsal bone in its distal half: the incision stops short of the metatarso-phalangeal joint. By a combination of knife dissection and stripping with an elevator, the periosteum is separated from the bone throughout the circumference of the metatarsal neck.

Curved bone levers—the Macdonald dissector is an appropriate instrument—are next inserted round the bone from either side to retract the soft tissues. Care should be taken to ensure that the metatarsal neck is cleared of periosteum right up to the attachment of the joint capsule. To expose this distal part of the neck adequately blunt button hooks should be inserted anteriorly in each corner of the wound.

Division of metatarsal neck. The first step is to divide the neck of the metatarsal cleanly. The line of osteotomy begins at the medial side of the neck immediately proximal to the point where the bone flares out to form the metatarsal head. From this point the line of division crosses the metatarsal neck obliquely, laterally and slightly distally (Fig. 575). The object of making the cut obliquely is to minimise shortening of the metatarsal; slight loss of length that will be entailed in notching and interlocking the two fragments is compensated by elongation as the head is displaced laterally across the inclined plane (Fig. 576). Ideally the osteotomy should be carried out with a cutting burr on a high-speed dental type drill or with a fine reciprocating power-operated saw blade. It is possible to use instead a fine bone-cutting forceps, but the operation then becomes much more difficult.

Shaping of bone fragments for interlocking fit. The object is to fashion a lateral peg from the cortex of the shaft fragment, with flanking notches cut in the adjacent cortex, and to drill a matching socket in the head fragment close to the medial margin. After displacement, the head fragment is then to be implanted on the peg while the adjacent parts of the cortex of each fragment interlock (Figs 575–580).

First the shaft fragment is delivered from the wound by placing a broad malleable retractor beneath it. The site of the proposed peg is marked on the bone: it should be mainly at the lateral margin of the cut surface of the metatarsal, but slightly towards the plantar aspect. The peg should be about 5 millimetres in diameter. The cortex adjacent to the peg plantarwards and dorsally is notched to a depth of 6 to 7 millimetres and the two notches are joined around the medial side of the peg at the expense of the cancellous bone (Fig. 580). This semicircular notch should be just wide enough to receive the medial cortex of the head fragment. This fragment is now delivered into the wound in place of the shaft fragment and the site of the proposed socket is marked. It should be in the medial extremity of the cut surface, slightly towards the dorsal aspect. The socket, 5 millimetres in diameter to match the peg on the shaft fragment, is cut with an appropriate dental burr or hand reamer. It should come close up to the medial cortex, which however must not be breached (Fig. 580).

Displacement of metatarsal head and impaction of fragments in interlocking fit. A strong bone hook is passed round the metatarsal shaft to allow it to be pulled medially. At the same time the big toe is grasped by the finger and thumb of the surgeon's other hand, and while the shaft is pulled medially

Bevelling of medial corner of shaft fragment. The prominent antero-medial corner of the shaft fragment is cut away to form a long bevel as shown in Figure 577. The bone thus obtained is saved for reimplanting at the lateral side of the metatarsal neck (Fig. 278).

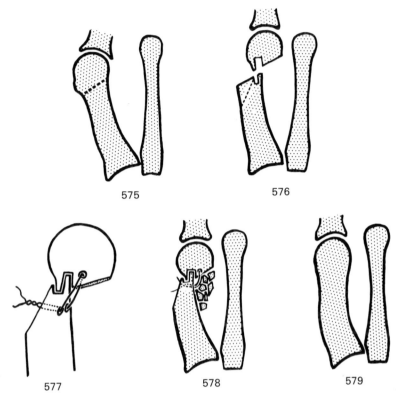

495

576

577

578

579

FIGS 575–579. Displacement osteotomy of neck of first metatarsal. Figure 575—Site and direction of osteotomy. Figure 576—The parts ready for assembly after shaping of the peg and socket. Interrupted line shows part of medial cortex to be bevelled off. Figure 577—The parts assembled: diagram shows detail of wire suture used to prevent redisplacement. Figure 578—Bone fragments removed from bevelled medial cortex transferred to lateral side. Figure 579—Appearance after remodelling: the axis of the metatarsal has been changed, with full correction of the original varus deviation.

the head is displaced laterally and distracted. In this way the peg on the shaft fragment is made to engage the socket in the head fragment. If the fragments have been fashioned correctly the two parts should then fit down into each other so that the medial cortex of the head fragment engages deeply in the semicircular notch in the shaft fragment (Fig. 577). In this way a stable position is gained.

Insertion of tie-wire. To guard against any possibility of accidental displacement of the fragments after operation a mattress stitch of stainless steel wire (gauge 28) is inserted. With the finest available drill a hole is made through the dorsal cortex of the head fragment about 3 millimetres from the cut edge. Wire is looped through this hole. Twin holes are then cut in the lateral cortex of the shaft fragment 3 or 4 millimetres proximal to the base of the peg. The ends of the wire are passed through the two holes and tied or twisted on the medial side of the metatarsal shaft where it has been bevelled (Fig. 577).

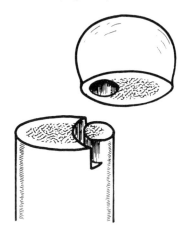

FIG. 580. "Exploded" diagram showing method of shaping the interlocking surfaces of the proximal and distal fragments.

Insertion of bone fragments. The bone fragments obtained from bevelling the antero-medial corner of the metatarsal shaft are replaced at the lateral side of the metatarsal, in the angle between the neck and the displaced head (Fig. 578).

Closure. The skin alone is sutured.

POST-OPERATIVE MANAGEMENT

A crepe bandage is applied spica fashion round the big toe and the foot with care not to make the dressing too bulky. The toe is then supported by a J-shaped plaster slab. This slab, about 20 centimetres long, is moulded to the medial border of the foot and its distal end is turned laterally over the end of the big toe and moulded to the lateral side of the toe almost as far as the web (Fig. 581). The plaster slab is held in place by a further covering of crepe bandage.

The patient is encouraged to walk within the confines of the ward, taking weight mainly upon the heel. After two weeks the sutures are removed and a below-knee plaster is applied, the plaster being extended forward to grip the toe. A

walking heel is added, high enough to ensure that the toes are held well clear of the ground. The plaster is retained until the end of the eighth week after operation, when union of the osteotomy is

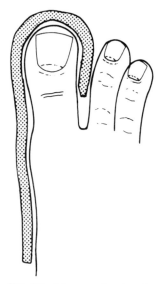

FIG. 581. Diagram showing the extent of the plaster splint.

usually sound enough to allow the plaster to be discarded. At that stage active exercises to mobilise the toe joints and to rehabilitate the intrinsic muscles are practised under the supervision of a physiotherapist.

Comment

This is an operation that must be carried out with precision. A close fit of the interlocking bone fragments is essential to ensure stability: all too often a hurried approach to this type of operation leads to technical faults that may cause instability, redisplacement of the fragments and a disappointing result.

The author's studies have shown that to ensure consistent success displacement of the head relative to the shaft of the metatarsal must be wide—not less than two-thirds of the diameter of the bone at the site of osteotomy. Wide displacement, with subsequent remodelling, ensures correction of metatarsus primus varus and lasting correction of the valgus deformity of the toe (Fig. 579). Since the metatarso-phalangeal joint is not disturbed, virtually a full range of movement is nearly always regained without difficulty. In this respect the operation has advantages over those that rely upon trimming of the exostosis or reefing of the capsule at the medial side of the joint. Wide displacement makes trimming of the exostosis unnecessary, for the prominence disappears automatically when the metatarsal head is shifted laterally.

Numerous techniques of displacement osteotomy of the neck of the first metatarsal have been described since the pioneer report of Hohmann (1923). Many of them give insufficient displacement or fail to ensure a stable position of the fragments. The variants that are most widely used are those of Mitchell *et al.* (1958) and of Wilson (1963). For details of these operations the original papers should be consulted.

EXCISION ARTHROPLASTY OF METATARSO-PHALANGEAL JOINT OF HALLUX

(KELLER'S ARTHROPLASTY)

This operation, described by Keller in 1904, is probably used more commonly than any other for hallux valgus and hallux rigidus. It combines excision of the base of the proximal phalanx with trimming of the medial prominence or "exostosis" of the head of the first metatarsal.

TECHNIQUE

Position of patient. The patient lies supine. A tourniquet may be used on the thickest part of the calf or on the upper thigh.

Incision. The skin incision is a longitidinal one just medial to the tendon of extensor hallucis longus. It lies over the distal 3 centimetres of the first metatarsal and over the proximal phalanx as far distally as its neck (Fig. 582). Usually the incision is 5 to 6 centimetres long.

Isolation and excision of base of proximal phalanx. The incision is deepened straight to bone and the skin edges are retracted with, on the lateral side, the tendon of extensor hallucis longus. By sharp dissection close to the bone, the periosteum and the margin of the joint capsule are stripped from the base of the proximal phalanx well round towards the plantar surface. Small well curved bone levers or Macdonald dissectors are inserted round the middle of the phalanx, one on each side. The phalanx is then freed by division of

the joint capsule. It is lifted up by the use of forceps such as those of Nissen or Verbrugge so that the flexor aspect of the phalanx can be well seen. The proximal half of the phalanx is then carefully freed from the flexor tendon before it is

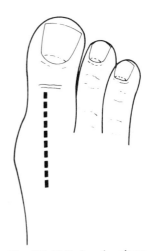

FIG. 582. Keller's arthroplasty.
The skin incision.

divided. The under surface of the phalanx is concave and the flexor tendon lies in the hollow. Unless the flexor tendon is freed it may be damaged when the phalanx is divided. After this preparation the phalanx is divided cleanly across in the middle of the shaft with a sharp-pointed bone-cutting forceps (Fig. 583).

A large button hook is now inserted into the medullary canal of the proximal fragment through the cut surface: this serves to control the fragment during the manoeuvres now required in order to mobilise the fragment and dissect it free. When this has been done it is well to inspect the cut surface of the distal fragment of the phalanx to make sure that the cut has been made cleanly and that no projecting spur of bone remains.

Trimming of exostosis. Attention is now turned to the proximal part of the wound, where the incision is deepened onto the head and neck of the first metatarsal. By dissection with blunt-pointed scissors or with a knife the soft tissues, including the adventitious bursa that lies over the "bunion", are freed from the underlying bone at the medial

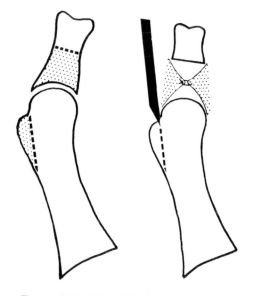

FIGS 583–584. Keller's arthroplasty. Figure 583—Stippled areas show the bone to be removed. Figure 584—The "exostosis" is best removed by a chisel directed proximally as shown. Note the soft-tissue curtain sewn between the bones.

side. The projecting medial prominence of the metatarsal—the so-called exostosis—is then cut away with a chisel, which is preferably driven in a proximal direction to enter the bone at the junction of articular surface and exostosis and to emerge on the medial surface of the neck of the metatarsal (Figs 583 and 584). The piece of bone

removed is wedge-shaped—broad anteriorly but tapering very obliquely to a point at its proximal extremity. It is usually unnecessary to interfere with the soft tissues of the bunion itself or with the medial sesamoid bone, which may be seen in the depth of the wound.

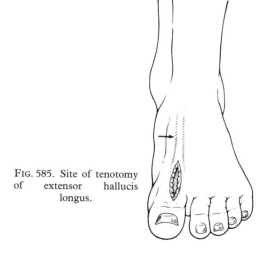

FIG. 585. Site of tenotomy of extensor hallucis longus.

Release of tight extensor hallucis longus. It is wise to tenotomise the tendon of extensor hallucis longus subcutaneously through a stab incision over the dorsum of the foot at about the level of the base of the first metatarsal. This tenotomy releases the springy tension of the extensor hallucis and prevents the stump of the proximal phalanx from being drawn up against the head of the first metatarsal. It is not recommended that the tendon be divided where it is visible in the lateral edge of the wound; subcutaneous tenotomy well proximal to the wound (Fig. 585) ensures that the tendon unites again, though with slight lengthening.

Interposition of soft tissues. A further step that should be taken to prevent contact between the stump of the phalanx and the metatarsal head is to suture a fold of adjacent fatty tissue between the bone ends with fine catgut (Fig. 584).

Closure. After removal of the tourniquet any bleeding points are controlled and the skin is sutured with interrupted everting mattress sutures.

POST-OPERATIVE MANAGEMENT

Light gauze dressings are held in place by a crepe bandage 7.5 centimetres wide which is applied spica fashion in order to hold the big toe straight. The foot should be kept slightly elevated for the first twelve to fourteen days. Removal of the sutures is preferably delayed until about that time. Thereafter, the patient may resume walking, at first in a slipper: swelling often prohibits the wearing of a slender shoe for six to eight weeks after the operation.

Exercises for the toes are practised from the beginning. At first the patient has no active control of movements of the big toe, but the joint should be put through a wide range of flexion and extension either by the physiotherapist or by the patient herself who, after removal of the sutures, may practise these movements in the bath.

Comment

Keller's operation generally gives pleasing results in elderly patients who are unlikely to make great demands upon their feet. On the other hand it leaves the toe far from normal, in that it is short, floppy and lacking in full voluntary control. It is therefore not generally to be recommended for young persons who aspire to resume running or active games. Displacement osteotomy should be considered instead for that group of patients.

The first point in technique that needs to be stressed is that excision of the base of the proximal phalanx should be generous: the authors believe that it is best to remove at least half of the phalanx. The second point is that steps should be taken to prevent retraction of the stump of the phalanx and contact between its cut surface and the head of the first metatarsal. The most important step towards prevention of retraction is to tenotomise the tendon of extensor hallucis longus, preferably by a subcutaneous stab cut proximal to the main wound. As a useful supplementary measure folds of fatty tissue should routinely be drawn together between the bone ends.

The patient should be warned that at first the big toe is likely to be jelly-like and to lack active movement. As the false joint tightens up in the succeeding weeks and months the power of active flexion and extension returns to some extent, though nothing approaching normal metatarso-phalangeal function is to be expected.

DORSAL WEDGE OSTEOTOMY FOR HALLUX RIGIDUS

This operation was described by Kessel and Bonney (1958) for hallux rigidus without severe arthritis in young patients with a moderate range of metatarso-phalangeal movement still preserved. It aims to change the arc of movement to give more extension at the expense of reduced flexion, and thus to make walking more comfortable.

PRELIMINARY STUDIES

The range of flexion and extension at the metatarso-phalangeal joint must be accurately measured. The aim should be to restore at least 30 degrees of extension (dorsiflexion). Thus if, for example, the range of movement before operation is 30 degrees of flexion and only 10 degrees of extension, removal of a 20 degrees dorsal wedge from the base of the proximal phalanx and closure of the gap would change the arc of movement to provide 10 degrees of flexion and 30 degrees of extension.

TECHNIQUE

Position of patient. The patient lies supine. A tourniquet may be used on the thickest part of the calf or on the upper thigh.

Incision. An L-shaped incision is made over the dorsum of the proximal phalanx of the hallux: its vertical limb lies medial to the extensor tendon and it curves smoothly into the transverse limb which crosses the toe at the level of the metatarso-phalangeal joint (Fig. 586).

Removal of wedge. The incision is deepened straight to the bone medial to the extensor tendon. Periosteum is stripped to expose the proximal half

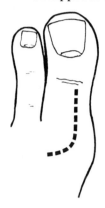

FIG. 586. Dorsal wedge osteotomy of proximal phalanx. The skin incision.

of the proximal phalanx, the extensor tendon being displaced laterally. The base of the wedge to be removed is next marked out on the dorsum of

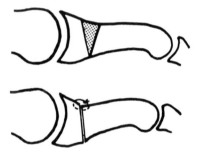

FIGS 587–588. Figure 587—Stippled area shows the wedge of bone to be removed. Figure 588—After closure of the gap the fragments are coapted with wire sutures inserted through fine drill holes.

the phalanx. Its proximal edge should cross the phalanx about 5 or 6 millimetres beyond the level of the joint, and its width should be calculated according to the angle of wedge required. The

wedge of bone is then removed with fine bone-cutting forceps or with a chisel (Fig. 587).

Closure of wedge-shaped gap. When the wedge of bone has been removed the next step is to make drill holes, each a millimetre in diameter, through the dorsal cortex on each side of the wedge and about 3 millimetres from its margin. Usually two drill holes in each fragment suffice. They serve to receive wire stitches designed to hold the fragments in apposition with the wedge-shaped gap fully closed. Closure is effected by forcibly extending the toe, and while it is held in this position the wire loops are tightened and tied (Fig. 588).

POST-OPERATIVE MANAGEMENT

If good fixation by wire sutures has been achieved plaster splintage may be dispensed with, but if there is doubt about the efficacy of the internal fixation a J-shaped plaster slab should be applied along the dorsum of the foot and hooked under the plantar aspect of the big toe. The plaster is bandaged on with a crepe bandage. The plaster is renewed after two weeks, when the sutures are removed: it should be retained for about six weeks in all.

Comment

This operation has a very limited application, because the circumstances to which it is suited seldom arise. Nevertheless it has worthwhile advantages over arthroplasty or arthrodesis when painful limitation of extension at the metatarsophalangeal joint is found without evidence of significant degenerative arthritis.

ARTHRODESIS OF METATARSO-PHALANGEAL JOINT OF HALLUX

The first metatarso-phalangeal joint may be fused by first rawing the articular surfaces and then transfixing the joint with a screw. The position at which the joint is fused is critical.

POSITION FOR ARTHRODESIS

It is best to fuse the joint in slight dorsiflexion to prevent excessive strain upon the interphalangeal joint during walking. The degree of dorsiflexion that is required depends to some extent upon the footwear that the patient is accustomed to use. In men dorsiflexion of 10 to 15 degrees is appropriate, but in a woman who is accustomed to wearing high heels and who intends to continue to do so dorsiflexion of 20 degrees may be recommended. In addition the normal angle of valgus—usually 10 to 15 degrees—should be preserved: if the toe is set in a direct line with the first metatarsal, without any valgus, the toe span will be too broad and fitting with shoes will be difficult.

TECHNIQUE

Position of patient. The patient lies supine. A tourniquet may be used on the thickest part of the calf or on the upper thigh.

Incision. The incision is a mainly vertical one just medial to the tendon of extensor hallucis

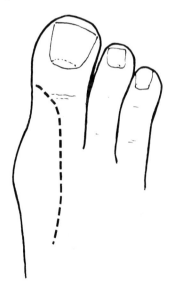

FIG. 589. Arthrodesis of meta-tarso-phalangeal joint of hallux. The skin incision.

longus. Proximally it lies over the distal third of the first metatarsal, and distally it extends forward over the proximal phalanx as far as its neck. At this point the incision curves medially and plantarwards to end on the medial border of the toe (Fig. 589).

Rawing of articular surfaces. The incision is deepened straight to bone. Periosteum is stripped from the neck and head of the first metatarsal and from the base of the proximal phalanx. At the same time the joint capsule and synovial membrane are dissected away from the joint margins at the dorsum of the toe. Acute flexion of the joint with division of the collateral ligaments now allows the joint surfaces to be dislocated and the head of the metatarsal may then be delivered from the wound. With sharp-pointed bone-cutting forceps or with a slender chisel the articular surface of the head of the metatarsal is pared away and the subchondral bone is removed sufficiently to expose raw spongy bone. The domed shape of the metatarsal head should be preserved.

When the metatarsal head has been thus dealt with the base of the proximal phalanx is delivered into the wound and the articular surface is similarly rawed either with bone-cutting forceps and nibbling forceps or with a suitable gouge. The raw surface should form a shallow cup to match the contour of the metatarsal head, so that when the two bones are fitted together there is intimate contact between them over the whole area of the former joint surface.

Internal fixation. The metatarsal head and the proximal phalanx are brought together and placed precisely at the predetermined position of dorsiflexion and valgus. Rotational deformity of the toe must not be allowed. With the toe held in this optimal position by an assistant, preparations are now made to drive a fixation screw obliquely across the joint. In order to hold the position more securely while the screw is inserted it may be advisable to transfix the joint temporarily with a Kirschner wire or guide wire.

In preparing the track for the fixation screw the surgeon should first expose the medial aspect of the proximal phalanx by turning plantarward the flap of skin outlined by the incision. When the periosteum has been stripped away from the bone a deep notch is cut into the medial surface of the phalanx about midway along its length (Fig. 590). The purpose of the notch is to allow a drill to be entered in the medullary canal of the phalanx and driven across the joint into the metatarsal. The notch serves also as a convenient recess to accommodate the head of the screw.

When the notch has been made sufficiently deep a drill track 3 millimetres in diameter is prepared in the base of the phalanx and head of the metatarsal. The drill should pass proximally and slightly

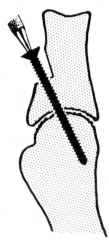

FIG. 590. Fixation by oblique screw after rawing of joint surfaces.

laterally to strike the lateral cortex of the neck of the first metatarsal from within: it is legitimate for the drill to penetrate through the cortex. The distal part of the drill track—that is, the part that traverses the base of the proximal phalanx— should be enlarged sufficiently to allow a sliding fit of the screw: this ensures that when the screw is driven home the two bones are compressed together. A screw 3.5 to 5 centimetres long is usually required. Care should be taken not to over-tighten it lest the screw head be sunk too far into the base of the proximal phalanx (Fig. 590).

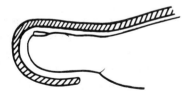

FIG. 591. The plaster-of-Paris splint used. The sides of the toe are left free.

Checking the position. Before the wound is closed the drapes should be removed from the foot so that a careful assessment may be made of the position of the big toe. If this is in any way

imperfect it is wise to remove the screw and adjust the position appropriately, and then to reinsert the screw in a new direction.

Closure. Only the skin needs to be closed.

POST-OPERATIVE MANAGEMENT

Even though internal fixation with a screw should afford good rigidity of the joint it is wise to reinforce the fixation by means of a plaster-of-Paris splint. Local splintage rather than a full below-knee plaster is usually adequate. A convenient plan is to take a long strip of plaster about 3 or 4 centimetres wide and about 15 layers thick, and to lay this along the dorsum of the foot and toe and to turn the anterior end under the pulp (Fig. 591). This dorsal plaster splint may be held in position by a crepe bandage.

After two weeks the initial splint and the dressings are removed to allow removal of the sutures. A new plaster is then applied; at this stage a full below-knee walking plaster is probably to be preferred. Plaster splintage is maintained until fusion is shown to be sound.

Comment

The most important part of this operation is to make sure that the metatarso-phalangeal joint is fused in the correct position. The position is critical and there is very little room for error. Although some dorsiflexion is required care must be taken not to over-do it; otherwise the skin over the dorsum of the interphalangeal joint is liable to impinge upon the upper of the shoe, with consequent soreness. Likewise it is a mistake to ignore the angle of valgus possessed by the normal hallux and to set the toe in a straight line with the metatarsal. If the other foot is normal the correct angle of valgus may be determined from it.

The only other point of difficulty is to direct the drill, and thus the screw, correctly into substantial bone so that it gains a good grip. Provided a sufficiently deep notch is cut in the medial border of the proximal phalanx the drill may be passed almost longitudinally, with only slight lateral inclination.

ARTHRODESIS OF INTERPHALANGEAL JOINT OF HALLUX

When the interphalangeal joint of the big toe is to be fused it should be placed in the straight position.

TECHNIQUE

It is possible, and usually satisfactory, to use the peg and socket type of arthrodesis such as is commonly used in the lesser toes for the correction of fixed flexion deformity (hammer toe) (p. 458). This has the effect of shortening the toe, however, and if it seems desirable to preserve full length the technique to be described, in which the opposing joint surfaces are rawed and then drawn together by a screw inserted at the distal end of the distal phalanx, is to be preferred.

Position of patient. The patient lies supine. A tourniquet may be used on the thickest part of the calf or on the upper thigh.

Incision. An elliptical incision is made transversely over the interphalangeal joint. If the toe shows a fixed flexion deformity at the interphalangeal joint a wide ellipse of skin may be excised.

Rawing of joint surfaces. The bone ends are mobilised by division of the collateral ligaments. The joint is then flexed acutely in order to subluxate the distal phalanx from the head of the proximal phalanx. The articular cartilage of the head of the proximal phalanx and of the base of the distal phalanx is cut away with a small chisel or gouge. Raw bone is thus exposed. The two surfaces must be so shaped that they fit together accurately with the toe straight.

Fixation by screw. A small skin incision is now made transversely across the distal end of the toe, through the pulp just below the nail. Through this incision the tip of the distal phalanx is identified and cleared.

A hole is next drilled longitudinally down the whole length of the distal phalanx. To do this it is easiest to enter the awl or drill at the joint surface—that is, at the centre of the articular aspect of the base of the phalanx—and to drill distally until the point of the instrument emerges through the terminal incision. The hole should be equal in diameter to the overall diameter of the screw to be used, to allow a sliding fit.

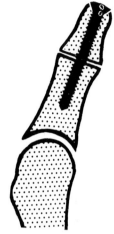

FIG. 592. Arthrodesis of interphalangeal joint of hallux. Fixation by screw driven in from the end of the toe. If the toe is short a Herbert scaphoid screw (see p. 213) may be used with advantage. (The longest Herbert screw at present available measures only 30 millimetres.)

With the toe now held straight at the interphalangeal joint a smaller drill—equal in diameter to the core diameter of the screw—is entered at the terminal incision and passed proximally along the track already prepared in the distal phalanx, and driven on into the proximal phalanx, almost to its base. A small-gauge screw, which should be long enough to penetrate at least three-quarters of the proximal phalanx, is driven home, compressing the two bones together (Fig. 592). The head of the screw should be well countersunk into the tip of the distal phalanx, to avoid any prominence under the skin.

As an alternative, a Herbert scaphoid screw (see p. 213) may be used. This has the advantage of having no head, so that the screw lies entirely within the bone. If the Herbert screw is used, the maker's recommendations for drill size should be observed.

Closure. Only the skin edges need be sutured.

POST-OPERATIVE MANAGEMENT

Provided secure fixation has been obtained with the screw, soft dressings only need be applied for the initial post-operative period. When walking is resumed about two weeks after the operation it may be wise to support the toe with a light plaster-of-Paris splint in the form of a broad strip laid upon the dorsum of the forefoot and hooked down over the tip of the toe to support the pulp (Fig. 591).

PEG ARTHRODESIS OF PROXIMAL INTERPHALANGEAL JOINT FOR HAMMER TOE

This is a peg-in-socket type of arthrodesis modified from the method described by Higgs (1931). It is applicable mainly to the lesser toes, but a similar technique is sometimes used for the big toe.

divided (Fig. 594). This manoeuvre allows the flexed middle phalanx to be pushed proximally and the head of the proximal phalanx to be delivered out of the wound (Fig. 595). The head is now shaped into a peg. First the articular cartilage

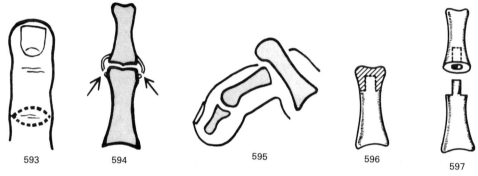

FIGS 593–597. Peg arthrodesis for hammer toe. Figure 593—The skin incision. Figure 594—Collateral ligaments divided to allow dislocation of joint. Figure 595—The joint dislocated and the head of the proximal phalanx delivered from the wound. Figure 596—Hatched area shows amount of bone to be removed from proximal phalanx to shape the peg. Figure 597—The parts ready for assembly.

TECHNIQUE

Position of patient. The patient lies supine. A tourniquet may be used on the thickest part of the calf or on the upper thigh.

Incision. The incision is a transverse ellipse across the whole width of the toe over the proximal interphalangeal joint (Fig. 593). The ellipse of skin is excised and discarded.

Fashioning of the peg and socket. Removal of the ellipse of skin exposes the extensor expansion, which is excised to expose the joint surfaces. The toe is now flexed acutely at the interphalangeal joint to bring the head of the proximal phalanx into prominence. With a fine knife (a size 15 blade is appropriate) inserted between the joint surfaces and then twisted onto the side of the head of the phalanx the collateral ligament on each side is

and subchondral bone of the distal surface of the condyle are removed with fine bone-cutting forceps. Then each side of the head of the phalanx is trimmed in a similar manner to form a parallel-

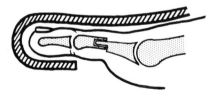

FIG. 598. The parts assembled. The diagram also shows the extent of the plaster strip splint.

sided peg about 6 millimetres long (Fig. 596). Finally, the plantar surface of the head is cut away parallel with the dorsal cortex. The main strength of the peg resides in this dorsal cortex, which should not be trimmed. The peg thus created is at present of square section. It may be rounded by shaving off the corners with a fine chisel used as a hand tool and not hammered.

A matching socket is now fashioned in the base of the middle phalanx. First the articular cartilage is cut away with fine bone-cutting forceps. The central cavity of the phalanx is entered with a Paton's burr or fine drill. It is then enlarged and the corners are squared off with a diamond plated rasp or a number 11 scalpel blade, until the socket is exactly equal in diameter to the peg on the proximal phalanx (Fig. 597).

Assembly and closure. When the peg and the socket have been shaped to a precise match the two parts are impacted firmly together (Fig. 598). The joint should now be rigidly immobile. The skin wound is closed with two or three interrupted mattress sutures.

POST-OPERATIVE MANAGEMENT
A strip of plaster-of-Paris about 10 centimetres long and 1.5 centimetres wide is laid over the front part of the forefoot and the dorsum of the toe and is hooked over the end of the toe to support the plantar surface (Fig. 598). The plaster is held in place by two or three turns of ribbon gauze. The initial plaster is worn for two weeks. Thereafter the sutures are removed and a further similar plaster is retained until the end of the sixth week from operation.

Comment

Provided the bones are shaped with care to ensure an accurate fit of the peg in the socket, this operation gives consistently reliable results. It is important that the ellipse of skin excised from the dorsum of the toe should be ample: suture of the edges then tightens the dorsal skin, which thus helps to splint the toe.

ARTHRODESIS OF DISTAL INTERPHALANGEAL JOINT OF LESSER TOE

Arthrodesis of the distal interphalangeal joint of a toe—usually for fixed flexion deformity—is required less commonly than that of the proximal interphalangeal joint. The operation to be described aims to promote fusion of the joint in the straight position.

TECHNIQUE

Position of patient. The patient lies supine. A tourniquet may be used on the thickest part of the calf or on the upper thigh.

Procedure. In the toe of a large foot it may be possible to use the peg-and-socket technique as described for arthrodesis of the proximal interphalangeal joint. Usually, however, the joint is too small for this to be practicable. The following simple technique is therefore recommended.

An elliptical incision is made across the full

width of the toe over the distal interphalangeal joint (Fig. 599). The ellipse of skin is discarded, as is a similar ellipse of underlying extensor tendon and joint capsule. The joint is thus exposed.

The joint is now flexed to its fullest extent to

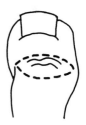
FIG. 599. Arthrodesis of distal interphalangeal joint of toe. The skin incision.

display the articular surfaces, and the ensheathing soft tissues are stripped away from the bone ends over a distance of 3 or 4 millimetres on either side of the joint. With fine-pointed bone-cutting forceps the articular surface of the head of the middle phalanx is cut off at right angles to the long axis of the phalanx, leaving a flat surface of cancellous bone. The articular surface of the distal phalanx is likewise cut away (Fig. 600). The two flat surfaces are now brought together and held in contact

POST-OPERATIVE MANAGEMENT
A small J-shaped plaster strip is applied as for arthrodesis of the proximal interphalangeal joint. It is usually sufficient to retain the plaster for three weeks.

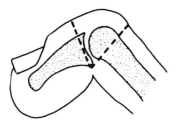 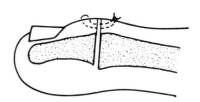

FIGS 600–601. Arthrodesis of distal interphalangeal joint of toe. Figure 600—The amount of bone and soft tissue to be removed. Figure 601—The rawed bones are held in apposition by mattress sutures through the skin edges.

simply by suturing the margins of the elliptical skin incision (Fig. 601). If the ellipse has been made of sufficient width, mattress sutures in the skin edges tighten the dorsal skin sufficiently to hold the fragments in position, and no other internal fixation is required.

Comment
The key feature of this operation is the removal of just enough skin in the elliptical incision to ensure that suture of the edges will tighten the dorsal skin sufficiently to splint the toe in extension but without excessive tension on the sutures.

TENDON TRANSFER: FLEXOR DIGITORUM LONGUS TO EXTENSOR EXPANSION

(FLEXOR TO EXTENSOR TRANSFER)

This operation, often referred to simply as flexor to extensor transfer, is associated with the name of Girdlestone. The technique was described by Taylor in 1951. It is applicable mainly to the correction of mobile claw toe. It may be used for a single toe, but more often the claw deformity is multiple and the operation is carried out on each of the four outer toes. It is not appropriate when there is fixed deformity. In essence the operation consists in transfer of the flexor digitorum longus tendon of each affected toe to the extensor expansion over the dorsum of the proximal phalanx (Fig. 602).

TECHNIQUE

Position of patient. The patient lies supine. A tourniquet may be used on the thickest part of the calf or on the upper thigh.

Incision. A separate incision is used for each toe. The incision begins at the level of the base of the proximal phalanx, immediately lateral to the extensor tendon. From this point it extends distally and plantarwards onto the lateral aspect of the toe (Fig. 603). Each incision is 2 centimetres long.

Mobilisation of long flexor tendon. The skin edges are retracted with slender hooks, and with fine dissecting scissors the incision is deepened towards the plantar surface of the proximal phalanx. When fatty tissue has been cleared the lateral

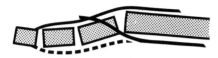

FIG. 602. Flexor-to-extensor tendon transfer for mobile claw toe. The flexor digitorum longus tendon has been detached from the distal phalanx and re-routed to pass through a slit in the extensor expansion, where it is sutured.

side of the fibrous flexor tendon sheath is brought into view. This is incised longitudinally with a fine knife to reveal the white glistening tendons within. At this point, under the proximal phalanx, three tendons will be found, namely the two lateral slips of flexor brevis on their way to their insertion at the base of the middle phalanx, and between these the long flexor tendon. This middle slip, the long tendon, is picked up with a blunt hook and pulled to test its action on the distal interphalangeal joint and thus to confirm its identity. The long flexor tendon is severed as far forwards as possible, either with curved scissors

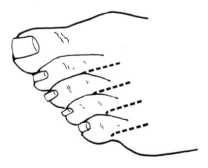

FIG. 603. Flexor-to-extensor transfer. The skin incisions.

or with a fine knife. It is probably wise to divide the two slips of flexor digitorum brevis as well, though only the long flexor is used for the transfer.

The freed long tendon is pulled upwards and delivered through the wound, being held by mos-

quito forceps. With moderate longitudinal tension applied to it, the tendon is re-routed round the lateral side of the toe towards the extensor expansion over the dorsum of the proximal phalanx (Fig. 602). To prevent sharp angulation of the tendon the sheath should be slit as far proximally as possible.

Re-insertion of transferred tendon. The extensor expansion over the proximal phalanx is cleaned so that its edges are clearly defined. Over the distal half of the proximal phalanx a horizontal slit is made through the expansion from side to side with a fine knife blade. A mosquito forceps is thrust through the slit from the medial to the lateral side and is used to draw the cut end of the long flexor tendon through the slit. With the toe held straight

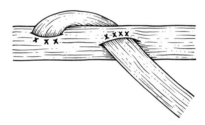

FIG. 604. Detail showing method of inserting the re-routed flexor tendon into the extensor expansion.

and the flexor tendon pulled moderately taut, two or three fine sutures of stainless steel wire are inserted through both tendons as they lie together at the point of intersection (Fig. 604). If there is sufficient length the free end of the flexor tendon may be passed through a second slit at right angles to the first and secured with further sutures; or it may be folded back upon itself and sutured to form a loop.

Closure. Each incision is closed with two or three fine skin sutures.

POST-OPERATIVE MANAGEMENT

The toes should be held straight for two weeks after operation by individual strips of plaster-of-Paris, each about 1.5 centimetres wide. Each strip is laid longitudinally upon the dorsum of the forefoot and toe, and hooked over the tip of the toe to be moulded snugly against the pulp of the distal segment (Fig. 598). The plaster strips are held in place by ribbon gauze round each toe and by a crepe bandage round the forefoot. After two weeks, when the sutures are removed, further external support is not required.

Comment

This is a delicate operation and the tissues must be handled with great gentleness. The inexperienced operator may find some difficulty in identifying the long flexor tendon and in severing it at the point of its insertion at the depth of the small incision.

Secondly, there is some difficulty in knowing when the tension on the transferred tendon is correct. Usually fault lies in suturing the tendon with too little tension rather than with too much. After suture of the tendons with wire, care should be taken to bury the ends of the wire; otherwise a sharp protruding end may enter the deep aspect of the skin and cause discomfort.

RE-ALIGNMENT OF ADDUCTED OVER-RIDING LITTLE TOE

Over-riding of the fifth toe upon the fourth is often evident at birth, but corrective operation is usually deferred until the child is 2 or 3 years old, or even longer if there is no complaint of discomfort or pain. The deformity is often obstinate and may recur unless a fairly radical operation is carried out. This fact was recognised by McFarland (1954), who had found the results of corrective operations so disappointing that he advocated syndactylisation of the fifth toe to the fourth.

The deformity comprises both adduction and extension. The skin and soft tissues must therefore be lengthened on the dorso-medial surface and shortened on the plantar-lateral surface.

TECHNIQUE
The operation comprises four elements: 1) relaxation of the tight medial skin by Z-plasty; 2) shortening of the proximal phalanx by excision of a length of bone from the shaft; 3) transfer of the flexor digitorum longus tendon of the fifth toe round the lateral side to the extensor expansion; and 4) shortening of the skin inferiorly and laterally by excision of an ellipse and closure of the gap.

Position of patient. The patient lies supine. A tourniquet may be used on the thickest part of the calf or on the thigh.

Skin incisions. The Z-plasty incision lies on the supero-medial aspect of the base of the toe and toe web. When the toe is held out in abduction it will be seen that the contracted skin lies obliquely in a line extending from the lateral side of the web and directed towards the navicular bone. The central

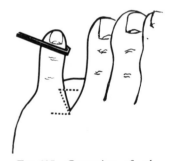

FIG. 605. Correction of adducted over-riding little toe. The medial Z-plasty incision.

limb of the Z incision lies along this tight skin (Fig. 605). The proximal limb, at 60 degrees to the central limb, extends laterally, and the distal limb,

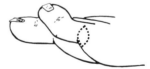

FIG. 606. The lateral incision. The ellipse of skin is excised.

also at 60 degrees, medially across the dorsal surface of the web (Fig. 605). The lateral incision is more or less transverse. It isolates an elliptical island of skin which should lie over the infero-lateral aspect of the base of the toe (Fig. 606). This ellipse of skin is removed. These two incisions suffice to allow the phalangeal osteotomy and the tendon transfer to be carried out without difficulty.

Isolation and distal division of flexor digitorum longus tendon. Through the lateral incision the lateral aspect of the proximal phalanx is exposed by blunt dissection. Immediately plantar to the phalanx will be found the fibrous flexor tendon sheath, which is opened longitudinally with a fine (number 15) knife blade. The flexor digitorum longus tendon is identified by its action in flexing the terminal phalanx when it is pulled, and with slender curved scissors within the tendon sheath it is severed from its attachment to the distal phalanx. The free tendon is withdrawn proximally and retracted with a holding stitch or mosquito forceps.

Shortening of proximal phalanx. Through the lateral incision the lateral aspect of the proximal phalanx is thoroughly cleared and the periosteum is incised longitudinally and reflected from the bone by Watson-Cheyne dissectors used as miniature bone levers. A section of bone 5 to 7 millimetres long according to the size of the patient (the excised part should represent about one-third of the total length of the phalanx) is removed after double osteotomy effected with fine bone-cutting forceps. The remaining cut ends of the bone are brought together into end-to-end apposition, but no attempt need be made to provide internal fixation.

Flexor-to-extensor tendon transfer. This stage of the operation is similar to the tendon transfer for mobile claw toes described on page 460. Through the medial (Z-plasty) incision the extensor expansion on the dorsum of the proximal phalanx is cleared by blunt dissection with scissors. A longitudinal slit through the tendon is made from side to side over the middle of the phalanx, by means of a fine (number 15) knife blade. A mosquito forceps is passed through the slit from the medial side, to emerge through the lateral incision, where the proximal cut end of the long flexor tendon is

delivered into the jaws of the forceps, which is then withdrawn, pulling the tendon through the slit in the extensor expansion (Fig. 604). While moderate tension is applied to the flexor tendon (still held in the mosquito forceps) a suture of fine stainless-steel tendon wire is inserted through the flexor tendon and through the recipient extensor expansion. The mosquito forceps is removed and a second suture may be inserted to hold the two tendons securely together.

Closure of elliptical lateral incision. The edges of the elliptical gap are approximated to tighten the infero-lateral skin sufficiently to hold the little toe in natural alignment. The ellipse may be enlarged if necessary by removal of further skin. The wound is then closed with everting mattress sutures.

Closure of Z-plasty incision. The triangular flaps are reversed, as in the standard Z-plasty procedure, and the re-aligned wound is closed with fine everting sutures.

POST-OPERATIVE MANAGEMENT

At the completion of the operation the toe lies in the fully corrected position. It is supported in this position by a J-shaped plaster-of-Paris splint similar to that shown in Figure 598, held in place by ribbon gauze and overlying strips of elastic adhesive bandage. The splint is discarded after three weeks.

Comment

This operation, simple in principle, must be effected with considerable precision. Less radical operations, such as Z-plasty combined with tendon transfer but without shortening of the phalanx, are liable to be followed by recurrence of the deformity. Shortening of the proximal phalanx is a useful component of the operation in that it helps to overcome the tightness of the medial tissues that is such an obstinate deforming force in these cases. Re-routing of the long flexor tendon to the extensor expansion from the lateral side of the toe helps to maintain correction, for the tendon now acts as an abductor of the toe and reinforces the intrinsic muscles as a flexor of the metatarso-phalangeal joint and an extensor of the interphalangeal joints. Excision of an ellipse of skin inferiorly and laterally helps further to maintain correction by tightening the skin on the outer side of the toe.

ABLATION OF NAIL OF BIG TOE

The operation to be described is designed to ablate the toe nail permanently by the method of Zadik (1950). The principle of the operation is to excise only the germinal epithelium—that is, the layer from which the nail grows, as represented by the lunula—and to close the gap by advancement of the proximal flap.

the nail fold, one at the medial side and one at the lateral, diverging slightly as shown in Figure 607. The anterior ends of these incisions are joined by a transverse incision along the free edge of the nail fold. The skin flap thus outlined is reflected proximally in the subcutaneous plane. A further incision divides the nail bed transversely

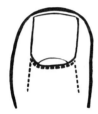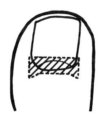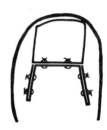

FIGS 607–609. Permanent ablation of nail of hallux. Figure 607—Outline of the skin incisions. Figure 608—Diagram showing the area of the nail bed to be removed (hatched). Figure 609—The proximal skin flap has been advanced to cover the raw area and sutured to the distal cut edge of the nail bed.

PRELIMINARY CARE

If the toe is infected—as for instance in a case of ingrowing toe nail—it is wise to allow a period of three or four weeks to clear up the sepsis before the operation is undertaken. The quickest way to clear the infection is to avulse the nail to ensure free drainage and then to apply mild antiseptic dressings as required.

TECHNIQUE

Position of patient. The patient lies supine. A tourniquet may be used on the thickest part of the calf or on the upper thigh.

Excision of germinal epithelium. If the nail has not already been removed it is avulsed as the first stage of the operation. Twin incisions 10 or 12 millimetres long are then made at the corners of

immediately distal to the whitish crescentic area known as the lunula (Fig. 608). This incision turns proximally along the nail fold at each side, to meet the anterior ends of the first incisions. A rectangular area of skin, bearing the germinal layer from which alone the nail is formed, is thus outlined and is now excised. It is reflected proximally by sharp dissection close to the underlying bone. Much care is required in excising the lateral and medial recesses, which form surprisingly deep pockets at each corner of the nail bed. It is essential to excise these pockets entire: otherwise small excrescences of nail will grow out from the remaining islands of germinal epithelium. It is wise to examine these pockets closely (this may be found easier if they are floated in a bowl of water) after they have been detached, in order to be sure that the epithelium is intact and that none has been left behind.

Closure of defect. At the completion of the excision a raw area 5 or 6 millimetres long remains. This is covered by advancement of the proximal skin flap, which is anchored distally and at the sides by fine interrupted sutures (Fig. 609).

POST-OPERATIVE MANAGEMENT

A dressing of dry gauze or of *tulle gras* is held in place by a narrow crepe bandage. The sutures are removed after seven days and light dressings are continued until the skin is stable.

Comment

The important essential is to excise the germinal epithelium in its entirety, to ensure that there is no regrowth of nail: this presents difficulty mainly at the corners of the nail, where it is all too easy to leave fragments of germinal epithelium in the deep recesses that extend proximally under the nail fold.

The Zadik operation has the disadvantage that tensing of the dorsal skin from advancement of the flap to cover the raw area tends to restrict flexion of the toe at the interphalangeal joint. In time, however, the skin stretches to restore reasonable movement. The operation is much to be preferred to that of shortening the distal phalanx and turning up a flap of skin from the pulp to cover the raw area created by excision of the nail bed. This leaves a shortened, bulbous and ugly toe. An acceptable alternative to the Zadik operation— though one that entails a longer convalescence—is to use a free skin graft instead of an advancement flap to cover the defect.

PARTIAL EXCISION OF NAIL BED FOR INGROWING TOE NAIL

(SEGMENTAL EXCISION OF GERMINAL MATRIX)

In severe cases of ingrowing toe nail, with ulceration of the nail wall on both sides, total excision of the germinal matrix as described above is appropriate; but in less severe cases in which only one nail wall is infected, the excision of the germinal matrix may be confined to an area about 5 millimetres wide. Only the germinal matrix needs to be removed; excision of a strip extending over the whole length of the nail bed—as often advocated—is unnecessary (Fowler 1958).

PRELIMINARY CARE

In nearly every case infection is present in the nail wall, and it is therefore necessary to clear up the infection before the definitive operation is undertaken. Infection is cleared by avulsing a strip of nail 5 millimetres wide, after the nail has been cut longitudinally with sharp-pointed scissors. It is well to wait at least three weeks, and preferably four, after avulsion of the strip of nail before the definitive operation is undertaken.

TECHNIQUE

Position of patient. The patient lies supine. A tourniquet may be used on the thickest part of the calf or, if preferred, a tourniquet may be applied round the base of the toe.

Procedure. On the affected side of the nail a longitudinal skin incision extends from a point on the nail fold close to its junction with the nail wall

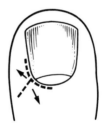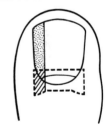

FIGS 610–611. Partial excision of nail bed. Figure 610—The incision. Triangular flaps are turned back as indicated. Figure 611—Hatched area shows extent of resection of germinal epithelium.

proximally for about 8 millimetres; by extending the distal end of this incision into the margin of the nail fold, triangular medial and lateral flaps are turned back (Fig. 610). These flaps include only the surface epidermis and dermis: the epidermal layer which forms the deep surface of the nail fold is left intact at this stage.

It remains now to define the extent of the germinal matrix and to excise it over a width of 5 millimetres at the proximal corner of the nail bed (Fig. 611). The excision extends distally just beyond the lunula and proximally to include the epidermal pocket formed by the germinal matrix and the under surface of the nail fold. It is important that this little pocket of skin be removed entire: otherwise growth of the relevant part of the nail will not be fully abolished.

Closure. It is possible to draw the triangular skin flaps distally sufficiently to cover the raw area almost, if not quite, fully.

POST-OPERATIVE MANAGEMENT

The first dressing is of tulle gras held in place by a narrow crepe bandage. This may be changed for a dry dressing after seven days, when the sutures may be removed.

BELOW-KNEE AMPUTATION OF LEG

Below-knee amputation of the leg is the commonest of all major amputations, mainly because of the frequency with which it is undertaken for arterial disease with ischaemia of the foot. In such cases special care has to be taken to preserve the viability of the skin edges. In cases of ischaemia primary healing is not always obtained, and in a proportion of cases re-amputation above the knee is required.

There has been much discussion on the planning of skin flaps to give the best prospect of their survival. Many surgeons now favour the method described by Burgess (1969) in which a long posterior flap and a very short anterior flap are used. Persson (1974), however, claimed good results from equal medial and lateral flaps.

In non-ischaemic cases the problem of necrosis of skin from inadequate blood supply does not arise. Consequently, there is much more latitude in the choice of flaps, as also in the length of the stump.

BELOW-KNEE AMPUTATION IN CASES OF ISCHAEMIA

The technique of Burgess is followed with minor modifications.

LEVEL OF AMPUTATION

As a general rule it is recommended that the bone section be made 14 centimetres below the upper margin of the tibia. A slightly shorter stump may have a marginally better chance of survival but it should never be less than 10 centimetres as measured from the upper margin of the tibia.

TECHNIQUE

Position of patient. The patient lies supine. In ischaemic cases a tourniquet should not be used.

Outlining the skin flaps. As a first step the proposed level of section of the tibia—say 14 centimetres from the upper margin of the tibia—is

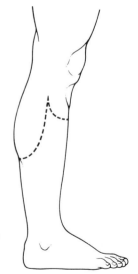

FIG. 612. Outline of long posterior flap and short anterior flap for below-knee amputation for ischaemia.

marked upon the skin surface. It is well to mark out the skin flaps carefully with ink before any incision is made (Fig. 612).

First a line is drawn transversely round the anterior two-fifths of the circumference of the leg, 15 centimetres below the upper margin of the tibia. From each end of this outline a vertical line is drawn in the long axis of the limb to extend 15 centimetres distal to the proposed level of bone section. The lower ends of these axial lines are then joined by a line drawn transversely round the posterior half of the circumference of the leg.

Division of anterior structures. First the anterior skin flap, about a centimetre long, is raised from the underlying muscles together with deep fascia. The anterior muscles are then divided transversely at the level of intended tibial section. During this stage the anterior main vessels are ligated by transfixion ligatures and divided.

Division of bones. The periosteum over the tibia is incised at the level of intended bone section and stripped up with an elevator on all its surfaces. The tibia is divided, preferably with a powered reciprocating saw. The distal fragment of the tibia is held steady by a large bone hook inserted into the medullary canal. The fibula is cleared two centimetres above the level of the tibial saw-cut and divided cleanly.

Preparation of posterior flap. While the distal fragment of the tibia is held slightly forwards with a strong bone hook the gastrocnemius and soleus muscles that will form part of the long posterior flap are dissected away from the distal fragments of the tibia and fibula. The main vessels are ligated and divided at the level of bone section and the tibial nerve is pulled distally, divided cleanly and allowed to retract. The posterior calf muscles are divided at the distal extremity of the long posterior flap to free the amputation specimen.

Bevelling and smoothing the tibial stump. The anterior corner of the tibial stump is bevelled off with a saw-cut beginning nearly a centimetre above the cut surface and directed at 45 degrees. The cut edges of the bone are then carefully smoothed with a file. The cut surface of the fibula is likewise made smooth.

Myoplasty. The sectioned posterior calf muscles are held out with tissue forceps to allow the muscle mass to be trimmed down with a large-bladed knife to leave a clean-cut flap of muscle that tapers to no more than a thin sheet at its distal extremity. The sides of the flap are also trimmed away to avoid excessive bulkiness.

After all bleeding points have been secured the posterior flap, composed of skin, fascia and muscle, is folded forwards to cover the ends of the bones. If the flap is too long it may be trimmed further to allow the aponeurosis of the gastrocnemius to be sutured to the periosteum at the anterior aspect of the tibial stump. A polythene tube for suction drainage is inserted deep to the posterior muscle flap.

Skin closure. The skin of the posterior flap is trimmed appropriately to ensure that it lies smoothly to allow suture of the edges without too much bagginess, yet without tension.

POST-OPERATIVE MANAGEMENT

Soft gauze dressings are held in place by a wide crepe bandage carefully applied to mould the stump evenly. A further bandage should be brought up over the knee. The bandages are anchored by strips of adhesive tape secured to the thigh. If desired, a light plaster-of-Paris shell may be moulded over the bandage to support and shape the stump. Suction drainage is discontinued after forty-eight hours but the dressings may be left undisturbed until ten or fourteen days after the operation.

Exercises for the quadriceps muscles should be practised from an early stage.

Comment

In ischaemic cases the incidence of failure of healing of the below-knee stump varies from centre to centre, but at its lowest it is probably in the region of 15 or 20 per cent. In other words, the success rate in attempts to preserve the knee is not more than 80 to 85 per cent. Several factors may contribute towards a better prognosis, of which the following are the most important: 1) avoidance of tourniquet; 2) a gentle technique with minimal handling of the tissues; 3) avoidance of a long anterior flap, which is particularly prone to necrosis; a posterior flap has a much better blood supply; 4) non-separation of the layers of the flap—the posterior muscles to be included with the posterior skin flap; 5) meticulous haemostasis to minimise the formation of a haematoma, which may make the difference between survival and necrosis; 6) careful suture of the muscle flap to the deep fascia and periosteum, and equally painstaking suture of the skin edges.

ALTERNATIVE TECHNIQUE

An alternative to the long posterior flap, suggested in 1966 by Tracy and advocated more recently by Persson (1974), is the use of equal lateral flaps so that the scar lies in the sagittal plane. It is claimed that equal lateral flaps have at least as good a potential for survival as a long posterior flap.

BELOW-KNEE AMPUTATION IN PATIENTS WITHOUT ISCHAEMIA

LEVEL OF AMPUTATION

In non-ischaemic cases there is some degree of latitude with regard to the level of the amputation. In traumatic cases the level may be dictated to some extent by skin damage or actual loss of skin. As a general rule a stump measuring about 15 centimetres from the upper margin of the tibia is satisfactory: it may be a little longer in a very tall person or shorter in one of short stature.

TECHNIQUE

Provided there is sufficient skin the technique outlined in the previous section, with a long posterior flap and a very short anterior flap, may be used. In traumatic cases, however, there is not always sufficient posterior skin to form a long flap. In this section therefore the use of equal anterior and posterior flaps, or preferably of a slightly longer anterior flap, will be described.

Position of patient. The patient lies supine. A sand-bag may be placed under the lower thigh.

The lower leg and foot should be draped separately up to a point just below the level of the proposed skin flaps. A tourniquet may be used on the upper thigh.

Marking out the skin flaps. It is well first to mark upon the skin the proposed level of tibial section. The diameter of the leg at this level is then measured in order to determine the length of the flaps. It is wise to allow 50 per cent of the diameter for the anterior flap and 70 per cent for the posterior flap: this allows some excess of skin which can be trimmed during closure. The outline of the flaps may be marked with ink upon the skin, the outline beginning in the mid-lateral line of the leg at the level of intended tibial section and ending in the mid-medial line.

Raising the flaps. Incisions are made in the outlines already drawn. The anterior flap is fashioned first. The incision extends only through skin and subcutaneous tissue. The flap is reflected proximally to the level of intended tibial section. The posterior skin flap is fashioned in like manner.

Division of anterior muscles. The anterior muscles are divided transversely one centimetre distal to the intended level of tibial section. The cut muscles tend to retract to about the level of bone section.

Fashioning of posterior muscle flap. While the limb is raised high by an assistant the skin of the distal part of the leg is pushed downwards to expose the aponeurosis covering the gastrocnemius muscle. The aponeurosis is divided low enough down in the leg to provide a flap that will fold forwards to cover the cut surfaces of muscles and bone. A substantial layer of gastrocnemius muscle is included in this flap: the remainder of the posterior muscles are severed transversely at the same level as the anterior muscles.

Division of tibia and fibula. When the level of tibial section has again been checked by measurement the tibia and fibula are sawn through transversely and the distal part of the limb is discarded. The tibial periosteum is stripped proximally to allow the anterior corner of the tibia to be bevelled at 45 degrees, the cut starting about a centimetre above the level of bone section and emerging on the cut surface just in front of the medullary canal. Next the fibula should be shortened so that the stump is about two centimetres shorter than the tibial stump. Finally the ends of the bones are smoothed and rounded with a file.

Haemostasis. Before the tourniquet is removed the major vessels are identified, transfixed and doubly ligated with catgut. The main nerves are identified, drawn distally, cut through cleanly and allowed to retract. After removal of the tourniquet time must be spent on securing full haemostasis before the wound is closed.

Closure. First the musculo-aponeurotic flap formed from the gastrocnemius and its overlying aponeurosis is folded forwards to cover the end of the stump: the flap is trimmed appropriately and the fresh edges are united to the cut edge of the deep fascia circumferentially. A polythene tube for suction drainage is inserted deep to the flap. Finally, the skin flaps are carefully trimmed and their edges approximated with interrupted everting mattress sutures.

POST-OPERATIVE MANAGEMENT

This is the same as described in the previous section.

SUPRA-MALLEOLAR AMPUTATION OF FOOT

(SYME'S AMPUTATION)

This amputation was first described by James Syme of Edinburgh, father-in-law of Lord Lister, in 1843. It gives an end-bearing stump, weight being taken upon the heel pad, which is folded forwards and applied to the under surface of the sawn-off tibia and fibula.

TECHNIQUE

Position of patient. The patient lies supine with a sand-bag or thick folded towel under the calf. A tourniquet may be used on the upper thigh.

Incision. Angled lateral and medial incisions meet over the front of the instep and below the heel (Fig. 613). The anterior part of the incision begins on the lateral side over the tip of the lateral malleolus, and runs upwards and forwards to cross the instep just above the level of the ankle joint. Thence it passes downwards and backwards on the medial side of the ankle to a point corresponding in level to the starting point on the lateral side—that is, about 2 centimetres below the tip of the medial malleolus. The inferior part of the incision is a U-shaped cut from the original starting point at the tip of the lateral malleolus, passing vertically underneath the heel to end where it

joins the anterior incision just below the medial malleolus (Fig. 613).

Disarticulation of talus and dissection of calcaneus from periosteum. The anterior incision in front of the ankle is deepened straight down to bone. The anterior capsule of the ankle joint is incised, and while the foot is forcibly plantarflexed the talus is shelled out from the ankle mortise by division of the capsule and the ligaments medially and laterally. The foot is gradually forced down into more plantarflexion as the talus is disarticulated, whereupon the upper surface of the calcaneal tuberosity is brought into view. This is cleared of soft tissue by dissection close to the bone, to enable the posterior aspect of the calcaneus to be reached.

The calcaneal tendon is severed close to its insertion and the calcaneus is shelled out from its covering of periosteum by sharp dissection. It is important that the separation of the bone from the heel pad should be close to the bone, and not at the expense of the specialised fibro-fatty tissue which serves an important function in weight bearing. The dissection is continued in this way until the entire calcaneus, and with it the foot, is separated and removed.

Supra-malleolar trimming of tibia and fibula. The skin flaps are drawn upwards to deliver the lower ends of the tibia and fibula out of the wound. The bones are then sawn cleanly across immediately proximal to the articular cartilage of the ankle joint. It is essential that this cut be made in such a way that with the patient standing the cut surface will be parallel with the ground both in the antero-posterior plane and in the lateral plane.

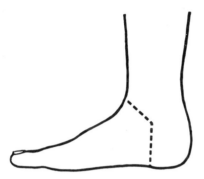

FIG. 613. Syme's amputation. Outline of the heel flap.

Approximation of heel flap to under surface of divided bones. The heel flap is turned upwards so that its anterior cut edge meets the proximal edge of the ankle incision. The flap is bulky and loose, but care must be taken to ensure that the weight-bearing part of the heel pad is applied accurately to the cut surface of the tibia and fibula.

Closure. The edges of the heel pad are united to the proximal edge of the ankle incision by interrupted sutures. A rubber drain should be inserted so as to emerge at each side of the wound; or alternatively suction drainage may be instituted.

POST-OPERATIVE MANAGEMENT

In bandaging the stump at the conclusion of the operation it is important that the weight-bearing heel pad be held in place beneath the cut surfaces of the tibia and fibula. If necessary strips of adhesive strapping may be used for this purpose. The stump should then be snugly bound with a crepe bandage over copious gauze dressings, with care to ensure that even pressure is exerted over the distal end. The drain should be removed after two days, when it is wise to re-dress the stump.

Comment

There are three important points to be observed. Firstly, the tibia and fibula should be sawn across as low as possible—that is, immediately above the articular cartilage of the ankle mortise. The saw must be so directed that the cut surface is parallel with the ground when the patient is standing. Secondly, the calcaneus must be dissected out subperiosteally in order to avoid damage to the specialised weight-bearing tissue of the heel flap and to facilitate rapid adherence of the heel flap to the under surface of the trimmed tibia and fibula. Thirdly, the heel flap must be so placed that its weight-bearing surface is accurately applied to the cut surfaces of the tibia and fibula.

The Syme amputation has advantages over the below-knee amputation (Harris 1956), notably when carried out for mutilating injuries of the foot and especially in men: the difficulty of fitting a cosmetically pleasing prosthesis makes it less acceptable to women.

AMPUTATION OF TOE

The descriptions that follow apply to ablation of the whole toe by disarticulation at the metatarsophalangeal joint. Similar principles apply to more conservative amputations either through bone or through an interphalangeal joint, the skin incisions being appropriately modified.

AMPUTATION OF BIG TOE

TECHNIQUE

Position of patient. The patient lies supine. A tourniquet may be used on the calf or on the upper thigh unless the amputation is being carried out for arterial disease, when the operation is best done without a tourniquet.

Incision. A modified racquet incision is used. The handle or apex of the racquet should lie over the distal 2 centimetres of the first metatarsal bone, medial to the extensor tendon of the big toe (Fig. 614). The periphery of the racquet forms a semi-circle round the plantar-medial aspect of the toe, immediately proximal to the interphalangeal

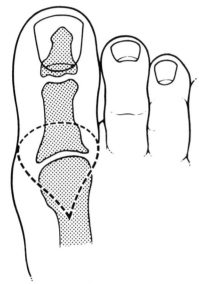

FIG. 614. Racquet incision for amputation of hallux at metatarso-phalangeal joint.

joint. In this way a plantar-medial flap that will be long enough to cover the metatarsal head without tension is fashioned.

Isolation of toe and division of metatarso-phalangeal joint capsule. The skin flap is dissected from the underlying tissues and the edges are reflected. Through the plantar part of the incision the long flexor tendon of the big toe is divided cleanly just proximal to the metatarso-phalangeal joint and allowed to retract. On the dorsum of the foot the long extensor tendon is likewise severed as far proximally as the incision will allow. The joint capsule and remaining tissues are then divided circumferentially around the joint to separate the toe.

Closure. If the head of the metatarsal bears protruding osteophytes it is well to smooth the surface of the bone with a sharp chisel before the skin is closed. The plantar-medial flap of skin is then brought over the metatarsal head towards the web between the hallux and the second toe. If there is an obvious excess of skin the flap may be trimmed appropriately, but it is a mistake to reduce the flap to the point at which the skin can be sutured only under tension: a reasonably lax covering is desirable. The skin closure should be performed meticulously with eversion mattress sutures. Special care must be taken to eliminate unsightly tags of skin or "dog ears". Drainage of the wound is not required.

POST-OPERATIVE MANAGEMENT
Rather copious gauze dressings are held snugly in place by a crepe bandage, which in turn should be secured by long strips of elastic adhesive bandage. Unless there is excessive matting of the dressings with dry blood the bandage may be left intact until the sutures are removed twelve to fourteen days after operation. If the dressings become unduly matted it is wise to change them on the second or third day.

Comment

In cases of skin damage from trauma it may be necessary to modify the skin incision in order to be able to fashion a flap from healthy skin. To this extent the technique of the operation must depend upon the circumstances of each individual case. It is important to secure full haemostasis before closure of the skin. To this end the tourniquet should be removed well in advance of wound closure.

AMPUTATION OF A LESSER TOE

TECHNIQUE
Position of patient. The patient lies supine. Except in ischaemic cases a tourniquet may be used on the calf or on the upper thigh.

Incision. A racquet-shaped incision is used, with the handle of the racquet at the dorsal aspect. At the plantar aspect the incision runs transversely across the toe at the level of the web. On each side of the toe the incision then curves dorsally and proximally so that the two limbs of the incision meet at an apex over the base of the proximal phalanx.

Isolation and separation of toe. At the plantar aspect the incision is deepened straight down to the bone of the proximal phalanx, the flexor tendons being divided cleanly and allowed to retract. The soft tissues are then stripped proximally from the base of the proximal phalanx until the metatarso-phalangeal joint is reached. The sides and the dorsum of the phalanx are likewise stripped back as far as the joint. At the apex of the incision dorsally the extensor tendon is severed well proximally. It then remains to divide the joint capsule circumferentially to separate the toe.

Closure. The skin edges are approximated to form a new web between the adjacent toes. Sur-plus skin is trimmed to give a smooth suture line without "dog ears". The closure is preferably made with eversion mattress sutures.

POST-OPERATIVE MANAGEMENT

Firm pressure should be maintained over the wound area by gauze dressings held snugly by a crepe bandage.

AMPUTATION OF LITTLE TOE

The technique of amputation of the fifth toe is basically the same as for the other lesser toes, but it may often be advisable to trim off the head of the metatarsal by an oblique cut through its neck. This is best done by placing the handle of the racquet incision over the supero-lateral aspect of the toe and prolonging it proximally over the metatarsal neck.

REFERENCES

ADAMS, J. C. (1943). Screw length in bone grafting. *Lancet*, **ii,** 415.

ADAMS, J. C. (1964). Vulnerability of the sciatic nerve in closed ischio-femoral arthrodesis by nail and graft. *Journal of Bone and Joint Surgery*, **46B,** 748.

ADAMS, J. C. (1966). *Ischio-femoral Arthrodesis*. Edinburgh: Livingstone.

ADKINS, E. W. O. (1955). Lumbo-sacral arthrodesis after laminectomy. *Journal of Bone and Joint Surgery*, **37B,** 208.

ALBEE, F. H. (1911). Transplantation of a portion of the tibia into the spine for Pott's disease. *Journal of the American Medical Association*, **57,** 885.

ALEXANDER, G. L. (1946). Neurological complications of spinal tuberculosis. *Proceedings of the Royal Society of Medicine*, **39,** 730.

ANDERSON, M., & GREEN, W. T. (1947). Experiences with epiphysial arrest in correcting discrepancies in length of the lower extremities in infantile paralysis. *Journal of Bone and Joint Surgery*, **29,** 659.

ANDERSON, R. (1932). A new method of treating fractures utilising the well leg for counter-traction. *Surgery, Gynecology & Obstetrics*, **54,** 207.

ATTENBOROUGH, C. G. (1978). The Attenborough total knee replacement. *Journal of Bone and Joint Surgery*, **60B,** 320.

AUSTIN, M. (1963). The Esmarch bandage and pulmonary embolism. *Journal of Bone and Joint Surgery*, **45B,** 384.

BARTON, N. J. (1973). Arthroplasty of the forefoot in rheumatoid arthritis. *Journal of Bone and Joint Surgery*. **55B,** 126.

BATCHELOR, J. S. (1951). In Symposium on congenital dislocation of the hip. *Journal of Bone and Joint Surgery*, **33B,** 288.

BAYLEY, I., & KESSEL, L. (1982). The Kessel total shoulder replacement. In *Shoulder Surgery* (ed. Bayley & Kessel). Berlin, Heidelberg, New York: Springer-Verlag.

BIRKELAND, I. W., & TAYLOR, T. K. F. (1969). Major vascular injuries in lumbar disc surgery. *Journal of Bone and Joint Surgery*, **51B,** 4.

BÖHLER, L. (1948). *Medullary Nailing of Kuntscher,* London: Bailliere, Tindall and Cox.

BOSWORTH, D. M. (1955). The role of the orbicular ligament in tennis elbow. *Journal of Bone and Joint Surgery*, **37A,** 527.

BOUCHER, H. H. (1959). A method of spinal fusion. *Journal of Bone and Joint Surgery*, **41B,** 248.

BROOKS, D. M. (1974). Personal Communication.

BROWN, A., & D'ARCY, J. C. (1971). Internal fixation for supracondylar fractures of the femur in the elderly patient. *Journal of Bone and Joint Surgery*, **53B,** 520.

BROWN, J. T., & ABRAMI, G. (1964). Transcervical femoral fracture. *Journal of Bone and Joint Surgery*, **46B,** 648.

BRUNER, J. M. (1973). Surgical exposure of flexor tendons in the hand. *Annals of Royal College of Surgeons of England*, **53,** 84.

BURGESS, E. M. (1969). The below-knee amputation. *Inter-Clinic Information Bulletin*, **8,** 1.

CAMPBELL, W. C. (1939). Reconstruction of the ligaments of the knee. *American Journal of Surgery*, **43,** 473.

CAPENER, N. (1954). Lateral rhachotomy. *Journal of Bone and Joint Surgery*, **36B,** 193.

CAPENER, N. (1966). The vulnerability of the posterior interosseous nerve of the forearm. *Journal of Bone and Joint Surgery*, **48B,** 770.

CARROLL, R. E., & Hill, N. A. (1973). Athrodesis of the carpo-metacarpal joint of the thumb. *Journal of Bone and Joint Surgery*, **55B,** 292.

CHARNLEY, J. (1948). Positive pressure in arthrodesis of the knee joint. *Journal of Bone and Joint Surgery*, **30B,** 478.

CHARNLEY, J. (1951). Compression arthrodesis of the ankle and shoulder. *Journal of Bone and Joint Surgery*, **33B,** 180.

CHARNLEY, J. (1960). Anchorage of the femoral head prosthesis to the shaft of the femur. *Journal of Bone and Joint Surgery*, **42B,** 28.

CHARNLEY, J. (1961). Arthroplasty of the hip: a new operation. *Lancet*, **ii,** 129.

CHARNLEY, J. (1964). A clean-air operating enclosure. *British Journal of Surgery*, **51,** 202.

CHARNLEY, J. (1970). Total hip replacement by low-friction arthroplasty. *Clinical Orthopaedics and Related Research*, **72,** 7.

CHARNLEY, J., & EFTEKHAR, N. (1969). Post-operative infection in total prosthetic replacement arthroplasty of the hip joint. *British Journal of Surgery*, **56,** 641.

CHIARI, K. (1955). Ergelonisse mit der Beckenosteotomie als Pfannendachplastik. *Zeitschrift fur Orthopadie und ihre Grenzgebiete*, **87,** 14.

CHIARI, K. (1970). Pelvic osteotomy for hip subluxation. *Journal of Bone and Joint Surgery*, **52B,** 174.

CHOLMELEY, J. A. (1958). Hallux valgus in adolescents. *Proceedings of the Royal Society of Medicine*, **51,** 903.

CHRISTENSEN, N. O. (1973). Kuntscher intramedullary reaming and nail fixation for non-union of fracture of the femur and the tibia. *Journal of Bone and Joint Surgery*. **55B,** 312.

CLARK, J. M. P. (1968). Surgical treatment of club foot. *Proceedings of the Royal Society of Medicine*, **61,** 779.

CONE, W., & TURNER, W. G. (1937). The treatment of fracture-dislocation of the cervical vertebrae by skeletal traction and fusion. *Journal of Bone and Joint Surgery*, **19,** 584.

COVENTRY, M. B., FINERMAN, A. M., RILEY, L. H., TURNER, R. H., & UPSHAW, J. E. (1972). A new geometric knee for total knee arthroplasty. *Clinical Orthopaedics*, **83,** 157.

DANDY, D. J. (1981). *Arthroscopic Surgery of the Knee.* Edinburgh & London: Churchill Livingstone.

DANIS, R. (1949). *Théorie et Pratique de l'osteosynthèse.* Paris: Masson et Cie.

DEBEYRE, J., PATTE, D., & ELMELIK, E. (1965). Repair of ruptures of the rotator cuff of the shoulder. *Journal of Bone and Joint Surgery,* **47B**, 181.

DEVAS, M., & HINVES, B. (1983). Prevention of acetabular erosion after hemiarthroplasty for fractured neck of femur. *Journal of Bone and Joint Surgery,* **65B**, 548.

DUMONT, F. (1887). Die Resektion des Haftgelenkes nach Kocher. *Correspondenz-Blatt fur Schweizer Aerzte,* **17**, 225.

DUNN, D. M. (1952). Anteversion of the neck of femur. *Journal of Bone and Joint Surgery,* **34B**, 181.

DUNN, D. M. (1964). The treatment of adolescent slipping of the upper femoral epiphysis. *Journal of Bone and Joint Surgery,* **46B**, 621.

DUNN, D. M., & ANGEL, J. C. (1978). Replacement of the femoral head by open operation in severe adolescent slipping of the upper femoral epiphysis. *Journal of Bone and Joint Surgery,* **60B**, 394.

DWYER, F. C. (1963). The treatment of relapsed club foot by the insertion of a wedge into the calcaneum. *Journal of Bone and Joint Surgery,* **45B**, 67.

EGGERS, G. W. N. (1952). Transplantation of hamstring tendons to femoral condyles in order to improve hip extension and to decrease knee flexion in cerebral spastic paralysis. *Journal of Bone and Joint Surgery,* **34A**, 827.

ELLIS, J. S. (1965). Smith's and Barton's fractures. *Journal of Bone and Joint Surgery,* **47B**, 724.

EVANS, D. (1961). Relapsed club foot. *Journal of Bone and Joint Surgery,* **43B**, 722.

EVANS, D. L. (1955). Wedge arthrodesis of the wrist. *Journal of Bone and Joint Surgery,* **37B**, 126.

FAIRBANK, H. A. T. (1942). The non-touch technique with special reference to the operative treatment of simple fractures. *British Medical Journal,* **ii**, 388.

FISK, G. R. (1944). The fractured femoral shaft. New approach to the problem. *Lancet,* **i**, 659.

FLYNN, M., & KELLY, J. P. (1976). Local excision of cyst of lateral meniscus of knee without recurrence. *Journal of Bone and Joint Surgery,* **58B**, 88.

FOWLER, A. W. (1958). Excision of the germinal matrix: A unified treatment for embedded toe-nail and onychogryposis. *British Journal of Surgery,* **45**, 382.

FOWLER, A. W. (1959). A method of forefoot reconstruction. *Journal of Bone and Joint Surgery,* **41B**, 507.

FREEBODY, D. (1964). Treatment of spondylolisthesis by anterior fusion via the transperitoneal route. *Journal of Bone and Joint Surgery,* **46B**, 788.

FREEBODY, D., BENDALL, R., & TAYLOR, R. D. (1971). Anterior transperitoneal lumbar fusion. *Journal of Bone and Joint Surgery,* **53B**, 617.

FREEMAN, M. A. R., & SWANSON, S. A. V. (1972). Total prosthetic replacement of the knee. In Proceedings of British Orthopaedic Association, September 1971. *Journal of Bone and Joint Surgery,* **54B**, 170.

GALWAY, R. D., BEAUPRÉ, A., & MACINTOSH, D. L. (1972). Pivot shift: a clinical sign of symptomatic anterior cruciate insufficiency. *Journal of Bone and Joint Surgery,* **54B**, 763.

GARDEN, R. S. (1961). Tennis elbow. *Journal of Bone and Joint Surgery,* **43B**, 100.

GARDEN, R. S. (1961). Low angle fixation in fractures of the femoral neck. *Journal of Bone and Joint Surgery,* **43B**, 647.

GIBSON, A. (1950). Posterior exposure of the hip joint. *Journal of Bone and Joint Surgery,* **32B**, 183.

GILLIES, H., & CHALMERS, J. (1970). The management of fresh ruptures of the tendo-achillis. *Journal of Bone and Joint Surgery,* **52A**, 337.

GIRDLESTONE, G. R. (1945). Discussion on treatment of unilateral osteoarthritis of the hip joint. *Proceedings of the Royal Society of Medicine,* **38**, 363.

GORDON-TAYLOR, G., & MONRO, R. S. (1952). Technique and management of hindquarter amputation. *British Journal of Surgery,* **39**, 536.

GRIFFITH, M. J. (1973). The morphology of slipped upper femoral epiphysis. *Journal of Bone and Joint Surgery,* **55B**, 653.

GRIFFITHS, D. LL., SEDDON, H. J., & ROAF, R. (1956). *Pott's Paraplegia.* Edinburgh: Livingstone.

GROVES, E. W. HEY. (1918). Ununited fractures with special reference to gunshot injuries and the use of bone grafting. *British Journal of Surgery,* **6**, 203.

HARRIS, N. H. (1965). A method of measurement of femoral neck anteversion. *Journal of Bone and Joint Surgery,* **47B**, 188.

HARRIS, R. I. (1956). Symes's amputation. *Journal of Bone and Joint Surgery,* **38B**, 614.

HAUSER, E. D. W. (1938). Total tendon transplant for slipping patella. *Surgery, Gynecology and Obstetrics,* **66**, 199.

HELAL, B. (1975). Metatarsal osteotomy for metatarsalgia. *Journal of Bone and Joint Surgery,* **57B**, 187.

HENRY, A. K. (1945). *Extensile Exposure Applied to Limb Surgery.* Edinburgh: Livingstone.

HERBERT, T. J., & FISHER, W. E. (1984). The management of the fractured scaphoid using a new bone screw. *Journal of Bone and Joint Surgery,* **66B**, 114.

HEYSE-MOORE, G. H., MacEACHERN, A. G., & JAMESON EVANS, D. C. (1983). Treatment of intertrochanteric fractures of the femur: A comparison of the Richards screw-plate with the Jewett nail-plate. *Journal of Bone and Joint Surgery,* **65B**, 262.

HIBBS, R. A. (1912). Operation for Pott's disease of the spine. *Journal of the American Medical Association,* **59**, 433.

HICKS, J. H. (1961). Fractures of the forearm treated by rigid fixation. *Journal of Bone and Joint Surgery,* **43B**, 680.

HIGGS, S. L. (1931). Hammer-toe. *Postgraduate Medical Journal,* **6**, 130.

HODGSON, A. R., & STOCK, F. E. (1960). Anterior spine fusion for the treatment of tuberculosis of the spine. *Journal of Bone and Joint Surgery,* **42A**, 295.

HODGSON, A. R., & WONG, S. K. (1968). A description of a technic and evaluation of results in anterior spinal fusion for deranged intervertebral disc and spondylolisthesis. *Clinical Orthopaedics,* **56**, 133.

HOFFMAN, T. (1912). An operation for severe grades of contracted or clawed toes. *American Journal of Orthopaedic Surgery,* **9**, 441.

HOHMANN, G. (1924). Zur Hallux valgus-operation. *Zentralblatt für Chirurgie,* **51**, 230.

HOHMANN, G. (1948). *Fuss and Bein.* München: J. F. Bergmann.

HUCKSTEP, R. L. (1972). Rigid intramedullary fixation of femoral shaft fractures with compression. *Journal of Bone and Joint Surgery,* **54B**, 204.

JACKSON, R. W., & DANDY, D. J. (1976). *Arthroscopy of the Knee*. New York: Grune & Stratton.

JEFFREYS, T. E. (1963). Recurrent dislocation of the patella due to abnormal attachment of the ilio-tibial tract. *Journal of Bone and Joint Surgery*, **45B**, 740.

JONES, K. G. (1963). Reconstruction of the anterior cruciate ligament. *Journal of Bone and Joint Surgery*, **45A**, 925.

JONES, R. (1916). Notes on military orphopaedics. III: The soldier's foot and the treatment of common deformities of the foot (part 2). *British Medical Journal*, **i**, 749.

JONES, R. (1921). Tendon transplantation in cases of musculo-spiral injury not amenable to suture. *American Journal of Surgery*, **35**, 333.

JUDET, J., & JUDET, R. (1950). The use of an artificial femoral head for arthroplasty of the hip joint. *Journal of Bone and Joint Surgery*, **32B**, 166.

JUDET, R., & JUDET, J. (1949). Essais de reconstruction prothètique de la hanche après resection de la tête femorale. *Journal de Chirurgie*, **65**, 17.

KAPLAN, E. B. (1959). Treatment of tennis elbow (epicondylitis) by denervation. *Journal of Bone and Joint Surgery*, **41A**, 147.

KATES, A., KESSEL, L., & KAY, A. (1967). Arthroplasty of the forefoot. *Journal of Bone and Joint Surgery*. **49B**, 552.

KEIM, H. A., & WEINSTEIN, J. D. (1970). Acute renal failure: a complication of spinal fusion in the tuck position. *Journal of Bone and Joint Surgery*, **52A**, 1248.

KELLER, W. L. (1904). The surgical treatment of bunions and hallux valgus. *New York Medical Journal*, **80**, 741.

KELLER, W. L. (1912). Further observations on the surgical treatment of hallux valgus and bunions. *New York Medical Journal*, **95**, 696.

KESSEL, L., & BONNEY, G. L. W. (1958). Hallux rigidus in the adolescent. *Journal of Bone and Joint Surgery*, **40B**, 668.

KEY, J. A. (1932). Positive pressure in arthrodesis for tuberculosis of the knee joint. *Southern Medical Journal*, **25**, 809.

KIRKALDY-WILLIS, W. H., & THOMAS, T. G. (1965). Anterior approaches in the diagnosis and treatment of infections of the vertebral bodies. *Journal of Bone and Joint Surgery*, **47A**, 87.

KIRWAN, E. O'G. (1977). Personal Communication.

KOCHER, T. (1887). Quoted by Dumont (q.v.)

KOCHER, T. (1907). *Chirurgische Operationslehre, 5th edition*. Jena: Gustav Fischer.

KOCHER, T. (1911). (translated Stiles, H. J.). *Textbook of Operative Surgery*. Edinburgh: A. & C. Black.

LAM, S. J. S. (1968). Reconstruction of the anterior cruciate ligament using the Jones procedure and its Guy's Hospital modification. *Journal of Bone and Joint Surgery*, **50A**, 1213.

LAMBOTTE, A. (1913). *Chirurgie Opératoire des Fractures*. Paris: Masson et Cie.

LAMBRINUDI, C. (1927). New operation in drop-foot. *British Journal of Surgery*, **15**, 193.

LAMBRINUDI, C. (1933). A method of correcting equinus and calcaneus deformities at the subastragaloid joint. *Proceedings of the Royal Society of Medicine*, **26**, 788.

LANE, W. A. (1914). *Operative Treatment of Fractures*. London: Medical Publishing Co.

LANGENBECK, B. V. (1874). Ueber die Schussverletzungen des Huftgelenke. *Archiv fur klinische Chirurgie*, **16**, 294.

LAURENCE, M. (1983). Ultra-clean air. *Journal of Bone and Joint Surgery*, **65B**, 375.

LAURENCE, M. (1991). Replacement arthroplasty of the rotator cuff deficient shoulder. *Journal of Bone and Joint Surgery*, **73B**, 916.

LAURENCE, M., FREEMAN, M. A. R., & SWANSON, S. A. V. (1969). Engineering considerations in the internal fixation of fractures of the tibial shaft. *Journal of Bone and Joint Surgery*, **51B**, 754.

LESLIE, J. T., & RYAN, T. J. (1962). The anterior axillary incision to approach the shoulder joint. *Journal of Bone and Joint Surgery*, **44A**, 1193.

LETTIN, A. W. F., COPELAND, S. A., & SCALES, J. T. (1982). The Stanmore total shoulder replacement. *Journal of Bone and Joint Surgery*, **64B**, 47.

LETTIN, A. W. F., DELISS, L. J., BLACKBURNE, J. S., & SCALES, J. T. (1978). The Stanmore hinged knee arthroplasty. *Journal of Bone and Joint Surgery*, **60B**, 327.

LEYSHON, A., IRELAND, J., & TRICKEY, E. L. (1984). The treatment of delayed union and non-union of the carpal scaphoid by screw fixation. *Journal of Bone and Joint Surgery*, **66B**, 124.

LIDWELL, O. M., LOWBURY, E. J. L., WHYTE, W., BLOWERS, R., STANLEY, S. J., & LOWE, D. (1982). Effect of ultraclean air in operating rooms on deep sepsis in the joint after total hip or knee replacement. *British Medical Journal*, **285**, 10.

LITTLEWOOD, H. (1922). Amputations at the shoulder and at the hip. *British Medical Journal*, **i**, 381.

MACEWEN, W. (1878). Antiseptic osteotomy for genu valgum, genu varum and other osseous deformities. *Lancet*, **ii**, 911.

McFARLAND, B. (1954). The treatment of dorsal adduction deformities of the fifth toe. *Journal of Bone and Joint Surgery*, **36B**, 146.

McFARLAND, B., & OSBORNE, G. (1954). Approach to the hip. *Journal of Bone and Joint Surgery*, **36B**, 364.

McGRAW, R. W., & RUSCH, R. M. (1973). Atlanto-axial arthrodesis. *Journal of Bone and Joint Surgery*, **55B**, 482.

MACINTOSH, D. L. (1958). Hemiarthroplasty of the knee using a space occupying prosthesis for painful varus and valgus deformities. In proceedings of the Joint Meeting of the Orthopaedic Associations of the English-speaking World. *Journal of Bone and Joint Surgery*, **40A**, 1431.

MACINTOSH, D. L. (1967). Arthroplasty of the knee in rheumatoid arthritis using the hemiarthroplasty prosthesis. In: *Synovectomy and Arthroplasty in Rheumatoid Arthritis: Second International Symposium* (Ed. G. Chapchal). Stuttgart: Thieme.

McKEE, G. K. (1951). Artificial hip joint. *Journal of Bone and Joint Surgery*, **33B**, 465.

McKEE, G. K. (1970). Development of total prosthetic replacement of the hip. *Clinical Orthopaedics and Related Research*, **72**, 85.

McKEE, G. K., & WATSON-FARRAR, J. (1966). Replacement of arthritic hips by McKee-Farrar prosthesis. *Journal of Bone and Joint Surgery*, **48B**, 245.

MacKenzie, I. G. (1959). Lambrinudi's arthrodesis. *Journal of Bone and Joint Surgery*, **41B**, 738.

McMURRAY, T. P. (1935). Osteoarthritis of the hip joint. *British Journal of Surgery*, **22**, 716.

MAGNUSON, P. B., & STACK, J. K. (1943). Recurrent dislocation of the shoulder. *Journal of American Medical Association*, **123**, 889.

MANKIN, H. J., LANGE, T. A., & SPANIER, S. S. (1982). The hazards of biopsy in patients with malignant primary bone and soft-tissue tumors. *Journal of Bone and Joint Surgery*, **64A**, 1121.

MAUDSLEY, R. H., & CHEN, S. C. (1972). Screw fixation in the management of the fractured carpal scaphoid. *Journal of Bone and Joint Surgery*, **54B**, 432.

MAZET, R., & HENNESSY, C. A. (1966). Knee disarticulation. A new technique and a new knee joint mechanism. *Journal of Bone and Joint Surgery*, **48A**, 126.

MENELAUS, M. B. (1966). Correction of leg length discrepancy by epiphysial arrest. *Journal of Bone and Joint Surgery*, **48B**, 336.

MILLER, A. J. (1974). Posterior malleolar fractures. *Journal of Bone and Joint Surgery*, **56B**, 508.

MILLESI, H. (1983). Microsurgery of peripheral nerves. In *Recent Advances in Orphopaedics* (4) (Ed. McKibbin). Edinburgh, London, New York: Churchill Livingstone.

MITCHELL, C. L., FLEMING, J. L., ALLEN, R., GLENNEG, C., & SANDFORD, G. A. (1958). Osteotomy-bunionectomy for hallux valgus. *Journal of Bone and Joint Surgery*, **40A**, 41.

MIXTER, W. J., & BARR, J. S. (1934). Rupture of the intervertebral disc with involvement of the spinal canal. *New England Journal of Medicine*, **211**, 210.

MOE, J. H. (1958). A critical analysis of methods of fusion for scoliosis. *Journal of Bone and Joint Surgery*, **40A**, 529.

MOORE, A. T. (1957). The self-locking metal hip prosthesis. *Journal of Bone and Joint Surgery*, **39A**, 811.

MOORE, J. R. (1947). Osteotomy-osteoclasis. *Journal of Bone and Joint Surgery*, **29**, 119.

MULDER, J. D. (1955). Activities and development in the field of orthopaedics. *Journal of Bone and Joint Surgery*, **37B**, 735.

MÜLLER, M. E. (1970). Total hip prostheses. *Clinical Orthopaedics and Related Research*, **72**, 46.

MÜLLER, M. E., ALLGÖWER, M., SCHNEIDER, R. & WILLENEGGER, H. (1991). *Manual of Internal Fixation*. Berlin, Heidelberg, New York: Springer-Verlag.

MYGIND, H. B. (1952). Operations for hallux valgus. *Journal of Bone and Joint Surgery*, **34B**, 529.

NAYLOR, A. (1979). Factors in the development of the spinal stenosis syndrome. *Journal of Bone and Joint Surgery*, **61B**, 306.

NEER, C. S., WATSON, K. C., & STANTON, F. J. (1982). Recent experience in total shoulder replacement. *Journal of Bone and Joint Surgery*, **64A**, 319.

NICOLL, E. A. (1956). Treatment of gaps in long bones by cancellous insert grafts. *Journal of Bone and Joint Surgery*, **38B**, 70.

NICOLL, E. A. (1963). Quadricepsplasty. *Journal of Bone and Joint Surgery*, **45B**, 483.

OSBORNE, R. P. (1931). The approach to the hip joint: a critical review and a suggested new route. *British Journal of Surgery*, **18**, 49.

OSMOND-CLARKE, H. (1948). Habitual dislocation of the shoulder. *Journal of Bone and Joint Surgery*, **30B**, 19.

PARTRIDGE, A. J., & EVANS, P. E. L. (1982). The treatment of fractures of the shaft of the femur using nylon cerclage. *Journal of Bone and Joint Surgery*, **64B**, 210.

PATRICK, J. (1962). Popliteal arterio-venous aneurysm as a complication of meniscectomy. *Journal of Bone and Joint Surgery*, **44B**, 744.

PEMBERTON, P. A. (1965). Pericapsular osteotomy of the ilium for treatment of congenital subluxation and dislocation of the hip. *Journal of Bone and Joint Surgery*, **47A**, 65.

PEMBERTON, P. A. (1974). Pericapsular osteotomy of the ilium for the treatment of congenitally dislocated hips. *Clinical Orthopaedics and Related Research*, **98**, 41.

PERKINS, G. (1958). *Fractures and Dislocations*. London: University of London, Athlone Press.

PERSSON, B. M. (1974). Sagittal incision for below-knee amputation in ischaemic gangrene. *Journal of Bone and Joint Surgery*, **56B**, 110.

PHEMISTER, D. B. (1947). Treatment of ununited fractures by onlay bone grafts without screw or tie fixation and without breaking down of the fibrous union. *Journal of Bone and Joint Surgery*, **29**, 1946.

POLLEN, A. G. (1965). Fallacies in the interpretation of radiographs during nailing of the neck of femur. *Proceedings of the Royal Society of Medicine*, **58**, 329.

PUGH, W. L. (1955). Self-adjusting nail-plate for fractures about the hip joint. *Journal of Bone and Joint Surgery*, **37A**, 1085.

PULVERTAFT, R. G. (1961). Tendon grafts. *Journal of Bone and Joint Surgery*, **43B**, 421.

PULVERTAFT, R. G. (1965). Problems of flexor tendon surgery of the hand. *Journal of Bone and Joint Surgery*, **47A**, 123.

RICHARDS, H. J. (1977). Digital flexor tendon repair and return of function. *Annals of Royal College of Surgeons of England*, **59**, 25.

ROBINSON, R. A. (1964). Anterior and posterior cervical spine fusions. *Clinical Orphopaedics*, **35**, 34.

ROBINSON, R. A., WALKER, E. A., FERLIC, D. C., & WIECKING, D. K. (1962). The results of anterior interbody fusion of the cervical spine. *Journal of Bone and Joint Surgery*, **44A**, 1569.

ROLES, N. C., & MAUDSLEY, R. H. (1972). Radial tunnel syndrome. *Journal of Bone and Joint Surgery*, **54B**, 499.

ROMANO, R. L., & BURGESS, E. M. (1971). Level selection in lower extremity amputations. *Clinical Orthopaedics*, **74**, 177.

ROMBOLD, C. (1966). Treatment of spondylolisthesis by postero-lateral fusion, resection of the pars interarticularis, and prompt mobilisation of the patient. *Journal of Bone and Joint Surgery*, **48A**, 1282.

RUSSE, O. (1960). Fracture of the carpal navicular. *Journal of Bone and Joint Surgery*, **42A**, 759.

SAID, G. Z. (1974). A modified tendon transference for radial nerve paralysis. *Journal of Bone and Joint Surgery*, **56B**, 320.

SALTER, R. B. (1961). Innominate osteotomy in the treatment of congenital dislocation and subluxation of the hip. *Journal of Bone and Joint Surgery*, **43B**, 518.

SALTER, R. B. (1969). An operative treatment for congenital dislocation and subluxation of the hip in the older child. In: *Recent Advances in Orthopaedics* (Ed. Apley). London: Churchill.

SCALES, J. T. (1983). Prosthetic replacement of the femoral head for femoral neck fracture: which design? *Journal of Bone and Joint Surgery*, **65B**, 530.

SCHANZ, A. (1905). Zur Behandlung der Schenkelhalsbrüche, *Archiv fur Klinische Chirurgie*, **83**, 336.

SCHANZ, A. (1907). Veber die nach Schenkelhalsbrüchen zuruckleibenden Gehstörungen. *Deutsche Medizinische Wochenschrift*, **51**, 730.

SCOTT, J. H. S. (1967). Intertransverse spinal fusion for spondylolisthesis. *Journal of Bone and Joint Surgery*, **49B**, 187.

SEDDON, H. J. (1975). *Surgical Disorders of the Peripheral Nerves*. Edinburgh: Churchill Livingstone.

SHEEHAN, J. M. (1978). Arthroplasty of the knee. *Journal of Bone and Joint Surgery*, **60B**, 333.

SHIERS, L. G. P. (1954). Arthroplasty of the knee. *Journal of Bone and Joint Surgery*, **36B**, 553.

SIMON, M. A. (1982). Biopsy of musculo-skeletal tumors. *Journal of Bone and Joint Surgery*, **64A**, 1253.

SLOCUM, D. B., & LARSON, R. L. (1968). Pes anserinus transplantation. *Journal of Bone and Joint Surgery*, **50A**, 226.

SMILLIE, I. S. (1957). Treatment of osteochondritis dissecans. *Journal of Bone and Joint Surgery*, **39B**, 248.

SMILLIE, I. S. (1960). *Osteochondritis Dissecans*. Edinburgh: Livingstone.

SMILLIE, I. S. (1980). *Diseases of the Knee Joint, 2nd edition*. Edinburgh: Churchill Livingstone.

SMITH-PETERSEN, M. N. (1940). A new approach to the wrist. *Journal of Bone and Joint Surgery*, **22**, 122.

SMITH-PETERSEN, M. N. (1949). Approach to and exposure of the hip joint for mold arthroplasty. *Journal of Bone and Joint Surgery*, **31A**, 40.

SMITH-PETERSEN, M. N., CAVE, E. F., & VAN GORDER, G. W. (1931). Intracapsular fractures of the neck of femur. *Archives of Surgery*, **23**, 715.

SMYTH, E. H. J. (1964). Triangle pinning of femoral neck fractures. *Journal of Bone and Joint Surgery*, **46B**, 156.

SMYTH, E. H. J., ELLIS, J. S., MANIFOLD, M. C., & DEWEY, P. R. (1964). Triangle pinning for fracture of the femoral neck. *Journal of Bone and Joint Surgery*, **46B**, 664.

SOMERVILLE, E. W. (1953). Open reduction in congenital dislocation of the hip. *Journal of Bone and Joint Surgery*, **35B**, 363.

SOMERVILLE, E. W. (1978). A long-term follow-up of congenital dislocation of the hip. *Journal of Bone and Joint Surgery*, **60B**, 25.

SOMERVILLE, E. W., & SCOTT, J. C. (1957). The direct approach to congenital dislocation of the hip. *Journal of Bone and Joint Surgery*, **39B**, 623.

STRACHAN, J. C. H., & Ellis, B. (1971). Vulnerability of the posterior interosseous nerve during radial head resection. *Journal of Bone and Joint Surgery*, **53B**, 320.

SYME, J. (1843). Amputation at the ankle joint. *London and Edinburgh Monthly Journal of Medical Sciences*, **3**, 93.

TAKAGI, K. (1933). Practical experience using Takagi's arthroscope. *Journal of the Japanese Orthopaedic Association*, **8**, 132.

TAYLOR, R. G. (1950). Pseudarthrosis of the hip joint. *Journal of Bone and Joint Surgery*, **32B**, 161.

TAYLOR, R. G. (1951). The treatment of claw toes by multiple transfer of flexor into extensor tendons. *Journal of Bone and Joint Surgery*, **33B**, 539.

TAYTON, K., JOHNSON-NURSE, C., McKIBBIN, B., BRADLEY, J., & HASTINGS, G. (1982). The use of semi-rigid carbon-fibre-reinforced plastic plates for fixation of human fractures. *Journal of Bone and Joint Surgery*, **64B**, 105.

THOMPSON, F. R. (1952). Vitallium intramedullary hip prosthesis: preliminary report. *New York State Journal of Medicine*, **52**, 3011.

THOMPSON, F. R. (1954). Two and a half years' experience with a Vitallium intramedullary hip prosthesis. *Journal of Bone and Joint Surgery*, **36A**, 489.

TRACY, G. D. (1966). Below-knee amputation for ischaemic gangrene. *Pacific Medicine and Surgery*, **74**, 251.

VALTANCOLI, G. (1925). Recurrent dislocation of the shoulder. *Chirurgia degli Organi Movimento*, **9**, 131.

VAN GORDER, G. W., & CHEN, C-M. (1959). The central-graft operation for fusion of tuberculous knees, ankles and elbows. *Journal of Bone and Joint Surgery*. **41A**, 1029.

VERBERNE, G. H. M. (1983). A femoral head prosthesis with a built-in joint. *Journal of Bone and Joint Surgery*, **65B**, 544.

WAINWRIGHT, D. (1976). The shelf operation for hip dysplasia in adolescence. *Journal of Bone and Joint Surgery*, **58B**, 159.

WALLDIUS, B. (1960). Arthroplasty of the knee using an endoprosthesis. *Acta Orthopaedica Scandinavica*, **30**, 137.

WATKINS, M. B. (1953). Postero-lateral fusion of the lumbar and lumbo-sacral spine. *Journal of Bone and Joint Surgery*, **35A**, 1014.

WESTH, R. N., & MENELAUS, M. B. (1981). A simple calculation for the timing of epiphysial arrest. *Journal of Bone and Joint Surgery*, **63B**, 117.

WHYTE, W., HODGSON, R., & TINKLER, J. (1982). The importance of airborne bacterial contamination of wounds. *Journal of Hospital Infection*, **3**, 123.

WILES, P. (1958). The surgery of the osteoarthritic hip. *British Journal of Surgery*, **45**, 488.

WILSON, J. N. (1963). Oblique displacement osteotomy for hallux valgus. *Journal of Bone and Joint Surgery*, **45B**, 552.

ZADIK, F. R. (1950). Obliteration of the nail bed of the great toe without shortening the terminal phalanx. *Journal of Bone and Joint Surgery*, **32B**, 66.

Index